TYPE 1 DIABETES – COMPLICATIONS, PATHOGENESIS, AND ALTERNATIVE TREATMENTS

Edited by **Chih-Pin Liu**

Type 1 Diabetes – Complications, Pathogenesis, and Alternative Treatments
Edited by Chih-Pin Liu

Published by InTech

Janeza Trdine 9, 51000 Rijeka, Croatia

Publishing Process Manager Sandra Bakic

Technical Editor Teodora Smiljanic

Cover Designer InTech Design Team

Additional hard copies can be obtained from orders@intechopen.com

Type 1 Diabetes – Complications, Pathogenesis, and Alternative Treatments,
Edited by Chih-Pin Liu
p. cm.
ISBN 978-953-307-756-7

For EU product safety concerns:
IN TECH d.o.o., Prolaz Marije Krucifikse Kozulić 3, 51000 Rijeka, Croatia,
info@intechopen.com or visit our website at intechopen.com.

Meet the editor

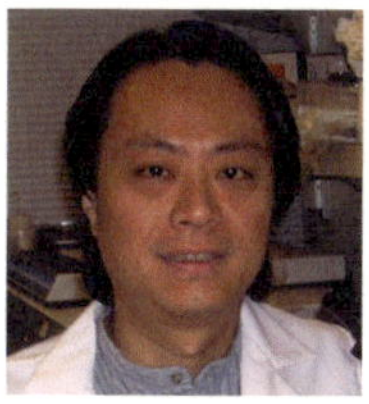

Dr. Chih-Pin Liu is a Professor, in Department of Diabetes and Metabolic Diseases and Department of Immunology, at Beckman Research Institute of City of Hope. He received his B.S. degree from National Taiwan University, and Ph.D. degree from University of Wisconsin-Madison, followed by postdoctoral fellowships at Beth Israel Hospital/Harvard Medical School in Boston and at National Jewish Medical and Research Center in Denver. He has had long-standing research interest in understanding the mechanisms that regulate immune tolerance induction during type 1 diabetes development. His recent work has focused on using genome-wide approaches to understand the molecular mechanisms responsible for modulating the function of regulatory T cells and identifying gene targets to improve regulatory T cell function for immunotherapy.

Contents

Preface

Diabetes is a leading cause of death in many countries affecting both the young and old at an alarming rate worldwide. Due to the destruction of insulin-producing beta islet cells by the body's own immune system, type 1 diabetes is the most common metabolic and endocrinal disease among children. Finding a cure for this disease has been a major challenge for both basic science and clinical investigators. Owing to rapid research progress in the field, we now have a better knowledge in understanding the cellular and molecular basis responsible for diabetes, the associated complications, and alternative treatments for this chronic inflammatory disease.

This book is intended as an overview of recent progress in type 1 diabetes research worldwide, with a focus on different research areas relevant to this disease. These include: diabetes mellitus and complications, psychological aspects of diabetes, perspectives of diabetes pathogenesis, identification and monitoring of diabetes mellitus, and alternative treatments for diabetes. In preparing this book, leading investigators from several countries in these five different categories were invited to contribute a chapter to this book. We have striven for a coherent presentation of concepts based on experiments and observation from the authors own research and from existing published reports. Therefore, the materials presented in this book are expected to be up to date in each research area.

Complications, such as those lead to severe cardiovascular diseases, caused by diabetes due to chronic inflammation have attracted intensive research in recent years. This section contains four chapters that discuss diabetes mellitus-caused complications due to the effect of glycative and oxidative stress, varied diet and life style, lipid disorders, and daily insulin doses. Better knowledge in these areas may help those who are affected by diabetes to reduce disease-associated long-term complications and to improve their life quality.

Type 1 disease usually occurs at young age and can have significant impact on those affected. Therefore, managing this disease becomes a very challenging daily task for the patients themselves and for their close family members. Frustration may occur while patients deal with their disease conditions, making adherence and proper glycemic control a challenge. To help address these challenges, four chapters discuss psychological aspects of diabetes, which provide updated and useful information regarding psychological factors related to diabetes in children and adolescents, how to avoid inadequate coping attitudes and maintain good eating behaviors, and how to improve adherence, metabolic control, and quality of life.

While many aspects of how type 1 diabetes may occur are discussed elsewhere, five chapters are included in this book to address some unique or alternative perspectives of diabetes pathogenesis. For example, a chapter discusses the effect of IRS-2 gene on fulminant type 1 diabetes in animal models. Another chapter discusses the role of obesity in the natural history of type 1 diabetes. Other factors, such as cytokines-induced beta cell death and the effect of L-Arg/L-Glu coupling on diabetes, are the topics of two other chapters respectively. Aided by recent progress in genomic studies, the fifth chapter discusses the use of meta-analysis of genome-wide association studies to better understand disease relatedness.

Due to the nature of the disease, it is not an easy task to identify disease risk or susceptibility early in life. The classification between type 1 vs. type 2 diabetes has also become less clear nowadays as increasing number of adults can develop symptoms of type 1 diabetes. Four chapters provide insightful discussion addressing this important issue. A chapter discusses evidence showing altering trends in the epidemiology of type 1 diabetes in children and adolescents. Thanks to recent research progress and better understanding of diabetes pathogenesis, a chapter discusses a more comprehensive list of phenotypic markers that may help clinical identification of families at risk. Another chapter suggests that genetic testing of newborns may also be a possibility to help identify disease susceptibility and distinguish different types of diabetes.

Finding a cure for type 1 diabetes remains a major challenge and ultimate goal for diabetes basic and clinical research. Currently, insulin injection is the gold standard for disease treatment. The use of insulin pump therapy has provided continuous subcutaneous insulin infusion for patients. A chapter provides an overview of mathematical modeling of using pump therapy as a management strategy for diabetes therapy. In seeking better treatments for this disease, recent studies suggest that it may be promising approaches using alternative medicine in therapies. Four chapters discuss findings in this area and suggest new aspects of using alternative medicine approaches to treat or ameliorate the disease conditions. These include the potential use of bile acid and probiotics, vitamin D, honey and fatty acids.

Finally, we would like to thank all the authors who have contributed to this book. While there is no doubt that this book may have omitted some important findings in diabetes field, we hope the information included in this book will be useful for both basic science and clinical investigators. We also hope that diabetes patients and their family will benefit from reading the chapters in this book.

Dr. Chih-Pin Liu
The Beckman Research Institute of the City of Hope,
Duarte, California,
USA

Part 1

Diabetes Mellitus and Complications

1

The Study of Glycative and Oxidative Stress in Type 1 Diabetes Patients in Relation to Circulating TGF-Beta1, VCAM-1 and Diabetic Vascular Complications

Vladimir Jakus[1], Jana Kostolanska[2], Dagmar Michalkova[1] and Michal Sapak[3]
[1]*Institute of Medical Chemistry, Biochemistry and Clinical Biochemistry, Faculty of Medicine, Comenius University, Bratislava*
[2]*Children Diabetological Center of the Slovak Republic, 1st Department of Pediatrics, Comenius University and University Hospital for Children, Bratislava*
[3]*Institute of Medical Immunology, Faculty of Medicine, Comenius University, Bratislava*
Slovakia

1. Introduction

Type 1 diabetes mellitus (T1DM) is one of most frequent autoimmune diseases and is characterized by absolute or nothing short of absolute endogenous insulin deficiency which results in hyperglycemia that is considered to be a primary cause of diabetic complications (DC) (Rambhade et al., 2010). T1DM leads to various chronic micro- and macrovascular complications. Diabetic nephropathy is a major cause of morbidity and mortality in patients with DM. Microvascular disease is the main determinant in the development of late complications in DM.

Persistent hyperglycemia is linked with glycation, glycoxidation, and oxidative stress (Aronson, 2008; Negre-Salvayre et al., 2009). During glycation and glycoxidation there are formed early, intermediate and advanced glycation products via Maillard reaction, glucose autoxidation and protein glycation. Accumulation of advanced glycation end products (AGEs) has several toxic effects and takes part in the development of DC, such as nephropathy (Kashihara et al, 2010), neuropathy, retinopathy and angiopathy (Peppa & Vlassara, 2005; Yamagishi et al., 2008; Goh & Cooper, 2008; Karasu, 2010). Higher plasma levels of AGEs are associated also with incident cardiovascular disease and all-cause mortality in T1DM (Nin et al., 2011). AGEs are believed to induce cellular oxidative stress through the interaction with specific cellular receptors (Ramasamy et al., 2005; Boulanger et al., 2006; Yamagishi, 2009; Mosquera, 2010). On the other side, carbonyl stress-induced tissue damage is caused by AGE precursors formed by hyperglycaemia, hyperlipidemia, nonenzymatic glycation, peroxidation of lipids and metabolic processes.

It has been suggested that the chronic hyperglycaemia in diabetes enhances the production of reactive oxygen species (ROS) from glucose autoxidation, protein glycation and glycoxidation, which leads to tissue damage (Son, 2007). Also, cumulative episodes of acute hyperglycaemia can be source of acute oxidative stress. A number of studies have summarized the relation between glycation and oxidation (Boyzel et al., 2010). The overproduction of ROS leads to oxidative modification of biologically important compounds and damage of them. Uncontrolled production of ROS often leads to damage of cellular macromolecules (DNA, lipids and proteins).

Some oxidation products or lipid peroxidation products may bind to proteins and amplify glycoxidation-generated lesions. Lipid peroxidation of polyunsaturated fatty acids, one of the radical reaction in vivo, can adequately reflect increased oxidative stress in diabetes. Advanced oxidation protein products (AOPP) are formed during oxidative stress by the action of chlorinated oxidants, mainly hypochlorous acid and chloramines. In diabetes the formation of AOPP is induced by intensified glycoxidation processes, oxidant-antioxidant imbalance, and coexisting inflammation (Piwowar, 2010a, 2010b). AOPP are supposed to be structurally similar to AGEs and to exert similar biological activities as AGEs, i.e. induction of proinflammatory cytokines in neutrophils, as well as in monocytes, and adhesive molecules (Yan et al., 2008). Accumulation of AOPP has been found in patients with chronic kidney disease (Bargnoux, et al., 2009). Further possible sources of oxidative stress are decreased antioxidant defenses, or alterations in enzymatic pathways.

Diabetes is associated also with inflammation (Navaro & Mora, 2006; Wautier et al., 2006; Devaraj et al., 2007; Hartge et al., 2007; Fawaz, et al., 2009 ; Van Sickle et al., 2009; Nobécourt et al., 2010). ROS are implicated also in the pathogenesis of the inflammatory response to ischemic-reperfusion which is exacerbated in diabetes. Oxidative stress during reperfusion is markedly balanced in diabetes and this appears to results from increased leukocyte recruitment and a higher capacity of diabetic leukocytes to generate ROS in response to stimulation. Several adhesion molecules are expressed on endothelial cells and participate in leukocyte adhesion to the endothelium. These molecules are important for monocyte-endothelium interaction in the initiation and progression of atherosclerosis. The monocyte-macrophage is a pivotal cell in atherogenesis. Cellular adhesion molecules mediate attachment and transmigration of leukocytes across the endothelial surface and are thought to play a crucial role in the early steps of atherogenesis (Seckin et al., 2006). Adhesion molecule VCAM-1 is not expressed under baseline conditions but is rapidly induced by proatherosclerotic conditions in rabbits, mice, and humans, including in early lesions. Initially, it is unclear whether VCAM-1 is simply a marker for atherogenesis or whether it acts in this disease pathway. AGEs promote VCAM-1 expression and atheroma formation in rabbits (Vlassara et al., 1995) and in cultured human endothelial cells (Schmidt et al., 1995). These results suggest the involvement of AGEs in the accelerated coronary atherosclerosis on diabetes (Zhang et al., 2003). Plasma concentrations of VCAM-1 are elevated also in T1DM patients with microalbuminuria and overt nephropathy (Schmidt et al., 1996; Clausen et al, 2000).

Diabetic nephropathy is characterized by specific morphological changes including glomerular basement membrane thickening, mesangial expansion and glomerular and tubulointersticial sclerosis. The first clinical manifestation of diabetic nephropathy is microalbuminuria, defined as a urinary albumin excretion rate of 20 to 200 microgram/min.

Growth factor TGF-beta1 is one of profibrotic cytokines and is important mediator in the pathogenesis of diabetic nephropathy (Goldfarb & Ziyadeh, 2001; Schrijvers et al., 2004; Wang et al., 2005; Wolf & Ziyadeh, 2007). TGF-beta1 stimulates production of extracellular

matrix components such as collagen-IV, fibronectin, proteoglycans (decorin, biglycan). TGF-beta1 may cause glomerulosclerosis and its one of the causal factor in myointimal hyperplasia after baloon injury of carotid artery. It mediates angiotensin-II modulator effect on smooth muscle cell growth. Besides profibrotic activity, TGF-beta1 has immunoregulatory function on adaptive immunity too. AGEs induce connective tissue growth factor-mediated renal fibrosis through TGF-beta1-independent Smad3 signalling (Zhou et al., 2004; Chung et al., 2010).
The present study investigates the relationship between diabetes complications presence, diabetes control (represented by actual levels of HbA1c (HbA1cA) and mean of HbA1c during the last 2 years (HbA1cP)), early glycation products (fructosamine (FAM)), serum advanced glycation end products (s-AGEs), lipid peroxidation products (LPO), advanced oxidation protein products (AOPP), profibrotic cytokines and adhesive molecules in patients with T1DM. We wanted to find a relationship of DC to glycative and oxidative stress parameters, circulating (serum) TGF-beta1 and soluble VCAM-1. Further, we aimed to compare measured parameters in groups -DC, one with DR, with DR combined with another DC and one with only DC another than DR and their combinations. The further aim of the present study was to evaluate if monitoring of circulating FAM, HbA1c, s-AGEs, AOPP, LPO in patients with T1DM could be useful to predict the diabetic complications development.

2. Study design and methods

2.1 Patients and design

The studied group consisted of 46 children and adolescents with T1DM regularly attending the 1st Department of Pediatrics, Children Diabetological Center of the Slovak Republic, University Hospital, Faculty of Medicine, Comenius University, Bratislava. They had T1DM with duration at least for 5 years. One of children was obese (BMIc 97 percentile) and three of them were of overweight (BMIc about 90 percentile). The file was divided into two subgroups: 20 persons without DC (-DC) and 46 those with them (+DC). Then the file of +DC patients was divided into several subgroups according to particular complications: the patients only with retinopathy, those with neuropathy combined with another kinds of DC and those with other than retinopathy to compare the parameters of glycative and oxidative stress and cytokines in each mentioned subgroups. The urine samples in our patients were collected 3 times overnight, microalbuminuria was considered to be positive when UAER was between 20 and 200 microgram/min in 2 samples. No changes (fundus diabetic retinopathy) were found by the ophtalmologist examining the eyes in subject without retinopathy. Diabetic neuropathy was confirmed by EMG exploration using the conductivity assessment of sensor and motor fibres of peripheral nerves. The controls file consists of 26 healthy children. The samples of EDTA capillary blood were used to determine of HbA1c and serum samples were used to determine of FAM, s-AGEs, AOPP and VCAM-1. The samples of serum were stored in -18°C/-80°C.

2.2 Parameter analysis

2.2.1 Determination of UAER

UAER was determined by means of immunoturbidimetric assay (Cobas Integra 400 Plus, Roche, Switzerland), using the commercial kit 400/400Plus. The assay was performed as a part of patients routine monitoring in Department of Laboratory Medicine, University Hospital, Bratislava.

2.2.2 Determination of fructosamine

For the determination of fructosamine we used a kinetic, colorimetric assay and subsequently spectrophotometrical determination at wavelength 530 nm. We used 1-deoxy-1-morpholino-fructose (DMF) as the standard. Serum samples were stored at -79°C and were defrost only once. This test is based on the ability of ketoamines to reduce nitroblue tetrazolium (NBT) to a formazan dye under alkaline conditions. The rate of formazan formation, measured at 530 nm, is directly proportional to the fructosamine concentration. Measurements were carried out in one block up to 5 samples. To 3 ml of 0.5 mmol/l NBT were added 150 microliters of serum and the mixture was incubated at 37°C for 10 minutes. The absorbance was measured after 10 min and 15 min of incubation at Novaspec analyzer II, Biotech (Germany).

2.2.3 Determination of glycated hemoglobin HbA1c

HbA1c was determined from EDTA capillary blood immediately after obtained by the low-pressure liquid chromatography (LPLC) (DiaSTAT, USA) in conjunction with gradient elution. Before testing hemolysate is heated at 62-68°C to eliminate unstable fractions and after 5 minutes is introduced into the column. Hemoglobin species elute from the cation-exchange column at different times, depending on their charge, with the application of buffers of increasing ionic strength. The concentration of hemoglobins is measured after elution from the column, which is then used to quantify HbA1c by calculating the area under each peak. Instrument calibration is always carried out when introducing a new column set procedure (Bio-RAD, Inc., 2003).

2.2.4 Determination of serum AGEs

Serum AGEs were determined as AGE-linked specific fluorescence, serum was diluted 20-fold with deionized water, the fluorescence intensity was measured after excitation at 346 nm, at emission 418 nm using a spectrophotometer Perkin Elmer LS-3, USA. Chinine sulphate (1 microgram/ml) was used to calibrate the instrument. Fluorescence was expressed as the relative fluorescence intensity in arbitrary units (A.U.).

2.2.5 Determination of serum lipoperoxides

Serum lipid peroxides were determined by iodine liberation spectrophotometrically at 365 nm (Novaspec II, Pharmacia LKB, Biotech, SRN). The principle of this assay is based on the oxidative activity of lipid peroxides that will convert iodide to iodine. Iodine can then simply be measured by means of a photometer at 365 nm. Calibration curves were obtained using cumene hydroperoxide. A stoichiometric relationship was observed between the amount of organic peroxides assayed and the concentration of I_3 produced (El-Saadani et al., 1989).

2.2.6 Determination of serum AOPP

AOPP were determined in the plasma using the method previously devised by Witko-Sarsat et al. (1996), modified by Kalousova et al. (2002). Briefly, AOPP were measured by spectrophotometry on a reader (FP-901, Chemistry Analyser, Labsystems, Finland) and were calibrated with chloramine-T solutions that in the presence of potassium iodide absorb at 340 nm. In standard wells, 10 microliters of 1.16 M potassium iodide was added to 200 microliters of chloramine-T solution (0–100 micromol/l) followed by 20 microliters of acetic acid. In test wells, 200 microliters of plasma diluted 1:5 in PBS was placed to cell of 9 channels, and 20 microliters of acetic acid was added. The absorbance of the reaction mixture is immediately read at 340 nm on the reader against a blank containing 200 microliters of PBS, 10 microliters of potassium iodide, and 20 microliters of acetic acid. The chloramine-T absorbance at 340 nm being linear within the range of 0 to 100 micromol/l, AOPP concentrations were expressed as micromoles per liter of chloramine-T equivalents.

2.2.7 Determination of TGF- beta1

Quantitative detection of TGF- beta1 in serum was done by enzyme linked immunosorbent assay, using human TGF-beta1 ELISA-kit (BMS249/2, Bender MedSystem).
Brief description of the method: into washed, with anti-TGF-beta1 precoated microplate were added prediluted (1:10) sera (100 microliters) and "HRP-Conjugate" (50 microliters) as a antihuman-TGF-beta1 monoclonal antibody and incubated for 4 hour on a rotator (100rpm). After microplate washing (3 times) "TMB Substrate Solution" (100 microliters) was added and was incubated for 10 minutes. Enzyme reaction was stopped by adding "Stop Solution" (100 microliters). The absorbance of each microwell was readed by HumaReader spectrophotometer (Human) using 450 nm wavelength. The TGF-beta1 concentration was determined from standard curve prepared from seven TGF-beta1 standard dilutions. Each sample and TGF-beta1 standard dilution were done in duplicate.

2.2.8 Determination of serum soluble form of adhesion molecule VCAM-1

For serum soluble form of VCAM-1 (sVCAM-1) estimating we used bead-based multiplex technology and Athena Multi-LyteTM Luminex 100 xMAP (multi-analyte profiling) analyser. We used RnD systems manufacturer kits: „Human Adhesion Molecule MultiAnalyte Profiling Base Kit" and „Fluorokine® MAP Human sVCAM-1/CD106 Kit".
Analyte-specific antibodies are pre-coated onto color-coded microparticles. Microparticles, standards and samples are pipetted into wells and the immobilized antibodies bind the analytes of interest. After washing away any unbound substances, a biotinylated antibody cocktail specific to the analytes of interest are added to each well. Following a wash to remove any unbound biotinylated antibody, streptavidin-phycoerythrin conjugate (Streptavidin-PE), which binds to the captured biotinylated antibody, is added to each well. A final wash removes unbound Streptavidin-PE and the microparticles are resuspended in buffer and read using the Luminex analyzer. One laser is microparticle-specific and determines which analyte is being detected. The other laser determines the magnitude of the phycoerythrin-derived signal, which is in direct proportion to the amount of analyte bound (R&D Systems, Inc. 2010).

2.2.9 Statistical analysis

Shapiro-Wilk test was performed to the test the distribution of all continuous variables. The variables with normal distribution were compared by one way ANOVA test followed by Bonferroni´s post-test and the results was expressed as mean ± SD. Since the evaluated variables did not have normal distribution, we compared them with Kruskal–Wallis non-parametric analysis of variance (ANOVA) followed by Bonferroni´s post-test and the results was expressed as median (1st quartile, 3rd quartile). The Fisher´s test was used to compare the subgroups in regard to diabetic retinopathy and other complications presence/absence. Pearson´s test with correlation coefficient r or Spearman´s one with Spearman's rank correlation coefficient R in case of small count of variables were then used to evaluate the association between parameters described within the text, in all studied patients and in diabetic and non-diabetic subgroups. P values less than 0.05 were accepted as being statistically significant. All statistical analyses were carried out using Excel 2003, Origin 8 and BioSTAT 2009.

3. Results

Clinical and biochemical characteristics of the patients with T1DM without and with diabetic complications and controls (CTRL) are reported in Table 1.

	CTRL	n	T1DM -DC	n	T1DM +DC	N
Age (yrs.)	9.0(6.1,14.0)	26	14.4(12.4, 17.9)[ab]	20	16.4(15.1, 17.6)[a]	26
DD (yrs.)	-	0	6(5.5, 8.1)[b]	20	10.0(7.9, 12.9)	26
HbA1cA (%)	5.0 ± 0.3	18	8.3 ± 1.4 [ab]	20	10.4 ± 1.4[a]	26
FAM (mmol/l)	1.67 ± 0.31	24	2.64 ± 0.38 [ab]	20	3.06 ± 0.48[a]	26
s-AGEs (A.U.)	54.9 ± 9.9	22	64.4 ± 10.1 [ab]	20	71.8 ± 11.6	24
AOPP (micromol/l)	58.8(52.0, 71.8)	11	43.3(42.6, 60.4)	17	78.2(49.5, 114.6)	20
LPO (nmol/ml)	100(88, 110)	10	106(105, 161)	19	127(109, 152)[a]	17
TGF-beta1 (ng/ml)	3.30 ± 3.41	8	5.9 ± 4.14[b]	10	10.49 ± 4.55[a]	16
VCAM-1 (ng/ml)	12.6 ± 3.7	15	17.1 ± 3.1	19	17.4 ± 3.3[a]	26

[a] significant difference in comparison with CTRL
[b] significant difference in comparison with +DC group T1DM

Table 1. Clinical and biochemical characteristics of the patients with T1DM and controls

As seen, HbA1c and FAM were significantly elevated in both diabetic groups in comparison with controls and also in +DC vs. -DC those. Serum AGEs were significantly elevated in +DC compared to -DC and also to controls, but the difference between -DC and controls was not significant. The levels of AOPP were evidently higher in +DC compared to controls, but the difference was not significant. The levels of LPO were significantly elevated in +DC vs. controls, the differences between both diabetic groups and between -DC vs. controls were not significant. The levels of TGF-beta1 similarly to s-AGEs were significantly elevated in +DC compared to -DC and also to controls, but the difference between -DC and controls was not significant (Fig. 1). In terms of the VCAM-1 values, only between +DC and controls there were found significant difference there (Fig. 2).
The levels of TGF-beta1 are significantly elevated in +DC compared to -DC (10.49 ± 4.55 vs. 5.9 ± 4.14 ng/ml, $p<0.05$) and also to controls (10.49 ± 4.55 vs. 3.30 ± 3.41ng/ml, $p<0.05$), but the difference between -DC and controls (5.9 ± 4.14 vs. 3.30 ± 3.41ng/ml, $p>0.05$) was not statistically significant.

3.1 The relationships between clinical and biochemical parameters

3.1.1 The subgroup of patients with T1DM without diabetic complications

The relationships characterized by Pearson´s correlation coefficient r or Spearman´s coefficient R between the parameters described within the text are reported in Table 2. As seen, we found significant linear correlations of FAM with HbA1cA (r=0.676), LPO with HbA1cP (r=-0.507) and AOPP (R=0.671). The relationship between LPO (y) and HbA1cP(x) is possible to describe by non-linear equation $y=19x^2-354x+1752$ ($R=0.632$, $R^2=0.400$, $p<0.05$). VCAM-1 significantly correlated with age (r=-0.478), HbA1cA (r=0.653, Fig. 3), HbA1cP (r=0.501) and with FAM (r=0.630, Fig. 4).

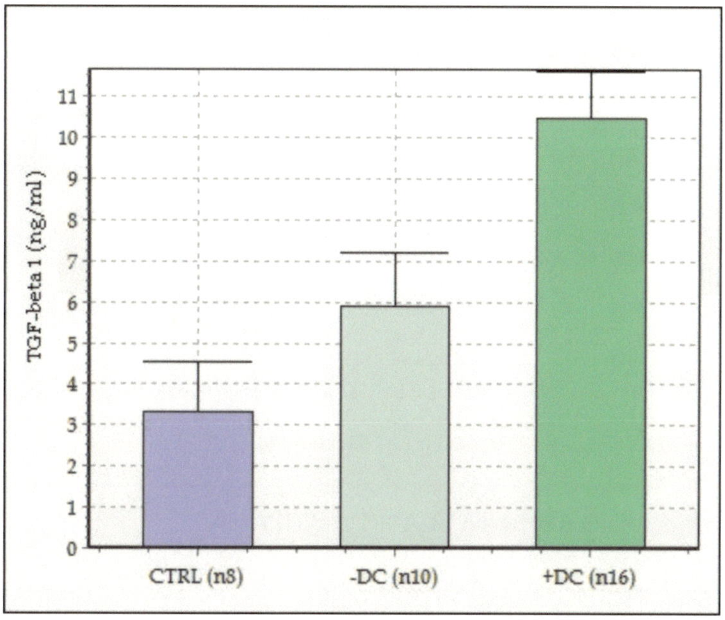

Fig. 1. Comparison of TGF-beta1 levels of patients with T1DM and controls

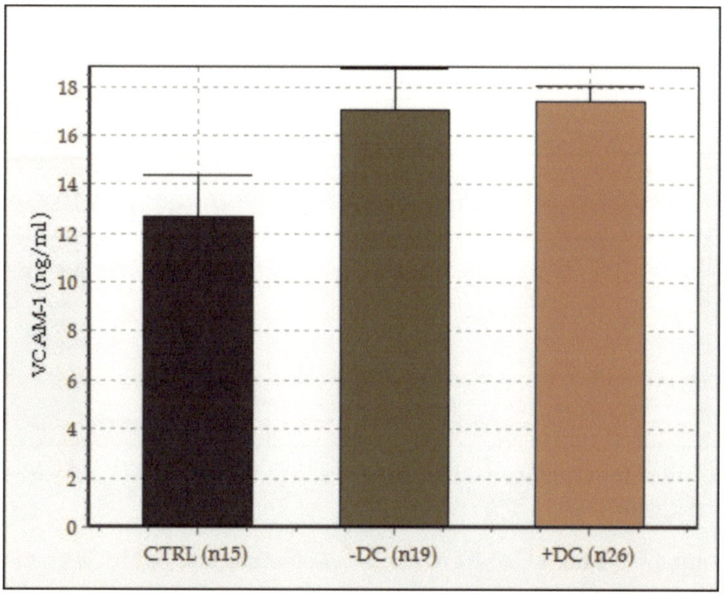

Fig. 2. Comparison of VCAM-1 levels of patients with T1DM and controls

The levels of VCAM-1 are significantly elevated in +DC compared to controls (17.4 ± 3.3 vs. 12.6 ± 3.7 ng/ml, $p<0.05$). The values of VCAM-1 in -DC subgroup differ obviously from those in controls, but the difference is non statistically significant (17.1 ± 3.1 vs. 12.6 ± 3.7 ng/ml, $p>0.05$). There are similar levels in both diabetic subgroups ((17.4 ± 3.3 vs. 17.1 ± 3.1 ng/ml, $p>>0.05$).

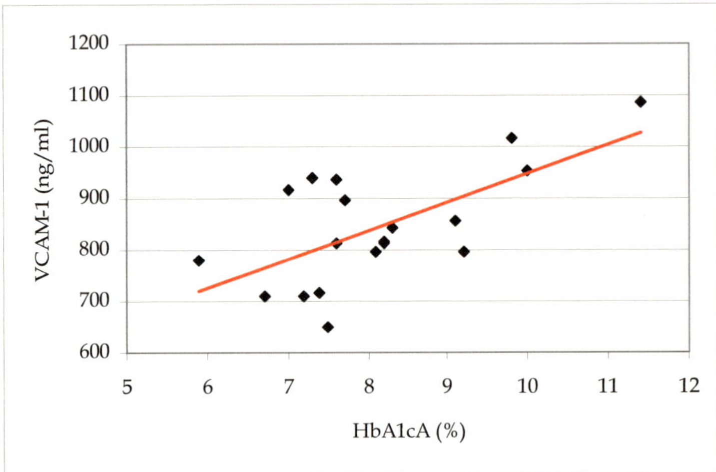

Fig. 3. The linear correlation between VCAM-1 and HbA1cA

	DD (yrs.)	HbA1cA	HbA1cP	FAM	s-AGEs	AOPP	LPO	TGF-beta1	VCAM-1
Age (yrs.)	0.205	-0.267	-0.232	-0.328	-0.030	0.130†	0.334	0.406†	-0.478$^{\Delta}$
DD (yrs.)	N	0.152	-0.008	0.326	-0.256	-0.193†	-0.001	0.036†	0.089
HbA1cA (%)		N	0.748$^{\Delta}$	0.676$^{\Delta}$	0.217	-0.298†	-0.398	-0.588†	0.653$^{\Delta}$
HbA1cP (%)			N	0.433	0.302	-0.400†	-0.507$^{\Delta}$	-0.042†	0.501$^{\Delta}$
FAM (mmol/l)				N	0.134	0.081†	-0.260	-0.224†	0.630$^{\Delta}$
s-AGEs (A.U.)					N	0.197†	0.270	0.006	0.068
AOPP (micromol/l)						N	0.671$^{\dagger\Delta}$	0.477†	-0.447†
LPO (nmol/ml)							N	0.200†	-0.404
TGF-beta1 (ng/ml)								N	-0.578†

Table 2. The relationships between the parameters in patients with T1DM without diabetic complications (†R, $^{\Delta}p<0.05$)

In this subgroup LPO and VCAM-1 were in association also with other parameters, but those were not statistically significant. Non linear statistically significant relationship with regression line equation $y=0.33x^2 - 4.10x + 28.26$ was found between VCAM-1(y) and HbA1cA(x) ($R=0.694$, $R^2=0.481$, $p<<0.05$).

3.1.2 The subgroup of patients with T1DM with diabetic complications

The relationships characterized by Pearson´s correlation coefficient r or Spearman´s coefficient R between the parameters described within the text are reported in Table 3.

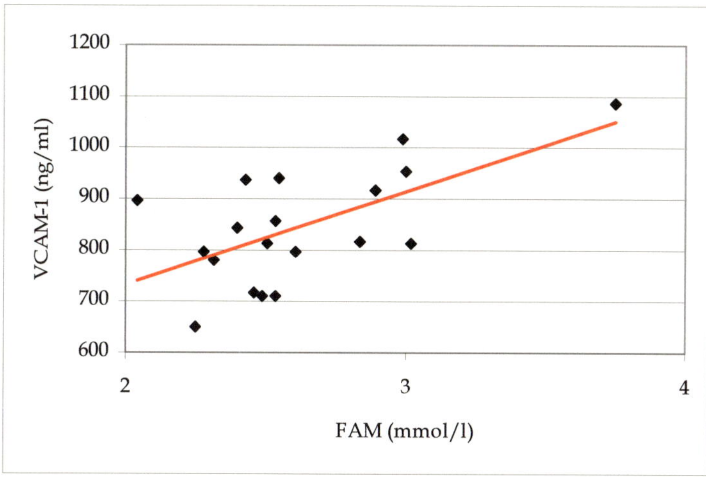

Fig. 4. The linear correlation between VCAM-1 and FAM

	DD (yrs.)	HbA1cA	HbA1cP	FAM	s-AGEs	AOPP	LPO	TGF-beta1	VCAM-1
Age (yrs.)	0.448Δ	-0.295	-0.422Δ	-0.023	-0.068	-0.165	-0.044†	0.541†Δ	0.067
DD (yrs.)	N	-0.070	-0.110	-0.170	-0.069	-0.034	-0.297†	0.247†	0.009
HbA1cA (%)		N	0.539Δ	0.581Δ	0.221	0.278	0.123†	-0.429†	0.006
HbA1cP (%)			N	0.3405	0.247	0.116	0.127†	-0.679†Δ	0.291
FAM (mmol/l)				N	0.479Δ	0.538Δ	0.471†	-0.708†Δ	0.183
s-AGEs (A.U.)					N	0.119†	0.125†	-0.356†	0.432Δ
AOPP (micromol/l)						N	0.355†	-0.545†	-0.026
LPO (nmol/ml)							N	-0.612†	-0.174†
TGF-beta1 (ng/ml)								N	-0.069†

(† R, Δ $p<0.05$)

Table 3. The relationships between parameters described within the text in patients with T1DM with diabetic complications

As seen, in +DC subgroup we found significant correlations of FAM with HbA1cA (r=0.581), s-AGEs with FAM (r=0.479) and AOPP with FAM (r=0.538). LPO correlated with FAM (r=0.471), but this relation is not statistically significant (p=0.056). TGF-beta1 correlated with age (R=0.541), HbA1cP (R=-0.679) and FAM (R=-0.708). Statistically significant moderate linear correlation was found between VCAM-1 and s-AGEs (r=0.432). Moderate relationships were found also between TGF-beta1 and oxidative stress parameters, but those were not statistically significant.

3.1.3 Controls

As seen in Table 4, there were found moderate negative relation on the border of significance between AOPP and FAM (R=-0.627, p=0.05) and strong relation between AOPP and s-AGEs (R=0.855) in controls. TGF-beta1 was in statistically significant relation with age (R=-0.838) and s-AGEs (R=-0.757) and moderate, but not significant relationship was found with LPO (R=0.478). Slight relationship were found between VCAM-1 and FAM (R=0.366) and also between VCAM-1 and s-AGEs (R=0.267).

	HbA1cA	FAM	s-AGEs	AOPP	LPO	TGF-beta1	VCAM-1
Age (yrs.)	0.354†	-0.249	-0.008	0.193†	0.026†	-0.838†Δ	-0.052†
HbA1cA (%)	N	0.109†	-0.133†	-0.022†	0.189†	-0.024†	-0.068†
FAM (mmol/l)		N	-0.143	-0.627†▪	-0.162†	0.276†	0.366†
s-AGEs (A.U.)			N	0.855†Δ	-0.382†	-0.757†Δ	0.267†
AOPP (micromol/l)				N	-0.286†	N	0.069†
LPO (nmol/ml)					N	0.478†	0.037†
TGF-beta1 (ng/ml)						N	0.152†

(† R, p<0.05, ▪ p=0.05)

Table 4. The relationships between the parameters in controls

3.2 The parameters of glycative and oxidative stress, TGF-beta1 and VCAM-1 with regard to presence/absence of retinopathy and/or other complications

We compared described parameters between subgroups with/without diabetic retinopathy. The results of Fisher´s post-test (p values) are reported in table 5.

Subgroups	FAM	HbA1cA	s-AGEs	AOPP	LPO	TGF-beta1	VCAM-1
DR vs. DR+O	NS	NS	NS	NS	NS	NA	NS
DR vs. ODC	0.055	NS	0.055	NS	<0.05	<0.05	NS
DR vs. -DC	NS	0,01	NS	NS	NS	<0.05	NS
DR+O vs. ODC	0.052	NS	0,05	NS	NS	NA	NS
DR+O vs. -DC	NS	<0.05	NS	NS	NS	NA	NS
ODC vs. -DC	<0.05	<0.05	<0.05	NS	NS	NS	NS

(DR – having diabetic retinopathy only, DR+ODC – having diabetic retinopathy and another complications, ODC – having only other diabetic complications except diabetic retinopathy-DC – having no complications, NS – non-significant difference, NA – not available)

Table 5. The differences in measured parameters between subgroups of patients with T1DM with regard to presence/absence of diabetic retinopathy and/or other (O) complications

FAM were significantly elevated in patients having diabetic complications only other than diabetic retinopathy compared to -DC (3.10(2.93, 3.54) vs. 2.54(2.42, 2.91) mmol/l, p<0.05, Fig. 5). HbA1c levels are elevated in patients having diabetic retinopathy against to -DC (9.8(9.6, 10.2) vs. (7.9(7.4, 9.1)%, p<0.05), in subgroup of patients having diabetic retinopathy with other complication/s compared to -DC (10.4(8.6, 11.2) vs. (7.9(7.4, 9.1) %, p<0.05, Fig.6) and also the subgroup of patients having diabetic complications only other than diabetic retinopathy compared to -DC (10.5(10.0, 11.1 vs. (7.9(7.4, 9.1) %, p<0.05, Fig. 6). Serum AGEs were significantly higher in subgroup with only other diabetic complications than diabetic retinopathy compared to -DC one (74.8(71.2, 76.5) vs. 61.9(58.9, 71.0) A.U., Fig. 7), and non-significantly higher in patients with retinopathy only than in those with others DC and also in patients with DR and another DC compared to ODC group, however, p-values were only slightly higher than 0.05 (Fig. 7). The values of LPO were significantly elevated in patients with complications other than retinopathy compared to those with retinopathy only (138(129, 165) vs. 101(93, 109) nmol/ml, Fig. 8). No significant differences were found between others in LPO. There were the significant differences between patients having only diabetic retinopathy vs. -DC in TGF-beta1 levels (14.17(13.32, 15.52) vs. 5.7(2.23, 8.71) ng/ml, p<0.05, Fig. 9) and also between subgroup of patients having only diabetic retinopathy and those having diabetic complications other than diabetic retinopathy (14.17(13.32, 15.52) vs. 9.05(5.29, 10.39) ng/ml, p=0.05, Fig. 9). Neither AOPP parameters nor VCAM-1 showed any significant differences between subgroups with regard to presence/absence diabetic retinopathy or other diabetic complications.

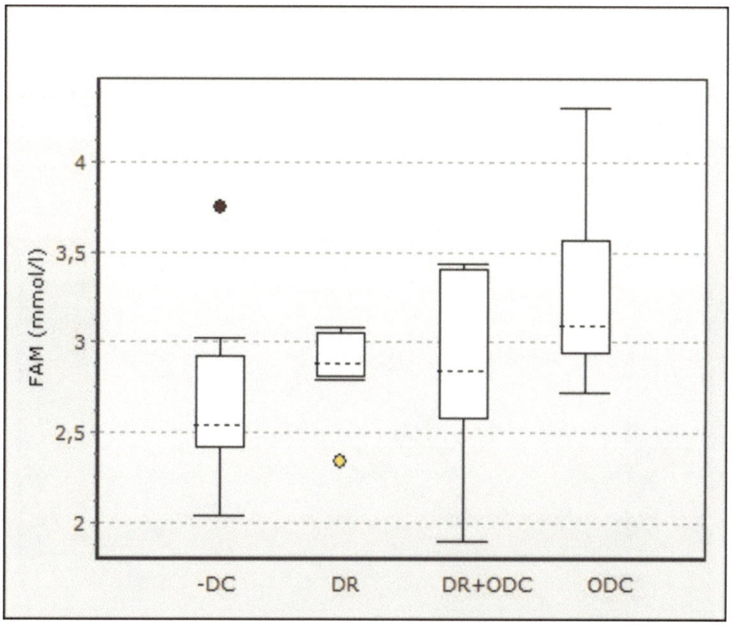

Fig. 5. The values of FAM in subgroups of patients with T1DM with regard to diabetic retinopathy presence/absence (DR – having diabetic retinopathy only, DR+ODC – having diabetic retinopathy and another complications, ODC – having only other diabetic complications except diabetic retinopathy, -DC – having no complications)

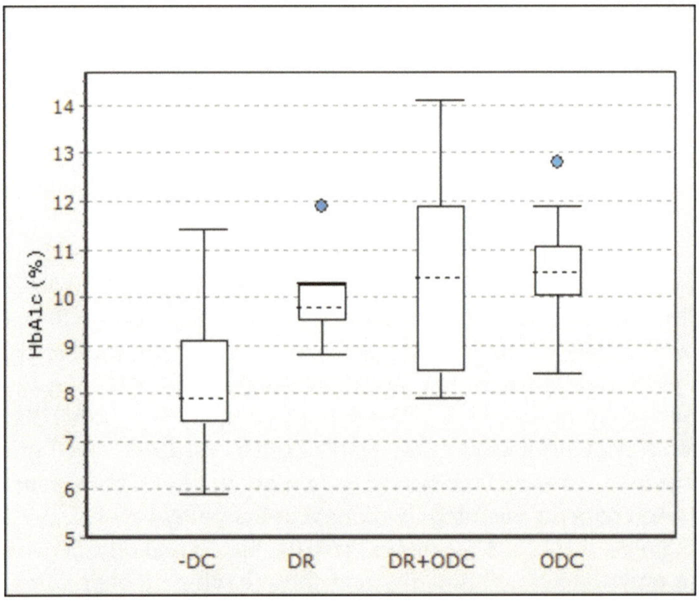

Fig. 6. The values of HbA1c in subgroups of patients with T1DM with regard to diabetic retinopathy presence/absence (DR – having diabetic retinopathy only, DR+ODC – having diabetic retinopathy and another complications, ODC – having only other diabetic complications except diabetic retinopathy, -DC – having no complications)

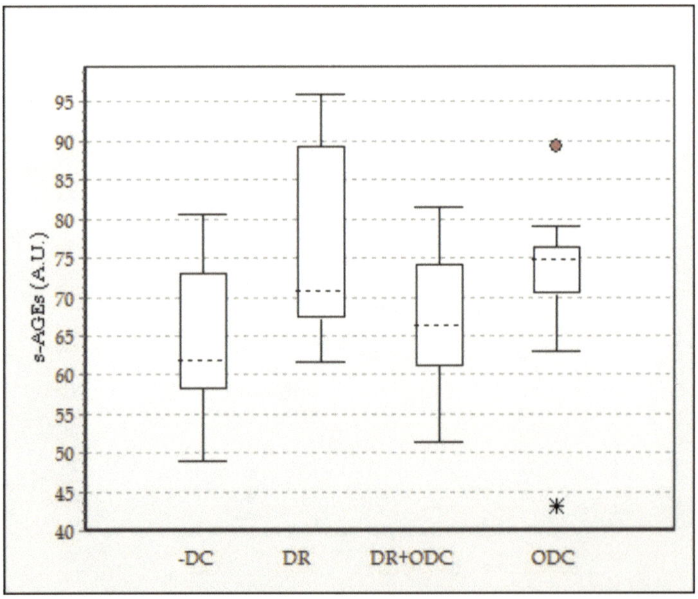

Fig. 7. The values of s-AGEs in subgroups of patients with T1DM with regard to diabetic retinopathy presence/absence (DR – having diabetic retinopathy only, DR+ODC – having diabetic retinopathy and another complications, ODC – having only other diabetic complications except diabetic retinopathy, -DC – having no complications)

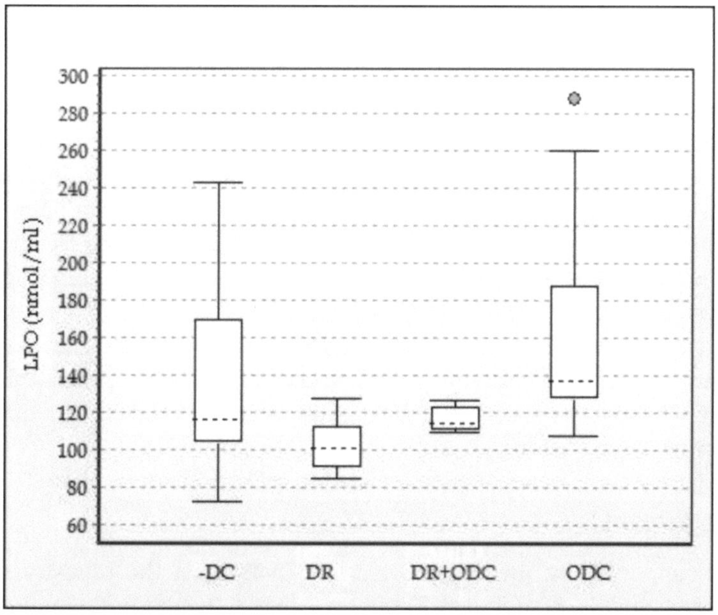

Fig. 8. The values of LPO in subgroups of patients with T1DM with regard to diabetic retinopathy presence/absence (DR – having diabetic retinopathy only, DR+ODC – having diabetic retinopathy and another complications, ODC – having only other diabetic complications except diabetic retinopathy, -DC – having no complications)

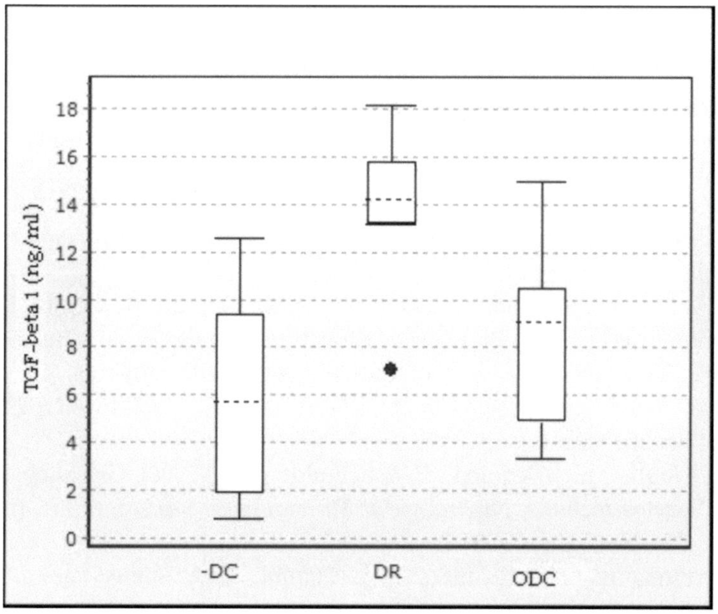

Fig. 9. The values of TGF-beta1 in subgroups of patients with T1DM with regard to diabetic retinopathy presence/absence (DR – having diabetic retinopathy only, ODC – having only other diabetic complications except diabetic retinopathy, -DC – having no complications)

4. Conclusion

Our results suggest the relation of glycation and oxidation to profibrotic cytokines, vascular molecules and diabetic complications. Serum AGEs were connected with complications other than retinopathy more than just with retinopathy, nevertheless, some relation of retinopathy and s-AGEs was found (p-values were only slightly higher than 0.05). Lipoperoxides showed some relation to DR since higher in patients with retinopathy than in those with other DC, whereas AOPP did not show any relation to any DC. It seems that in our patients TGF-beta1 and VCAM-1 are linked with the development of DC, but only TGF-beta1 showed some linkage to diabetic retinopathy.

We ought to keep in mind the fact our investigation concerns the children and adolescents. Maybe the study of older patients with T1DM would show more, especially about VCAM-1 and its relation to glycative and oxidative stress and consequently to development of retinopathy/other complications.

5. Acknowledgment

This work is supported by the Vega Grant 1-0375-09 from the Ministry of Education, Sciences, Research and Sport of Slovak Republic. Authors thank Mr. Ľ. Barak, M.D., Mrs. E. Jancova, M.D., Mrs. A. Stanikova, M.D., Mrs. D. Tomcikova, M.D. for assistance with subject recruitment and assessment and Mrs. J. Kalninova, RN.D. and Mrs. E. Tomeckova for technical assistance.

6. References

Bio-Rad, a.s. (2003). *DiaSTAT Hemoglobin A1c Program.* Bio-Rad laboratories Inc., Hercules CA, USA retrieved from http://www.embeediagnostics.com/equip/glycol/diastat.htm April 28th 2009.

R&D Systems, a.s. (2010). Fluorokine MAP. Human Adhesion Molecule MultiAnalyte Profiling Base K. retrieved from http://www.rndsystems.com/product_results.aspx?m=2246&c=87 March 1th 2011.

Aronson, D. (2008). Hyperglycemia and pathobiology of diabetic complications. *Advances in Cardiology,* Vol. 45, pp. 1-16, ISSN 0065-2326

Bargnoux, A.S., Morena, M., Badiou, S., Dupuy, A.M., Canaud, B., Cristol, J.P. & Groupe de travail de la SFBC: Biologie des fonctions renales et de l' insuffisance renale (2009). Carbonyl stress and oxidatively modified proteins in chronic renal failure. *Annales de Biologie Clinique (Paris),* Vol.67, No.2, (March 2009), pp. 153-158, ISSN 0003-3898

Boulanger, E., Wautier, J.L., Dequiedt, P. & Schmidt, A.M. (2006). Glycation, glycoxidation and diabetes mellitus. *Nephrologie et Therapeutique,* Vol.2, Suppl.1, (January 2006), pp. S8-S16, ISSN 1769-7255

Boyzel, R., Bruttmann, G, Benhamou, P.Y., Halimi, S. & Stanke-Labesque, F. (2010). Regulation of oxidative stress and inflammation by glycaemic control: evidence for reversible activation of the 5-lipoxygenase pathway in type 1 diabetes, but not in diabetes 2. *Diabetologia,* Vol.53, No.9, pp. 2068-2070, ISSN 0012-186X

Clausen, P., Jacobsen, P., Rossing, K., Jensen, J.S., Parving, H.H. & Feldt-Rasmussen, B. (2000). Plasma concentration of VCAM-1 and ICAM-1 are elevated in patients with Type 1 diabetes mellitus with microalbuminuria and overt nephropathy. *Diabetic Medicine*, Vol.17, No.9, pp. 644-649, ISSN 0742-3071

Devaraj, S., Cheung, A.T., Jialal, I., Griffen, S.C., Nguyen, D., Glaser, N., & Aoki, T. (2007). Evidence of increased inflammation and microcirculatory abnormalities in patients with type 1 diabetes and their role in microvascular complications. *Diabetes*, Vol.56, No.11, (November 2007), pp. 2790-2796, ISSN 0012-1797

El-Saadani, M., Esterbauer, H., el-Sayed, M., Goher, M., Nassar, A.Y. & Jürgens, G. (1989). A spectrophotometric assay for lipid peroxides in serum lipoproteins using a commercially available reagent. *Journal of Lipid Research*, Vol.30, No.4, (April 1989), pp. 627-630, ISSN 0022-2275

Fawaz, L., Elwan, A.E., Kamel, Y.H., Farid, T.M., Kamel, A. & Mohamed, W.A. (2009). Value of C-reactive protein and IL-6 measurements in type 1 diabetes mellitus. *Archives of Medical Science*, Vol.5, No.3, pp. 383-390, ISSN 1734-1922

Goh, S.Y. & Cooper M.E. (2008). Clinical review: The role of advanced glycation end products in progression and complications of diabetes. *Journal of Clinical Endocrinology and Metabolism*, Vol.93, No.4, (January 2008), pp.1143-1152, ISSN 0021-972X

Goldfarb, S. & Ziyadeh, F.N. (2001). TGF-beta: a crucial component of the pathogenesis of diabetic nephropathy. *Transactions of the American Clinical and Climatological Association*, Vol.112, pp.27-33 , ISSN 0065-7778

Hartge, M.M., Unger, T. & Kintscher, U. (2007). The endothelium and vascular inflammation in diabetes. *Diabetes and Vascular Disease Research*, Vol.4, No.2, (June 2007), pp. 84-88, ISSN 1479-1641

Chung, A.C.K., Zhang, H., Kong, Y.Z., Tan, J.J., Huang, X.R., Kopp, J.B. & Lan, H.Y. (2010). Advanced glycation end-products induce tubular CTGF via TGF-beta-independent Smad3 signalling. *Journal of the American Society of Nephrology*, Vol.21, No.2, (February 2010), pp. 249-260, ISSN 1046-6673

Kalousova, M., Škrha, J. & Zima, T. (2002). Advanced glycation end-products and advanced oxidation protein products in patients with diabetes mellitus. *Physiological Research*, Vol.51, No.6, pp. 597–604, ISSN 0862-8408

Karasu, C. (2010). Glycoxidative stress and cardiovascular complications in experimentally-induced diabetes: effects of antioxidant treatment. *The Open Cardiovascular Medicine Journal*, Vol.4, (Nov 2010), pp. 240-256, ISSN 1874-1924

Kashihara, N., Haruna, Y., Kondeti, V.K. & Kanvar, Y.S. (2010). Oxidative stress in diabetic nephropathy. *Current Medicinal Chemistry*, Vol.17, No.34, (December 2010), pp. 4256-4269, ISSN 0929-8673

Mosquera, J.A. (2010). Role of the receptor for advanced glycation end products (RAGE) in inflammation. *Investigación Clinica*, Vol.51, No.2, (June 2010), pp. 257-268, ISSN 0535-5133

Navarro, J.F., & Mora, C. (2006). Diabetes, inflammation, proinflammatory cytokines, and diabetic nephropathy. *The Scientific World Journal*, pp. 6908-6917, ISSN 1537-744X

Negre-Salvayre, A., Salvayre, R., Auge, N., Pamplona, R. & Portero-Otin, M. (2009). Hyperglycemia and glycation in diabetic complications. *Antioxidants & Redox Signaling*, Vol. 11, No.12, (December 2009), pp. 3071-3109, ISSN 1523-0864

Nin, J.W., Jorsai, A., Ferreira, J., Schalwijk, C.G., Prins, M.H., Parving, H.H., Tarnow, L., Rossing, P. & Stehouwer, C.D. (2011). Higher plasma levels of advanced glycation end products are associated with incident cardiovascular disease and all-cause mortality in type 1 diabetes: A 12-year follow-up study. *Diabetes Care*, Vol.34, No.2, (February 2011), pp. 442-447, ISSN 0149-5992

Nobécourt, E., Tabet, F., Lambert, G., Puranik, R., Bao, S., Yan, L., Davies, M.J., Brown, B.E., Jenkins, A.J., Dusting, G.J., Bonnet, D.J., Curtiss, L.K., Barter, P.J. & Rye, K.A. (2010). *Arteriosclerosis, Thrombosis, and Vascular Biology*, Vol.30, No.4, (April 2010), pp. 766-772, ISSN 1079-5642

Peppa, M. & Vlassara, H. (2005). Advanced glycation end products and diabetic complications: A General overview. *Hormones*, Vol.4, No.1, pp. 28-37, ISSN 1109-3099

Piwovar, A. (2010a). Advanced oxidation products. Part I. Mechanism of the formation, characteristics and property. *Polski Merkuriusz Lekarski*, Vol.28, No.164, (February, 2010), pp. 166-169, ISSN 1426-9686

Piwovar, A. (2010b). Advanced oxidation products. Part II. The significance of oxidation protein products in the pathomechanism of diabetes and its complications. *Polski Merkuriusz Lekarski*, Vol.28, No.165, (March, 2010), pp. 227-230, ISSN 1426-9686

Ramasamy, R., Vannucci, S. J., Yan, S. S., Herold, K., Yan, S. F. & Schmidt A. M. (2005). Advanced glycation end products and RAGE: a common thread in aging, diabetes, neurodegeneration, and inflammation. *Glycobiology*, Vol.15, No.7, pp. 16R–28R, ISSN 0959-6658

Rambhade, S., Chakraborty, A.K., Patil, U.K., & Rambhade, A. (2010). Diabetes mellitus- Its complications, factors influencing complications and prevention - An Overview. *Journal of Chemical and Pharmaceutical Re*search, Vol.2, No.6, pp. 7-25, ISSN 0975-7384

Seckin, D, Ilhan, N., Ilhan, N. & Ertugrul, S. (2006). Glycaemic control, markers of endothelial cell activation and oxidative stress in children with type 1 diabetes mellitus. *Diabetes Research and Clinical Practice*, Vol.73., (August 2006), pp. 191-197, ISSN 0168-8227

Schmidt, A.M., Hori, A., Jing, X.C., Jian, F.L., Crandall, J. Zhang, J., Cao, R., Shi, D.Y., Brett, J. & Stern, D. (1995). Advanced glycation endproducts interacting with their endothelial receptor induce expression of vascular cell adhesion molecule-1 (VCAM-1) in cultured human endothelial cells and in mice: A potential mechanism for the accelerated vasculopathy of diabetes. *Journal of Clinical Investigation*, Vol.96, No.3, pp.1395-1403, ISSN 0021-9738

Schmidt, A.M., Crandall, J., Hori, O., Cao, R. & Lakatta, E. (1996). Elevated plasma levels of vascular adhesion molecule (VCAM-1) in diabetic patients with microalbuminuria: A marker of vascular dysfunction and progressive vascular disease. *British Journal of Haematology,* Vol.92, No.3, pp. 747-750, ISSN 0007-1048

Schrijvers, B.F., De Vriese, A.S. & Flyvbjerg, A. (2004). From hyperglycemia to diabetic kidney disease: The role of metabolic, hemodynamic, intracellular factors and growth factors/cytokines. *Endocrine Reviews,* Vol.25, No.6, (December 2004), pp. 971-1010, ISSN 0163-769X

Son, S.M. (2007). Role of vascular reactive oxygen species in development of vascular abnormalities in diabetes. *Diabetes Research and Clinical Practice,* Vol. 77, Suppl. 1, pp. S65–S70, ISSN 0168-8227

Van Sickle, B.J., Simmons, J., Hall, R., Raines, M., Ness, K. & Spagnoli, A. (2009). Increased circulating IL-8 is associated with reduced IGF-1 and related to poor metabolic control in adolescents with type 1 diabetes mellitus. *Cytokine,* Vol.48, No.3, pp. 290-294, ISSN 1043-4666

Vlassara, H., Fuh, H., Donnelly, T. & Cybulsky, M. (1995). Advanced glycation endproducts promote adhesion molecule (VCAM-1, ICAM-1) expression and atheroma formation in normal rabbits. *Molecular Medicine (Cambridge, Mass.),* Vol.1, No.4, (May 1995), pp. 447-456, ISSN 1076-1551

Wang, W., Koka, V. & Lan, H.Y. (2005). Transforming growth factor-β and Smad signalling in kidney diseases. *Nephrology,* Vol.10, No.1, (February 2005), pp. 48-56, ISSN 1320-5358

Wautier, J.L., Boulanger, E. & Wautier, M.P. (2006). Postprandial hyperglycemia alters inflammatory and hemostatic parameters. *Diabetes and Metabolism,* Vol.32, No.HS2, (September 2006), pp. 2S34-2S36, ISSN 1262-3636

Witko-Sarsat, V., Friedlander, M., Capeillère-Blandin, C., Nguyen-Khoa, T., Nguyen, A. T., Zingraff, J., Jungers, P. & Descamps-Latscha, B. (1996). Advanced oxidation protein products as a novel marker of oxidative stress in uremia. *Kidney Internatinal,* Vol. 49, No.5, (May 1996), pp. 1304-1313, ISSN 0085-2538

Wolf, G. & Ziyadeh, F.N. (2007). Cellular and molecular mechanisms of proteinuria in diabetic nephropathy. *Nephron-Physiology,* Vol.106, No.2, (June 2007), pp. 26-31, ISSN 1660-2137

Yamagishi, S. Ueda, S. Matsui, T., Nakamura, K. & Okuda, S. (2008). Role of advanced glycation end products (AGEs) and oxidative stress in diabetic retinopathy. *Current Pharmaceutial Design,* Vol.14, No.10, pp. 962-968, ISSN 1381-6128

Yamagishi, S. (2009). Advanced glycation end products and receptor-oxidative stress system in diabetic vascular complications. *Therapeutic Apheresis and Dialysis,* Vol.13, No.6, (December 2009), pp. 534-539, ISSN 1744-9979

Yan S.F., Ramasamy, R. & Schmidt, A.M. (2008). Mechanisms of disease: advanced glycation end products and their receptors in inflammation and diabetes complications. *Nature Clinical Practice Endocrinology Metabolism,* Vol.4, No.5, (May 2008), pp. 285-293, ISSN 1745-8366

Zhang, L., Zalewski, A., Liu, Y., Mazurek, T., Cowan, S., Martin, J.L., Hofmann, S.M., Vlassara, H. & Shi, Y. (2003). Diabetes induced oxidative stress and low-grade inflammation in porcine coronary arteries. *Circulation,* Vol.108, No.4, (July 2003), pp. 472-478, ISSN 0009-7322

Zhou, G., Li C. & Cai, L. (2004). Advanced glycation end-products induce connective tissue growth factor-mediated renal fibrosis predominantly through transforming growth factor β-independent pathway. *American Journal of Pathology,* Vol.165, No.6, (December 2004), pp. 2033-2043, ISSN 0002-9440

2

Diet, Lifestyle and Chronic Complications in Type 1 Diabetic Patients

S. S. Soedamah-Muthu[1], S. Abbring[1] and M. Toeller[2]
[1]*Division of Human Nutrition, Wageningen University, Wageningen*
[2]*Department of Endocrinology, Diabetology and Rheumatology*
Heinrich-Heine-University Duesseldorf
[1]*Netherlands*
[2]*Germany*

1. Introduction

Diabetes mellitus is with 220.000 deaths per year the eighth leading cause of death in high income countries (World Health Organization (WHO) 2008). In 2007, over 740.000 people in the Netherlands were suffering from diabetes and this number is expected to grow to 1.3 million people in 2025 (National Institute for Public Health and the Environment (RIVM) 2010). Worldwide approximately 285 million people had the disease in 2010 and this number will increase till 438 million in 2030 (World Diabetes Foundation (WDF) 2010). In 2000, diabetes was most prevalent in India with 31.7 million cases. China (20.8 million cases) and the United States (17.7 million cases) were on the second and third place. Diabetes also has a great economic impact on the individual, nation healthcare system and economy (International Diabetes Federation (IDF) 2010).

Type 1 diabetes accounts for 5% of all cases of diabetes worldwide. Of this 5% the vast majority are children. In type 1 diabetes the body does not produce insulin (American Diabetes Association (ADA) 2010).The disease has a strong genetic component, inherited mainly through the HLA complex but the exact cause is unknown. Most likely there is an environmental trigger in genetically susceptible people that causes an immune reaction. The body's white blood cells mistakenly attack the insulin-producing pancreatic β-cells (U.S. National Library of Medicine 2011). Putative environmental triggers include viruses (e.g. enteroviruses), environmental toxins (e.g. nitrosamines) or foods (e.g. early exposure to cow's milk proteins, cereals or gluten) (Daneman D 2006). This 'food' trigger explains why type 1 diabetes is less common in people who were breastfed and in those who first ate solid foods at later ages (Sadauskaitė-Kuehne V et al. 2004; American Diabetes Association (ADA) 2010).

People with type 1 diabetes also have an increased risk of developing some serious and life threatening complications. This involves acute complications, like hyperglycaemia and hypoglycaemia which can lead to a coma, but also chronic complications (National Institute for Public Health and the Environment (RIVM) 2007). Chronic complications can be subdivided into macrovascular and microvascular complications. Cardiovascular disease is the major macrovascular complication and includes mainly myocardial infarction and stroke (American Diabetes Association (ADA) 2010). The risk for cardiovascular disease, is 4-8 times higher for people with type 1 diabetes (Soedamah-Muthu SS et al. 2006). The major microvascular complications are diabetic nephropathy, diabetic neuropathy and diabetic retinopathy (American Diabetes Association (ADA) 2010). Of the patients with type 1 diabetes approximately 29% develop persistent microalbuminuria (urinary albumin excretion rate between 30 and 300 mg/24 h) after 20 years. Of these 29%, 34% progressed further to persistent macroalbuminuria (urinary albumin excretion rate > 300 mg/24 h). Persistent microalbuminuria is a risk factor for the development of diabetic nephropathy. Microalbuminuria can be seen as an early marker of diabetic kidney disease (Hovind P 2004). Also retinopathy is a common microvascular complication. The 25-year cumulative incidences of any visual impairment and severe visual impairment are 13% and 3%, respectively. Diabetic retinopathy is an important cause of visual impairment (Klein R et al. 2010). Finally the high incidence of lower extremity amputations also stresses how serious the complications of type 1 diabetes are. The overall 25-year incidence of lower extremity amputations is 10.1% in 943 American type 1 diabetic patients (Sahakyan K et al. 2011). These complications account for the major morbidity and mortality associated with type 1 diabetes, so it is very important to treat them (Daneman D 2006).

In type 1 diabetes, special attention is paid to balancing the insulin dose with episodes of activity and the quantity and timing of food intake to prevent acute episodes of hypoglycaemia and hyperglycaemia (Franz MJ et al. 2003). This is important because these acute complications can lead to a coma, but also because a high blood glucose concentration (glycosylated hemoglobin (HbA1c) ≥ 7%) in people with diabetes increases the risk for macrovascular as well as microvascular complications. Other risk factors for these chronic complications are smoking, obesity, physical inactivity, high blood pressure and high cholesterol levels. Also people with a longer history of diabetes have a higher risk (National Institute for Public Health and the Environment (RIVM) 2007). Furthermore it is important to realise that the microvascular complications lie on the pathway between diabetes and cardiovascular disease. Nephropathy for example is an important risk factor for cardiovascular disease in people with type 1 diabetes (Jensen T et al. 1987).

Recent studies have shown that people with type 1 diabetes eat a more atherosclerosis-prone diet. This includes a high intake of energy from saturated fat and a low intake of fiber, fruits and vegetables, which could increase the risk of the development of atherosclerosis. An atherogenic diet may contribute to the risk of cardiovascular disease (Øverby NC et al. 2006; Snell-Bergeon JK et al. 2009). It has been demonstrated that 80%-90% of type 2 diabetes and coronary heart disease cases can be prevented by healthy lifestyle behavior with a focus on healthy diet and exercise.(Stampfer et al. 2000; Hu et al. 2001; Yusuf et al. 2004) These studies suggest that there could be a potential role for diet in type 1 diabetes to reduce the risk of cardiovascular disease.

There are more studies suggesting that diet (including alcohol) can play an important role in treating the complications of diabetes (Franz MJ et al. 2003; Franz et al. 2010). Several studies have reviewed nutritional recommendations for people with diabetes (Franz MJ et al. 2003; Toeller M July 2010). But most of these recommendations combine both type 1 as well as type 2 diabetes. Furthermore they are general and not always specific for the different type of complications. An overview of the relationship between diet (including alcohol) and complications in type 1 diabetic patients is lacking. Also the effect of lifestyle (including physical activity and dietary patterns) on complications is still not elucidated for type 1 diabetic patients. Lack of physical activity together with an atherogenic diet could enhance development of complications especially in high risk type 1 diabetic patients.

In the following paragraphs of this bookchapter the literature on associations between diet (including alcohol) and lifestyle and chronic complications in type 1 diabetic patients will be summarized. Since 'diet' and 'lifestyle' are broad terms the focus will be on macronutrients (carbohydrates (including fiber), proteins and fats (including cholesterol), alcohol, physical activity and dietary patterns. The paragraphs are divided by nephropathy, retinopathy and CVD. In the final paragraphs all recommendations on diet and lifestyle in patients with type 1 diabetes will be put in perspective with the current literature.

2. Diet, lifestyle and nephropathy

Eighteen studies reported an association between macronutrients and type 1 diabetic nephropathy. Of these, thirteen reported results for the association between protein and nephropathy. The other five focussed on other dietary macronutrients such as fat, cholesterol or carbohydrate in relation with nephropathy. There were also three studies that reported results for protein as well as carbohydrate or fats and nephropathy. Furthermore one study reported an association between alcohol consumption and nephropathy in type 1 diabetic patients and one study reported an association between physical activity and nephropathy in type 1 diabetic patients. No studies were found examining the effect of glycaemic index/glycaemic load on nephropathy in type 1 diabetic patients.

2.1 Macronutrients

2.1.1 Protein

Of the thirteen studies that reported an association between protein and nephropathy there were three cross-sectional studies (Toeller M et al. 1997; Riley MD& Dwyer T 1998; O'Hayon BE et al. 2000), one case control study (Möllsten AV et al. 2001), two cohort studies (Jibani MM et al. 1991; Barsotti G et al. 1998), six randomized controlled trials (Brouhard BH& LaGrone L 1990; Zeller K et al. 1991; Dullaart RP et al. 1993; Raal FJ et al. 1994; Hansen HP et al. 1999; Hansen HP et al. 2002) and a pilot study (Percheron C et al. 1995). These will be discussed in the following paragraphs by study design.

The three cross-sectional studies were not consistent in their conclusions on the effect of protein on diabetic nephropathy. O'Hayon et al. (O'Hayon BE et al. 2000) failed to show a significant relationship between dietary protein intake and markers of early nephropathy, other than creatinine clearance. Toeller et al. (Toeller M et al. 1997) found a significant relationship between dietary protein intake and urinary albumin excretion rate (AER). A higher AER was particularly found in people consuming more than 20% of their dietary food energy as protein. Riley et al. (Riley MD& Dwyer T 1998) even found the opposite, a decreased prevalence of microalbuminuria at high relative intakes of protein.

In the case-control study (Möllsten AV et al. 2001) total protein intake was not associated with the presence of microalbuminuria, but a diet including a high amount of fish protein seemed to decrease the risk. Furthermore they could not confirm an association between a high total animal protein intake and having microalbuminuria. In contrast to this finding , Jibani et al. (Jibani MM et al. 1991) found in their cohort study that a predominantly vegetarian diet (low in animal protein) may have an important beneficial effect on diabetic nephropathy without the need for a heavily restricted total protein intake. But they were not able to determine if the reduction in total protein intake rather than the reduction in the fraction of animal origin was primarily responsible for the fall in the fractional albumin clearance. Another (Barsotti G et al. 1998) cohort study showed that a low protein diet has a protective effect on the residual renal function in type 1 diabetic patients.

In conclusion, these studies were not consistent in their conclusions on the effect of protein restriction on type 1 diabetic nephropathy. Furthermore there is not enough evidence for recommendations about the preferred type of dietary protein.

Of the six randomized controlled trials reporting an association between protein and nephropathy (**Table 1**), four have reported a decline in glomerular filtration rate (GFR) during the low protein diet (protein intake of approximately 0.8 g/kg/day) (Brouhard BH& LaGrone L 1990; Dullaart RP et al. 1993; Hansen HP et al. 1999; Hansen HP et al. 2002). In one of these four this decline was greater in the low protein diet group than in the usual protein diet group, but this difference was not significant (Hansen HP et al. 1999). In two studies this decline was greater in the usual protein diet group than in the low protein group (Brouhard BH& LaGrone L 1990; Hansen HP et al. 2002). Among these 2 studies, one (Brouhard BH& LaGrone L 1990) found a decline that was significantly greater in the usual protein group. Another study showed a decline in GFR in the low protein diet group, but did not directly compare this with the usual protein group (Dullaart RP et al. 1993). Only one study(Raal FJ et al. 1994) reported an increase in GFR during the low protein diet, but this increase was not significant. Zeller et al. (Zeller K et al. 1991) used iothalamate clearance and creatinine clearance to assess renal function. The rates of decline in both iothalamate and creatinine clearence were significantly slower in the patients in the study-diet group than in those in the control-diet group.

Five trials reported an effect of protein on albuminuria (Brouhard BH& LaGrone L 1990; Dullaart RP et al. 1993; Raal FJ et al. 1994; Hansen HP et al. 1999; Hansen HP et al. 2002). In three of these five trials there was a decline in albuminuria in the low protein diet group as well as in the usual protein diet group (Dullaart RP et al. 1993; Hansen HP et al. 1999; Hansen HP et al. 2002). Two of these three showed a significant greater decline in albuminuria in the low protein diet group than in the usual protein diet group (Dullaart RP et al. 1993; Hansen HP et al. 1999). The other two trials showed a decline in albuminuria in the low protein diet group and an increase in the usual diet protein group (Brouhard BH& LaGrone L 1990; Raal FJ et al. 1994). One of these (Brouhard BH& LaGrone L 1990) found a significant difference between the diet groups. Furthermore, another (pilot) study (Percheron C et al. 1995) also found a decline in albuminuria and in creatinine clearance. They conclude that moderately (protein intake of approximately 1.2 g/kg/day) rather than severely protein restricted diets (protein intake of approximately 0.8 g/kg/day) should be recommended, because of the lack of compliance with severely protein restricted diets. The only trial (Hansen HP et al. 2002) that determined the effect of dietary protein restriction on survival and progression to end stage renal disease (ESRD) in diabetic nephropathy reported a relative risk of 0.23 (95% CI: 0.07-0.72) for ESRD in patients assigned to a low-protein diet compared with patients assigned to a usual protein diet.

In conclusion, protein restriction (protein intake of approximately 0.8 g/kg/day, **Table 1**) had a positive significant effect on albuminuria, but no effect on GFR was found.

2.1.2 Carbohydrate

Two cross-sectional studies (Watts GF et al. 1988; Riley MD& Dwyer T 1998) examined the association between carbohydrates and nephropathy. In one study (Watts GF et al. 1988) type 1 diabetic patients with microalbuminuria consumed a significantly smaller percentage of total energy as carbohydrate compared with patients with normal albumin excretion. In the other study (Riley MD& Dwyer T 1998) no significant association between energy adjusted carbohydrate intake and microalbuminuria was found. This could be due to their

Ref.	Study pop.	Age (mean or range)	Study duration	Exposure	Results		
					Mean protein intake (g/kg/day)	GFR	Albuminuria
Hansen (2002) (Hansen HP et al., 2002)	n=82	18-60	4 years	LPD (0.6 g/kg/day) vs. UPD	LPD: 0.89 UPD: 1.02	LPD: mean decline 3.8 ml/min/yr UPD: mean decline 3.9 ml/min/yr	LPD: mean decline 148 mg/24 h UPD: mean decline 107 mg/24 h
Hansen (1999) (Hansen HP et al., 1999)	n=29	18-60	8 weeks	LPD (0.6 g/kg/day) vs. UPD	LPD: 0.8 UPD: 1.1	LPD: mean decline 8.6 ml/min/1,73m² UPD: mean decline 2.5 ml/min/1,73m²	LPD: mean decline 28.7% UPD: mean decline 0.0%
Raal (1994) (Raal FJ et al., 1994)	n=22	20-41	6 months	Unrestricted protein diet (>1,6 g/kg/day) vs. moderately protein-restricted diet (0,8 g/kg/day)	LPD: 0.87 UPD: 2.00	LPD: mean increase 3 ml/min/1,73m² UPD: mean decline 8 ml/min/1,73m²	LPD: mean decline 1.02 g/day UPD: mean increase 0.34 g/day
Dullaart (1993) (Dullaart RP et al., 1993)	n=30	40,8	2 years	LPD (0.6 g/kg/day) vs. UPD	LPD: 0.79		LPD: mean decline 26%* UPD: mean decline 5%*
Zeller (1991) (Zeller K et al., 1991)	n=35	18-60	mean: 34.7 months	LPLP (0.6g/kg/day protein; 500-1000 mg phosphorus) vs. Control diet (1.0 g/kg/day protein; 1000 mg phosphorus)	LPLP: 0.72 Control: 1.08	LPLP: IC: decline of 0.0043 ml/s/mo CC: 0.0055 ml/s/mo Control: IC: decline of 0.0168 ml/s/mo CC: 0.0135 ml/s/mo	
Brouchard (1990) (Brouhard BH& LaGrone L 1990)	n=15	18-49	12 months	LPD (0.6 g/kg/day) vs. UPD	LPD: 1.3 UPD: 1.5	LPD: decline 0.28 ml/min/1.73m²/mo UPD: decline 0.68 ml/min/1.73m²/mo	LPD: mean decline 407 µg/min UPD: mean increase 1055 µg/min

* after adjustment for MAP (mean arterial pressure) and diabetes duration
GFR: glomerular filtration rate; LPD: low protein diet; UPD: usual protein diet; LPLP: low protein, low phosphorus; IC: iothalamate clearance; CC: creatinine clearance

Table 1. Randomized controlled trials; protein and diabetic nephropathy

study design (cross-sectional), due to a substantial measurement error in the food frequency questionnaires (FFQs) and due to the low response rate (61.2%) for participation.

2.1.3 Fat/cholesterol

Four cross-sectional studies reported an association between fat and/or cholesterol and nephropathy (Watts GF et al. 1988; Bouhanick B 1995; Riley MD& Dwyer T 1998; Toeller M et al. 1999 [1]). One study (Riley MD& Dwyer T 1998) found no significant association between energy adjusted monounsaturated fat intake or energy adjusted polyunsaturated fat intake and microalbuminuria, but reported a positive association between usual dietary saturated fat intake and microalbuminuria. Another study (Watts GF et al. 1988) found a significant positive association between total fat intake and microalbuminuria. Another study (Bouhanick B 1995) examined the relationship between fat intake and glomerular hyperfiltration (GFR > 173 ml/min/1.73m^2), a marker for diabetic nephropathy, in type 1 diabetic patients. They found that excess fat intake may contribute to hyperfiltration in type 1 diabetic patients. Finally the fourth study(Toeller M et al. 1999 [1]) found a higher intake of cholesterol, total fat and saturated fat in Eastern Europe compared to Southern or North-Western Europe. They also found more frequent acute and chronic complications (including nephropathy) in Eastern Europe people. Since it was a cross-sectional study they could not conclude if this was due to the high intake of cholesterol, total fat and/or saturated fat.

These cross-sectional studies show that there seems to be a detrimental effect of total dietary fat intake as well as saturated fat intake on type 1 diabetic nephropathy. No association between energy adjusted MUFA and energy adjusted PUFA and microalbuminuria was found.

In a case-control study (Möllsten AV et al. 2001), no association between total fat intake and microalbuminuria was found. In a prospective study (Cárdenas C et al. 2004) a progression of nephropathy with greater saturated fatty acid (SFA) consumption and lesser polyunsaturated fatty acid consumption (PUFA) was demonstrated. Specifically with higher SFA-to-PUFA and SFA-to-MUFA ratios. Another prospective cohort study (Lee CC et al. 2010) found an association between PUFA and microalbuminuria. They found that dietary n-3 PUFAs (eicosapentaenoic acid and docosahexaenoic acid) are inversely associated with the degree but not with the incidence of albuminuria in type 1 diabetes (Lee CC et al. 2010).

In conclusion these prospective studies are consistent with the cross-sectional studies about the detrimental effect of saturated fat on type 1 diabetic nephropathy. The effect of total fat intake on nephropathy is still not elucidated. The cross-sectional study of Watts et al. (Watts GF et al. 1988) and the case control study of Möllsten et al. (Möllsten AV et al. 2001) were in contrast with each other. Also the effect of PUFAs on nephropathy is still doubtful, but there seems to be an inverse association between n-3 PUFAs and the degree of albuminuria.

2.1.4 Alcohol

In the EURODIAB Prospective Complications Study (Beulens et al. 2008) the association between alcohol and nephropathy was analysed cross-sectionally. They found that moderate alcohol consumers (30-70 g alcohol per week) had a lower risk of diabetic nephropathy, with an odds ratio of 0.36 (95% CI: 0.18-0.71). This association was most pronounced for the consumption of wine.

2.1.5 Physical activity

There were no prospective studies on physical activity and type 1 diabetic nephropathy. One cross-sectional study (Kriska AM et al. 1991) found the lowest occurrence of diabetic nephropathy in people being 7^{+} hours a week physically active (sports and leisure physical activity).

3. Diet, lifestyle and retinopathy

Only two studies reported results for the association between macronutrients and type 1 diabetic retinopathy. Furthermore two studies reported an association between alcohol consumption and diabetic retinopathy and one study reported an association between physical activity and diabetic retinopathy. No studies were found examining the effect of glycaemic index/glycaemic load on retinopathy in type 1 diabetic patients.

3.1 Macronutrients

In post-hoc analyses (Cundiff DK& Nigg CR 2005) a positive association between total dietary fat, saturated fat and MUFA with retinopathy progression and retinopathy risk factors (mean arterial pressure, LDL/HDL cholesterol ratio, serum triglycerides, HbA1c, body mass index, and insulin utilization) was found. Furthermore, a negative association between carbohydrates and dietary fiber with retinopathy progression and risk factors was found. In addition to this, another cross-sectional study(Toeller M et al. 1999 [1]) reported a higher intake of cholesterol, total fat and saturated fat in Eastern Europe compared to Southern or North-Western Europe. They also found more frequent acute and chronic complications (including retinopathy) in Eastern European people. As with nephropathy, they could not conclude if this was due to the high intake of cholesterol, total fat and/or saturated fat.

In conclusion there is limited research on the effect of diet on diabetic retinopathy. The results of the post hoc analyses should be interpreted carefully, since it is a retrospective analysis which can generate hypotheses but not prove them.

3.1.2 Alcohol

In cross-sectional analyses of the EURODIAB Prospective Complications Study (Beulens et al. 2008) moderate alcohol consumers (30-70 g alcohol per week) had a lower risk of diabetic proliferative retinopathy, with an odds ratio of 0.60 (95% CI: 0.37-0.99). This association was most pronounced for the consumption of wine. Another cross-sectional study (Moss SE et al. 1992) examined whether alcohol consumption was associated with type 1 diabetic retinopathy. They found that moderate alcohol consumption was inversely associated with the prevalence of retinopathy (OR=0.49, 95% CI: 0.27-0.92) in patients with type 1 diabetes.

3.1.3 Physical activity

One cross-sectional study (Kriska AM et al. 1991) examined the relationship between physical activity and the occurrence of retinopathy in type 1 diabetic patients. They found no association between physical activity (sports and leisure physical activity) and occurrence of retinopathy.

4. Diet, lifestyle and cardiovascular disease

Eight studies reported an association between macronutrients and CVD in type 1 diabetic patients. Of these eight, six are cross-sectional studies (Toeller M et al. 1999 [1,2,3]; Helgeson 2006; Øverby NC et al. 2006; Snell-Bergeon JK et al. 2009). Only Strychar et al. (Strychar I et al. 2009) and Georgopoulos et al. (Georgopoulos A et al. 2000) performed a randomized controlled trial. One study reported an association between lifestyle risk factors (including alcohol) and atherosclerosis, which is often the underlying cause of CVD (Bishop et al. 2009). Eight studies reported an association between physical activity and CVD risk factors (Kriska AM et al. 1991; Lehmann R et al. 1997; Fuchsjäger-Mayrl G et al. 2002; Herbst A et al. 2007; Valerio G et al. 2007; Bishop et al. 2009; Trigona B et al. 2010; Seeger JPH et al. 2011), and two studies reported an association with dietary patterns (Gunther ALB et al. 2008; Liese AD et al. 2011). Furthermore no studies were found examining the effect of glycaemic index/glycaemic load on CVD in type 1 diabetic patients.

4.1 Macronutrients

Data on the relationship between macronutrients and incident CVD is lacking in patients with type 1 diabetes. Limited information on macronutrients is available from cross-sectional studies. Main focus was on fat, in particularly saturated fat, and fiber and CVD risk factors were used as a proxy for CVD events.

4.2 Cross-sectional studies on fat and fiber in relation to CVD

In more detail, one cross-sectional study (Øverby NC et al. 2006) found a higher than recommended percentage of energy intake from fat and saturated fat among type 1 diabetic patients compared with healthy same-age control subjects and a lower than recommended intake of fiber. They conclude that this higher intake of energy from saturated fat and this lower intake of energy from dietary fiber, vegetables and fruits could increase the risk of atherosclerosis, which is often the underlying cause of CVD. Another study (Helgeson 2006) reported a higher than recommended percentage of energy intake from fat and saturated fat among type 1 diabetic patients, but they did not study associations with CVD or CVD risk factors. Another cross-sectional study (Toeller M et al. 1999 [2]) found similar associations between dietary fiber and CVD. Higher fiber intake had a protective significant effect against CVD in type 1 diabetic women but not in men. In type 1 diabetic men it leads to positive changes of the serum cholesterol pattern (higher HDL, lower LDL, lower ratio total cholesterol:HDL cholesterol). In another study (Toeller M et al. 1999 [3]) a significant increase in energy adjusted total and LDL-cholesterol levels was associated with higher intakes of total fat, saturated fat and cholesterol. This was associated with a higher prevalence of CVD, although after adjusting for dietary fiber intake, these associations were attenuated. A third study by Toeller et al. (Toeller M et al. 1999 [1]) found a higher intake of cholesterol, total fat and saturated fat in Eastern Europe compared to Southern or North-Western Europe. They also found more frequent acute and chronic complications (including CVD) in Eastern European people. However, since it was a cross-sectional study they could not conclude if this was due to the high intake of cholesterol, total fat and/or saturated fat. In the CACTI study (Snell-Bergeon JK et al. 2009) found an increased risk of CVD in type 1 diabetic patients eating high amounts of fat and saturated fat. Carbohydrates were negatively correlated with CHD risk factors (higher total cholesterol, LDL cholesterol, obesity, poorer glycaemic control). Furthermore higher intakes of fat and protein were associated with greater odds of coronary artery calcium (CAC), which is a strong predictor for coronary events approximating CVD risk. The opposite was true for carbohydrate intake, higher intake was associated with a reduced odds of CAC.

In conclusion a higher intake of total fat as well as saturated fat is positively correlated with CVD or CVD risk factors (atherosclerosis and CAC in these studies) and a higher intake of carbohydrate is negatively correlated with CVD or CVD risk factors. Furthermore dietary fiber is independently related to a lower risk for CVD in type 1 diabetic women. Since all these studies were cross-sectional, they could only look at the intake of certain nutrients and the prevalence of CVD or CVD risk factors at a certain time point. They could not conclude if these are related to each other and if the nutrients are responsible for the lower or higher prevalence of CVD.

4.3 Randomized controlled trials

Two randomized controlled trials reported an association between macronutrients and CVD (**Table 2**), but demonstrated conflicting conclusions. In one trial (Strychar I et al. 2009), the authors concluded that a diet lower in carbohydrate and higher in MUFA might be preferable to a diet higher in carbohydrate and lower in MUFA for type 1 diabetic patients. This was solely based on the positive effect on triglyceride (TG) levels and plasminogen activator inhibitor 1 levels (PAI-1) in the first diet. A significant decrease in PAI-1 was found after 6 months in the lower carbohydrate and higher MUFA diet. In the other diet there was a significant increase after 6 months of follow up. PAI-1 is an inhibitor of fibrinolysis, a process that degrades blood clots. A lower level of PAI-1 means less inhibition and more degradation of blood clots, which means a lower chance of developing atherosclerosis. Also a decrease in TG levels was found after 6 months following the low carbohydrate/high MUFA diet, although this decrease was not significant. In the other diet group there was an increase in TG levels, also this increase was not significant. Furthermore they conclude that the lower carbohydrate/higher MUFA diet was only a proper choice for nonobese individuals with weight control since this diet had induced a weight gain of 2% (1.6 kg) after 6 months. The other trial (Georgopoulos A et al. 2000) found exactly the opposite using a crossover design. They found that a diet high in carbohydrates might be preferable to a diet high in MUFA. Mainly because of the higher atherosclerotic risk due to more and bigger very low-density lipoprotein (VLDL) particles in the last diet. Furthermore the TG levels did not significantly differ between the two diets in this study.

In conclusion, these trials show that the effect of carbohydrate or MUFA on cardiovascular disease risk factors in type 1 diabetic patients is still not elucidated. Although they recommend exactly the opposite (higher intake of MUFA preferable vs. higher intake of carbohydrate preferable) they both found that a high MUFA or a high carbohydrate diet did not affect the TG levels. Their conclusions are based on PAI-1 and VLDL levels, which are not such a good predictors for atherosclerosis (and by extension CVD) as TG levels are. Furthermore none of these randomized controlled trials examined the potential positive effect of dietary fiber on CVD or the potential negative effect of saturated fat found in cross-sectional studies.

4.4 Alcohol

One cross-sectional study (Bishop et al. 2009) reported findings on the association between alcohol and cardiovascular disease. No significant association was found between alcohol consumption (±13.8 drinks/month) and CAC, a marker of coronary artery atherosclerosis (adjusted OR=0.9, 95% CI: 0.8-1.1, p=0.15). The positive effect of moderate alcohol

Ref.	Study pop.	Age (mean or range)	Study duration	Exposure	Results PAI-1 (ng/ml) (mean ± SD)	TG (mmol/l) (mean ± SD)	VLDL (mg/l) (mean ± SEM)
Strychar (2009) (Strychar I et al., 2009)	n=30	37.9	6 months	diet high in CH/low in fat* vs. diet low in CH/high in fat**	HCLF: change after 6 mo: -12.8 ± 27.0 LCHF: change after 6 mo: + 14.2 ± 24.5	HCLF: change after 6 mo: -0.03 ± 0.22 LCHF: change after 6 mo: +0.14 ± 0.46	
Georgopoulos (2000) (Georgopoulos A et al., 2000)	n=19	22-47	4 weeks	diet high in MUFA*** vs. diet high in CH****		High MUFA: 0.89 ± 0.39 High CH: 0.90 ± 0.36	High MUFA: 31.4 ± 7.4 High CH: 20.0 ± 3.8

* 54-57% CH, 27-30% total fat (10% MUFA)
** 43-46% CH, 37-40% total fat (20% MUFA)
*** 40% total fatty acids (25% MUFA, 6% PUFA, 9% saturated), 45% CH and 15% protein
**** 24% total fatty acids (9% MUFA, 6% PUFA, 9% saturated), 61% CH and 15% protein
PAI-1: plasminogen activator inhibitor 1; TG: triglycerides; VLDL: very low-density lipoprotein; SD: standard deviation; SEM: standard error of mean; CH: carbohydrate; MUFA: monounsaturated fatty acid; HCLF: high carbohydrate, low fat; LCHF: low carbohydrate, high fat

Table 2. Randomized controlled trials; diet and cardiovascular disease

consumption on CVD as in the general population is not confirmed for type 1 diabetic patients in this study. However, this could also be due to the kind of study (cross-sectional) and the fact that markers for CVD were used instead of CVD as endpoint. There are no prospective studies which have addressed the relation between alcohol and CVD in type 1 diabetic patients.

4.5 Physical activity

Of the eight studies that reported an association between physical activity and CVD there were five cross-sectional studies (Kriska AM et al. 1991; Herbst A et al. 2007; Valerio G et al. 2007; Bishop et al. 2009; Trigona B et al. 2010) and three trials (Lehmann R et al. 1997; Fuchsjäger-Mayrl G et al. 2002; Seeger JPH et al. 2011). No prospective cohort studies were found. The studies will be discussed in the following paragraphs by study design.

One study (Kriska AM et al. 1991) examined the relationship between physical activity and the occurrence of CVD in type 1 diabetic patients. They found the lowest occurrence of CVD in people being 4-7 hours a week physical active (sports and leisure physical activity). The other four cross-sectional studies examined an association between physical activity and CVD risk factors. They all found a positive association. Another two studies (Herbst A et al. 2007; Valerio G et al. 2007) found that increased frequency of regular physical activity was associated with lower TG levels. One of these (Herbst A et al. 2007) found besides the positive association with TG levels also a positive significant association between regular physical activity and HDL cholesterol levels. Another study (Trigona B et al. 2010) found that 60 min/day of moderate-to-vigorous physical activity was associated with an enhanced endothelial function in type 1 diabetic patients. Impaired endothelial function is considered as an early sign of atherosclerosis, which is often the underlying cause of CVD. And finally, (Bishop et al. 2009) a significant inverse association between physical activity and CAC, a marker of coronary artery atherosclerosis, was demonstrated.

In conclusion all these studies found a beneficial effect of physical activity on cardiovascular risk factors. However, since all these studies were cross-sectional, they could only look at physical activity and the prevalence of CVD or CVD risk factors at a certain time point. They could not conclude if these are related to each other and if physical activity was responsible for the lower prevalence of CVD.

The three trials reporting an association between physical activity and cardiovascular disease risk factors (**Table 3**) were consistent in their conclusions. They all emphasize an important role for physical activity in type 1 diabetic patients. Two studies (Fuchsjäger-Mayrl G et al. 2002; Seeger JPH et al. 2011) examined the association between physical activity and brachial artery flow-mediated dilation (FMD). Endothelial dysfunction is reflected by an impaired FMD response and is an early sign of atherosclerosis. An increase in FMD was found in type 1 diabetic patients following an exercise training program (endurance sports; on average 2 times a week 60 minutes, **Table 3**). In both trials this increase was significant ($p=0.038$ and $p=0.040$ respectively). Two studies (Lehmann R et al. 1997; Fuchsjäger-Mayrl G et al. 2002) examined the impact of physical activity on lipid related cardiovascular risk factors (LDL cholesterol, HDL cholesterol and TG). They both found a decrease in LDL cholesterol levels in the training group, but only in one of these (Lehmann R et al. 1997) this decrease was significant ($p=0.02$). An additional effect was reported in one of these studies (Lehmann R et al. 1997) with a significant increase in HDL cholesterol levels ($p=0.03$) in the training group. No effect of physical activity on TG levels

Ref.	Study pop.	Age (mean)	Study duration	Exposure	Results				
					VO_{2max}	FMD (%)	Triglycerides (mmol/L)	LDL cholesterol (mmol/L)	HDL cholesterol (mmol/L)
Seeger (2011) (Seeger JPH et al., 2011)	n=7	10.9	18 weeks	18 week exercise training program*	Mean increase: 2.0 ml/kg/min	Mean increase: 4.9			
Fuchsjäger-Mayrl (2002) (Fuchsjäger-Mayrl G et al., 2002)	n=23	37.5	4 months	TrGr: 4 mo exercise training program** C: type 1 diabetic patients following usual lifestyle	TrGr: mean increase: 7.6 ml/kg/min C: mean increase: 0.1 ml/kg/min	TrGr: mean increase: 3.3 C: mean increase: 0.7	TrGr: mean decline: 0.2 C: mean increase: 0.2	TrGr: mean decline: 0.3 C: mean decline: 0.2	TrGr: mean decrease: 0.2 C: mean decrease: 0.2
Lehmann (1997) (Lehmann R et al., 1997)	n=20	33.0	3 months	3 month exercise training program***	Mean increase: 178 ml/min		Mean increase: 0.09	Mean decline: 0.4	Mean increase: 0.16

* two times a week: first day: 30 min running exercise (intervals) and 30 min group-based activities such as ball games, short relay races, running techniques and stretching; second day: individual exercise session at home involved 30 min of interval running and a 10-min warm-up and cooling down (including stretching)
** first 2 weeks: two times a week 1 hour stationary cycling, during the remaining study period three times a week 1 hour stationary cycling
*** 135 min per week endurance sports (biking, long-distance running, or hiking)
VO_{2max}: peak oxygen uptake; FMD: flow mediated dilation; LDL: low-density lipoprotein; HDL: high-density lipoprotein; TrGR; training group; C: control group

Table 3. Randomized controlled trials; physical activity and cardiovascular disease risk factors

was found in both studies. Furthermore all three studies (Lehmann R et al. 1997; Fuchsjäger-Mayrl G et al. 2002; Seeger JPH et al. 2011) assessed physical fitness by VO_{2max} (peak oxygen uptake). They all found a positive significant association between physical activity and VO_{2max}. The relation between physical fitness and CVD was not examined.

In conclusion the three trials show that physical activity improves physical fitness as well as endothelial function in type 1 diabetic patients. A positive effect on lipid related cardiovascular risk factors was only found in one study (Lehmann R et al. 1997).

4.6 Dietary patterns

Two cross-sectional studies reported an association between dietary patterns, in this case the 'Dietary Approaches to Stop Hypertension' (DASH) diet, and CVD risk factors (Gunther ALB et al. 2008; Liese AD et al. 2011). No cross-sectional or prospective studies were found examining the effect of a Mediterranean diet or a Western diet on CVD in type 1 diabetic patients.

One study (Gunther ALB et al. 2008) reported an association between adherence to the DASH diet and hypertension in type 1 diabetic patients. They found that a higher adherence to this diet amongst type 1 diabetic patients was inversely related to hypertension (OR=0.6, 95% CI: 0.4-0.9, p=0.007). They did not investigate a possible association between the DASH diet and CVD, but used hypertension as the main risk factor for CVD. Another study (Liese AD et al. 2011) reported a possible association between the DASH diet and other CVD risk factors (total cholesterol, LDL cholesterol, HDL cholesterol, TG, LDL particle density, apolipoprotein B, body mass index (BMI), waist circumference, and adipocytokines) than blood pressure. A significant and inverse association between the DASH diet and LDL/HDL ratio was found. An estimated 0.07 lower LDL/HDL ratio was found in the highest adherence group compared with the lowest adherence group. No significant association was found between LDL particle density, BMI, waist circumference, adipocytokines, or TG and the DASH diet.

In conclusion a positive effect of adherence to the DASH diet on hypertension and LDL/HDL ratio, which are important risk factors for CVD, was found. Unfortunately there were no studies found examining the effect of dietary patterns on CVD events.

5. Current recommendations on diet and lifestyle in patients with type 1 diabetes put in perspective

Overall, fiber and saturated fat intake play an important role in type 1 diabetic patients, with a beneficial and detrimental effect on the chronic complications respectively. Many researchers have shown the inappropriate intake of these nutrients in patients with type 1 diabetes. A protein restriction diet helped reduce micro/macro albuminuria in known type 1 diabetic patients with nephropathy, however, the compliance was low. Also moderate alcohol intake and physical activity may have beneficial effects in type 1 diabetic patients. Most of the findings are consistent with the guidelines for type 1 diabetic patients (**Table 4**). The main limitations are the lack of prospective studies on diet and lifestyle in type 1 diabetics, lack of randomized controlled trials and the limited number of studies on dietary cholesterol, protein, carbohydrates, fat, fiber and no cardiovascular morbidity data. The available studies, with their limitations, all indicate that diet and lifestyle play an important role in preventing chronic complications of type 1 diabetes. To put the findings in the literature in perspective, current nutritional recommendations are evaluated in the

	Evidence grade A*	Evidence grade B**	Evidence grade C-E***
Carbohydrate[1]	Metabolic characteristics suggest the most appropriate intake: vegetables, legumes, fruits, wholegrain foods, naturally occurring foods rich in fiber Fiber intake should be ideally ≈ 20 g/1000 kcal/day Low glycaemic index foods provided other attributes of these foods are appropriate Moderate amounts of free sugars (up to 50 g/day)	There is no justification for the recommendation of very low carbohydrate diets in persons with diabetes Cereal-based foods should, whenever possible, be wholegrain and high in fiber	Consider quantity, sources and distribution of CHO to facilitate near-normal long-term glycaemic control Timing and dosage of insulin or hypoglycaemic agents should match quantity and nature of CHO Daily consumption of 5 servings of fiber-rich vegetables or fruits and 4 servings of legumes per week help to achieve recommended fiber intake Total free sugars should not exceed 10% total energy
Dietary fat[1]	Saturated and trans-unsaturated fatty acids <10% total energy (<8% if LDL cholesterol is elevated) Dietary cholesterol <300 mg/day (further reduction of LDL is elevated)	Oils rich in mono-unsaturated fatty acids are encouraged (10-20% total energy), total fat <35% total energy 2-3 servings of oily fish/week and plant sources of n-3 fatty acids (e.g. rapeseed oil, soybean oil, nuts) are recommended	Polyunsaturated fatty acids should not exceed 10% total daily energy Total fat intake should not exceed 35% total energy
Protein[1]	0.8 g/kg normal body weight in patients with type 1 diabetes and established nephropathy	10-20% total energy in patients with no evidence of nephropathy	Insufficient evidence for recommendations about the preferred type of dietary protein For type 1 diabetes with incipient nephropathy and type 2 diabetes with incipient or established nephropathy no firm recommendations regarding protein restriction
Alcohol[1]		Moderate use up to 10 g/day for women and up to 20 g/day for men is possible In patients treated with insulin or insulin secretagogues alcohol should be taken with carbohydrate to avoid hypoglycaemia	Intake should be limited in overweight, hypertensive, hypertriglyceridemic individuals as well as during pregnancy and in advanced neuropathy
Physical[2] Activity	90 to 150 minutes of accumulated moderate-intensity aerobic physical activity per week as well as resistance/strength training three times per week is recommended		

[1] obtained from DNSG EASD: Diabetes and Nutrition Study Group of the European Association for the Study of Diabetes(Toeller M July 2010);
[2]obtained from ADA: American Diabetic Association(American Diabetes Association (ADA) 2011)
* Evidence grade A: evidence obtained from meta-analyses of randomized controlled trials or at least one randomized controlled trial
** Evidence grade B: evidence obtained from at least one well designed and controlled study without randomization, well-designed quasi-experimental or non-experimental descriptive study
*** Evidence grade C-E: evidence obtained from expert committee reports or opinions and/or clinical experiences of respected authorities

Table 4. Nutritional recommendations for persons with type 1 and type 2 diabetes

following paragraphs at a macronutrient level. **Table 4** summarizes the nutritional recommendations as well as the lifestyle recommendations for type 1 and type 2 diabetic patients. These recommendations are for all diabetic patients in general, based in the majority of cases on evidence from type 2 diabetic patients.

5.1 Carbohydrates

The 'Diabetes and Nutrition Study Group of the European Association for the Study of Diabetes' (DNSG EASD) guidelines for persons with type 1 and type 2 diabetes (**Table 4**) recommend that the most appropriate intake of carbohydrates consists of vegetables, legumes, fruits, wholegrain foods and naturally occurring foods rich in fiber. The fiber intake should be ideally ≈ 20 g/1000 kcal/day. Cross-sectional data of the EURODIAB Complications Study showed an inverse association between fiber and LDL cholesterol and a positive association between fiber and HDL cholesterol. In addition dietary fiber was inversely and significantly related to CVD (Toeller M et al. 1999 [2]). This effect was already found with a fiber intake of approximately 8.1 g/1000 kcal, which is below the recommended intake. The average fiber intake in type 1 diabetic patients is 8.1 g/1000 kcal, but the recommended intake is 20 g/1000 kcal. Recommendation was only achieved in 0.4% of the type 1 diabetic population (Toeller M et al. 1996). Data from the EURODIAB Prospective Complication Study on fiber intake measured at baseline by 3-day food diaries and presented by each center is given in **Figure 1**. As seen in this figure, even the 10 g/1000 kcal recommended fiber intake by the 'American Diabetes Association' (ADA) was hardly achieved by type 1 diabetic patients. Only Finnish type 1 diabetic patients achieved the ADA fiber recommendation of 10 g/1000 kcal **Figure 1**). Keeping in mind that these samples are clinic based and not population based and that these figures may not exactly reflect the current nutritional intake, however it gives an indication of the status on fiber intake. Although positive effects were already found on CVD with a fiber intake of 8.1 g/1000 kcal, we assume that effects could be probably even higher when recommended levels of fiber intake are reached. Unfortunately, this positive effect of fiber on CVD and CVD risk factors was only found in cross-sectional studies. This makes it very difficult to distinguish cause and effect. Further research in prospective studies or randomized controlled trials is needed to ascertain the role of fiber in CVD.

DNSG EASD do not recommend a low carbohydrate diet for type 1 and type 2 diabetic patients (**Table 4**). A low carbohydrate diet does not produce beneficial health effect. It is more acceptable to avoid too much foods high in fast available carbohydrates, foods high in fat and cholesterol. An earlier quote (Helgeson 2006) expressed this precisely: 'families of adolescents with diabetes may be more concerned that the sugar in candy is going to translate into high blood glucose levels today than that the fat in potato chips will translate into cardiovascular disease in 10 years'.

5.2 Fat

The DNSG EASD guidelines for dietary fat for persons with type 1 and type 2 diabetes recommend a saturated and trans-unsaturated fatty acid consumption of <10% of the total energy intake (<8% if LDL cholesterol is elevated). Total fat intake should not exceed 35% of total energy and dietary cholesterol should be <300 mg/day (**Table 4**). Saturated fat is an important risk factor for diabetic nephropathy, diabetic retinopathy as well as CVD (Riley

MD& Dwyer T 1998; Toeller M et al. 1999 [3]; Cárdenas C et al. 2004; Cundiff DK& Nigg CR 2005). The recommended intake is <10% of the total energy intake which was only achieved by a small minority (14%) (Toeller M et al. 1996). Data from the EURODIAB Prospective Complication Study on saturated fatty acid intake measured at baseline by 3-day food diaries and presented by each center is given in **Figure 2**. The even lower saturated fatty acid recommendation of <7% total energy of the ADA was not achieved by any of the centers (**Figure 2**). All centers indicated in F**igure 2** exceed the recommendation of <7% saturated fat of the total energy intake. Type 1 diabetic patients from Italy had the lowest intake of saturated fatty acids, but this intake was still too high (F**igure 2**). Again, keeping in mind that these samples are clinic based and not population based and that these figures may not exactly reflect the current nutritional intake.

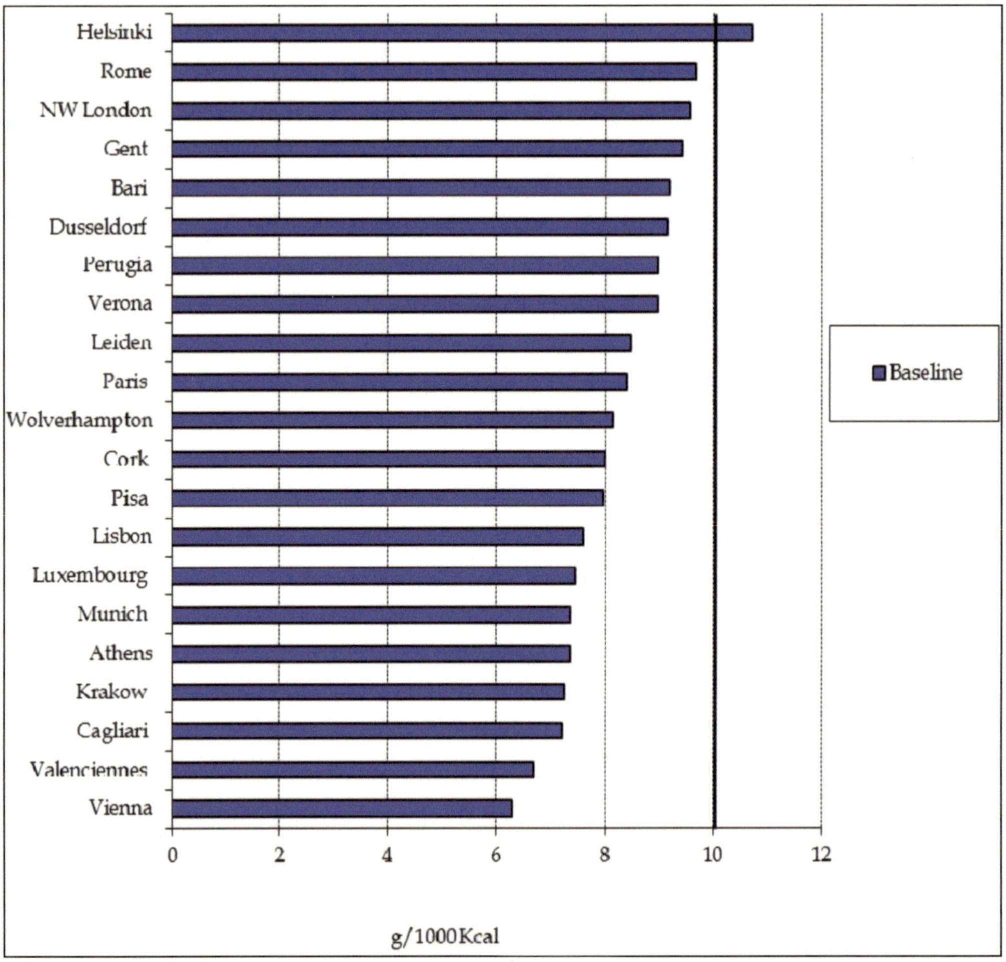

Fig. 1. Mean fiber intake in 1102 individuals with type 1 diabetes across Europa (Toeller M, Soedamah-Muthu 2011)

Furthermore the DNSG EASD guidelines recommend oils rich in MUFA (10-20% total energy) and that PUFA should not exceed 10% of total energy intake (T**able 4**). There were only a few studies examining the effect of MUFA or PUFA on chronic complications in type 1 diabetic patients. A positive association was found between MUFA and retinopathy (Cundiff DK& Nigg CR 2005) but no association was found between MUFA and PUFA and microalbuminuria (Riley MD& Dwyer T 1998). These conclusions are based on post-hoc analyses and a cross-sectional study respectively and should therefore be interpreted carefully. Also the conclusion of Strychar et al. (Strychar I et al. 2009) to recommend a diet higher in MUFA and lower in carbohydrate for nonobese type 1 diabetic individuals to reduce CVD risk factors is doubtful. Their conclusion is based on PAI-1 and VLDL levels, which are not such a good predictors for atherosclerosis (and by extension CVD) as TG levels are. And a high MUFA diet did not alter TG levels. Furthermore, the small study population of 30 subjects limits the power of their conclusions. In order to make accurate recommendations concerning MUFA and PUFA intake for type 1 diabetic patients more research with more participants (preferably in a prospective study) is needed.

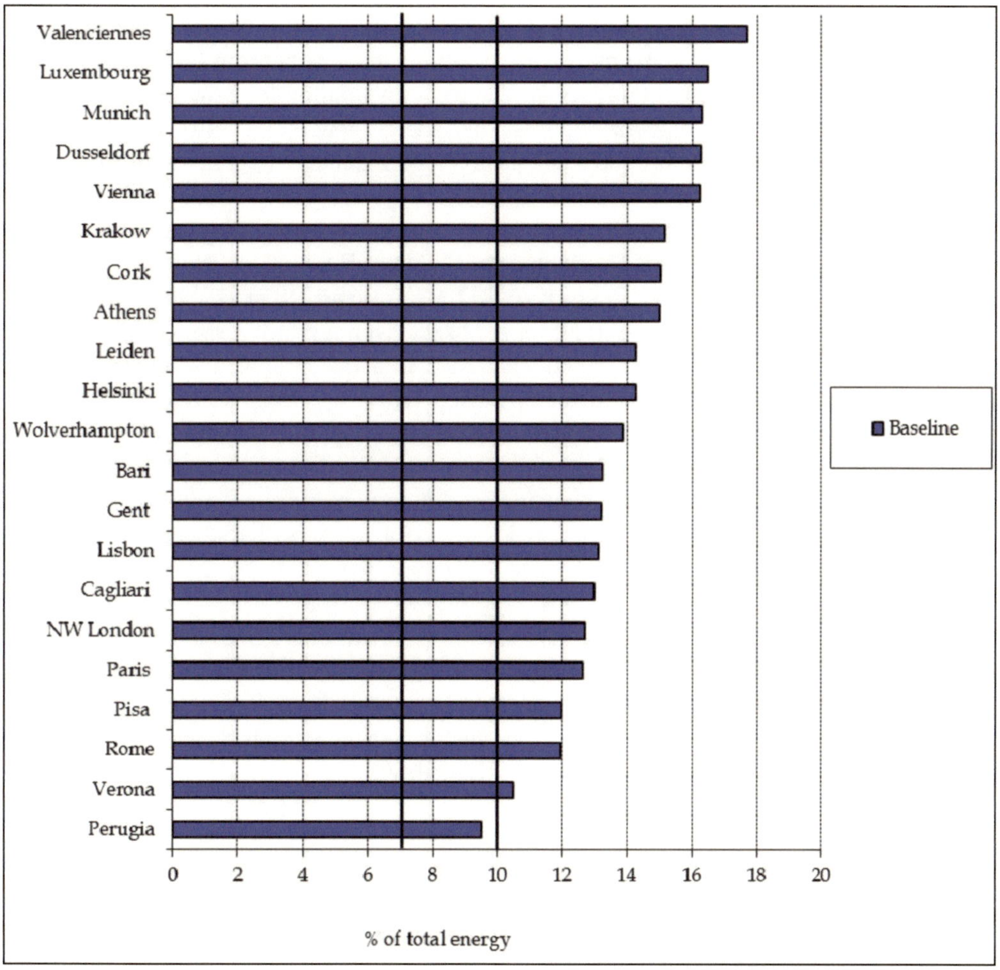

Fig. 2. Mean saturated fatty acid intake in 1102 individuals with type 1 diabetes across Europe (Toeller M, Soedamah-Muthu 2011)

The recommendation of the DNSG EASD to consume 2-3 servings of oily fish/week and plant sources of n-3 fatty acids (**Table 4**) is consistent with the findings in studies specific for type 1 diabetes. The prospective cohort study of Lee et al. (Lee CC et al. 2010) found that dietary n-3 PUFAs (eicosapentaenoic acid and docosahexaenoic acid) are inversely associated with the degree but not with the incidence of albuminuria in type 1 diabetes. A hypothesis is that n-3 PUFAs decrease urinary AER via anti-inflammatory mechanisms. It decreases lipopolysaccharide-induced nuclear factor-kB (NF-kB) activation and monocyte chemoattractant protein (MCP)-1 expression in human renal tubular cells (Lee CC et al. 2010). Further prospective studies and randomized controlled trials are needed to confirm this hypothesis.

5.3 Protein

With regards to protein, the DNSG EASD guidelines recommend an intake of 0.8 g/kg normal body weight in patients with type 1 diabetes and established nephropathy. There are no firm recommendations regarding protein intake for type 1 diabetic patients with incipient nephropathy. An intake of 10-20% of total energy is recommended for patients with no evidence of nephropathy (**Table 4**). The recommendation for protein intake is most important for patients with diabetic nephropathy. The guideline of a restricted protein diet which contains 0.8 g/kg normal body weight for type 1 diabetic patients with established nephropathy was demonstrated by previous research. Several randomized controlled trials showed that protein normalization (protein intake of approximately 0.8 g/kg/day, **Table 1**) had a positive significant effect on albuminuria, although no effect on GFR was found (Brouhard BH& LaGrone L 1990; Zeller K et al. 1991; Dullaart RP et al. 1993; Raal FJ et al. 1994; Hansen HP et al. 1999; Hansen HP et al. 2002). Even a relative risk of 0.23 (95% CI: 0.07-0.72) was found for ESRD in patients assigned to a low protein diet compared with patients assigned to a usual protein diet (Hansen HP et al. 2002). A hypothesis is that excessive protein intake causes renal vasodilatation and glomerular excessive perfusion leading to a raised glomerular transcapillary hydraulic pressure gradient ending in proteinuria and glomerular damage, conversely, will prevent kidney damage (Percheron C et al. 1995). So, indeed protein restriction is beneficial for type 1 diabetic patients with established nephropathy. However, we have to mention that although this beneficial effect of a restricted protein intake was found in randomized controlled trials, the sample size of these trials were really small (maximum of 82 people). Furthermore, we have to consider the feasibility of a protein intake of 0.8 g/kg/day. Percheron et al. (Percheron C et al. 1995) showed that even with this intake the compliance is poor. Further studies with a larger sample size are needed to find a cutoff point for protein intake which would still have a positive effect on diabetic nephropathy and its feasibility.

Alcohol

The DNSG EASD guidelines for alcohol for persons with type 1 and type 2 diabetes recommend a moderate use up to 10 g/day for women and up to 20 g/day for men (**Table 4**). In prior studies, moderate alcohol consumers (30-70 g alcohol per week) had a lower risk of diabetic nephropathy (OR=0.36, 95% CI: 0.18-0.71) and diabetic retinopathy (OR=0.60, 95% CI: 0.37-0.99) in patients with type 1 diabetes (Beulens et al. 2008). Alcohol has favourable effects on HDL-cholesterol, inflammation and inhibition of platelet aggregation

(Beulens et al. 2008). Because of this favourable effects we expect a beneficial effect on CVD, however to date no association was found between alcohol and CVD in type 1 diabetes patients (Bishop et al. 2009). In this cross-sectional study, markers for CVD were used instead of CVD as endpoint. Also the association between alcohol and diabetic nephropathy and diabetic retinopathy was only observed in cross-sectional studies. So the current recommendations for alcohol are confirmed by research in type 1 diabetes, but only based on cross-sectional studies, and especially for the association between alcohol and CVD in type 1 diabetic patients more research is needed.

5.4 Physical activity

There are no specific guidelines concerning physical activity for type 1 diabetic patients. The guidelines mentioned in **Table 4** are only for type 2 diabetic patients. However, it was shown that the guidelines for type 2 diabetic patients are also applicable for type 1 diabetic patients. Several randomized controlled trials (**Table 3**) showed that physical activity (endurance sports; on average 2 times a week 60 minutes) improves physical fitness as well as endothelial function in type 1 diabetic patients (Lehmann R et al. 1997; Fuchsjäger-Mayrl G et al. 2002; Seeger JPH et al. 2011). Especially the improvement in endothelial function is important since endothelial dysfunction is an early sign of atherosclerosis, which is often the underlying cause of CVD. Also a positive effect on lipid related cardiovascular risk factors was found in one study (Lehmann R et al. 1997). However, also this conclusion should be interpreted carefully. Although the evidence is gained from randomized controlled trials, the conditions of these trials are really disappointing. They had a maximum sample size of 23 people, and a minimum sample size of only 9 people. The follow-up period was relatively short, up to four months. The studies of Lehman et al. (Lehmann R et al. 1997) and Seeger et al. (Seeger JPH et al. 2011) not even used a control group. Furthermore CVD risk factors were used instead of CVD as endpoint. So the studies are in agreement with the guidelines but more research in better performed randomized controlled trials is needed to confirm this positive effect of physical activity on CVD in type 1 diabetic patients.

6. Conclusion

A diet high in fiber, low in saturated fat, moderate in protein intake with moderate alcohol consumption as well as physical activity can be recommended for type 1 diabetic patients to prevent complications. Inspite of the lack of large robust prospective studies, using the available evidence, we can conclude that diet as well as lifestyle could play an important role in preventing longterm complications of type 1 diabetes.

7. References

American Diabetes Association (ADA). (2010). "Diabetes Basics." Retrieved 24 March, 2011, from http://www.diabetes.org/diabetes-basics/.

American Diabetes Association (ADA). (2011). "Recommendations Summary Diabetes Mellitus (DM): Physical Activity." Retrieved 19 April, 2011, from http://www.adaevidencelibrary.com/template.cfm?template=guide_summary&key=2062.

Barsotti G, Cupisti A, et al. (1998). "Dietary treatment of diabetic nephropathy with chronic renal failure." Nephrology, dialysis, transplantation 13(8): 49-52.

Beulens, J. W. J., J. S. Kruidhof, et al. (2008). "Alcohol consumption and risk of microvascular complications in type 1 diabetes patients: the EURODIAB Prospective Complications Study." Diabetologia 51(9): 1631-1638.

Bishop, F. K., D. M. Maahs, et al. (2009). "Lifestyle risk factors for atherosclerosis in adults with type 1 diabetes." Diabetes and Vascular Disease Research 6(4): 269-275.

Bouhanick B, S. S., Berrut G, Bled F, Simard G, Lejeune JJ, Fressinaud P, Marre M. (1995). "Relationship between fat intake and glomerular filtration rate in normotensive insulin-dependent diabetic patients." Diabète and Métabolisme 21(3): 168-172.

Brindisi MC, Bouillet B, et al. (2010). "Cardiovascular complications in type 1 diabetes mellitus: review." Diabetes & Metabolism.

Brouhard BH and LaGrone L (1990). "Effect of dietary protein restriction on functional renal reserve in diabetic nephropathy." The American Journal of Medicine 89(4): 427-431.

Cárdenas C, Bordiu E, et al. (2004). "Polyunsaturated fatty acid consumption may play a role in the onset and regression of microalbuminuria in well-controlled type 1 and type 2 diabetic people: a 7-year, prospective, population-based, observational multicenter study." Diabetes Care 27(6): 1454-1457.

Colhoun HM, Otvos JD, et al. (2002). "Lipoprotein subclasses and particle size and their relationship with coronary artery classification in men and women with and without type 1 diabetes " Diabetes 51: 7.

Cundiff DK and Nigg CR (2005). Diet and Diabetic Retinopathy: Insights From the Diabetes Control and Complications Trial (DCCT). Medscape General Medicine. 7.

Daneman D (2006). "Type 1 diabetes." The Lancet 367(9513): 847-858.

Dullaart RP, Beusekamp BJ, et al. (1993). "Long-term effects of protein-restricted diet on albuminuria and renal function in IDDM patients without clinical nephropathy and hypertension." Diabetes Care 16(2): 483-492.

Franz MJ, Bantle JP, et al. (2003). "Evidence-based nutrition principles and recommendations for the treatment and prevention of diabetes and related complications." Diabetes Care 26(1): S51-S61.

Franz, M. J., M. A. Powers, et al. (2010). "The Evidence for Medical Nutrition Therapy for Type 1 and Type 2 Diabetes in Adults." Journal of the American Dietetic Association 110(12): 1852-1889.

Fuchsjäger-Mayrl G, Pleiner J, et al. (2002). "Exercise training improves vascular endothelial function in patients with type 1 diabetes." Diabetes Care 25(10): 1795-1801.

Georgopoulos A, Bantle JP, et al. (2000). "A high carbohydrate versus a high monounsaturated fatty acid diet lowers the atherogenic potential of big VLDL particles in patients with type 1 diabetes." The journal of nutrition 130(10): 2503-2507.

Gunther ALB, Liese AD, et al. (2008). "Association Between the Dietary Approaches to Hypertension Diet and Hypertension in Youth With Diabetes Mellitus." Hypertension 53(1): 6-12.

Hansen HP, Christensen PK, et al. (1999). "Low-protein diet and kidney function in insulin-dependent diabetic patients with diabetic nephropathy." Kidney International 55(2): 621-628.

Hansen HP, Tauber-Lassen E, et al. (2002). "Effect of dietary protein restriction on prognosis in patients with diabetic nephropathy." Kidney International 62(1): 220-228.

Helgeson, V. S. (2006). "Diet of Adolescents With and Without Diabetes: Trading candy for potato chips?" Diabetes Care 29(5): 982-987.

Herbst A, Kordonouri O, et al. (2007). "Impact of Physical Activity on Cardiovascular Risk Factors in Children With Type 1 Diabetes: A multicenter study of 23,251 patients." Diabetes Care 30(8): 2098-2100.

Hovind P (2004). "Predictors for the development of microalbuminuria and macroalbuminuria in patients with type 1 diabetes: inception cohort study." Bmj 328(7448): 1105-1100.

Hu, F. B., J. E. Manson, et al. (2001). "Diet, lifestyle, and the risk of type 2 diabetes mellitus in women." N Engl J Med. 345(11): 790-797.

International Diabetes Federation (IDF). (2010). "IDF Diabetes Atlas: The Economic Impacts of Diabetes." Retrieved 21 March, 2011, from http://www.diabetesatlas.org /content/economic-impacts-diabetes.

Jensen T, Borch-Johnsen K, et al. (1987). "Coronary heart disease in young type 1 (insulin-dependent) diabetic patients with and without diabetic nephropathy: incidence and risk factors." Diabetologia 30(3): 144-148.

Jibani MM, Bloodworth LL, et al. (1991). "Predominantly vegetarian diet in patients with incipient and early clinical diabetic nephropathy: effects on albumin excretion rate and nutritional status. ." Diabetic Medicine 8(10): 949-953.

Klein R, Lee KE, et al. (2010). "The 25-Year Incidence of Visual Impairment in Type 1 Diabetes MellitusThe Wisconsin Epidemiologic Study of Diabetic Retinopathy." Ophthalmology 117(1): 63-70.

Kornerub K, Nordestgaard BG, et al. (2003). "Increased transvascular low density lipoprotein transport in insulin dependent diabetes: a mechanistic model for development of atherosclerosis." Atherosclerosis 170: 163-168.

Kriska AM, LaPorte RE, et al. (1991). "The association of physical activity and diabetic complications in individuals with insulin-dependent diabetes mellitus: the Epidemiology of Diabetes Complications Study." Journal of Clinical Epidemiology 44(11): 1207-1214.

Lee CC, Sharp SJ, et al. (2010). "Dietary Intake of Eicosapentaenoic and Docosahexaenoic Acid and Diabetic Nephropathy: Cohort Analysis of the Diabetes Control and Complications Trial." Diabetes Care 33(7): 1454-1456.

Lehmann R, Kaplan V, et al. (1997). "Impact of physical activity on cardiovascular risk factors in IDDM." Diabetes Care 20(10): 1603-1611.

Liese AD, Bortsov A, et al. (2011). "Association of DASH Diet With Cardiovascular Risk Factors in Youth With Diabetes Mellitus: The SEARCH for Diabetes in Youth Study." Circulation 123(13): 1410-1417.

Möllsten AV, Dahlquist GG, et al. (2001). "Higher intakes of fish protein are related to a lower risk of microalbuminuria in young Swedish type 1 diabetic patients." Diabetes Care 24(5): 805-810.

Moss SE, Klein R, et al. (1992). "Alcohol consumption and the prevalence of diabetic retinopathy." Ophthalmology 99(6): 926-932.

National Institute for Public Health and the Environment (RIVM). (2007). "Diabetes in Nederland. Omvang, risicofactoren en gevolgen, nu en in de toekomst." Retrieved 22 March, 2011, from http://www.rivm.nl/bibliotheek/rapporten/260322001.pdf.

National Institute for Public Health and the Environment (RIVM). (2010). "Nationaal Kompas Volksgezondheid: Diabetes mellitus samengevat." Retrieved 21 March, 2011, from http://www.nationaalkompas.nl/gezondheid-en-ziekte/ziekten-en-aandoeningen/endocriene-voedings-en-stofwisselingsziekten-en-immuniteitsstoornissen/diabetes-mellitus/diabetes-mellitus-samengevat/.

O'Hayon BE, Cummings EA, et al. (2000). "Does dietary protein intake correlate with markers suggestive of early diabetic nephropathy in children and adolescents with Type 1 diabetes mellitus?" Diabetic Medicine 17(10): 708-712.

Øverby NC, Flaaten V, et al. (2006). "Children and adolescents with type 1 diabetes eat a more atherosclerosis-prone diet than healthy control subjects." Diabetologia 50(2): 307-316.

Percheron C, Colette C, et al. (1995). "Effects of moderate changes in protein intake on urinary albumin excretion in type I diabetic patients." Nutrition 11(4): 345-349.

Raal FJ, Kalk WJ, et al. (1994). "Effect of moderate dietary protein restriction on the progression of overt diabetic nephropathy: a 6-mo prospective study." The American Journal of Clinical Nutrition 60(4): 579-585.

Riley MD and Dwyer T (1998). "Microalbuminuria is positively associated with usual dietary saturated fat intake and negatively associated with usual dietary protein intake in people with insulin-dependent diabetes mellitus." The American Journal of Clinical Nutrition 67(1): 50-57.

Roper NA, Bilous RW, et al. (2002). "Cause-specific mortality in a population with diabetes." Diabetes Care 25(1): 43-48.

Sadauskaitė-Kuehne V, Ludvigsson J, et al. (2004). "Longer breastfeeding is an independent protective factor against development of type 1 diabetes mellitus in childhood." Diabetes/Metabolism Research and Reviews 20(2): 150-157.

Sahakyan K, Klein BEK, et al. (2011). "The 25-Year Cumulative Incidence of Lower Extremity Amputations in People With Type 1 Diabetes." Diabetes Care 34(3): 649-651.

Seeger JPH, Thijssen DHJ, et al. (2011). "Exercise training improves physical fitness and vascular function in children with type 1 diabetes." Diabetes, Obesity and Metabolism 13(4): 382-384.

Snell-Bergeon JK, Chartier-Logan C, et al. (2009). "Adults with type 1 diabetes eat a high-fat atherogenic diet that is associated with coronary artery calcium." Diabetologia 52(5): 801-809.

Soedamah-Muthu SS, Fuller JH, et al. (2006). "High risk of cardiovascular disease in patients with type 1 diabetes in the U.K.: a cohort study using the general practice research database." Diabetes Care 29(4): 798-804.

Stampfer, M. J., F. B. Hu, et al. (2000). "Primary prevention of coronary heart disease in women through diet and lifestyle." N Engl J Med. 343(1): 16-22.

Strychar I, Cohn JS, et al. (2009). "Effects of a Diet Higher in Carbohydrate/Lower in Fat Versus Lower in Carbohydrate/Higher in Monounsaturated Fat on Postmeal Triglyceride Concentrations and Other Cardiovascular Risk Factors in Type 1 Diabetes." Diabetes Care 32(9): 1597-1599.

Toeller M: Lifestyle Issues: Diet. In: Textbook of Diabetes. Holt RIG, Cockram CS, Flyvbjerg A, Goldstein BJ (eds). 4th edition, Wiley-Blackwell Chichester U.K. 2010, pp 346-357

Toeller M, Buyken A, et al. (1997). "Protein intake and urinary albumin excretion rates in the EURODIAB IDDM Complications Study." Diabetologia 40(10): 1219-1226. [1]

Toeller M, Buyken AE, et al. (1999). "Prevalence of chronic complications, metabolic control and nutritional intake in type 1 diabetes: comparison between different European regions. EURODIAB Complications Study group." Hormone and Metabolic Research 31(12): 680-685. [2]

Toeller M, Buyken AE, et al. (1999). "Fiber intake, serum cholesterol levels, and cardiovascular disease in European individuals with type 1 diabetes. EURODIAB IDDM Complications Study Group." Diabetes Care 22(2): B21-B28. [3]

Toeller M, Buyken AE, et al. (1999). "Associations of fat and cholesterol intake with serum lipid levels and cardiovascular disease: the EURODIAB IDDM Complications Study." Experimental and Clinical Endocrinology & Diabetes 107(8): 512-521.

Toeller M, Klischan A, et al. (1996). "Nutritional intake of 2868 IDDM patients from 30 centres in Europe. EURODIAB IDDM Complications Study Group." Diabetologia 39(8): 929-939.

Trigona B, Aggoun Y, et al. (2010). "Preclinical Noninvasive Markers of Atherosclerosis in Children and Adolescents with Type 1 Diabetes Are Influenced by Physical Activity." The Journal of Pediatrics 157(4): 533-539.

U.S. National Library of Medicine. (2011). "Type 1 diabetes." Retrieved 24, 2011, from http://www.nlm.nih.gov/medlineplus/ency/article/000305.htm.

Valerio G, Spagnuolo M, et al. (2007). "Physical activity and sports participation in children and adolescents with type 1 diabetes mellitus." Nutrition, Metabolism and Cardiovascular Diseases 17(5): 376-382.

Watts GF, Gregory L, et al. (1988). "Nutrient intake in insulin-dependent diabetic patients with incipient nephropathy." European Journal of Clinical Nutrition 42(8): 697-702.

Weis U, Turner B, et al. (2001). "Long-term predictors of coronary artery disease and mortallity in type 1 diabetes." QJM 94: 623-630.

World Diabetes Foundation (WDF). (2010). "Diabetes facts " Retrieved 21 March, 2011, from http://www.worlddiabetesfoundation.org/composite-35.htm.

World Health Organization (WHO). (2008). "Fact sheet N°310 The top 10 causes of death." Retrieved 21 March, 2011, from http://www.who.int/mediacentre/factsheets/fs310/en/index.html

Yusuf, S., S. Hawken, et al. (2004). "Effect of potentially modifiable risk factors associated with myocardial infarction in 52 countries (the INTERHEART study): case-control study." Lancet. 364(9438): 937-952.

Zeller K, Whittaker E, et al. (1991). "Effect of restricting dietary protein on the progression of renal failure in patients with insulin-dependent diabetes mellitus." The New England Journal of Medicine 324(2): 78-84.

3

Lipid Disorders in Type 1 Diabetes

Bruno Vergès
Service Endocrinologie, Diabétologie et Maladies Métaboliques
Dijon University Hospital
France

1. Introduction

Cardiovascular disease is the major cause of death in persons with type 1 diabetes (Libby et al., 2005). Dyslipidemia has been shown to be a significant coronary heart disease risk factor in type 1 diabetes (Soedamah-Muthu et al., 2004; Grauslund et al., 2010). Thus, it seems important to pay attention to lipid abnormalities, in patients with type 1 diabetes, in order to reduce cardiovascular disease in this population.
Patients with type 1 diabetes show lipid disorders, mostly qualitative abnormalities of lipoproteins, which may promote atherogenesis. The pathophysiology of these lipid abnormalities is not totally explained, but hyperglycemia and peripheral hyperinsulinemia, due to the subcutaneous route of insulin administration, are likely to play a role. After a brief review of lipoprotein metabolism and some information on the role of insulin on lipid metabolism, quantitative abnormalities then qualitative abnormalities of lipoproteins, in type 1 diabetes, will be discussed.

2. Brief review of lipoprotein metabolism

Lipoproteins, which transport non-water soluble cholesterol and triglycerides in plasma, are spherical particles composed of a central core of non-polar lipids (cholesterol esters, triglycerides) and a surface monolayer of phospholipids, free cholesterol and apolipoproteins. Lipoproteins are generally classified according to their density as chylomicron, Very Low Density Lipoprotein (VLDL), Intermediate Density Lipoprotein (IDL), Low Density Lipoprotein (LDL) and High Density Lipoprotein (HDL). An overview of lipoprotein metabolism is shown in Figure 1.

2.1 Chylomicrons

Chylomicrons, the largest lipoprotein particles, are responsible for the transport of dietary triglycerides and cholesterol. Chylomicrons are composed of triglycerides (85-90%), cholesterol esters, phospholipids and apolipoproteins (mainly apoB48 but also apoA-I and apoA-IV). The formation of chylomicrons takes place in the enterocytes, and the process associating the lipid components (triglycerides, cholesterol esters, phospholipids) and the apoB48 is performed by the MTP (Microsomal Tranfer Protein). Chylomicrons are secreted into the lymphatic circulation before entering the bloodstream. In plasma, triglycerides of chylomicrons are hydrolyzed by the lipoprotein lipase leading to the formation of smaller, triglyceride-poorer particles known as chylomicron-remnants. Chylomicron-remnants are cleared by the liver through LDL B/E receptor or LRP receptor (LDL-receptor related protein).

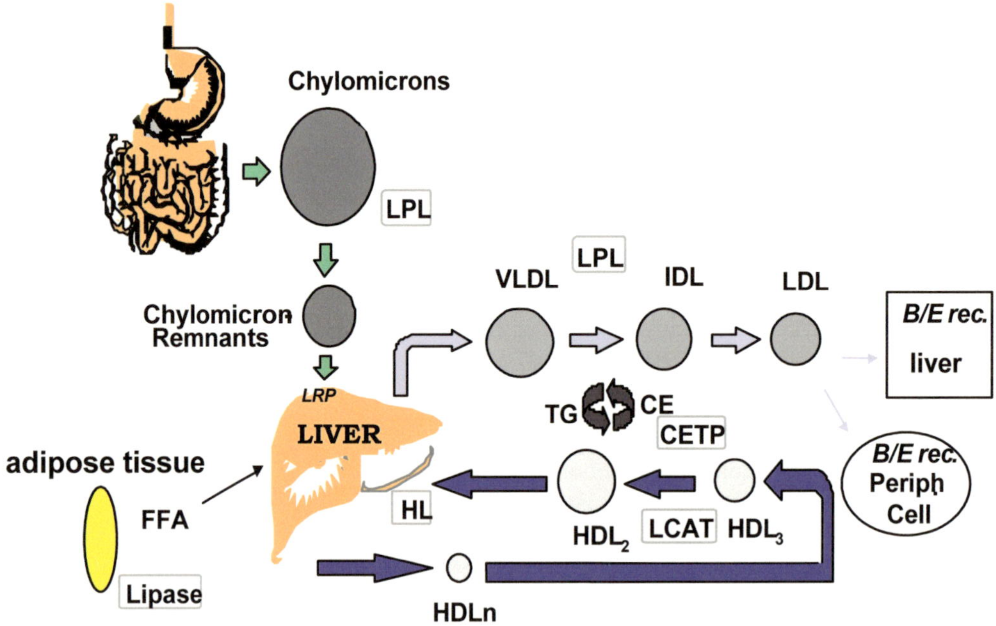

VLDL: Very Low Density Lipoprotein; *IDL*: Intermediate Density Lipoprotein, *LDL*: Low Density Lipoprotein; *HDL*: High Density Lipoprotein; *LPL*: LipoProtein Lipase; *HL*: Hepatic Lipase; *CETP*: Cholesteryl Ester Transfer Protein; *LCAT*: Lecithin-Cholesterol Acyl Transferase; *FFA*: Free Fatty Acids ; *B/E rec.*: B/E receptor (LDL receptor); *TG*: Triglycerides; *CE*: Cholesterol Esters; *ABCA1*: ATP Binding Cassette A1 transporter.

Fig. 1. Human lipoprotein metabolism.

2.2 VLDLs and IDLs

VLDL particles, which are secreted by the liver, consist of endogenous triglycerides (55% to 65%), cholesterol, phospholipids and apolipoproteins (apoB100 as well as apoCs and apoE). In the hepatocyte, the formation of VLDL occurs in two major steps. In the first step, which takes place in the rough endoplasmic reticulum, apoB is co-translationally and post-translationally lipidated by the MTP (Microsomal Tranfer Protein). MTP transfers lipids (mainly triglycerides but also cholesterol esters and phospholipids) to apoB. This first step leads to the formation of pre-VLDL (Olofsson et al., 2000). In the second step, pre-VLDL is converted to VLDL in the smooth membrane compartment. This step is driven by ADP ribosylation factor-1 (ARF-1) and its activation of phospholipase D, needed for the formation of VLDL from pre-VLDL (Olofsson , 2000).

In plasma, triglycerides of VLDLs are hydrolyzed by the lipoprotein lipase. As VLDLs become progressively depleted in triglycerides, a portion of the surface including phospholipids and apolipoproteins C and E is transferred to HDLs. This metabolic cascade leads to the formation of IDL particles, which are either cleared by the liver through LDL B/E receptor or further metabolized to form LDLs. The enzyme, hepatic lipase, which has both triglyceride lipase and phospholipase activities, is involved in this metabolic process generating LDL particles from IDLs.

2.3 LDLs

LDL is the final product of the VLDL-IDL-LDL cascade. LDL is the main cholesterol-bearing lipoprotein in plasma. Each LDL particle contains one molecule of apoB100, which plays an important role in LDL metabolism, particularly recognition of its dedicated LDL B/E receptor. Clearance of LDL is mediated by the LDL B/E receptor. Seventy percent of LDL B/E receptors are located on hepatic cells and 30% on the other cells of the body.

2.4 HDLs

HDL particles are secreted by the hepatocytes as small lipid-poor lipoproteins, containing mostly apoA-I, which receive, in the circulation, phospholipids, apoCs and apoE from chylomicrons and VLDLs. Nascent or lipid-poor HDLs get from peripheral cells free cholesterol and phospholipids through ABCA1 transporter (ATP Binding Cassette A1 transporter), allowing the transport of free cholesterol and phospholipids from the cell cytoplasm into the HDL particles (Oram & Lawn, 2001). Within HDL particles, free cholesterol is esterified by LCAT (Lecithin Cholesterol AcylTransferase) leading to the formation of HDL_3 particles. The fusion of 2 HDL_3 particles, which is promoted by PLTP (PhosphoLipid Transfer Protein), leads to the formation of one larger size HDL_2 particle. HDL_2 lipoproteins, rich in cholesterol ester, are degraded by the hepatic lipase and the endothelial lipase, leading to the formation of HDL remnant particles that are cleared by the liver after recognition by SR-B1 receptor (Scavenger Receptor class B type 1) (Jian et al., 1998).

2.5 Lipid transfer proteins

Lipoprotein metabolism is largely influenced by lipid transfer proteins. Among these, two play an important role: CETP (Cholesteryl Ester Transfer Protein) and PLTP (PhosphoLipid Transfer Protein). CETP facilitates the transfer of triglycerides from triglyceride-rich lipoproteins (mainly VLDLs) toward HDLs and LDLs and the reciprocal transfer of cholesteryl esters from HDLs and LDLs toward VLDLs (Lagrost, 1994). PLTP facilitates the transfer of phospholipids and α-tocopherol between lipoproteins. PLTP is also involved in the formation of HDL_2 lipoproteins from HDL_3 particles (Lagrost et al., 1998). Any modification of CETP or PLTP activities is likely to promote significant qualitative abnormalities of lipoproteins.

3. Insulin and lipoprotein metabolism

Insulin plays a central role in the regulation of lipid metabolism (Vergès, 2001). The main sites of action of insulin on lipoprotein metabolism are shown in Figure 2.

In adipose tissue, insulin inhibits the hormone-sensitive lipase. Thus, insulin has an anti-lipolytic action, promoting storage of triglycerides in the adipocytes and reducing release of free fatty acids from adipose tissue in the circulation.

Insulin inhibits VLDL production from the liver. In normal subjects, it has been shown that insulin induces a 67% decrease of VLDL-triglyceride production and a 52% decrease of VLDL-apoB production (Lewis et al., 1993; Malmström et al., 1998). Insulin reduces VLDL production by diminishing circulating free fatty acids (due to its antilipolytic effect), which are substrates for VLDL, but also by a direct inhibitory effect in the hepatocyte (Malmström et al., 1998). Insulin is a potent activator of lipoprotein lipase (LPL), promoting the catabolism of triglyceride-rich lipoproteins and reducing, as a consequence, plasma triglyceride level. Insulin not only enhances LPL activity (Brunzell et al., 1998), but has also a direct positive effect on LPL gene, promoting LPL synthesis (Fried etal., 1993). Insulin promotes the clearance of LDL, by increasing LDL B/E receptor expression and activity (Chait et al., 1979, Mazzone et al., 1984).

Insulin acts also on HDL metabolism by activating LCAT and hepatic lipase activities (Ruotolo et al., 1994).

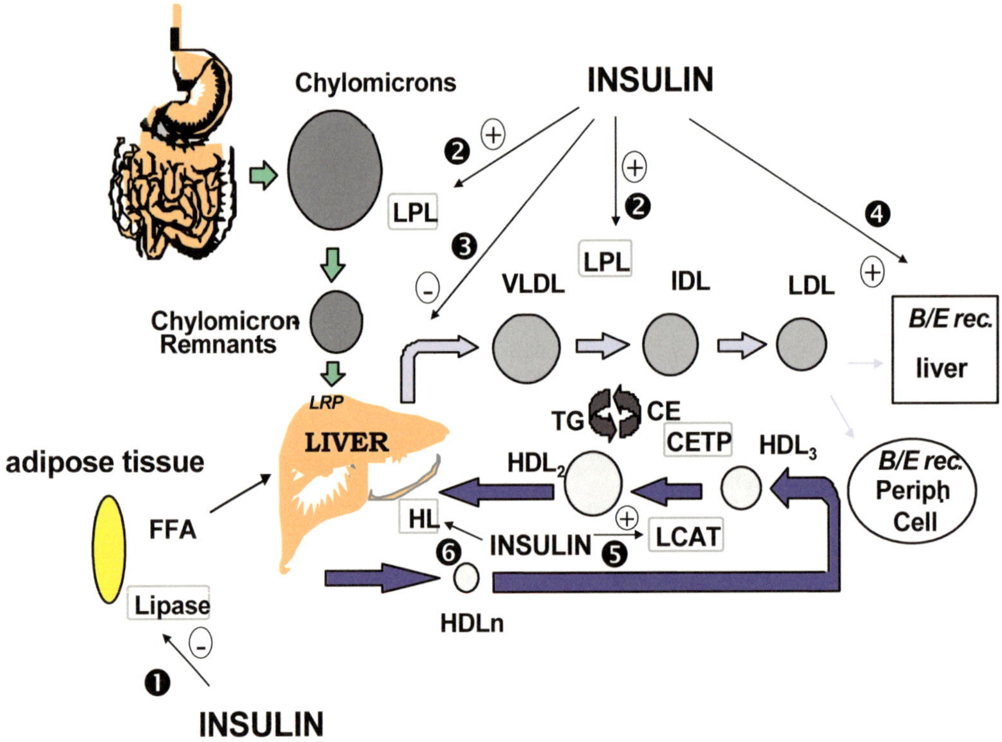

VLDL: Very Low Density Lipoprotein; *IDL*: Intermediate Density Lipoprotein, *LDL*: Low Density Lipoprotein; *HDL*: High Density Lipoprotein; *LPL*: LipoProtein Lipase; *HL*: Hepatic Lipase; *CETP*: Cholesteryl Ester Transfer Protein; *LCAT*: Lecithin-Cholesterol Acyl Transferase; *FFA*: Free Fatty Acids ; *B/E rec.*: receptor B/E (LDL receptor); *TG*: Triglycerides; *CE*: Cholesterol Esters. **1**: insulin inhibits hormone-sensitive lipase. **2** : insulin activates LipoProtein Lipase (LPL). **3**: insulin inhibits hepatic VLDL production. **4**: insulin increases LDL B/E receptor expression. **5**: insulin activates LCAT. **6**: insulin activates Hepatic Lipase (HL).

Fig. 2. Main effects of insulin on lipoprotein metabolism.

4. Quantitative lipid abnormalities in type 1 diabetes

4.1 Untreated (diabetic ketoacidosis) type 1 diabetes

In type 1 diabetic patients with diabetic ketoacidosis, quantitative lipid abnormalities are observed, due to insulin deficiency.

Triglyceride-rich lipoproteins (chylomicrons, VLDLs) are increased leading to hypertriglyceridemia. This is mainly due to decreased lipoprotein lipase activity (Vergès, 2001; Dullaart, 1995). Diabetic ketoacidosis is a situation of severe insulin deficiency with reduced lipoprotein lipase activity as a consequence, because insulin usually stimulates its activity. Decreased lipoprotein lipase activity leads to profound reduction of triglyceride-rich lipoprotein catabolism (Taskinen, 1987). In this condition of severe insulin deficiency, reduced catabolism of triglyceride-rich lipoproteins is, by far, the main factor involved in hypertriglyceridemia. This hypertriglyceridemia resolves rapidly after well titrated insulin therapy (Weidman et al., 1982).

LDL-cholesterol is decreased during diabetic ketoacidosis (Weidman et al., 1982). This fall in plasma LDL-cholesterol level is the direct consequence of the reduction of triglyceride-rich lipoprotein catabolism, due to decreased lipoprotein lipase activity (see above).

In diabetic ketoacidosis, HDL-cholesterol level is significantly decreased (Weidman et al., 1982). This is a consequence of hypertrigliceridemia observed in this condition. Indeed, the augmented level of plasma triglyceride-rich lipoproteins drives, through CETP, the transfer of triglycerides from triglyceride-rich lipoproteins to HDLs leading to the formation of triglyceride-rich HDL particles. HDLs enriched in triglycerides become very good substrate for hepatic lipase, leading to increase their catabolism and, thus, to decrease plasma HDL-cholesterol level. This low HDL-cholesterol condition resolves rapidly after well titrated insulin therapy (Weidman et al., 1982).

4.2 Treated type 1 diabetes

Patients with treated type 1 diabetes may show quantitative lipid disorders. In a prospective study performed in 895 young subjects with type 1 diabetes, 20.1% had plasma triglycerides above 1.7 mmol/l, 9.6% had LDL-cholesterol above 3.4 mmol/l and 25.9% had non-HDL cholesterol above 3.4 mmol/l (Marcovecchio et al., 2009). It has been shown that abnormal lipid levels, in type 1 diabetes, predict worse cardiovascular outcomes (Soedamah-Muthu et al., 2004). HbA1c has been shown to be independently correlated with LDL-cholesterol, non-HDL cholesterol and triglyceride levels, indicating that these disorders were mostly observed in patients with poor glycemic control (Marcovecchio et al., 2009). In a British follow-up study of 229 children with type 1 diabetes, LDL cholesterol and non-HDL cholesterol values increased with duration of diabetes (Edge et al., 2008). In that study, total cholesterol, triglycerides and non-HDL cholesterol were positively correlated with HbA1c and around 10% of the patients had lipid values outside recommendations (Edge et al., 2008). In a large study performed in 29 979 patients with type 1 diabetes, multivariate analyses showed a significant positive association between HbA1c and total cholesterol ($p<0.0001$), LDL cholesterol ($p<0.0001$) and a significant negative association between HbA1c and HDL cholesterol ($p<0.0001$) (Schwab et al., 2009). In the Diabetes Control and Complications Trial (DCCT), HbA1c correlated positively with total cholesterol, LDL-cholesterol and triglycerides at baseline (The DCCT Research Group, 1992). Data from the Coronary Artery Calcification in type 1 diabetes (CACTI) study, which examined 652 patients with type 1 diabetes, have shown, in patients not using hypolipidemic agents, that a higher HbA1c was associated with significantly higher levels of total cholesterol, triglycerides, LDL cholesterol and non-HDL cholesterol (Maahs et al., 2010). In that study, 1% change in HbA1c was associated with an increase of 0.101 mmol/l (4 mg/dl) for total cholesterol, of 0.052 mmol/l (4.5 mg/dl) for triglycerides, of 0.103 mmol/l (4 mg/dl) for LDL cholesterol and of 0.129 mmol/l (5 mg/dl) for non-HDL cholesterol (Maahs et al.,

2010). In a recent study, performed in 512 young patients with type 1 diabetes and in 188 healthy age-matched controls, patients with suboptimal control (HbA1c ≥ 7.5%) had much more lipid quantitative disorders than patients with optimal control (HbA1c<7.5%) (Guy et al., 2009). All these data suggest that quantitative lipid abnormalities are more frequent, when type 1 diabetes is not well controlled.

In addition, some patients with type 1 diabetes may have insulin resistance, in situation of abdominal obesity and/or family history of type 2 diabetes. Such patients have been shown to have greater dyslipidemia (Purnell et al., 2003). In a recent study performed in 60 young type 1 diabetic patients and 40 adults with type 1 diabetes, it has been shown, using hyperinsulinemic clamp studies, that lower glucose infusion (more insulin resistance) was associated with lower levels of HDL cholesterol in youths with type 1 diabetes and with higher levels of triglycerides and higher triglyceride/HDL ratio in both youths and adults (Maahs et al., 2011). These data indicate that insulin resistance may be an additional factor that could induce quantitative lipid abnormities in some type 1 diabetic patients with a background of insulin resistance (abdominal obesity, family history of type 2 diabetes). In this chapter we will consider only the typical situation of type 1 diabetes without insulin resistance.

4.2.1 Treated type 1 diabetes with poor or suboptimal glycemic control

In case of poor or suboptimal control, patients with type 1 diabetes may show increased plasma triglyceride levels (Dullaart,1995). This hypertriglyceridemia is due to increased production of VLDL, promoted by elevated circulating free fatty acids secondary to the relative insulin deficiency (Nikkilä & Kekki, 1973).

Type 1 diabetic patients with poor or suboptimal glycemic control show increased LDL-cholesterol levels as compared to non-diabetic individuals and type 1 diabetic patients with optimal glycemic control (Dullaart, 1995; Guy et al., 2009). Indeed, in this condition, VLDL production is increased (see above), when catabolism of triglyceride-rich lipoproteins is not importantly decreased, which leads to increase LDL production (Dullaart, 1995).

4.2.2 Treated type 1 diabetes with optimal glycemic control

In well controlled type 1 diabetes, the lipid profile is totally different than in poorly controlled type 1 diabetes (Dullaart, 1995; Nikkilä & Kekki, 1973).

Plasma triglycerides are normal or slightly decreased (Dullaart, 1995; Nikkilä & Kekki, 1973). This slight decrease in plasma triglycerides may be observed with intense insulin therapy because of increased down control of VLDL production by augmented plasma insulin levels as a consequence of the subcutaneous route of insulin delivery (Dashti & Wolfbauer, 1987; Taskinen, 1992). Furthermore, in patients with well controlled type 1 diabetes, peripheral hyperinsulinemia has been shown to be associated with increased lipoprotein lipase activity that could be an additional factor responsible for decreased plasma triglycerides (Nikkilä et al., 1977).

Plasma LDL-cholesterol level is normal or slightly decreased (Winocour et al., 1986). This slight decrease in plasma LDL-cholesterol may be observed with intense insulin therapy as a consequence of decreased VLDL production by peripheral hyperinsulinemia (see above).

Plasma HDL-cholesterol level is normal or slightly increased in well controlled type 1 diabetic patients (Dullaart, 1995). Some studies have shown an increase in HDL subfraction 2 (Eckel et al., 1981; Kahri et al., 1993), when others have found an increase in HDL subfraction 3 (Winocour et al., 1986). It has also been reported that elevation of HDL in type 1 diabetic patients with good glycemic control was caused by an increase of HDL particles containing only apoA-I (LpA-I) (Kahri et al., 1993). This increase in plasma HDL-cholesterol could be the consequence of the elevated Lipoprotein Lipase/Hepatic Lipase ratio that is observed in patients with well controlled type 1 diabetes (increased Lipoprotein Lipase activity and normal Hepatic Lipase activity) (Kahri et al., 1993). The increased Lipoprotein Lipase activity observed in these patients is likely to be due to peripheral hyperinsulinemia as a consequence of the subcutaneous route of insulin administration (Kahri et al., 1993).

4.2.3 Subcutaneous insulin therapy versus intraperitoneal insulin therapy

Intensive subcutaneous insulin therapy results in normalization of plasma glucose, but at the expense of peripheral hyperinsulinemia, which is likely to modify lipoprotein metabolism (as discussed above). Implantable insulin pumps with intraperitoneal insulin administration mimic the physiologic route of insulin delivery and are likely to restore the normal portal-peripheral insulin gradient. For this reason, several studies have been performed to analyze the modification of lipoprotein metabolism after replacement of subcutaneous insulin therapy by intraperitoneal insulin therapy. Plasma triglycerides have been found increased in one study (Selam et al., 1989) and unchanged in three other studies (Bagdade & Dunn, 1996; Ruotolo et al., 1994; Duvillard et al., 2005). Total cholesterol and apoB were found unchanged (Bagdade & Dunn, 1996; Ruotolo et al., 1994; Duvillard et al., 2005). HDL-cholesterol has been found decreased (Selam et al., 1989) or not modified (Bagdade & Dunn, 1996; Ruotolo et al., 1994; Duvillard et al., 2007). The discrepancies of these studies that may be due to confounding factors such as degree of glycemic control and peripheral insulin levels during subcutaneous insulin therapy. Further studies are needed to clearly evaluate the effect of intraperitoneal insulin administration on lipoprotein metabolism.

4.2.4 Type 1 diabetes with nephropathy

In type 1 diabetic patients with nephropathy and overt albuminuria, elevated plasma levels of total cholesterol, triglycerides and LDL-cholesterol are observed whereas HDL-cholesterol is decreased due to a fall in HDL_2 (Dullaart ,1995; Taskinen, 1992; Jensen et al., 1987). In the EURODIAB IDDM Complications study, macroalbuminuria was associated with significantly increased plasma triglycerides, cholesterol, LDL-cholesterol and LDL/HDL ratio in both sexes and decreased HDL-cholesterol in women (Mattock et al., 2001).

Some quantitative lipid modifications are also observed in type 1 diabetic patients with microalbuminuria. Microalbuminuric patients compared with normoalbuminuric patients show increased plasma apoB (Jones et al., 1989, Dullaart et al, 1989a; Jay et al., 1991), LDL cholesterol (Jones et al., 1989, Dullaart et al, 1989a) and apoB/apoA1 ratio (Dullaart et al, 1989a; Jay et al., 1991). A positive correlation has been found between urinary albumin excretion rate and plasma apoB and apoB/apoA1 ratio (Dullaart et al, 1989a). In the EURODIAB IDDM Complications study, microalbuminuria was associated with increased plasma triglycerides (Mattock et al., 2001). In a prospective study performed in 895 young subjects with type 1 diabetes, total cholesterol and non-HDL cholesterol were independently related to longitudinal changes in albumin-to-creatinine ratio (Marcovecchio et al., 2009). The mechanisms responsible for these lipoprotein abnormalities in type 1 diabetic patients with microalbuminuria remain unclear.

Moreover, serum lipids have been shown to be associated with the progression of nephropathy in type 1 diabetes. In a prospective study performed in 152 patients with type 1 diabetes followed for 8-9 years, LDL-cholesterol was an independent factor associated with progression of nephropathy (Thomas et al., 2006).

5. Qualitative lipid abnormalities in type 1 diabetes

Several qualitative abnormalities of lipoproteins are observed in patients with type 1 diabetes, even in those with good metabolic control, who do not have significant quantitative lipid changes. These qualitative lipid abnormalities are not totally reversed by optimal glycemic control and are likely to be atherogenic.

5.1 VLDLs

VLDLs from patients with type 1 diabetes are frequently enriched in esterified cholesterol at the expense of triglycerides leading to an increased VLDL cholesterol/triglyceride ratio (Rivellese et al., 1988; Bagdade et al., 1991a). It has been suggested that this compositional changes may be due to increased cholesteryl ester transfer between lipoproteins (Bagdade et al., 1991a). It has been shown that the VLDL cholesterol/triglyceride ratio was significantly reduced with intraperitoneal insulin therapy (Dunn, 1992). Furthermore, the free cholesterol /lecithin ratio within the peripheral layer of VLDL particles is increased (Dullaart, 1995; Bagdade et al., 1991a). Such increase in the free cholesterol /lecithin ratio within the peripheral layer of lipoproteins has been shown to raise the risk for cardiovascular events possibly by reducing fluidity and stability of lipoproteins (Kuksis, 1982). Moreover, VLDLs from patients with type 1 diabetes have been shown, in vitro, to induce abnormal response of cellular cholesterol metabolism in human macrophages (Klein et al., 1989).

5.2 LDLs

In patients with type 1 diabetes, LDLs are often enriched in triglycerides and increased number of small dense LDL particles is observed (Guy et al., 2009; Lahdenperä et al., 1994; James & Pometta, 1990; Skyrme-Jones et al., 2000). In a study performed in 2657 patients with type 1 diabetes, it has been shown that dense LDL increased with HbA1c with buoyant LDL shifting toward dense LDL for HbA1c values above 8% (Albers et al., 2008). It has been shown that the presence of small dense LDL particles is associated with increased cardiovascular risk (Austin et al., 1990). Many data indicate that small dense LDL particles have atherogenic properties. Indeed, small dense LDL particles have reduced affinity for the LDL B/E receptor and are preferentially taken up by macrophages, through the scavenger receptor, leading to the formation of foam cells. Small dense LDL particles have higher affinity for intimal proteoglycans than large LDL particles which may favor the penetration of LDL particles into the arterial wall (Chapman et al., 1998). It has been shown that subjects with small dense LDL particles show an impaired response to endothelium dependent vasodilator acetylcholine (Vakkilainen et al., 2000). Moreover, small dense LDL particles show an increased susceptibility to oxidation (Tribble et al., 1992). A reduction of the proportion of small dense LDL particles has been reported after optimization of glycemic control in patients with type 1 diabetes (Caixàs et al., 1997).
The free cholesterol /lecithin ratio within the peripheral layer of LDL particles is increased (Dullaart, 1995; Bagdade et al., 1991a). In patients with type 1 diabetes, glycation of ApoB

occurs within LDL in parallel with plasma hyperglycemia. It has been shown that apoB glycation reduces significantly LDL binding to the B/E receptor even when apoB glycation is moderate (Witztum et al., 1982; Steinbrecher et al, 1984). Furthermore, glycated LDLs are preferentialy taken up by macrophages through the scavenger receptor, leading to the formation of foam cells in the arterial wall. In patients with type 1 diabetes, advanced glycation end products-modified LDL have been shown to be positively associated with increased intima media thickness (IMT) (Lopes-Virella et al., 2011).

Moreover, patients with type 1 diabetes may show an increased oxidation of LDL which is promoted by glycemic excursions (de Castro et al., 2005). Increased urinary excretion of malondialdehyde, reflecting enhanced lipid peroxidation, has been reported in patients with type 1 diabetes (Hoeldtke et al., 2009). Oxidative modification of LDL results in rapid uptake by macrophages, leading to foam cell formation. Oxidized LDLs produce chemotactic effects on monocytes by increasing the synthesis of adhesion molecules, such as ICAM-1 (intercellular adhesion Molecule 1) by endothelial cells. Oxidized LDLs stimulate the formation by macrophages of cytokines, such as TNFα or IL1, which amplify the inflammatory atherosclerotic process. It has recently been shown that oxidized LDL particles were significantly associated with progression and increased levels of IMT in type 1 diabetes (de Castro et al., 2005).

5.3 HDLs

HDL particles from patients with type 1 diabetes are often enriched in triglycerides (Dullaart, 1995; Bagdade et al., 1991a). This modification has been attributed to increased cholesteryl ester transfer between lipoproteins (Bagdade et al., 1991a). In HDL particles from patients with type 1 diabetes, sphingomyelin/lecithin ratio within the peripheral layer is augmented, which may increase HDL rigidity (Bagdade & Subbaiah, 1989). These alterations are not totally reversed after achievement of optimal glycemic control (Bagdade et al., 1991b). ApoA-I within HDL is glycated in patients with type 1 diabetes, which may impair the HDL-mediated reverse cholesterol pathway. Indeed, it has been shown that HDL particles containing glycated apoA-I were less effective to promote cholesterol efflux from the cells (Fievet et al., 1992).

In addition to their role in the reverse cholesterol pathway, HDLs have anti-oxidative, anti-inflammatory, anti-thrombotic and vasorelaxant properties, potentially anti-atherogenic (Link et al., 2007). Some of these properties have been shown to be reduced in patients with type 1 diabetes. Indeed, a significant reduction of the activity of paraoxonase, an anti-oxidative enzyme associated with HDLs, is observed in patients with type 1 diabetes (Boemi et al., 2001; Ferretti et al., 2004). As a consequence, HDLs from patients with type 1 diabetes protect less efficiently erythrocyte membranes and LDL particles against oxidative damage than HDLs from normal individuals (Boemi et al., 2001; Ferretti et al., 2004). Furthermore, using rabbit aorta rings, it has been shown that HDL from patients with type 1 diabetes are no more able to prevent the endothelium dependent vasoconstriction induced by oxidized LDL, whereas HDL from normal individuals can prevent it (Perségol et al., 2007).

5.4 Lipid transfer proteins

In some studies, an increased cholesteryl ester transfer between lipoproteins (Bagdade et al., 1991a; Bagdade et al., 1994) or an augmented activity of CETP (Colhoun et al., 2001) have been found in normolipidemic patients with type 1 diabetes. In some other studies, increased CETP activity has been reported only in type 1 diabetic patients that smoke or

those having microalbuminuria (Dullaart et al., 1989b; Dullaart et al., 1991). This augmented CETP activity may explain the increase in free cholesterol/ triglycerides ratio within VLDL and its decrease within HDL. Some studies have shown a positive correlation between CETP activity and hyperglycemia (Ritter & Bagdade, 1994; Chang et al., 2001). However, the main factor which is likely to be responsible for increased CETP activity, in type 1 diabetes, could be peripheral hyperinsulinemia secondary to the subcutaneous route of insulin administration. Indeed, peripheral hyperinsulinemia has been shown to be responsible for increased lipoprotein lipase activity in patients with type 1 diabetes (Nikkilä et al., 1977) and it has been reported that lipoprotein lipase, in presence of VLDL, enhances CETP activity (Sammett & Tall,1985; Pruneta et al., 1999). Moreover, it has been shown, in patients with type 1 diabetes, that the increase in both lipoprotein lipase and CETP activities was abolished when insulin was administrated intraperitoneously with implantable insulin pumps, mimicking the physiologic portal route or after pancreatic graft (Bagdade et al., 1994; Bagdade et al., 1996).
Increased PLTP activity has been reported in patients with type 1 diabetes (Colhoun et al., 2001). In this study, PLTP activity was positively correlated with CETP activity, LDL-cholesterol and HDL-cholesterol (Colhoun et al., 2001). The reasons and consequences of this increased PLTP activity are not clear.

6. Conclusion

In conclusion, quantitative lipid abnormalities are observed in patients with poorly controlled type 1 diabetes (increased triglyceride and LDL-cholesterol levels) or with micro- or macroalbuminuria (increased triglycerides and LDL-cholesterol, decreased HDL-cholesterol). Patient with optimally controlled type 1 diabetes show normal or slightly decreased triglycerides and LDL-cholesterol levels and sometimes increased HDL-cholesterol levels. Qualitative abnormalities of lipoproteins are observed in patients with type 1 diabetes, even in good glycemic control. These abnormalities are not fully explained by hyperglycemia and may partly be due to peripheral hyperinsulinemia associated with the subcutaneous route of insulin administration. The exact consequences of these qualitative lipid changes on the development of cardiovascular disease in type 1 diabetes are still unknown.

7. References

Albers JJ, Marcovina SM, Imperatore G, Snively BM, Stafford J, Fujimoto WY, Mayer-Davis EJ, Petitti DB, Pihoker C, Dolan L & Dabelea DM. (2008). Prevalence and determinants of elevated apolipoprotein B and dense low-density lipoprotein in youths with type 1 and type 2 diabetes. *J Clin Endocrinol Metab.*; 93: 735-42

Austin MA, King MC, Vranizan KM & Krauss RM. (1990). Atherogenic lipoprotein phenotype : a proposed genetic marker for coronary heart disease risk. *Circulation*; 82, 495-506.

Bagdade JD & Subbaiah PV. (1989). Whole-plasma and high-density lipoprotein subfraction surface lipid composition in IDDM men. *Diabetes*; 38: 1226-30.

Bagdade JD, Ritter MC & Subbaiah PV. (1991a). Accelerated cholesteryl ester transfer in plasma of patients with insulin dependent diabetes mellitus. *Eur J Clin Invest*, 21, 161-167.

Bagdade JD, Helve E & Taskinen MR. (1991b). Effects of continuous insulin infusion therapy on lipoprotein surface and core lipid composition in insulin-dependent diabetes mellitus. *Metabolism*; 40: 445-9.

Bagdade JD, Dunn FL, Eckel RH & Ritter MC. (1994). Intraperitoneal insulin therapy corrects abnormalities in cholesteryl ester transfer and lipoprotein lipase activities in insulin-dependent diabetes mellitus. *Arterioscler Thromb*; 14: 1933-9.

Bagdade JD & Dunn FL. (1996). Improved lipoprotein surface and core lipid composition following intraperitoneal insulin delivery in insulin-dependent diabetes mellitus. *Diabetes Metab*; 22: 420-6.

Bagdade JD, Ritter MC, Kitabchi AE, Huss E, Thistlethwaite R, Gabfr O et al. (1996). Differing effects of pancreas-kidney transplantation with systemic versus portal venous drainage on cholesteryl ester transfer in IDDM subjects. *Diabetes Care*; 19:1108-12.

Boemi M, Leviev I, Sirolla C, Pieri C, Marra M & James RW. (2001). Serum paraoxonase is reduced in type 1 diabetic patients compared to non-diabetic, first degree relatives; influence on the ability of HDL to protect LDL from oxidation. *Atherosclerosis*; 155: 229-35.

Brunzell JD, Schwartz RS, Eckel RH & Goldberg AP. (1981). Insulin and adipose tissue lipoprotein lipase activity in humans. *Int J Obes*; 5: 685-94.

Caixàs A, Ordóñez-Llanos J, de Leiva A, Payés A, Homs R & Pérez A. (1997). Optimization of glycemic control by insulin therapy decreases the proportion of small dense LDL particles in diabetic patients. *Diabetes*; 46: 1207-13.

Chait A, Bierman EL & Albers JJ. (1979). Low-density lipoprotein receptor activity in cultured human skin fibroblasts. Mechanism of insulin-induced stimulation. *J Clin Invest*; 64:1309-19.

Chang CK, Tso TK, Snook JT, Huang YS, Lozano RA & Zipf WB. (2001). Cholesteryl ester transfer and cholesterol esterification in type 1 diabetes: relationships with plasma glucose. *Acta Diabetol*, 38: 37-42.

Chapman MJ, Guerin M & Bruckert E. (1998). Atherogenic, dense low-density lipoproteins. Pathophysiology and new therapeutic approaches. *Eur Heart J*; 19 (Suppl A): A24-30.

Colhoun HM, Scheek LM, Rubens MB, Van Gent T, Underwood SR, Fuller JH et al. (2001). Lipid transfer protein activities in type 1 diabetic patients without renal failure and nondiabetic control subjects and their association with coronary artery calcification. *Diabetes*; 50: 652-9.

Dashti N, Wolfbauer G. (1987). Secretion of lipids, apolipoproteins, and lipoproteins by human hepatoma cell line, HepG2: effects of oleic acid and insulin. *J Lipid Res*; 28: 423-36.

de Castro SH, Castro-Faria-Neto HC & Gomes MB. (2005). Association of postprandial hyperglycemia with in vitro LDL oxidation in non-smoking patients with type 1 diabetes--a cross-sectional study. *Rev Diabet Stud*; 2: 157-64.

Dullaart RP, Dikkeschei LD & Doorenbos H. (1989a). Alterations in serum lipids and apolipoproteins in male type 1 (insulin-dependent) diabetic patients with microalbuminuria. *Diabetologia;* 32: 685-9.

Dullaart RP, Groener JE, Dikkeschei LD, Erkelens DW & Doorenbos H. (1989b). Increased cholesteryl ester transfer activity in complicated type 1 (insulin-dependent) diabetes mellitus--its relationship with serum lipids. *Diabetologia;* 32:14-9.

Dullaart RP, Groener JE, Dikkeschei BD, Erkelens DW & Doorenbos H. (1991). Elevated cholesteryl ester transfer protein activity in IDDM men who smoke. Possible factor for unfavorable lipoprotein profile. *Diabetes Care;* 14: 338-41.

Dullaart RP. (1995). Plasma lipoprotein abnormalities in type 1 (insulin-dependent) diabetes mellitus. *Neth J Med;* 46: 44-54.

Dunn FL. (1992). Plasma lipid and lipoprotein disorders in IDDM. *Diabetes,* 41 (Suppl 2): 102-6.

Duvillard L, Florentin E, Baillot-Rudoni S, Lalanne-Mistrich ML, Brun-Pacaud A, Petit JM, Brun JM, Gambert P & Vergès B (2005). Comparison of apolipoprotein B100 metabolism between continuous subcutaneous and intraperitoneal insulin therapy in type 1 diabetes. *J Clin Endocrinol Metab;* 90: 5761-4.

Duvillard L, Florentin E, Baillot-Rudoni S, Lalanne-Mistrich ML, Brun-Pacaud A, Petit JM, Brun JM, Gambert P & Vergès B. (2007). No change in apolipoprotein AI metabolism when subcutaneous insulin infusion is replaced by intraperitoneal insulin infusion in type 1 diabetic patients. *Atherosclerosis;* 194: 342-7.

Eckel RH, Albers JJ, Cheung MC, Wahl PW, Lindgren FT & Bierman EL. (1981). High density lipoprotein composition in insulin-dependent diabetes mellitus. *Diabetes;* 30: 132-8.

Edge JA, James T & Shine B. (2008). Longitudinal screening of serum lipids in children and adolescents with Type 1 diabetes in a UK clinic population. *Diabet Med.;* 25: 942-8.

Ferretti G, Bacchetti T, Busni D, Rabini RA & Curatola G. (2004). Protective effect of paraoxonase activity in high-density lipoproteins against erythrocyte membranes peroxidation: a comparison between healthy subjects and type 1 diabetic patients. *J Clin Endocrinol Metab;* 89: 2957-62.

Fievet C, Theret N, Shojaee N, Duchateau P, Castro G, Ailhaud G et al. (1992). Apolipoprotein A-I-containing particles and reverse cholesterol transport in IDDM. *Diabetes;* 41 (Suppl 2): 81-5.

Fried SK, Russell CD, Grauso NL & Brolin RE. (1993). Lipoprotein lipase regulation by insulin and glucocorticoid in subcutaneous and omental adipose tissues of obese women and men. *J Clin Invest;* 92: 2191-8.

Grauslund J, Jørgensen TM, Nybo M, Green A, Rasmussen LM & Sjølie AK. (2010). Risk factors for mortality and ischemic heart disease in patients with long-term type 1 diabetes. *J Diabetes Complications;* 24: 223-8.

Guy J, Ogden L, Wadwa RP, Hamman RF, Mayer-Davis EJ, Liese AD et al. (2009). Lipid and lipoprotein profiles in youth with and without type 1 diabetes: the SEARCH for Diabetes in Youth case-control study. *Diabetes Care;* 32: 416-20.

Hoeldtke RD, Bryner KD, Corum LL, Hobbs GR & Van Dyke K. (2009). Lipid peroxidation in early type 1 diabetes mellitus is unassociated with oxidative damage to DNA. *Metabolism*; 58: 731-4.

James RW & Pometta D. (1990). Differences in lipoprotein subfraction composition and distribution between type I diabetic men and control subjects. Diabetes; 39: 1158-64.

Jay RH, Jones SL, Hill CE, Richmond W, Viberti GC, Rampling MW et al. (1991). Blood rheology and cardiovascular risk factors in type 1 diabetes: relationship with microalbuminuria. *Diabet Med*; 8: 662-7.

Jensen T, Borch-Johnsen K, Kofoed-Enevoldsen A & Deckert T. (1987). Coronary heart disease in young type 1 (insulin-dependent) diabetic patients with and without diabetic nephropathy: incidence and risk factors. *Diabetologia*; 30:144-8.

Jian B, de la Llera-Moya M, Ji Y, Wang N, Phillips MC, Swaney JB et al. (1998). Scavenger receptor class B type I as a mediator of cellular cholesterol efflux to lipoproteins and phospholipid acceptors. *J Biol Chem*; 273:5599-606.

Jones SL, Close CF, Mattock MB, Jarrett RJ, Keen H & Viberti GC. (1989). Plasma lipid and coagulation factor concentrations in insulin dependent diabetics with microalbuminuria. *BMJ*; 298: 487-90.

Kahri J, Groop PH, Viberti G, Elliott T & Taskinen MR. (1993). Regulation of apolipoprotein A-I-containing lipoproteins in IDDM. *Diabetes*; 42:1281-8.

Klein RL, Lyons TJ & Lopes-Virella MF. (1989). Interaction of very-low-density lipoprotein isolated from type I (insulin-dependent) diabetic subjects with human monocyte-derived macrophages. *Metabolism*; 38:1108-14.

Kuksis A, Myher JJ, Geher K, Jones GJ, Breckenridge WC, Feather T et al. (1982). Decreased plasma phosphatidylcholine/free cholesterol ratio as an indicator of risk for ischemic vascular disease. *Arteriosclerosis*; 2: 296-302.

Lagrost L, Desrumaux C, Masson D, Deckert V & Gambert P. (1998). Structure and function of the plasma phospholipid transfer protein. *Curr Opin Lipidol*; 9: 203-9.

Lagrost L. (1994). Regulation of cholesteryl ester transfer protein (CETP) activity: review of in vitro and in vivo studies. *Biochim Biophys Acta*; 1215: 209-36.

Lahdenperä S, Groop PH, Tilly-Kiesi M, Kuusi T, Elliott TG, Viberti GC et al. (1994). LDL subclasses in IDDM patients: relation to diabetic nephropathy. *Diabetologia*; 37: 681-8.

Lewis GF, Uffelman KD, Szeto LW, Weller B & Steiner G. (1993). Effects of acute hyperinsulinemia on VLDL triglyceride and VLDL apo B production in normal weight and obese individuals. *Diabetes*; 42: 833-42.

Libby P, Nathan DM, Abraham K, Brunzell JD, Fradkin JE, Haffner SM, Hsueh W, Rewers M, Roberts BT, Savage PJ, Skarlatos S, Wassef M, Rabadan-Diehl C & National Heart, Lung, and Blood Institute; National Institute of Diabetes and Digestive and Kidney Diseases Working Group on Cardiovascular Complications of Type 1 Diabetes Mellitus. (2005). Report of the National Heart, Lung, and Blood Institute-National Institute of Diabetes and Digestive and Kidney Diseases Working Group on Cardiovascular Complications of Type 1 Diabetes Mellitus. *Circulation*; 111: 3489-93.

Link JJ, Rohatgi &, de Lemos JA. (2007). HDL cholesterol: physiology, pathophysiology, and management. *Curr Probl Cardiol*; 32: 268-314.

Lopes-Virella MF, Hunt KJ, Baker NL, Lachin J, Nathan DM, Virella G & Diabetes Control and Complications Trial/Epidemiology of Diabetes Interventions and Complications Research Group. (2011). Levels of oxidized LDL and advanced glycation end products-modified LDL in circulating immune complexes are strongly associated with increased levels of carotid intima-media thickness and its progression in type 1 diabetes. *Diabetes*; 60: 582-9

Maahs DM, Ogden LG, Dabelea D, Snell-Bergeon JK, Daniels SR, Hamman RF & Rewers M. (2010). Association of glycaemia with lipids in adults with type 1 diabetes: modification by dyslipidaemia medication. *Diabetologia*; 53: 2518-25.

Maahs DM, Nadeau K, Snell-Bergeon JK, Schauer I, Bergman B, West NA, Rewers M, Daniels SR, Ogden LG, Hamman RF & Dabelea D. (2011). Association of insulin sensitivity to lipids across the lifespan in people with Type 1 diabetes. *Diabet Med.*; 28:148-55.

Malmström R, Packard CJ, Caslake M, Bedford D, Stewart P, Yki-Jarvinen H et al. (1998). Effects of insulin and acipimox on VLDL1 and VLDL2 apolipoprotein B production in normal subjects. *Diabetes*; 47: 779-87.

Marcovecchio ML, Dalton RN, Prevost AT, Acerini CL, Barrett TG, Cooper JD et al. (2009). Prevalence of Abnormal Lipid Profiles and the Relationship with the Development of Microalbuminuria in Adolescents with Type 1 Diabetes. *Diabetes Care*; 32: 658-663.

Mattock MB, Cronin N, Cavallo-Perin P, Idzior-Walus B, Penno G, Bandinelli S et al. (2001). EURODIAB IDDM Complications Study. Plasma lipids and urinary albumin excretion rate in Type 1 diabetes mellitus: the EURODIAB IDDM Complications Study. *Diabet Med*; 18: 59-67.

Mazzone T, Foster D & Chait A. (1984). In vivo stimulation of low-density lipoprotein degradation by insulin. *Diabetes*; 33: 333-8.

Nikkilä EA & Kekki M. (1973). Plasma triglyceride transport kinetics in diabetes mellitus. Metabolism; 22:1-22.

Nikkilä EA, Huttunen JK & Ehnholm C. (1977). Postheparin plasma lipoprotein lipase and hepatic lipase in diabetes mellitus. Relationship to plasma triglyceride metabolism. *Diabetes*; 26:11-21.

Olofsson SO, Stillemark-Billton P & Asp L. (2000). Intracellular assembly of VLDL: two major steps in separate cell compartments. *Trends Cardiovasc Med*; 10: 338-45.

Oram JF & Lawn RM. ABCA1. (2001). The gatekeeper for eliminating excess tissue cholesterol. *J Lipid Res*; 42:1173-9.

Perségol L, Foissac M, Lagrost L, Athias A, Gambert P, Vergès B & Duvillard L. (2007). HDL particles from type 1 diabetic patients are unable to reverse the inhibitory effect of oxidised LDL on endothelium-dependent vasorelaxation. *Diabetologia*; 50: 2384-7.

Pruneta V, Pulcini T, Lalanne F, Marçais C, Berthezène F, Ponsin G et al. (1999). VLDL-bound lipoprotein lipase facilitates the cholesteryl ester transfer protein-mediated transfer of cholesteryl esters from HDL to VLDL. *J Lipid Res*; 40:2333-9.

Purnell JQ, Dev RK, Steffes MW, Cleary PA, Palmer JP, Hirsch IB, Hokanson JE & Brunzell JD. (2003). Relationship of family history of type 2 diabetes, hypoglycemia, and autoantibodies to weight gain and lipids with intensive and conventional therapy in the Diabetes Control and Complications Trial. *Diabetes*; 52: 2623-9.

Ritter MC & Bagdade JD. (1994). Contribution of glycaemic control, endogenous lipoproteins and cholesteryl ester transfer protein to accelerated cholesteryl ester transfer in IDDM. *Eur J Clin Invest*; 24: 607-14.

Rivellese A, Riccardi G, Romano G, Giacco R, Patti L, Marotta G et al. (1988). Presence of very low density lipoprotein compositional abnormalities in type 1 (insulin-dependent) diabetic patients; effects of blood glucose optimisation. *Diabetologia*; 31: 884-8.

Ruotolo G, Parlavecchia M, Taskinen MR, Galimberti G, Zoppo A, Le NA et al. (1994). Normalization of lipoprotein composition by intraperitoneal insulin in IDDM. Role of increased hepatic lipase activity. *Diabetes Care*; 17: 6-12.

Sammett D & Tall AR. (1985). Mechanisms of enhancement of cholesteryl ester transfer protein activity by lipolysis. *J Biol Chem*; 260: 6687-97.

Schwab KO, Doerfer J, Naeke A, Rohrer T, Wiemann D, Marg W, Hofer SE, Holl RW & German/Austrian Pediatric DPV Initiative. (2009). Influence of food intake, age, gender, HbA1c, and BMI levels on plasma cholesterol in 29,979 children and adolescents with type 1 diabetes--reference data from the German diabetes documentation and quality management system (DPV). *Pediatr Diabetes.*; 10: 184-92.

Selam JL, Kashyap M, Alberti KG, Lozano J, Hanna M, Turner D et al. (1989). Comparison of intraperitoneal and subcutaneous insulin administration on lipids, apolipoproteins, fuel metabolites, and hormones in type I diabetes mellitus. *Metabolism*; 38: 908-12.

Skyrme-Jones RA, O'Brien RC, Luo M & Meredith IT. (2000). Endothelial vasodilator function is related to low-density lipoprotein particle size and low-density lipoprotein vitamin E content in type 1 diabetes. *J Am Coll Cardiol*; 35: 292-9.

Soedamah-Muthu SS, Chaturvedi N, Toeller M, Ferriss B, Reboldi P, Michel G, Manes C, Fuller JH & EURODIAB Prospective Complications Study Group. (2004). Risk factors for coronary heart disease in type 1 diabetic patients in Europe: the EURODIAB Prospective Complications Study. *Diabetes Care*; 27: 530-7.

Steinbrecher UP & Witztum JL. (1984). Glucosylation of low-density lipoproteins to an extent comparable to that seen in diabetes slows their catabolism. Diabetes; 33:130-4.

Taskinen MR. (1987). Lipoprotein lipase in diabetes. *Diabetes Metab Rev*; 3:551-70.

Taskinen MR. (1992). Quantitative and qualitative lipoprotein abnormalities in diabetes mellitus. *Diabetes*; 41 (Suppl 2):12-7.

The DCCT Research Group. (1992). Lipid and lipoprotein levels in patients with IDDM diabetes control and complication. Trial experience. *Diabetes Care*; 15: 886-94.

Thomas MC, Rosengård-Bärlund M, Mills V, Rönnback M, Thomas S, Forsblom C et al. (2006). Serum lipids and the progression of nephropathy in type 1 diabetes. *Diabetes Care*; 29: 317-22.

Tribble DL, Holl LG, Wood PD & Krauss RM. (1992). Variations in oxidative susceptibility among six low density lipoprotein subfractions of differing density and particle size. *Atherosclerosis*; 93: 189-99.

Vakkilainen J, Makimattila S, Seppala-Lindroos A, Vehkavaara S, Lahdenpera S, Groop PH et al. (2000). Endothelial dysfunction in men with small LDL particles. *Circulation*; 102: 716-21.

Vergès B. (2001). Insulin sensitiviy and lipids. *Diabetes Metab*; 27: 223-7.

Weidman SW, Ragland JB, Fisher JN Jr, Kitabchi AE & Sabesin SM.J. (1982). Effects of insulin on plasma lipoproteins in diabetic ketoacidosis: evidence for a change in high density lipoprotein composition during treatment. *J Lipid Res*; 23: 171-82.

Winocour PH, Durrington PN, Ishola M & Anderson DC. (1986). Lipoprotein abnormalities in insulin-dependent diabetes mellitus. *Lancet*; 1: 1176-8.

Witztum JL, Mahoney EM, Branks MJ, Fisher M, Elam R & Steinberg D. (1982). Nonenzymatic glucosylation of low-density lipoprotein alters its biologic activity. *Diabetes*; 31: 283-91.

4

Prevalence of Type 1 Diabetes Correlates with Daily Insulin Dose, Adverse Outcomes and with Autoimmune Process Against Glutamic Acid Decarboxylase in Adults

Mykola Khalangot[1], Vitaliy Gurianov[2], Volodymir Kovtun[1], Nadia Okhrimenko[1], Viktor Kravchenko[1] and Mykola Tronko[1]

[1]Komisarenko Institute of Endocrinology and Metabolism Academy of Medical Sciences, Kiev

[2]National Medical University, Donetsk, Ukraine

1. Introduction

The territorial differences in the prevalence of type 1 diabetes mellitus (T1D) around the world were previously reported (Amos et al., 1997; Green & Patterson, 2001; Lévy-Marchal, 2001), but the data were based on the study of juvenile T1D epidemiology, i.e., in patients diagnosed with T1D before the age of 15 years. These data became the basis for the epidemiological evaluation of the whole T1D patient population. With the relatively limited number of children with T1D within the current territory, less effort is required for data gathering. Besides, as the age increases, it becomes more difficult to relate a diabetic condition to a certain diabetes type (Keen, 1998), thus, making it impossible to directly use the diabetes-type data obtained from Primary Care. In modern epidemiological studies, the key data concern the age at the time of the diagnosis—patients who were diagnosed before the age of 30 years and are insulin-treated, are considered to suffer from T1D.

1.1 T1D epidemiology in adults

European researchers have proved that the epidemiological characteristics of T1D in children significantly differ from that in young adults (Kyvik et al., 2004). Therefore, studying the peculiarities of T1D in adults is a major concern. Furthermore, data on the number of diabetic patients usually found in the reports of the healthcare system are unstructured according to the history of the disease, and cannot be a source of epidemiological information on patients suffering from T1D. Owing to the development of the Diabetes Register in Ukraine, it has become possible to conduct analytical comparisons and further studies on almost all the T1D adult populations.

1.2 Diabetes Register

The Diabetes Register contains individual, structured information on the disease history, and has already been used in some epidemiological studies (Khalangot et al., 2009[a];

Khalangot et al., 2009[b]; Vaiserman et al., 2009; Khalangot et al., 2009[d]; Vaiserman & Khalangot, 2008). Until recently there was no evidence on age and gender structure of patients diagnosed with diabetes mellitus in Ukraine. Neither is there any information on risk factors that may influence main aetiological diabetes mellitus type's incidence, as well as development of diabetic complications in Ukraine. Diabetes register is recognized as an important tool of diabetes research: it is a fully functioning diabetes register created in Ukraine. It includes over 620 000 diabetes patients (2010) and gives a unique possibility to analyze the structure of aetiological types, gender and age features, prevalence, trends of incidence, risk factors of non-fatal events and mortality among Ukrainian diabetes patients. Observational cross-sectional (distribution of diabetes types and treatment, trends of life span) and cohort (assessment of mortality risks) epidemiological studies using national patient register based on data provided by primary care doctors became possible. The register included most of Ukraine's insulin treated patients, as well as significant part of patients receiving oral glucose lowering drugs (OGLD). The insulin-treated patient data covers 24 out of 25 Ukrainian regions, meaning that at least nearly all of Ukraine's T1D population is included in the register. According to the Health Ministry data, the total amount of patients with known diabetes is 1 048375 (2006), which means that nearly half of type 2 diabetes (T2D) patients have yet to be included in the register, which consists of 509 933 patients, including 37 406 death cases.

1.3 Register-based diabetes epidemiology studies

Systematic epidemiological study of main diabetes mellitus (DM) types through analysis of electronic population registers has been lasting for over 10 years. Usage of DM population registers has become quite advanced in the UK, in particular in Scotland, where by the end of 2004, 161 946 diabetics have been included into local diabetic registers which is equal to 3.2% of the general population. In Scotland, 14 out of 15 healthcare institutions are involved in controlling treatment of DM patients. An important aspect is that Scottish DM registers include all DM patients, unlike others, that only include patients receiving certain kind of treatment. It seems that at the moment, the most advanced and successful Scottish local register is Tayside (Boyle et al., 2001; Leese et al., 2006; Morris et al., 1997). It should be noted that this relatively small, but constantly functioning register became a source of not just "traditional" epidemiologic information concerning prevalence and annual incidence of T1D and T2D, dynamics of DM complications frequency, and quality of treatment, which is a generalization of routine data from active GPs working in the region, and can be accessed through the register's website (http://www.diabetes-healthnet.ac.uk/), but also of purely scientific fundamental data (Doney et al., 2003, 2005; Evans et al., 2005, 2006; Schofield et al., 2006). A few of these papers have entirely clinically-epidemiological nature, comparing mortality among patients with limb amputations depending on presence of DM (Schofield et al., 2006), or mortality risks depending on certain type of treatment (Evans et al., 2005, 2006), while others use the register to study genetic characteristics among different categories of DM patients (Doney et al., 2003, 2005). One of the researchers of Belgian Diabetic Register (BDR) Prof. Frans K. Gorus (Diabetes Research Center, Vrije Universiteit Brussel) indicated the possibility of such scientific use of diabetic registers (Gorus, 1996). Important epidemiologic, immunologic, and genetic studies of T1D in children and adolescents were carried out using BDR (Gorus, 1996; Vandewalle et al., 1997; Weets et al., 2001, 2002).

1.3.1 Register-based T2D epidemiology studies

Some results obtanied by means of studying electronic registers may at first seem unusual or paradoxic. In particular our studies of T2D patients (Khalangot et al., 2009[b]) indicate that Hazard Ratios (HRs) of cardiovascular disease (CVD) mortality among extremely obese patients [body mass index (BMI) ≥ 35 kg/m^2] adjusted for age, smoking and alcohol consumption were higher than for overweight patients [BMI 25-29 kg/m^2]: HR=1.54 (95% CI 1.16-2.05) and 1.35 (95% CI 1.15-1.59) among men an women respectively, $p<0.01$. Furthermore, the graph that shows risks of general and CVD mortality for T2D patients depending on BMI has the shape of an asymmetric parabola: HRs associated with low and normal BMI were significantly higher comparing to those, related to overweight or moderate obesity. The above phenomenon partially corresponds to "obesity paradox" that has been recently discovered among patients suffering from CVD (Gruberg et al., 2002; Curtis et al., 2005) , however in our study this effect concerns T2D patients. An observational study that included 25 361 T2D patients showed that glibenclamide treatment is associated with much higher risk of general and CVD mortality, comparing to treatment with another derivative of sulfonylurea - gliclazide. HRs for total and CVD mortality within the glibenclamide patient cohort were 2.57 (95% CI 1.73–3.82) and 2,93 (95%CI 1.83–4.71) respectively; ($p < 0,001$). These data correspond to changes of OGLD distribution and trends of life duration among DM patients that we have revealed as well (Khalangot et al., 2009 [e]). Previously, there had been only one study where similar results concerning total mortality associated with the use of glibenclamide or gliclazide in a cohort of 568 T2D patients were obtained (Monami et al., 2007). Our study broadens this tendency onto CVD mortality.

1.3.2 Register-based T1D epidemiology studies

T1D incidence among Ukrainian adults from 1994 till 2004, that we have evaluated retrospectively according to the register data, had a decreasing tendency (Khalangot, 2009). Our assessment of T1D incidence dynamics among adults does not confirm the information about steady increase of global T1D incidence (Green et al., 2001; Gale, 2002), however these studies only concerned child incidence. As Ukraine is also experiencing a rise of DM incidence among children, our data can be easily explained by earlier DM manifestation among people, who carry the genotype predisposing to T1D. Researchers of Danish DM register have recently reported a decrease of DM incidence among young adults. National diabetic register of Denmark has collected data on 359 000 DM cases between 1995 and 2006, and it includes the total population, diagnosed with DM. This register has recorded a clear tendency towards reduction of mortality among DM patients, which has been observed since 2003 (Carstensen et al., 2008). We have recently conducted a series of studies as well that focused on factors influencing mortality and territorial heterogeneity of T1D in Ukraine (Khalangot, 2008; Khalangot et al., 2009 [c]; 2010). The purpose of these studies (Khalangot et al., 2009 [d]) was also to determine whether the insulin requirement can change systematically in T1D patients, and whether this requirement depends on the same factors that determine its prevalence. This chapter is mainly a review of these studies.

2. Methods

A database with 282,988 records of diabetic patients was developed on the basis of epidemiological analysis conducted during the 2005-2006 register verification (01.12.2006). To evaluate the completeness of the register data, we compared it to the official 2005

Ministry of Health statistical data (Anonymous, 2006). The integrity of the register, i.e., the data on the number of patients who have received insulin, was assessed based on the information provided by the primary care doctors (district endocrinologists) to the regional diabetic registers. Consequently, the regional endocrinologists were responsible for updating the data and endorsing it to the central level. Accordingly, by assuming that the data were encoded into the regional registers with various degrees of completeness, significant limitations were noted in the assessment of the prevalence of insulin-dependent diabetes as well as in further epidemiological evaluations. Considering the fact that Ukraine has a national, free-of-charge insulin supply to the patients who require it, the Ministry of Health data reflect the number of these patients to the fullest extent. However, the Ukrainian Ministry of Health receives only non-personalized data that are difficult to verify. A comparison of the data from the 2006 Diabetes Register with the 2005 data on the insulin-treated patients from the Ministry of Health (considered 100%) revealed certain similarities: the fraction of the patients included in the register was 91.1%, based on the number of the patients according to the Ministry of Health data. However, in the Kharkiv region, only 58.6% of the Ministry of Health patients were in the register. It was assumed that the Kharkiv region data in the register could be incomplete, and hence, was not used in the analysis of T1D prevalence among adults.

2.1 T1D cases selection

Therefore, the analysis was carried out using the T1D criteria used by the epidemiologists–researchers for the European diabetes population databases (Kyvik et al., 2004; Soedamah-Muthu, 2006). The patients were selected based on the following conditions: T1D primary care diagnosis; age at the time of being included in the register ≥15 years; place of residence and gender; and data on diagnoses before the age of 30 years.

2.2 T1D prevalence assessment

The prevalence of T1D in the Ukrainian regions was determined as of the end of 2004. The T1D prevalence was calculated using the official data on the adult population of the corresponding regions (Anonymous, 2006), and 95% confidence interval (CI) was determined using arcsine transformation (Altman et al., ed-s., 2003). Multiple comparisons of T1D regional prevalence were subsequently carried out using the modified (Liakh & Gurianov, 2004) L. Marascuilo mathematical procedure (Marascuilo, 1966). The MedStat statistical package was used for the calculations (Liakh & Gurianov, 2004). Logistic regression analysis was used to determine the influence of the explanatory variables on the resulting variable (Bland, 2000). For each input variable, we evaluated the estimated logistic regression coefficient with the standard error, estimated as the odds ratio (OR) with a CI for its actual value and associated p value, and performed a Wald test (testing the null hypothesis on the congruency of the OR of the "disease" associated with the increase of this variable by 1). We used this information to determine whether each variable was related to the outcome of interest, and to quantify the extent of such a relationship (Bland, 2000). The Statistica 5.5 (StatSoft Inc., 1999) package was used in this set of calculations.

2.3 T1D outcomes assessment

We have evaluated the prevalence of proliferative retinopathy (PR), arterial hypertension (AH), and mortality risks in the retrospective cohort of T1D (27,896 patients); these data was published elsewhere (Khalangot et al., 2009[c] ; 2010). In brief, mortality was assessed using the Cox regression model, determining hazard ratios (HRs) and corresponding 95% confidence intervals (95% CI). We calculated odds ratios (ORs), and used a logistic regression to compare PR and AH.

2.4 Diabetes-associated antibodies and c-peptide measurements

A total of 86 T1D patients (42 males and 44 females), with a mean age of 27.5 years (0.86) and mean diabetes duration of 10.3 (0.72) years (SE), were randomly selected from four regional diabetes-mellitus registers: Chernihivska, Zaporizka; Ivano-Frankivska, and Chernivetska. The glutamic acid decarboxylase 65 antibody (GADA), insulin antibody (IA), and plasma c-peptide levels were determined using radioimmunoassay (RIA) kits (IMMUNOTECH™) after obtaining the patients' informed consent. The model of the logistic regression was used for the multifactor data analysis of GADA, IA, c-peptide persistence, OR, and the 95% CI that were determined. The plasma was considered GADA- or IA-positive, if GADA >1 U/ml or IA >0.4 U/ml, and low c-peptide, if its level was <32.6 pmol/l.

3. Register analysis results and discussion

The analysis of the register of diabetic patients has allowed for the first time to assess the adult prevalence of T1D in Ukraine in comparison with important clinical (daily insulin dose, mortality, and complications) and some paraclinical (GADA) characteristics of the disease (Khalangot et al., 2009 [c]; Khalangot et al., 2009 [d]; 2010).

3.1 T1D territorial dissimilarity and clusterization

The data on adult T1D prevalence in 24 Ukrainian regions (Table 1) indicated territorial dissimilarity: chi-square = 648.30, degree of freedom, k =23 (p< 0.001).

Further multiple comparisons using the modified Marascuilo procedure (Marascuilo, 1966) allowed conducting a pairwise assessment of each region. This assessment enabled clustering of the regions according to T1D prevalence. The flagged regions that did not statistically differ from the minimal level according to prevalence were considered as a cluster. This procedure was repeated for the remaining regions as well. The following regional clusters were distinguished according to the T1D prevalence:

Minimal prevalence cluster = AR Crimea, Ivano-Frankivska, Mykolaivska, Odeska, Chernivetska, and Luganska regions.

Intermediate prevalence cluster = Vinnitska, Volynska, Dnipropetrovska, Donetska, Zhytomyrska, Zakarpatska, Kirovogradska, Lvivska, Rivnenska, Kievska, Sumska, Ternopilska, Poltavska, Khersonska, and Cherkaska regions.

Maximal prevalence cluster = Zaporizka, Khmelnytska, and Chernigivska regions.

Cases of T1D in each regional cluster were unified and the prevalence was calculated for the actual clusters. The T1D prevalence was found to be 6 (5–6), −7 (6–7), and −9 (8–9) per 10,000 adults, for the minimal, intermediate, and maximal prevalence clusters respectively. A comparison of the differences between these groups indicated a high level of confidence (χ^2 = 214.4; p< 0.001), as shown in figure 1.

Region (oblast′)	Gender		Number of type1 adult diabetic patients		Total adult population
	males	females	total, n	per 10 000 adults (95 % CI)	
AR Crimea	564	513	1077	5 (5-6)	2 032 600
Vinnitska	600	464	1064	7 (7-8)	1 440 600
Volynska	354	271	625	7 (7-8)	844 300
Dnipropetrovska	1107	1017	2124	7(6-7)	2 992 000
Donetska	1477	1282	2759	7 (6-7)	4 071 100
Zhytomyrska	387	339	726	6 (6-7)	1 122 300
Zakarpatska	354	264	618	6(6-7)	1 000 700
Zaporizka	732	712	1444	9 (8-9)	1 619 200
Ivano-Frankivska	351	274	625	5 (5-6)	1 137 500
Kievska	1476	1514	2990	8 (7-8)	3 804 900
Kirovogradska	334	327	661	7 (7-8)	913 500
Luganska	604	623	1227	6 (5-6)	2 127 900
Lvivska	802	700	1502	7 (6-7)	2 136 000
Mykolaivska	292	279	571	5 (5-6)	1 041 600
Odeska	470	438	908	4 (4-5)	2 037 900
Poltavska	552	464	1016	7 (7-8)	1 345 600
Rivnenska	355	316	671	7 (7-8)	930 000
Sumska	408	321	729	7 (6-7)	1 071 700
Ternopilska	411	297	708	8 (7-8)	925 000
Kharkivska	*597*	*493*	*1090*		*2 479 700*
Khersonska	303	286	589	6 (6-7)	957 000
Khmelnitska	510	468	978	8 (8-9)	1 163 000
Cherkaska	408	366	774	7 (6-7)	1 154 600
Chernivetska	267	177	444	6 (5-6)	746 000
Chernigyvska	473	403	876	9 (8-9)	1 020 300
Total	14188	12608	26796		40 115 000

Table 1. Prevalence of Type 1 Diabetes Mellitus in Adults Diagnosed Before the Age of 30 in Ukrainian Regions (Khalangot et al., 2009d)

3.2 T1D gender assessment

The fraction of males among the 26,796 adults diagnosed before the age of 30 years corresponded to 52.95%, and varied from 49.2% in Luganska to 60.1% in Chernivetska regions. In the majority (23 out of 25) of the regions, this fraction was >50%. Comparison of the 25 regions with the fraction of T1D males revealed a certain variation according to the territorial attribute (chi-square = 67.70, the degrees of freedom, k =24; p <0.001). However, multiple comparisons failed to reveal any distinctions according to the fraction of T1D males between the specific regions. Furthermore, it must be noted that there was no increase in the female fraction among T1D adults, which is common in the general population.

It is possible that an increase in the male fraction in this population reflects the epidemiological peculiarities of this disease, which have not yet been described by the identified (as well as the unknown) factors that could lead to the increase in the mortality among males.

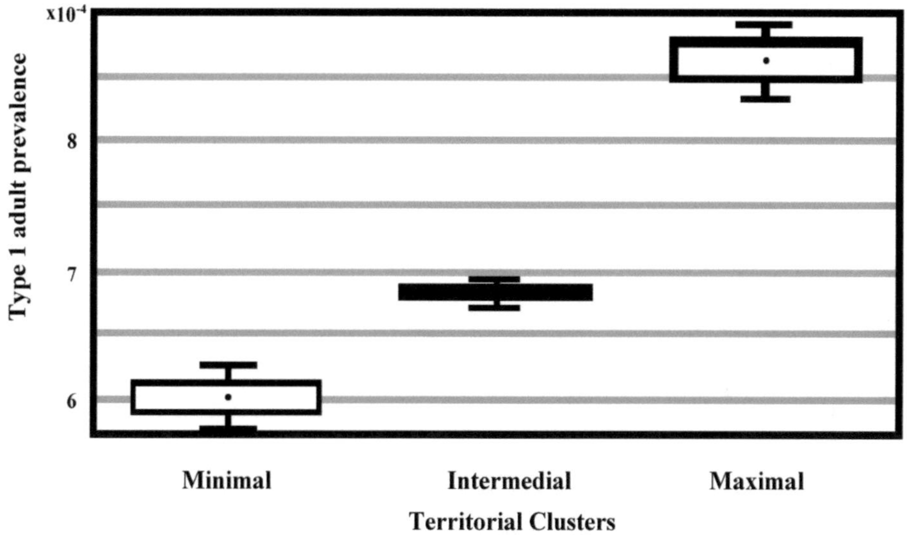

Note: given Means ± SE (the dot within the box and height of boxes respectively), 95% CI (lines that emerge above and below the boxes)

Fig. 1. Prevalence of Type 1 Diabetes Mellitus Diagnosed in Patients Under the Age of 30 in Territorial Clusters of Ukrainian Regions (per 10 000 adults, 95% CI) (Khalangot et al., 2009 [d])

3.3 T1D insulin doses assessment

The data analysis of the 23,633 T1D patients (Table 2) from the register, who were classified according to insulin dose, age, and disease duration, indicated that women have a higher average age and disease duration, but lower daily insulin dose, when compared with men.

Number of T1D patients (n)	Mean age, yrs(SD)	Mean diabetes duration, yrs(SD)	Mean insulin dose, U/day (SD)
Man (12364)	32.48 (11.60)	14.11 (10.47)	52.03 (18.56)
Women (11269)	33.38 (12.43)	15.69 (10.99)	49.50 (17.98)
Total (23633)	32.91 (12,01)	14.86 (10.75)	50.83 (18.33)

Note: P (man/women) < 0.001

Table 2. Average Age, Disease Duration, and Daily Insulin Dose of Type 1 Diabetes Mellitus Patients in Ukraine According to the Diabetes Register data (Khalangot et al., 2009 [d])

3.3.1 T1D insulin doses and diabetes duration

As the average duration of the disease was found to be 14.86 years, the average daily insulin doses were calculated for each year of the duration, from 0 (<1) to 15 years.

The regression analysis (figure 2) indicated that in this range, the insulin dose rises with the increase in the disease duration:

Insulin (units/day) = 0.7326 × duration (years) + 43.74 (coefficient of linear correlation, R = 0.899, $p < 0.001$).

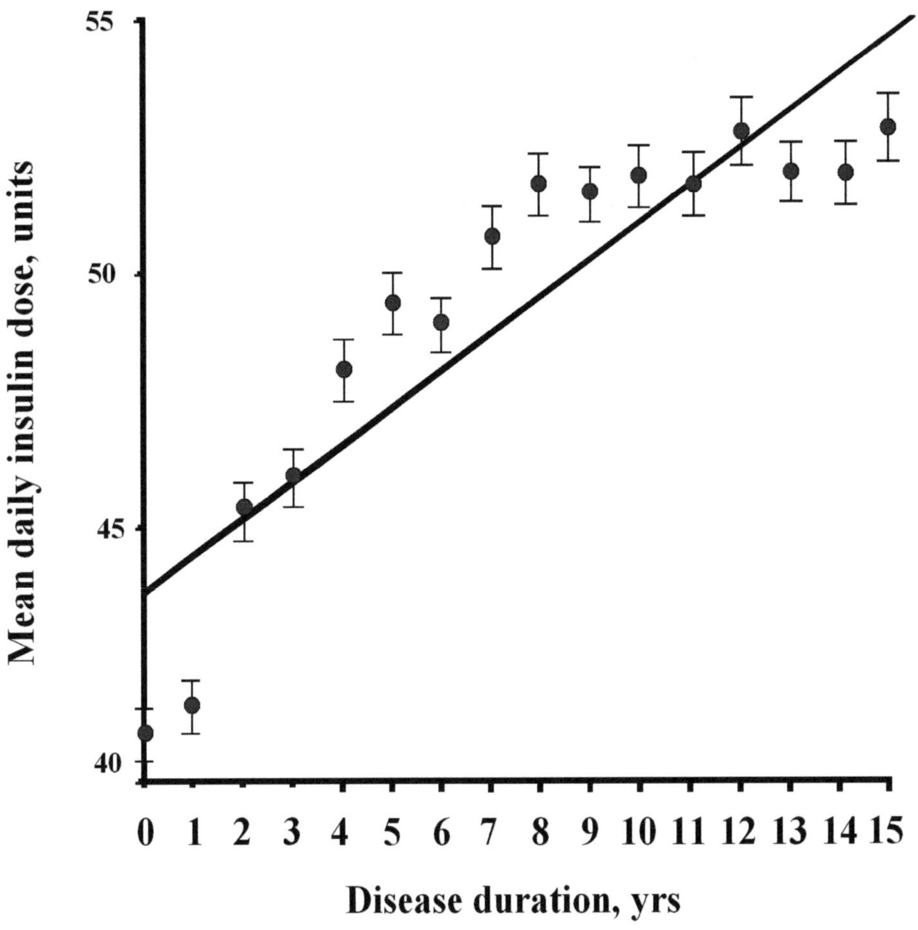

Fig. 2. Average (Mean ± SE) daily insulin doses of type 1 diabetes mellitus patients depending on the disease duration in the range of 0-15 years (Khalangot et al., 2009 [d])

A further increase in the disease duration in the range of 16–31 years was not accompanied by regular changes in the insulin dose. The regular rise of insulin dose, observed with the increase in the duration of T1D in adults diagnosed before the age of 30 years, is still an unknown phenomenon. However, this phenomenon was observed to correspond to the observation that T1D patients have long-standing insulin secretion at times (the study of c-peptide level), which was proven by Bonora (Bonora et al., 1984) and confirmed by the Diabetes Control and Complications Trial (DCCT). These research efforts uncovered the diverse influence of different insulin-therapy patterns on the process described (*The DCCT Research Group,* 1987; 1998). The confirmation of this data with the prospective observation was undertaken in Germany (Linn et al., 2003). Our results could be viewed as an indirect confirmation of the extended continuation of the β-cell secretion, obtained through the cross-sectional treatment data analysis of almost the entire population of T1D patients in Ukraine. The standardization of the daily insulin doses, depending on the disease duration, enables the necessary quantitative comparisons of the treatments for T1D adult patients.

3.3.2 T1D insulin doses in territorial clusters

It would be logical to consider that the rate of decrease in insulin secretion among the T1D patients that differs according to the prevalence of such autoimmune disease, as T1D will also vary. Table 3 presents the comparisons of the daily insulin doses (median) in all the three clusters of the regions selected according to the prevalence of T1D in adults.

Type 1 diabetes prevalence cluster	Insulin doses standardized according to diabetes duration, median, U/day	95%CI	P
1. minimal	45.89	45.28 - 47.19	< 0.01 (1 vs 3)
2. intermediate	52	47.61 - 52.78	< 0.05 (1 vs 2)
3. maximal	56.59	53.33 -57.88	< 0.05 (2 vs 3)

Note: Number of diabetes duration yearly groups (n) in all clusters is 16.

Table 3. Comparison of daily insulin doses standardized for every year of disease duration in the range of 0-15 years in clusters of regions singled out according to prevalence of diabetes mellitus type 1 (Khalangot et al., 2009 [d]).

Insulin doses standardized according to the disease duration within the range of 0–15 years in the minimal prevalence cluster of T1D prevalence were significantly lower, when compared with the intermediate and maximal prevalence clusters. The values in the intermediate prevalence cluster were lower than those in the maximal prevalence cluster (figure 3, table 3).

By evaluating the data presented in table 3, it should be noted that the probability coefficients (*P*), in this case, reflect a relatively small number of the "yearly" groups (n=16) in each cluster. If we were to assess the individual data on the insulin dose in each cluster without yearly grouping, then the number of cases (n) corresponding to the number of patients would greatly increase: 4,658; 14,712 and 2,879 in the minimal, intermediate, and maximal prevalence clusters, respectively. The unstandardized according to the diabetes duration average doses and their standard deviations (SD) in each of the three clusters, were observed to be 46.62 (19.38); 51.54 (17.57); and 55.94 (19.46) units/day, respectively, which was found to increase ($p < 0.0001$) in the clusters with higher T1D prevalence. However, the correlation of the insulin dose and the T1D prevalence found in this current region needs to be explained. One of the explanations for the difference in the daily insulin doses could be that in different Ukrainian regions, the doctors administer different levels of diabetes control: the lower dose is explained not only by the lower requirement of insulin by patients, but rather by the lower quality of treatment. An alternative explanation could be the higher intensity of the autoimmune process in patients residing in a territory with higher T1D prevalence.

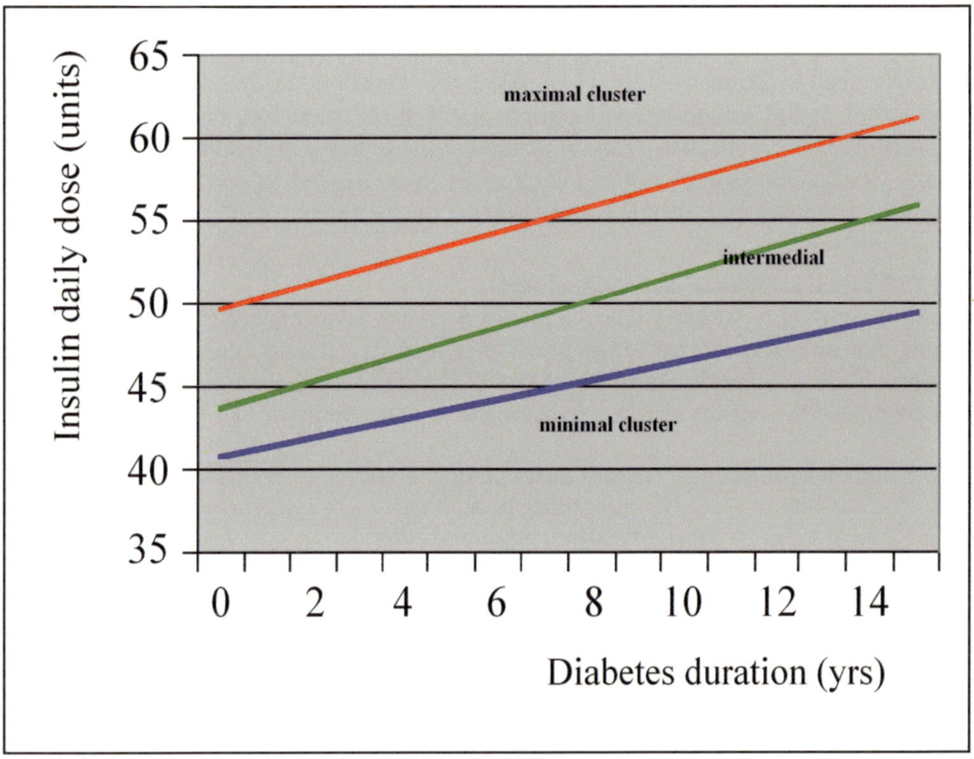

Fig. 3. Average daily insulin doses of diabetes mellitus type 1 patients depending on the disease duration (in the range of 0-15 years) as well as on the territorial cluster, selected according to disease prevalence (Khalangot et al., 2009 d)

3.3.3 Quality of glucose lowering treatment and mean insulin doses in T1D prevalence clusters

Glycated hemoglobin (HbA1c) is considered as the most evident criteria in determining the quality of glucose-lowering treatment. We have analyzed and compared the levels of HbA1c of 1,288 T1D patients, included in the register. Table 4 shows the average HbA1c levels and the daily insulin doses according to the T1D prevalence clusters.

Type1 diabetes prevalence cluster	N	Mean HbA1c level, % (SD)	Mean insulin dose, U/day (SD)
1. Minimal	111	8.57 (3.29)	40.91(16.24)
2. Intermediate	778	8.24 (2,3)	51.5 (14.8)
3. Maximal	240	9.52 (2.24)	54.79 (18.05)
P (1 vs 3)		< 0.01	< 0.001

Table 4. Average levels of HbA1c (%) and insulin doses (units/day) considering territorial clusters with various diabetes type 1 prevalence (Khalangot et al., 2009 d)

The level of HbA1c in the maximal prevalence cluster was significantly greater than that in the minimal prevalence cluster, which does not support the assumption of lower treatment quality in the regions with lower T1D prevalence. Therefore, the alternative explanation using the discovered phenomenon remains rather the most likely one. Its confirmation may include c-peptide determination as well as the determination of antibodies associated with diabetes in patients residing in the Ukrainian territories with different T1D prevalence. However, the reason for the heterogenic prevalence of T1D is still unknown.

3.4 GADA, IA and c-peptide levels in plasma of T1D patients from different prevalence clusters

The GADA and IA levels in children recently diagnosed with T1D are observed to be higher in countries with a greater incidence of this disease, such as Sweden, when compared with those where the T1D incidence is lower, such as Lithuania (Holmberg et al., 2006). In our study, the GADA levels and persistence in patients from the maximal T1D prevalence cluster (n=38), were higher than that in patients from the minimal prevalence cluster (n=48): 14.1±4.6 and 3.2±1.2 U/ml, respectively, mean ± SE = 0.028; OR = 9.66 (3.31–28.17), p< 0.001. Adjusting for age, gender, and duration of diabetes affected the results only slightly: OR = 7.91 (2.44–25.57), p< 0.001. However, the IA and c-peptide levels and their persistence were not observed to be associated with T1D prevalence. It should be noted that persistence of IA is common only for children with T1D (reviewed by Dib & Gomes, 2009), when our study analyzed adults. These data was obtained in 2007 and published earlier elsewhere (Khalangot et al., 2009 [d]). In another series of our studies (unpublished data) conducted in 2010 on T1D patients (11 from Minimal cluster and 18 from Maximal one) selected in the same way, the GADA levels also differed significantly: 0.92 (0.61-3.04) and 24.43 (3.28-61.42) U/l, Me , 95% CI, p = 0.003; adjusted for diabetes duration OR = 8.6 (1.1-65.7), p=0.036.
That is, the chance to have high GADA levels is almost 9 times higher for patients from the Maximal cluster as compared to the Minimal cluster, and this ratio was stable during repeated trials in these populations of T1D. Thus, the phenomenon of stable GADA persistence was discovered among adult T1D patients, residing in Ukraine within the maximal prevalence cluster.

3.5 T1D outcomes assessment in territorial prevalence clusters

The obtained results allow us to assume that there may be differences in the incidence of adverse outcomes of the disease among populations with varying prevalence of T1D. The gathered large cohort (29 708 T1D patients) may be viewed as almost complete data on this category of patients in Ukraine (Khalangot et al., 2009 [c], 2010). It should be noted, that the average duration of T1D is low (17.32 years). According to the data from a cross sectional study of Swedish National Diabetic Register (NDR), in 1997 the duration of T1D was 23.1 years and in 2004 it increased to 26.1 years. The criteria for T1D in the NDR study were treatment by insulin only and diagnosis before the age of 30 (Eeg-Olofsson et al., 2007), which corresponds to criteria used by us. According to the data from one of the regional diabetic registers in the US, the average T1D duration in a cohort of patients who were diagnosed before 19 years of age exceeded 25 years (Nishimura et al., 2001).

3.5.1 Main characteristics of T1D patients from the cohort studied

The number of men in this cohort is greater than the number of women. Men have shorter disease duration (P <0,001) and higher levels of blood pressure (BP) (p <0,001), whereas women have slightly higher levels of fasting glycemia (P <0,05). Blindness, cataracts and proliferative retinopathy more common for women (P <0,001). During 122,656.9 person-years (median observation period 4.7 years) 1958 deaths were recorded. The main cause of death was kidney failure. Cancer was very insignificant among other causes of death (table 5) . Possible reason for this phenomenon may be a short life expectancy of patients with diabetes.

Characteristics	Men	Women	All
Number of patients, n	15738	13970	29 708
Mean age, years (SD)	34.35(12.55)	34.61(13.30)	34.47(12.91)
Body mass index, kg/m² (SD)	23.01(3.84) n=14331	23.34(4.37) n=12729	23.16(4.10)
BP systolic, mm Hg (SD)	126.29(18.75)	125.48(20.81)	125.91(19.75)
BP diastolic, mm Hg. (SD)	78.57(10.53) n=14298	77.66(11.38) n=12654	78.15(10.94)
Fasting blood glucose, mmol/l (SD)	9.23(2.82) n=13747	9.30(2.87) n=12174	9.26(2.85)
HbA1c, % (SD)	8.68(2.53) n=1784	8.83(2.61) n=1789	8.75(2.57)
Smoking, n (%)*	3223 (20.48)	414(2.96)	3637(12.24)
Mean T1D duration, years	16.73	17.98	17.32
Nephropathy treatment, n (%)*	4627(31.42)	4921(37.59)	9548(34.32)
Cataract, n (%) *	1573(10.68)	2041(15.59)	3614(12.99)
Proliferative retinopathy, n (%) *	1187(8.06)	1297(9.91)	2484(8.93)
Blindness, n (%) *	459(3.1)	506(3.9)	965(3.47)
Follow up period, median, years	4.7	4.73	4.71
Total mortality cases, n (%)	1149 (100)	809(100)	1958(100)
CVD mortality, n (%)	266(23.15)	182(22.5)	448(22.88)
Cancer mortality, n (%)	16(1.39)	7(0.87)	23(1.17)
Renal failure, n (%)	295(25.67)	262(32.39)	557(28.45)
DKA and Coma	25(2.18)	36(4.45)	61(3.12)
Other reasons (%)	344(29.94)	174(21.51)	518(26.46)
Unknown	203(17.68)	148(18.29)	351(17.93)

Notes. BP – blood pressure, DKA – diabetic ketoacydosis;
* - data concerned to 14723 man and 13092 women

Table 5. Same characteristics of T1D patients' cohort (Khalangot et al., 2010)

Life expectancy of T1D patients in Ukraine in 2007, assessed according to age at the time of death did not exceed 40.2 yrs (Khalangot, 2008). In UK, according to similar cohort study this value is 55 yrs (Soedamah-Muthu et al., 2006), however the British cohort also included children, which could influence the assessment of average T1D duration and age at the time of death. Renal failure is the leading cause of death (28.4%) in T1D patient cohort, whereas according to a British study of DM patient register containing primary care data, the leading cause of death among T1D patients was CVD (Laing et al., 1999). Similar results were obtained by a European study EURODIAB (Soedamah-Muthu et al., 2008). Comparison of main causes of death according to EURODIAB data and Ukrainian Diabetes Register (UDR) data is shown in figure 4. Apparently death from renal failure among T1D patients in Ukraine prevails several times over other causes, while in other parts of Europe the main cause of death is CVD. It was previously noted by epidemiologists that the main cause of death for T1D patients is renal failure (Dorman et al., 1984), however these data were relevant in 1960s-1970s. Today's experts believe that the shift in mortality structure towards CVD happened due to intensification of hypotensive therapy and insulin treatment (Maahs et al., 2006), therefore the mortality structure of T1D patients that we have revealed when analyzing UDR can be assumed to conform to earlier time period of clinical practice.

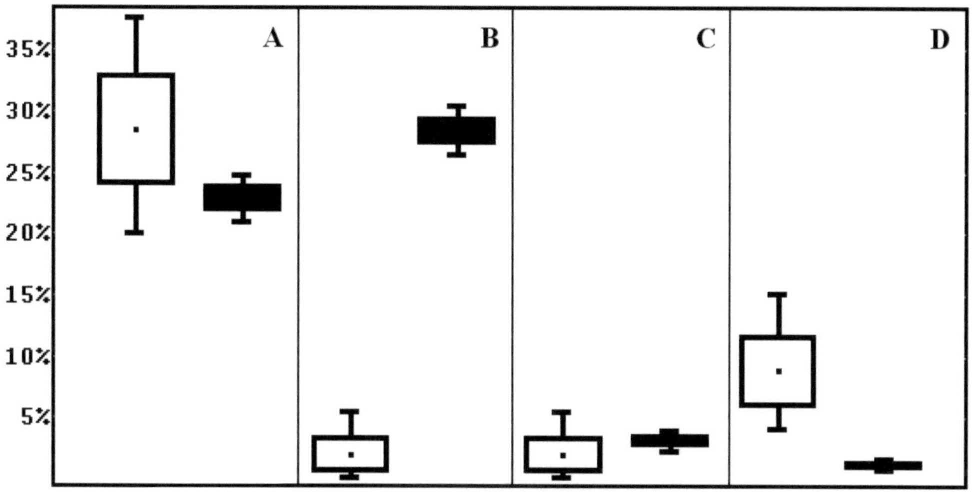

Note: given Means (%) ± SE (the dot within the box and height of boxes respectively), 95% CI (lines that emerge above and below the boxes). Data from Ukrainian Diabetes Register given according to Khalangot et al., 2010; EURODIAB given according to Soedamah-Muthu et al., 2008.

Fig. 4. Interval estimation of structure (%) of the main death causes among T1D patients, diagnosed before 30 years of age according to EURODIAB data (white boxes) and Ukrainian Diabetes Register (black boxes). Death causes: CVD (A); renal failure (B); DKA or coma (C); cancer (D).

3.5.2 Mortality assesment in territorial T1D prevalence clusters

To build the regression model we used 1925 deaths recorded among 27 896 patients. We have found that the patients living on the territory belonging to the maximal T1D prevalence cluster associated with increased risk of total mortality compared with the minimal prevalence cluster. In the minimal territorial cluster mortality was 15.68, and in the maximal -- 22.64 cases per 1000 person-years of follow up, $p < 0.001$. The risk (hazard ratio - HR) of death from all-cause mortality in patients from maximal in relation to the the minimal cluster was 1.5 (95% CI 1.31-1.79). Adjusting for gender had almost no effect on this risk: HRs standardized according to age, gender, and T1D duration for all cause mortality in the maximal T1D prevalence cluster compared to the minimal made up 1.56 (95 % CI 1.33-1.81), p<0.001, whereas the same value for diabetes-related mortality was 1.5 (95 % CI 1.14-1.96), p<0.001. The risk of total mortality for patients from the intermediate cluster did not differ from the minimal one (fig. 5, 6).

During the whole period of observation, 57 cases of death from acute T1D complications among 27510 patients have been recorded. It has been established, that prevalence of T1D is directly associated with the increase of mortality from acute T1D complications (table 6, figure 7). Hazard ratios, determined using Cox model of regression, and standartized according to gender, duration, and age in maximal territorial cluster of T1D prevalence comparing to the minimal cluster, exceeded 5 : HR= 5.25 (95% CI 1.76-15.63), p<0.001.

T1D prevalence cluster	Patients, n	Follow up period, person years	Mean Follow up, years	SD	Death cases, n	Death cases per 1000 person-years
Minimal	5 769	20 079,52	3.48	1.74	4	0.2
Intermedial	17 898	77 323,3	4.3	1.69	36	0.47
Maximal	3 919	17 974,66	4.59	1.79	17	0.95

Table 6. Mortality related to acute T1D complications (Khalangot et al., 2010)

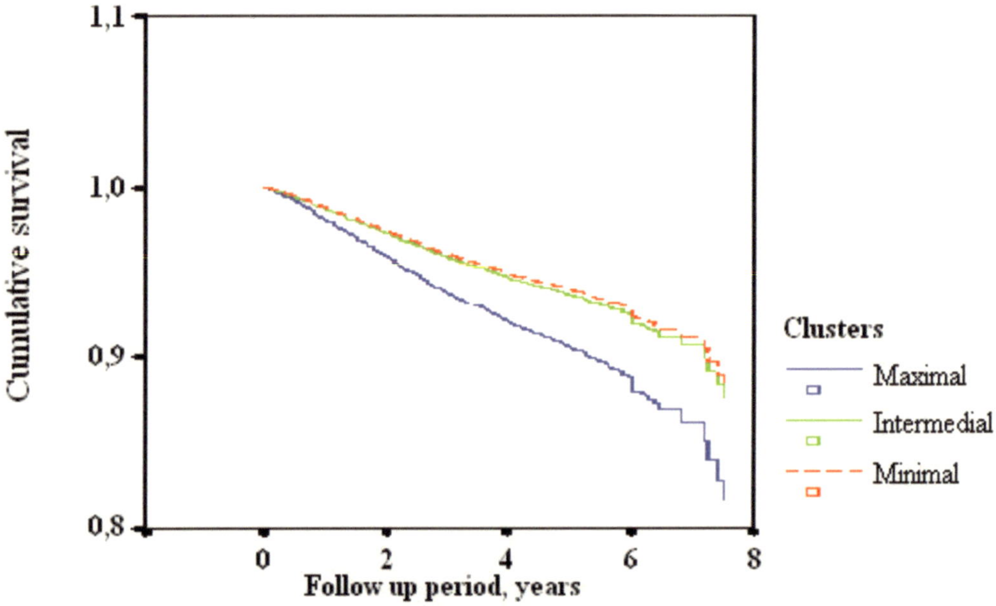

Fig. 5. All cause mortality represented by survival function in minimal, intermediate, and maximal clusters of T1D prevalence (Khalangot et al., 2009c)

3.5.3 Assesment of high blood pressure and proliferative retinopathy prevalence in territorial T1D prevalence clusters

Assessment of arterial hypertension (AH) incidence among patients in regional clusters was performed using the same cohort of 27 896 patients. A total of 4159 hypertension cases, or

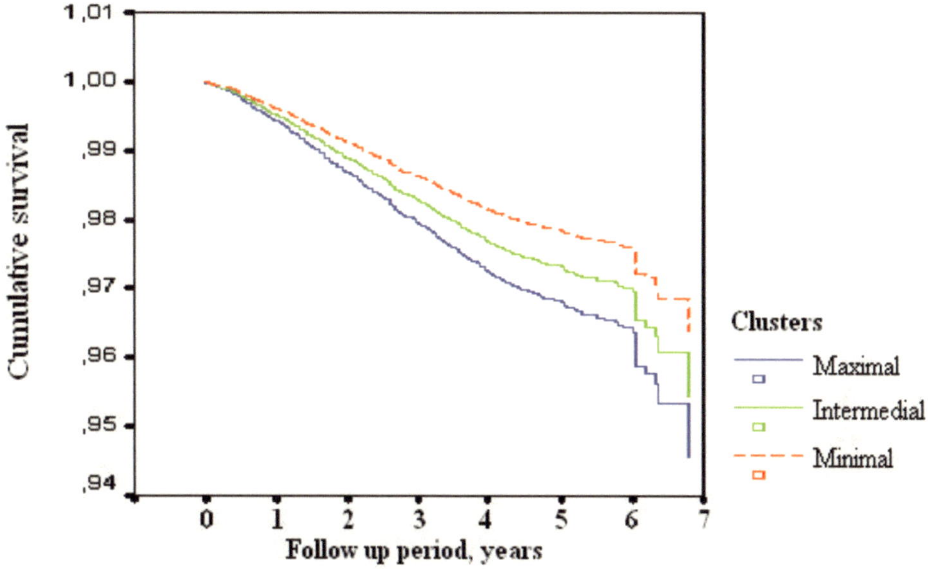

Fig. 6. DM-related mortality represented by survival function in minimal, intermediate, and maximal clusters of T1D prevalence (Khalangot et al., 2009c)

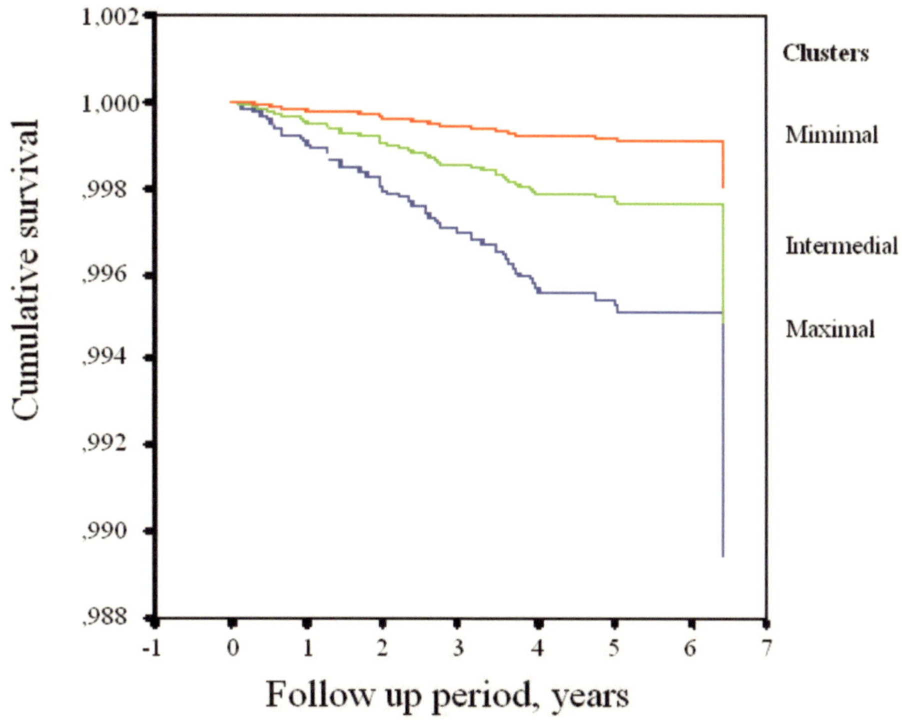

Fig. 7. Mortality related to acute T1D complications (cumulative survival) in different territorial clusters (Khalangot et al., 2010)

14.91%, were recorded. The minimal cluster included 691 AH cases (11.79%), maximal cluster had 570 cases (14.46%), and intermediate cluster included 2898 AH cases (16.02%). The prevalence of AH or proliferative retinopathy (PR) in the maximal or intermediale clusters is greater in relation to the minimal one (Table 7, Fig. 8). Hazard ratios were 1.36 and 1.46 for maximal and intermediale clusters in relation to the minimal cluster, the HR of which was considered as 1. Each year the T1D duration increases the risk of having hypertension. Adjusting according to gender, age and diabetes duration did not significantly change the risk of AH (table 6). Corresponding ORs for AH and PR were 1.36 (95% CI 1.2-1.54), p<0,001 and 2.04 (95 % CI 1.72-2.41), p<0.001. It was revealed that T1D prevalence is directly linked to the increase of all-cause and diabetes-related mortality risks, as well as to PR and AH prevalence.

T1D prevalence cluster	Patients, n	Cases of Arterial Hypertension, n	%	95 % CI
Minimal	5860	691	11.8	11.0-12.6
Intermedial	18095	2898	16.0	15.5-16.6
Maximal	3941	570	14.5	13.4-15.6

Table 7. Prevalence of arterial hypertension in T1D patients in different territorial clusters (Khalangot et al., 2009c)

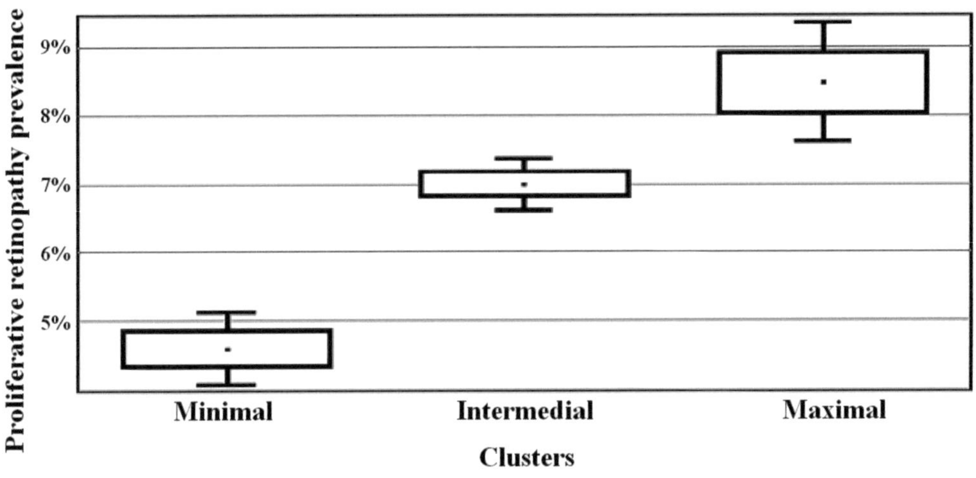

Fig. 8. Fraction (%) of patients with proliferative retinopathy (PR) in different clusters of T1D prevalene. The levels of PR prevalence (the dot within the box), its standart errors (the box height) and 95% CI (lines that emerge) are shown (Khalangot et al., 2009c).

We have found only one study that compared mortality between populations that differ in prevalence of T1D. This was a joint study of epidemiologists from Finland and Japan (Asao et al., 2003). Previously it was known that the incidence and prevalence of T1D in Finland is several times higher than in Japan, however mortality is higher among Japanese patients. The researchers explain this phenomenon by the fact that Finland was "disturbed" by its world's highest incidence of T1D, and because of that the Finnish health care system has long been implementing public programs of relevant quality for treating diabetes (Asao et al., 2003). Comparison of our mortality data among patients with T1D in Ukraine (from 15.7 to 22.6 per 1000 person-years, respectively, in the minimal and maximal prevalence clusters) with mortality among patients with juvenile T1D in Japan and Finland (6.07 and 3.52 per 1000 person-years, respectively), demonstrates a considerably higher mortality in Ukraine and the presense of an opposing relationship between the frequency of T1D in compared countries and mortality in cohorts of patients with juvenile diabetes. Please note that cited Asao et al. study (2003) compared the mortality in cohorts of patients with infantile T1D from different countries, while our study compares T1D that develops in patients before the age of 30 in the same country.

4. T1D sybtype may be responsible for the T1D territorial heterogenity in Ukraine

Currently, researchers (eg. Dib & Gomes, 2009) distinguish such subtypes of T1D, as T1A (characterized by selective destruction of beta-cells by an autoimmune process that quickly leads to absolute insulin deficiency; most common among caucasians), LADA (Latent Autoimmune Diabetes in Adults with an onset usually after 35 years of age and characterized by slowly developing insulin deficit), and T1B, also called idiopathic (clinical course is similar to T1A, but without the autoimmune component). Fulminant diabetes is one of the subtypes of T1B. Its is common in asian countries, such as Japan, China, and Korea. It is characterized by a very quick progression of acute metabolic decompensation, damage of alpha and beta cells of pancreas, and absence of autoimmune disorders. The discovered positive relationship between T1D prevalence, exogenic insulin requirement level, development of diabetes complications, and mortality does not allow us to associate T1D territorial heterogenity with LADA. Furthermore, the increase of GADA persistence in T1D patients who reside in regions with higher prevalence of this disease does not allow to consider T1B as responsible for this phenomenon. Thus, T1A rather than T1B subtype of T1D determines the territorial differences in the risk of developing T1D as well as course severity of this autoimmune disease.

5. Future studies

Causal link between the territorial distribution of autoimmune T1D in adults and the severity of its course and outcomes remains unknown. The recently discovered antibodies to the type 8 zinc transporter (ZnT8As) have substantially improved the clinical stratification of autoimmune diabetes in adults, demonstrating the link to a more severe insulin deficiency (Lampasone et al., 2010). Swedish researchers point out the possibility of low zinc content in drinking water as a possible T1D risk factor in children (Samuelsson et al., 2010; Haglund et al., 1996). Interestingly, in accordance with our preliminary results (unpublished data), there is no shortage of zinc in blood plasma in adults without diabetes, residing on territories with high prevalence of T1D, and we have even observed an increase of plasma zinc levels among adults with T1D comparing to similar patients from the minimal cluster. Plasma zink levels may be low (T2D) or high (T1D), zink supplementation may improve glycemic control in the two major types of diabetes, however the underlying molecular mechanisms have been elucidated very insignificantly (revieved by Jansen et al. , 2009). It is possible that the study of ZnT8As in comparison to the levels of zinc in the environment and human body will provide new information about the cause of territorial heterogeneity of T1D.

6. Conclusions

We have shown, that the prevalence of T1D in the Ukrainian regions differs substantially. The daily insulin dose was found to increase regularly with the duration of the disease. This study also revealed a positive relation between T1D prevalence and the daily insulin doses, and observed a difference in the blood GADA levels among the T1D adults residing in territories with different T1D prevalence.

A unique feature of this study is that instead of examining the incidence, the prevalence of T1D was examined. This can be attributed to the relatively recent development of the Ukrainian diabetes-mellitus register (Khalangot & Tronko, 2007). Nevertheless, we believe that such an approach enabled us to study virtually the entire Ukrainian T1D population, and reveal a positive correlation between T1D prevalence, intensity of insulin treatment, hyperglycemia (HbA1c), and GADA levels, and its prevalence in adults. However, an earlier study of GADA in children recently diagnosed with T1D did not find any relation between GADA positivity and the clinical parameters of the disease (Holmberg, 2006).

7. Acknowledgements

The authors of this work acknowledge the efforts of all Ukrainian endocrinologists, who have contributed data about their patients to the diabetes mellitus register. Special thanks to Novo Nordisk A/C, Ukraine, for helping to promote the manuscript.

8. References

Altman D.G., Machin D., Bryant T.N., Gardner M.J. (Ed(s)). (2003). Statistics with confidence. Confidence intervals and statistical guidelines. Edited by Bristol.- BMJ Books. Second edition.-240 p.

Amos A.F., McCarty D.J., Zimmet P. (1997). The rising global burden of diabetes and its complications: estimates and projections to the year 2010. Diabet Med. Vol. 14, suppl 5, pp. S1-85.

Anonymous. (2006) Main indicators of endocrinologicalcare of Ukraine for 2005: review. Kiev: V.P. Komisarenko Institute of Endocrinology and Metabolism (Acad Med Sci, Ukraine Ministry of Health) Press Limited, (in Ukrainian).

Asao K., Satri C., Forsen N. et al. (2003). Long-term mortality in nationwide cohorts of childhood-onset type 1 diabetes in Japan and Finland. Diabetes Care. Vol. 26, pp. 2037-2042.

Bland M. (2000). An introdaction to medical statistics. New York. Oxford University Press. Third edition. 405 p.

Bonora E., Coscelli C., Butturini U. (1984). Residual B-cell function in type 1 (insulin-dependent) diabetes mellitus: its relation to clinical and metabolic features. *Acta Diabetol. Lat.* Vol. 21, № 4, pp. 375 - 383.

Boyle D.I., Cunningham S., Sullivan F.M., Morris A. (2001). Technology integration for the provision of population-based equitable patient care: The Tayside Regional Diabetes Network--a brief description. *Diabetes Nutr Metab.* Vol. 14, pp. 100-103.

Carstensen B., Kristensen J.K., Ottosen P., Borch-Johnsen K. (2008). On behalf of the steering group of the National Diabetes Register. The Danish National Diabetes Register: trends in incidence, prevalence and mortality. *Diabetologia.* Vol. 51, pp. 2187-2196.

Curtis J.P., Selter J.G., Wang Y., et al. (2005). The obesity paradox: body mass index and outcomes in patients with heart failure. *Arch Intern Med.* Vol. 165, pp. 55-61.

Dib SA, Gomes MB. (2009). Etiopathogenesis of type 1 diabetes mellitus: prognostic factors for the evolution of residual beta cell function. *Diabetol Metab Syndr.* Vol. 4, № 1, 25 p.

Doney A.S., Fischer B., Cecil J.E., Cohen P.T., Boyle D.I., Leese G., Morris A.D., Palmer C.N. (2003). Male preponderance in early diagnosed type 2 diabetes is associated with the ARE insertion/deletion polymorphism in the PPP1R3A locus. *BMC Genet.* Vol. 4, p.11.

Doney A.S.F., Lee S., Leese G.P., Morris A.D., Palmer C.N.A. (2005). Increased cardiovascular morbidity and mortality in type 2 diabetes is associated with the glutathione S transferase theta-null genotype: A Go-DARTS Study *Circulation.* Vol. 111, pp. 2927–2934.

Dorman J.S., Laporte R.E., Kuller L.H., Cruickshanks K.J., Orchard T.J., Wagener D.K., Becker D.J., Cavender D.E., Drash A.L. (1984). The Pittsburgh insulin-dependent diabetes mellitus (IDDM) morbidity and mortality study. Mortality results. *Diabetes.* Vol. 33, № 3, pp. 271 -276.

Eeg-Olofsson K., Cederholm J., Nilsson P.M., Gudbjörnsdóttir S., Eliasson B. (2007). Steering Committee of the Swedish National Diabetes Register. Glycemic and risk factor control in type 1 diabetes: results from 13,612 patients in a national diabetes register. *Diabetes Care.* Vol. 30, № 3, pp. 496-502.

Evans J.M., Donnelly L.A., Emslie-Smith A.M. et al. (2005). Metformin and reduced risk of cancer in diabetic patients *BMJ.* Vol. 330, pp. 1304–1305.

Evans J.M., Ogston S.A., Emslie-Smith A., Morris A.D. (2006). Risk of mortality and adverse cardiovascular outcomes in type 2 diabetes: a comparison of patients treated with sulfonylureas and metformin. *Diabetologia.* Vol. 49, pp. 930–936.

Gale E.A.M. (2002) The rise of childhood type 1 diabetes in the 20th Century. *Diabetes.* Vol. 51, pp. 3353 - 3361.

Gorus FK. (1996). The importance of diabetes registries and clinical biology for the study and treatment of type1 diabetes mellitus. *Verh K Acad Geneeskd Belg.* V. 58, pp. 539 - 586.

Green A., Patterson C.C. (2001). EURODIAB TIGER Study Group. Europe and Diabetes.Trends in the incidence of childhood-onset diabetes in Europe 1989-1998. *Diabetologia.* Vol. 44, suppl 3, pp. B3-8.

Gruberg L., Weissman N.J., Waksman R., et al. (2002). The impact of obesity on the short-term and long-term outcomes after percutaneous coronary intervention: the obesity paradox? *Am Coll Cardiol.* Vol. 39, pp. 578-584.

Haglund B., Ryckenberg K., Selinus O., Dahlquist G. (1996). Evidence of a relationship between childhood-onset type I diabetes and lowgroundwater concentration of zinc. *Diabetes Care.* Vol. 19, № 8, pp. 873-875.

Holmberg H., Vaarala O., Sadauskaite-Kuehne V., Ilonen J., Padaiga Z., Ludvigsson J. (2006). Higher prevalence of autoantibodies to insulin and GAD65 in Swedish compared to Lithuanian children with type 1 diabetes. *Diabetes Res Clin Pract.* Vol. 72, № 3, pp. 308-314.

Jansen J., Karges W., Rink L. (2009). Zinc and diabetes--clinical links and molecular mechanisms. *J Nutr Biochem.* Vol. 20, № 6, pp. 399-417.

Keen H. (1988). Limitations and problems of diabetes classification from an epidemiological point of view. In: M. Vranic, C. H. Hollenberg, G. Steiner (Ed.) *Comparison of type I and type II diabetes.* New York, Plenum Press.

Khalangot M, Tronko M. (2007). Primary care diabetes in Ukraine. *Primary Care Diabetes.* № 1, pp. 203-205.

Khalangot, 2008 . [Age and sex-related pecularietes of mortality in type 1 diabetes mellitus patients]. (Article in Ukrainian) Problemy starenia I dolgoletia. 2008. 17(1): 75-82. http://www.nbuv.gov.ua/portal/Chem_Biol/PSD/2008_1.

Khalangot M. D. (2009) Epedemiologic characteristics of diabetes mellitus type1 and 2 according to data from national population-based patient register. Manuscript. Thesis for the Degree of Doctor of Medical Sciences. V.P.Komisarenko Institute of Endocrinology and Metabolism AMS of Ukraine, Kiev.

Khalangot M., Hu G., Tronko M., Kravchenko V., Guryanov V. (2009a January-February). Gender risk of nonfatal stroke in type 2 diabetic patients differs depending on the type of treatment. *J Womens Health (Larchmt).* Vol. 18, № 1, pp. 97-103.

Khalangot M., Tronko M., Kravchenko V., Kulchinska J., Hu G. (2009b, March). Body mass index and the risk of total and cardiovascular mortality among patients with type 2diabetes: a large prospective study in Ukraine. *Heart.* Vol. 95, № 6, pp. 454-560.

Khalangot M. D., Kravchenko V. I., Okhrimenko N. V., Kovtun V.A., Tronko E. M. (2009c). [Analysis of mortality, proliferative retinopathy prevalence, and arterial hypertension among type 1 diabetic patients residing in areas that differ in prevalence of this disease] *Endocrinologia.* Vol. 14 , № 1, pp. 77-85 (Article in Ukrainian).

Khalangot M., Kravchenko V., Tronko M., Gur'ianov V. (2009 [d], Octoвer). Correlation between the prevalence of type 1 diabetes with the daily insulin dose and the autoimmuneprocess against glutamic acid decarboxylase in adults. *Eur J Intern Med.* Vol. 20, № 6, pp. 611-615.

Khalangot M., Tronko M., Kravchenko V., Kovtun V. (2009 e, December) Glibenclamide-related excess in total and cardiovascular mortality risks: data from large Ukrainian observational cohort study. *Diabetes Res ClinPract.* Vol. 86, № 3, pp. 247-253.

Khalangot M. D., Tronko M.D., Kravchenko V. I., Kovtun V.A., Okhrimenko N. V., Bolgarska S.V. (2010) [Some mortality risk factors for type 1 diabetes mellitus patients in Ukraine evaluated according to data from National Register] *Endocrinologia.* Vol. 15 , № 1, pp. 62-70 (Article in Ukrainian).

Kyvik K.O., Nystrom L., Gorus F., Songini M., Oestman J., Castell C., Green A, Guyrus E., Ionescu-Tirgoviste C., McKinney P.A., Michalkova D., Ostrauskas R., Raymond N.T. (2004, Mar.) The epidemiology of Type 1 diabetes mellitus is not the same in young adults as in children. *Diabetologia.* Vol. 47, № 3, pp. 377-384.

Laing S.P., Swerdlow A.J., Slater S.D., Botha J.L., Burden A.C., Waugh N.R., Smith A.W., Hill R.D., Bingley P.J., Patterson C.C., Qiao Z., Keen H. (1999). The British Diabetic Association Cohort Study, II: cause-specific mortality in patients with insulin-treated diabetes mellitus. *Diabet Med.* Vol. 16, № 6, pp. 466-471.

Lampasona V., Petrone A., Tiberti C., Capizzi M., Spoletini M., di Pietro S., Songini M., Bonicchio S., Giorgino F., Bonifacio E., Bosi E., Buzzetti R. (2010). Non Insulin

Requiring Autoimmune Diabetes (NIRAD) Study Group. Zinc transporter 8 antibodies complement GAD and IA-2 antibodies in the identification and characterization of adult-onset autoimmune diabetes: Non Insulin Requiring Autoimmune Diabetes (NIRAD) 4. *Diabetes Care.* Vol. 33, № 1, pp. 104-108.

Leese G., Boyle D., Morris A. (2006). The Tayside Diabetes Network . *Diabetes Research and Clinical Practice* . Vol. 74, suppl. 2, pp. 197 - 199.

Lévy-Marchal C., Patterson C.C., Green A. (2001). EURODIAB ACE Study Group. Europe and Diabetes. Geographical variation of presentation at diagnosis of type I diabetes in children: the EURODIAB study. *Diabetologia.* Vol. 44, suppl. 3, pp. B75-80.

Liakh Yu.E., Gurianov V.G. (2004). Data Analysis of Biomedical Researches and Clinical Trials by Means of Statistical Program MedStat.*Vestn. Hyg. Epid.* Vol. 8, № 1, pp. 155 - 167.

Linn T., Mann M., Mann M., Bretzel R.G., Boedeker R.H. (2003). Randomised prospective study for the effect of therapy on residual beta cell function in type-1 diabetes mellitus. *BMC Endocr. Disord.* Vol. 3, № 1, 5 p.

Maahs DM, Rewers M. Editorial: (2006). Mortality and renal disease in type 1 diabetes mellitus—progress made, more to be done. *J Clin Endocrinol Metab.* Vol. 91, № 10, pp. 3757 - 3759.

Marascuilo, L. (1966) Large-Sample Multiple Comparisons. *Psychological Bulletin.* V. 65, № 4, pp. 289-299.

Monami M., Balzi D., Lamanna C., Barchielli A., Masotti G., Buiatti E., Marchionni N., Mannucci E. (2007). Are sulphonylureas all the same? A cohort study on cardiovascular and cancer-related mortality. *Diabetes Metab Res Rev.* Vol. 23, pp. 479-484.

Morris A.D., Boyle D.I., MacAlpine R. et al. (1997). The diabetes audit and research in Tayside Scotland (DARTS) study: electronic record linkage to create a diabetes register (DARTS/MEMO Collaboration). *BMJ.* Vol. 315, pp. 524–528.

Nishimura R., LaPorte R.E., Dorman J.S., Tajima N., Becker D., Orchard T.J. (2001). Mortality trends in type 1 diabetes. The Allegheny County (Pennsylvania) Registry 1965-1999. *Diabetes Care.* Vol. 24, № 5, pp. 823-827.

Samuelsson U., Oikarinen S., Hyöty H.,Ludvigsson J. (2010). Low zinc in drinking water is associated with the risk of type 1 diabetes in children. *Pediatr Diabetes.*, 7. doi: 10.1111/j.1399-5448.2010.00678.x.

Schofield C.J., Libby G., Brennan G.M., MacAlpine R R., Morris A.D., Leese G.P. (2006). (DARTS/MEMO Collaboration). Mortality and hospitalization in patients after amputation: A comparison between patients with and without diabetes. *Diabetes Care.* Vol. 29, pp. 2252–2256.

Soedamah-Muthu S.S., Fuller J.H., Mulnier H.E., Raleigh V.S., Lawrenson R.A., Colhoun H.M. (2006). All-cause mortality rates in patients with type 1 diabetes mellitus compared with a non-diabetic population from the UK general practice research database, 1992-1999. *Diabetologia.* Vol. 49, № 4, pp. 660-666.

Soedamah-Muthu S.S., Chaturvedi N., Witte D.R., Stevens L.K., Porta M., Fuller J.H. (2008). EURODIAB Prospective Complications Study Group. Relationship between risk factors and mortality in type 1 diabetic patients in Europe: the EURODIAB Prospective Complications Study (PCS). *Diabetes Care.* Vol. 31, № 7, pp. 1360-1366.

The DCCT Research Group. (1987). Effects of age, duration and treatment of insulin-dependent diabetes mellitus on residual beta-cell function: observations during eligibility testing for the Diabetes Control and Complications Trial (DCCT). *J Clin Endocrinol Metab.* Vol. 65, № 1, pp. 30 – 36.

The Diabetes Control and Complications Trial Research Group. (1998). Effect of intensive therapy on residual beta-cell function in patients with type 1 diabetes in the diabetes control and complications trial. A randomized, controlled trial. *Ann Intern Med.* Vol. 128, № 7, pp. 517 – 523.

Vaiserman A., Khalangot M. (2008). Similar seasonality of birth in type 1 and type 2 diabetes patients: a sign for common etiology? *Med Hypotheses.* Vol. 71, № 46, pp. 604-605.

Vaiserman A.M., Khalangot M.D., Carstensen B., Tronko M.D., Kravchenko V.I., Voitenko V.P., Mechova L.V., Koshel N.M., Grigoriev P.E. (2009) Seasonality of birth in adult type 2 diabetic patients in three Ukrainian regions. *Diabetologia.* Vol. 52, № 12, pp. 2665-2667.

Vandewalle C.L., Coeckelberghs M.I., De Leeuw I.H., Du Caju M.V., Schuit F.C., Pipeleers D.G., Gorus F.K. (1997). Epidemiology, clinical aspects, and biology of IDDM patients under age 40 years. Comparison of data from Antwerp with complete ascertainment with data from Belgium with 40% ascertainment. The Belgian Diabetes Registry. *Diabetes Care.* Vol. 20, pp. 1556-1561.

Weets I., Van Autreve J., Van der Auwera B.J., Schuit F.C., Du Caju M.V., Decochez K., De Leeuw I.H., Keymeulen B., Mathieu C., Rottiers R., Dorchy H., Quartier E., Gorus F.K. (2001). Belgian Diabetes Registry. Male-to-female excess in diabetes diagnosed in early adulthood is not specific for the immune-mediated form nor is it HLA-DQ restricted: possible relation to increased body mass index. *Diabetologia.* Vol. 44, pp. 40-47.

Weets I., Siraux V., Daubresse J.C., De Leeuw I.H., Féry F., Keymeulen B., Krzentowski G., Letiexhe M., Mathieu C., Nobels F., Rottiers R., Scheen A., Van Gaal L., Schuit F.C., Van der Auwera B., Rui M., De Pauw P., Kaufman L., Gorus F.K. (2002). Belgian Diabetes Registry. Relation between disease phenotype and HLA-DQ genotype in diabetic patients diagnosed in early adulthood. *Clin Endocrinol Metab.* Vol. 87, pp. 2597-2605.

Part 2

Psychological Aspects of Diabetes

5

Type I Diabetes in Children and Adolescents

Laura Nabors[1], Phillip Neal Ritchey[2],
Bevin Van Wassenhove[3] and Jennifer Bartz[3]
[1]*School of Human Services, College of Education, Criminal Justice, and Human Services, University of Cincinnati,*
[2]*Department of Sociology, College of Arts and Sciences, University of Cincinnati,*
[3]*Department of Psychology, College of Arts and Sciences, University of Cincinnati, Cincinnati, Ohio*
USA

1. Introduction

Type I Diabetes is characterized by pancreatic failure. Daily exogenous insulin replacement is necessary for the child's survival. Insulin typically is administered by injections before lunch and dinner. Type I diabetes affects approximately 1 in every 400 to 600 children (Centers for Disease Control and Prevention, 2003). Rates of Type I diabetes are increasing (Chisholm et al., 2007). This is concerning as this disease has long-term health care consequences including problems with circulation, vision, and cardiovascular issues (Frey et al., 2006). The care of children with Type I diabetes involves complex procedures including daily blood glucose testing, dietary monitoring, intensive insulin therapy, and increased physical activity to maintain metabolic control (Anderson et al., 2007). Several studies have shown that children as well as adolescents have difficulty adhering to diet, exercise, blood glucose testing, and insulin regimens (e.g., Chang et al., 2007; Frey et al., 2006). Patterns of diabetes care are established early in the disease course, and therefore understanding factors related to child adherence is a mechanism for generating strategies to improve diabetes management for children. This, in turn, may positively influence health outcomes in adolescence and adulthood (Bui et al., 2005).

Children's management of their diabetes is often measured by assessment of blood glucose or HbA1c levels (i.e., measure of diabetic control). Monitoring blood glucose levels has become an increasingly important self-management task for children who have diabetes (Bui et al., 2005). Psychosocial factors, such as attitudes about one's diabetes, support from others, and stress, have been related to HbA1c levels or other factors serving as proxy variables for diabetes management (Chisholm et al., 2007; Nabors et al., 2010). This chapter reviews the relationship between psychosocial factors, chiefly children's attitudes, support from others, stress, and diabetes management. This chapter will provide suggestions for improving children's attitudes and reducing their stress to improve their diabetes management. The next section of this chapter reviews ways in which children's attitudes, namely health locus of control and stress, influence children's diabetes management.

2. Diabetes management and children

2.1 Attitude and diabetes

Health locus of control, a concept originating from Rotter's (1966) theory, is a belief about whether an individual might receive positive outcomes resulting from a particular health behavior. Thus, a child may estimate that eating "healthy" (e.g., "low carbohydrate" foods), drinking water, engaging in mild exercise, and reducing his or her stress will result in good diabetes management. The relations among beliefs, such as locus of control, and health actions have been illustrated in theoretical models, including the Health Belief Model (Rosenstock, 1974). Research supports relationships between locus of control beliefs and diabetes management (Bennett-Murphy et al., 1997). Locus of control may influence self-confidence, such that children with an internal locus of control, or an "I can do it" attitude, may do a better job of assisting with their diabetes management (Nabors et al., 2010).

Children's perceptions of their diabetes are related to regimen adherence and their HbA1c levels (Edgar & Skinner, 2003). For example, Lehmkuhl and Nabors (2008) found that feelings of sadness and feeling that having the disease was unfair were related to higher HbA1c levels for children. Others have reported that confidence in the ability to improve one's health was an indicator of good diabetes management for children (Skinner & Hampson, 1998). Similarly, Nabors et al. (2010) found that children with a higher level of an internal locus of control over (their health) disease were more likely to have lower HbA1c levels, indicating better glycemic control, than children with lower levels of an internal locus of control. Consequently, it may be that a myriad of attitudinal factors, including locus of control (Nabors et al., 2010), beliefs about the seriousness of one's illness (Edgar & Skinner, 2003), and beliefs about being able to compensate for different behaviors that might negatively influence diabetes management (Rabiau et al., 2009) contribute to self-management behaviors.

2.2 Stress and diabetes

Another psychological factor influencing diabetes management is stress (Beveridge et al., 2006; Seiffge-Krenke & Stemmler, 2003). Research has demonstrated that stress is indirectly related to HbA1c levels (Aiken et al., 1992). Balfour and colleagues (1993) proposed that stress is directly related to dietary control, which then influences glycemic control. Likewise, Helgeson et al. (2010) reported that stress may be related to poor self-care, which in turn negatively influences metabolic control. One type of stress that might be particularly salient for children with Type I Diabetes is fear of hypoglycemic episodes. These episodes can cause seizures, resulting in a coma and even death (Green et al., 1990). When a child is fearful of hypoglycemic episodes, he or she may ignore a medical regimen and administer insulin as he or she deems necessary. This can result in poor control. Over time, this can lead to negative health outcomes and elevated stress for the child. Then again, this "worry" is not a universal experience for all children who have diabetes. Marrero et al. (1997) assessed parent perceptions of child reactions to hypoglycemic episodes. Their results indicated that youth who had experienced a hypoglycemic event were experiencing higher levels of worry and anxiety. This was not necessarily related to diabetes management, however, which is a positive finding in that the worry was not appearing to translate into poor disease management. On the other hand, these authors have found that children also can worry about experiencing hyperglycemia or feeling "high." Thus, the medical team should carefully assess child or parent fears about these types of episodes and explain ways to treat these episodes and make referrals for counseling as necessary.

Children may experience stress related to feeling different from peers due to having Type I Diabetes. They also may have difficulty talking to teachers about how to manage their disease at school (Nabors et al., 2003). Coaching for these children, in addition to written care plans may assist them in communicating important information to teachers and other professionals in the school setting. But, not all children and adolescents with diabetes may face significant diabetes-related stressors. For example, Hema et al. (2009) discovered that children and adolescents with diabetes reported daily stressors similar to youth without chronic illnesses; interestingly, they did not report significant diabetes-related stressors as being hassles. Consequently, health care professionals need to consider the social and emotional needs of children with diabetes to determine whether recommendations for stress management or referral for counseling is appropriate (Chisholm et al., 2007).

Children with diabetes also can experience stress related to negative school experiences. Storch et al. (2006) found a link between bullying of children with diabetes and self-management behaviors. If children with diabetes experienced teasing or negative reactions from peers for testing their blood glucose or other self-management behaviors, they were less likely to engage in self-care. In addition, these researchers proposed that children who are depressed because of having diabetes may be less likely to monitor their glucose levels. They concluded that assessment of bullying experiences by peers is an important component of clinical interviews with school-age children, because bullying can be an indicator of poor self-management and higher HbA1c levels.

In another study, Peters et al. (2008) assessed the relationship between experiences of teachers being unsupportive and adherence and self-management in one hundred and sixty-seven children, between the ages of eight to seventeen years, with Type 1 Diabetes. Their findings indicated that perceptions of teachers as being unsupportive of the child's self-management were related to poorer adherence behaviors for younger children, between the ages of eight and eleven years, but not for older children (ages twelve through seventeen). Thus, a poor teacher-student relationship, often characterized by teachers misunderstanding the importance of adherence to the medical regimen, may be detrimental to diabetes management for elementary or primary school-age youth, who depend on teacher support and guidance to facilitate their efforts at managing their diabetes at school.

3. Systems-level factors and diabetes management

3.1 Support from others

Diabetes management can be very difficult and children may not be able to independently manage their treatment regimen (Allen et al., 1983). Additionally, children have reported that they benefit from support from teachers, peers, and nurses in school settings (Nabors et al., 2003). A key factor influencing diabetes management is support from friends and family. LaGreca et al. (1995) reported that support from parents and friends were protective factors for adolescents with diabetes. Greco and her colleagues (2001) found that support from a best friend was perceived as beneficial for diabetes management by adolescents. Skinner and Hampson (1998) also discovered that family support is a critical component of diabetes management for adolescents.

Arguably, the most important support for diabetes management may come from children's parents. Hanna and Guthrie (2001) reported that when parents acted as supervisors, providing guidance to assist their child in diabetes management, both parents and their child who had diabetes felt more comfortable about managing the child's disease. Guidelines of the American Diabetes Association (Silverstein et al., 2005) suggest that parent and child teamwork, or shared responsibility, for diabetes management tasks facilitates diabetes management. Thus, a partnership between the child and parent, synonymous with joint ownership of diabetes management and care, may be one strategy that doctors can emphasize to promote child wellness (Beveridge et al., 2006). We believe that the supportive role of parents can be influenced by other family and disease related factors; consequently, these factors also are an area of inquiry for clinical interviews and possible intervention.

3.2 Family adjustment model

John Rolland (1987) presented a conceptual framework for viewing family adjustment to a child's chronic illness. He suggested that the family's developmental stage, the child's own developmental stage, and factors related to the child's illness influence family members' adjustment to a child's chronic illness. Rolland proposed that these factors interact and influence child and family adjustment at different points in the child's life. This theory has explanatory "validity" when one reviews literature on parents' and children's adjustment to childhood diabetes. For example, literature reviewed for this chapter indicated that parents respond differently, in terms of helping the child manage his or her diabetes, based on the child's age or the duration of his or her diabetes (Fielding & Duff, 1999; Hanna & Guthrie, 2001). Others have shown that child age and health status (e.g., diabetes "control") can have a significant influence on diabetes management (Lewin et al., 2006). Furthermore, parents' roles change based on whether the child has good "control" (i.e., glycemic control) of his or her diabetes (Davis et al., 2000). Thus, the supportive role of parents and family is influenced by parent or family factors, disease-related factors, and the stage of the child's development.

Different points in the child or family lifecycle may influence adherence behaviors, such that education or counseling may be needed at various phases of the child's life (Rolland, 1987). For this reason, we recommend that mental health professionals play a supportive role. The analogy of a "band of support" may illuminate this role. The mental health professional plays an educational or counseling role as needed and offers more or less support based on an assessment of child and family stress as well as anxiety. Because both parents and children often experience stress related to disease management, collaboration between counselors and the child's medical team remains an important part of clinical practice. This collaboration can provide critical information for the child's doctor and other members of their medical team, who also can support the use of stress management techniques, education and therapy to decrease parent or child stress, and dietary and medication changes to manage the waxing and waning symptoms of this disease.

Thus far, we have presented literature highlighting issues for children. Nevertheless, as mentioned, parents experience significant stress too. Consequently, the next section of our chapter presents research related to parental stress and adjustment to a child's diabetes. We begin with a discussion of the association between parenting style and diabetes management. Next, we highlight adolescence as a critical period, as this is a time in the child's life where parental care and support often play a pivotal role in diabetes management. At the same time, due to the developmental changes and struggles experienced by some adolescents, this may be a time of heightened stress for parents. We conclude this section with a review of research related to parental adjustment and needs for counseling and education.

4. Diabetes management and parents

4.1 Parental interactions

Parental "style" or method of interacting with their child may be related to positive diabetes management and adherence to the child's medical regimen. For example, studies have shown that parental warmth and supportiveness are related to "good" glycemic control and adherence to diabetes regimens and fewer instances diabetic ketoacidosis (DKA; Geffken et al., 2008). Davis et al. (2000) assessed parenting styles of parents whose children had diabetes. They discovered that parental warmth and an emphasis on child self-management were related to positive health outcomes. They also reported that a more restrictive parenting style was correlated with relatively poorer management and higher stress levels for children.

Geffken and colleagues (2008) found that negative parental attitudes were related to instances of DKA in children with Type I Diabetes. These researchers assessed the relationship between child and caregiver opinions about family behavior and they also assessed episodes of diabetic ketoacidosis. Participants were one hundred children with Type I Diabetes and their caregivers. Study results indicated that children who perceived their parents attitudes toward them as being warm and caring were less likely to have reported episodes of ketoacidosis and were more likely to have better diabetes management than those who thought that their parents did not use warm and caring parenting styles.

Parenting style may change, based on child and parent/family stage of development (Rolland, 1987). Parents of young children may exhibit higher levels of control to assist the child in following his or her treatment regimen. As children enter adolescence and become more autonomous, parents often become more non-directive and are "available as needed" to provide guidance (Hanna & Guthrie, 2000; 2001). This non-directive stance may change, if the adolescent is managing his or her disease in a manner that results in *poor* glycemic control. If this occurs parent-adolescent conflict can ensue, as parents begin to provide more direct assistance and move away from an advisory role (Nabors et al., 2010). Being able to move between a supportive and directive stance based on the situation and the adolescent's needs may be particularly important as parents provide assistance to their teenager.

4.2 Parental adjustment

Parents may experience significant stress and anxiety related to their child's disease and its management (Driscoll et al., 2010). Parents may experience symptoms of stress similar to those experienced by individuals with Post-traumatic Stress Syndrome (PTSD). These symptoms can include hypervigilance, resulting in an over-monitoring of their child's disease management or conversely, avoidance resulting in under-monitoring. Research has demonstrated that 10% of mothers of children who had diabetes met criteria for a diagnosis of PTSD, while another 15% of mothers displayed some of the symptoms, partially meeting the criteria for this diagnosis (Horsch et al., 2007). Symptoms related to parental experiences of "PTSD" may increase, when the child has mental health problems in addition to his or her diabetes. Researchers have found that parents of children who have diabetes experience increased anxiety and depression if their children are experiencing mental health problems (Driscoll et al., 2010).

Parents may have a difficult time adjusting to their child's diabetes if they or their child do not feel confident about being able to manage the child's diabetes. Similarly, parents whose children have recently been diagnosed or are "newly" diagnosed also may experience high stress. Often a diagnosis occurs with little forewarning and parents may feel shock and grief related to learning about their child's illness. Parents in either of the aforementioned situations may benefit from education about disease management and counseling to improve their abilities to cope with stress as well as co-occurring symptoms of depression or anxiety (Streisand et al., 2008).

Poor parental adjustment and parental stress may be related to becoming overwhelmed with caretaking responsibilities and disease management for a significant period of time, leading to classic symptoms of "burnout. " Parents who are "burned out" may not assist their child with disease management, and feel apathetic about assisting their child in coping with his or her diabetes (Lindstrom et al., 2010). Other variables that may be related to parental stress are uncertainty about the treatment of the child's diabetes and uncertainty about health outcomes related to diabetes (Carpentier et al., 2006). Health care providers should informally assess parental stress and uncertainty associated with their child's illness on a regular, ongoing basis. Counseling should be recommended when parental stress is high, as lowering parental stress can have a positive influence on parents, which leads to improved diabetes management for their child. Parents experiencing high levels of trauma because their child has diabetes may require counseling to avoid symptoms of depression and anxiety (Horsch et al., 2007; Streisand et al., 2008).

5. Adolescence: A critical period

Parental support may be critical to diabetes management during adolescence, as children begin to take a more active role in managing their diabetes (Silverstein et al., 2005). Adherence is a very important area of study for adolescents with diabetes because managing IDDM involves multiple strategies including, diet, exercise, and glucose monitoring as well as administering medication (Helgeson et al., 2010). The early teenage years are a difficult time to manage insulin levels, because adolescents may have decreased insulin sensitivity and poor self-management skills (Shroff-Pendley et al., 2002). Difficulties in managing diabetes may also occur in late adolescence, especially when adolescents experience stressful life events (e.g., change in a romantic relationship, parental divorce; Helgeson et al., 2010). Self-care may be compromised for a period of time as the child copes with the event, and during this period the adolescent may require counseling or additional support from family or friends to manage his or her diabetes. Previous research (Weissberg-Benchell, 2007) and guidelines of the American Diabetes Association (Silverstein et al., 2005) suggest that parent and child teamwork, or shared responsibility, for diabetes management tasks facilitates diabetes management. Thus, a partnership between the adolescent and his or her parents may be one strategy that doctors can emphasize to promote the development of a relationship that is supportive and allows parents to move between doing more to assist with diabetes management when needed and doing less when the adolescent is doing a good job managing on his or her own.

Skinner and Hampson (1998) found that family support, such as high levels of connectedness among family members, is a critical component of diabetes management for teenagers. On the other hand, family conflict and a lack of cohesion in family relationships has been related to with poor metabolic control (higher glycosated hemoglobin levels or HgbA1C levels; Hauser, Jacobson, Lavori, et al., 1990). Strong, constructive family relationships may have a positive influence on adherence (Skinner at al., 2000; Lewin et al., 2006). Family functioning is related to adolescents' adherence, management, and metabolic control (Wysocki et al., 2001). In general, we believe that a positive parent-teenager relationship will lead to family cohesion and will improve diabetes management. For this reason, we recommend that members of the child's medical team encourage a team-based approach to diabetes management and in other aspects of the child's life as a "family-level" intervention when an adolescent is having difficulty with diabetes management.

6. Conclusion

Our review of the literature indicated that child and parent adjustment influence diabetes management. Moreover, the phase of the child's life and phase in the family's own life-cycle impacts disease management and glycemic control (Chisholm et al., 2007; Rolland, 1987). We recommend that health and mental health professionals provide support as needed to children and parents, providing education based on child and parent needs. This type of patient- and family-centered approach may improve child and parent efficacy for disease management. A child- or patient-focused approach to adherence will ensure that health care professionals and school personnel "meet children where they are" and offer patient-centered care that will promote diabetes management and wellness for youth (Bauman, 2000). Counseling for children may improve their ability to cope with difficult psychosocial and developmental issues. Existing studies (e.g., Cohen et al., 2004) indicate that children's emotional and behavioral problems and low family cohesion are related to regimen adherence as well as glycemic control. Interventions which provide education about stress management and increase peer support (i.e., support from close friends) may improve adjustment to diabetes (Boardway et al., 1993; Greco et al., 2001). Health and mental health professionals working with children with diabetes should also work with children and their parents to reduce barriers, such as a lack of support from teachers or friends, to child illness management. Working to strengthen positive attitudes about disease management and illness trajectories and reduce stress also may be related to patient and parent satisfaction with the child's medical care and adherence to the child's medical regimen. More research on ways that group and individual counseling can assist children with diabetes and their parents and other family members will provide more information about the success of these support-based interventions. In conclusion, strengthening child and parent resilience, working with children and parents to develop strategies to facilitate diabetes management, and helping children and parents adjust to diabetes-related stress are elements of successful care that will optimize care and health outcomes for children with diabetes.

7. References

Aiken, J., Wallender, J., Bell, D., & Cole, J. (1992). Daily stress variability, learned resourcefulness, regimen adherence, and metabolic control in Type 1 diabetes mellitus: Evaluation of a path model. *Journal of Consulting and Clinical Psychology*, Vol.60, pp. 113-118, ISSN 0022-006X

Allen, D. A., Tennen, H., McGrade, B. J., Affleck, G., & Ratzan, S. (1983). Parent and child perceptions of the management of juvenile diabetes. *Journal of Pediatric Psychology*, Vol.8, pp. 129-141, ISSN 0146-8693

Anderson, B. J., Svoren, B., & Laffel, L. (2007). Initiatives to promote effective self-care skills in children and adolescents with diabetes mellitus. *Disease Management and Health Outcomes*, Vol.15, pp. 101-108, ISSN 1173-8790

Balfour, L., White, D., Schiffrin, A., Daugherty, G., & Dufresne, J. (1993). Dietary disinhibition, perceived stress, and glucose control in young Type I diabetic women. *Health Psychology*, Vol.12, pp. 33-38, ISSN 0887-0446

Bauman, L. J. (2000). A patient-centered approach to adherence: Risks for non-adherence. In D. Drotar (Ed.). *Promoting adherence to medical treatment in chronic childhood illness: Concepts, methods, and interventions*. Mahwah, N.J.: Lawrence Erlbaum, ISBN 978-8058-3348-5

Bennett-Murphy, L. M., Thomson, R. J., & Morris, M. A. (1997). Adherence behavior among adolescents with type 1 insulin-dependent diabetes mellitus: The role of cognitive appraisal processes. *Journal of Pediatric Psychology,* Vol.22, pp. 811-825, ISSN 0146-8693

Beveridge, R. M., Berg, C. A., Wiebe, D. J., & Palmer, D. L. (2006). Mother and adolescent representations of illness ownership and stressful events surrounding diabetes. *Journal of Pediatric Psychology,* Vol.31, pp. 818-827, ISSN 0146-8693

Boardway, R. H., Delamater, A.M., Tomakowsky, J., & Gutai, J. P. (1993). Stress management training for adolescents with diabetes. *Journal of Pediatric Psychology,* Vol.52, pp. 685-716, ISSN 0146-8693

Bui, H., Perlman, K., & Daneman, D. (2005). Self-monitoring of blood glucose in children and teens with diabetes. *Pediatric Diabetes,* Vol.6, pp. 50-62, ISSN 1399-543X

Carpentier, M. Y., Mullins, L. L., Chaney, J. M., & Wagner, J. L. (2006). The relationship of illness uncertainty and attributional style to long-term psychological distress in parents of children with type 1 diabetes mellitus. *Children's Health Care,* Vol.35, No.2, pp. 141-154, ISSN 0273-9615

Centers for Disease Control and Prevention. (2003). *National diabetes fact sheet: General information and national estimates on diabetes in the United States, 2002.* Atlanta, GA. U.S. Department of Health and Human Services, Centers for Disease Control and Prevention, Government Doc. No. HE 20.7002:D 54/6

Chang, C.-W., Yeh, C.-H., Lo, F.-S., & Shih, Y.-L. (2007). Adherence behaviors in Taiwanese children and adolescents with type 1 diabetes mellitus. *Journal of Nursing and Healthcare of Chronic Illness* in association with *Journal of Clinical Nursing,* Vol.16, No.7b, pp. 207-214, ISSN 0962-1067

Chisholm, V., Atkinson, L., & Donaldson, C., Noyes, K., Payne, A., & Kelnar, C. (2007). Predictors of treatment adherence in young children with Type I diabetes. *Journal of Advanced Nursing,* Vol.57, pp. 482-493, ISSN 0309-2402

Cohen, D. M., Lumley, M. A., Naar-King, S., Partridge, T., & Cakan, N. (2004). Child behavior problems and family functioning as predictors of adherence and glycemic control in economically disadvantaged children with type 1 diabetes: A prospective study. *Journal of Pediatric Psychology,* Vol.29, No.3, pp. 171-184, ISSN 0146-8693

Davis, C., Delameter, A., Shaw, K., La Greca, A., Edison, M., Perez-Rodriguez, J., & Nemery, R. (2000). Parenting styles, regimen adherence, and glycemic control in 4- to 10-year-old children with diabetes. *Journal of Pediatric Psychology,* Vol.26, No. 2, pp. 123-129, ISSN 0146-8693

Driscoll, K. A., Johnson, S. B., Barker, D., Quittner, A. L., Deeb, L. C., Geller, D. E. (2010). Risk factors associated with depressive symptoms in caregivers of children with type 1 diabetes or cystic fibrosis. *Journal of Pediatric Psychology,* Vol.35, No.8, pp. 814-822, ISSN 0146-8693

Edgar, K. A., & Skinner, T. C. (2003). Illness representations and coping as predictors of emotional well-being in adolescents with type 1 diabetes. *Journal of Pediatric Psychology,* Vol.28, pp. 485-493, ISSN 0146-8693

Fielding, D., & Duff, A. (1999). Compliance with treatment protocols: Interventions for children with chronic illness. *Archives of Disease in Childhood,* Vol.80, pp. 196-200, ISSN 0003-9888

Frey, M. A., Ellis, D., Templin, T., Naar-King, S., & Gutai, J. P. (2006). Diabetes management and metabolic control in school-age children with Type 1 diabetes. *Children's Health Care,* Vol.35, pp. 349-363, ISSN 1532-6888

Geffken, G. R., Lehmkuhl, H., Walker, K.N., Storch, E., A., Heidgerken, A. D., Lewin, A. et al. (2008). Family functioning processes and diabetic ketoacidosis in youths with Type I Diabetes. *Rehabilitation Psychology*, Vol.53, No.2, pp. 231-237, ISSN 0090-5550

Greco, P., Pendley, J. S., McDonell, K., & Reeves, G. (2001). A peer group intervention for adolescents with type 1 diabetes and their best friends. *Journal of Pediatric Psychology*, Vol.26, pp. 485-490, ISSN 0146-8693

Green, L., Wysocki, T., & Reineck, B. (1990). Fear of hypoglycemia in children and adolescents with diabetes. *Journal of Pediatric Psychology*, Vol.15, pp. 633-641, ISSN 0146-8693

Hanna, K. M., & Guthrie, D. (2000). Adolescents' perceived benefits and barriers related to diabetes self-management - part 1. *Issues in Comprehensive Pediatric Nursing*, Vol.23, pp. 165-174, ISSN 0146-0862

Hanna, K.M., & Guthrie, D. W. (2001). Health-compromising behavior and diabetes management among adolescents and young adults with diabetes. *Diabetes Educator*, Vol.27, No.2, 223- 230, ISSN 0145-7217

Hauser, S. T., Jacobson, A. M., Lavori, P., Wolfsdorf, J. I., Herskowitz, R. D., Milley, J. E., Bliss, R., & Gelfand, E. (1990). Adherence among children and adolescents with insulin dependent diabetes mellitus over a 4-year longitudinal follow-up: II. Immediate and long-term linkages with family milieu. *Journal of Pediatric Psychology*, Vol.15, pp. 527-542, ISSN 0146-8693

Helgeson, V. S., Escobar, O., Siminerio, L., & Becker, D. (2010). Relation of stressful life events to metabolic control among adolescents with diabetes: 5-year longitudinal study. *Health Psychology*, Vol.29, pp. 153-159, ISSN 0887-0446

Hema, D. A., Roper, S. O., Nehring, J. W., Call, A., Mandleco, B. L., & Dyches, T. T. (2009). Daily stressors and coping responses of children and adolescents with Type I diabetes. *Child Care, Health and Development*, Vol.35, pp. 330-339, ISSN 1365-2214

Horsch, A., McManus, F., Kennedy, P., & Edge, J. (2007). Anxiety, depressive, and posttraumatic stress symptoms in mothers of children with type 1 diabetes. *Journal of Traumatic Stress*, Vol.20, No.5, pp. 881-891, ISSN 1573-6598

LaGreca, A. M., Auslander, W. F., Greco, P., Spetter, D., Fisher, E. B., & Santiago, J. V. (1995). I get by with a little help from my family and friends: Adolescents support for diabetes care. *Journal of Pediatric Psychology*,Vol.20, pp. 449-476, ISSN 0146-8693

Lehmkuhl, H. D., & Nabors, L. A. (2008). Children with diabetes: Satisfaction with school support, illness perceptions, and HbA1C levels. *Journal of Developmental and Physical Disabilities*, Vol.20, pp. 101-114, ISSN 1573-3580

Lewin, A.B., Heidgerken, A. D., Geffken, G. R., Williams, L. B., Storch, E. A., Gelfand, K. M. et al. (2006). The relation between family factors and metabolic control: The role of diabetes adherence. *Journal of Pediatric Psychology*, Vol.31, No.2, pp. 174-183, ISSN 0146-8693

Lindstrom, C., Aman, J., & Norberg, A. L. (2010). Increased prevalence of burnout symptoms in parents of chronically ill children. *Acta Paediatrica*, Vol.99, No.3, pp. 427-432, ISSN 1651-2227

Marrero, D. G., Guare, J. C., Vandagriff, J. L., & Fineberg, N. S. (1997). Fear of hypoglycemia in the parents of children and adolescents with diabetes: Maladaptive or healthy response? *Diabetes Educator*, Vol.23, No.3, pp. 281-286, ISSN 0145-7217

Nabors, L. A., McGrady, M. E., & Kichler, J. (2010). Children's attitudes toward their diabetes, locus of control, and HbA1c levels. *Journal of Developmental and Physical Disabilities*, Vol.22, pp. 475-484, ISSN 1056-263X

Nabors, L., Lehmkuhl, H., Christos, N., & Andreone, T. L. (2003). Children with diabetes: Perceptions of supports for self-management at school. *Journal of School Health*, Vol.73, pp. 216-221, ISSN 1746-1561

Peters, C. D., Storch, E. A., Geffken, G. R., Heidgerken, A. D., & Silverstein, J. H. (2008). Victimization of youth with type-1 diabetes by teachers: Relations with adherence and metabolic control. *Journal of Child Health Care*, Vol.12, No.3, pp. 209-220, ISSN 1367-4935

Rabiau, M. A., Knuper, B., Nguyen, T-K, Sufrategui, M., & Polychronakos, C. (2009). Compensatory beliefs about glucose testing are associated with low adherence to treatment and poor metabolic control in adolescents with Type I diabetes. *Health Education Research*, Vol.24, pp. 890-896, ISSN 0012-3692

Rolland, J. S. (1987). Chronic illness and the life cycle: A conceptual framework. *Family Process*, Vol.26, pp. 203-221, ISSN 0014-7370

Rosenstock, I. M. (1974). Historical origins of the Health Belief Model. *Health Education Monographs*, Vol.2, pp. 328-335, ISSN 0073-1455

Rotter, J. B. (1966). Generalized expectancies of internal versus external control of reinforcements. *Psychological Monographs*, Vol.80 (whole no. 609), ISSN 0096-9753

Shroff-Pendley, J., Kasmen, L. J., Miller, D. L., Donze, J., Swenson, C., & Reeves, G. (2002). Peer and family support in children and adolescents with type I diabetes. *Journal of Pediatric Psychology*, Vol.27, No.5, pp. 429-438, ISSN 0146-8693

Seiffge-Krenke, I., & Stemmler, M. (2003). Coping with everyday stress and links to medical and psychosocial adaptation in diabetic adolescents. *Journal of Adolescent Health*, Vol.33, pp. 180-188, ISSN 1054-139X

Silverstein, J., Klingensmith, G., Copeland, K., Plotnick, L., Kaufman, F., Laffel, L., et al.(2005). Children and adolescents with Type 1 diabetes. *Diabetes Care*, Vol.28, pp. 186-212, ISSN 0149-5992

Skinner, T. C., John, M., & Hampson, S. E. (2000). Social support and personal needs models of diabetes as predictors of self-care and well-being: A longitudinal study of adolescents with diabetes. *Journal of Pediatric Psychology*, Vol.25, pp. 257-267. ISSN 0146-8693

Skinner, T. C., & Hampson, S. E. (1998). Social support and personal models of diabetes in relation to self-care and well-being in adolescents with type 1 diabetes mellitus. *Journal of Adolescence*, Vol.21, pp. 703-715, ISSN 0140-1971

Storch, E.A., Heidgerken, A.D., Geffken, G.R., Lewin, A.B., Ohleyer, V., et al. (2006). Bullying, regimen self-management, and metabolic control in youth with Type I Diabetes, *Journal of Pediatrics*, Vol.148, No.6, pp. 784-787, ISSN 0022-3476

Streisand, R., Mackey, E. R., Elliot, B. M., Mednik, L., Slaughter, I. M., Turek, J. et al. (2008). Parental anxiety and depression associated with caring for a child newly diagnosed with type 1 diabetes: Opportunities for education and counseling. *Patient Education and Counseling*, Vol.73, pp. 333-338, ISSN 0738-3991

Weissberg-Benchell, J., Goodman, S. S., Lomaglio, J. A., & Zebracki, K. (2007). The use of continuous subcutaneous insulin infusion (CSII): Parental and professional perceptions of self-case mastery and autonomy in children and adolescents. *Journal of Pediatric Psychology*, Vol.32, No.10, pp. 1196-1202, ISSN 0146-8693

Wysocki, T., Greco, P., Harris, M. A., Bubb, J., & White, N. H. (2001). Behavior therapy for families of adolescents with diabetes: Maintenance of treatment effects. *Diabetes Care*, Vol.24, pp. 441-446, ISSN 0149-5992

6

Inadequate Coping Attitudes, Disordered Eating Behaviours and Eating Disorders in Type 1 Diabetic Patients

Ricardo V. García-Mayor and Alejandra Larrañaga
Eating Disorders Section, Endocrinology, Diabetes, Nutrition and Metabolism Department, University Hospital of Vigo
Spain

1. Introduction

Diabetes mellitus has been found to be the sixth leading cause of death for those living in the United States affecting the young and old at an alarming rate (National Center for Health Statistics, 2011). Type 1 diabetes typically has an early onset in life, but can occur at any age. It primarily develops when the body's own immune system attacks and destroys pancreatic beta cells, which produce the hormone insulin that regulates blood glucose levels. This type of diabetes accounts for 5 to 10 % of all diagnosed cases. Type 2 diabetes affects mainly adult subjects, its prevalence around the world has increased in relationship with the increase of the prevalence of overweight and obesity, attributed to lifestyle changes such as sedentary habits and overeating. Consequently, diabetes is one of the most challenging and burdensome chronic diseases of the 21st century, and it is a growing threat to the world's public health (King et al, 1995; King et al, 1998). Diabetes mellitus, especially type 1 form represent a very hard experience that requires subsequent psychological adaptation. Unfortunately, this often does not occur and it is followed by frustration and the non-acceptance of the disease. Problems with coping are one of the important consequences of the disease and the cause of uncountable problems in the future.

The management of type1 diabetes and its associated health-risk factors are often complex and require considerable patient education and frequent medical monitoring (Koopmanschap, 2002). The participation of the patients is basic in order to obtain a correct degree of metabolic control; however, this carries as a consequence considerable amount of stress. People on insulin must learn how to regulate their blood sugars by monitoring blood glucose levels daily while carefully attending to their food intake and an exercise regimen. Careful blood glucose monitoring is necessary to prevent wide variations in blood sugars that affect both short term and long term health and functioning. Hypoglycaemia reactions are a concern in the short run not only because they are frightening and disruptive, but also because, when severe, they can lead to unconsciousness, coma and death (Cox & Gonder-Frederick, 1992). The constant stress of maintaining tight glycaemia control can result in two types of psychological distress (a) subclinical emotional distress, and (b) diagnosable psychological disorders (Rubin & Payrot, 2001). Additionally, psychiatric conditions can

occur independently without being a consequence of diabetes. It has been shown that individuals with diabetes have a disproportionately higher rate of psychiatric disorders (Bogner et al, 2007; Llorente & Urrutia, 2006), with affective and anxiety disorders being more commonly diagnosed than in the general population (De Mont-Marin et al, 1995). This is evidenced by research showing high rates of psychiatric disorders, particularly depression and anxiety, for example, Fettahoglu et al., (Fettahoglu et al, 2007) found over 40% increased risk in having any type of psychiatric disorder in patients with diabetes, and Gülseren et al. (Gülseren et al, 2001) found that depression and anxiety account for 45% of psychiatric disorders in patients with diabetes. These results show the negative impact that diabetes can have on an individual's psychosocial adjustment, and the need for research to determine the most appropriate and common coping strategies to deal with the stress of illness.
Other psychological problems of these patients are Eating Disorders (ED). The classical ED are anorexia nervosa (AN) and bulimia nervosa (BN), but recently another entity was recognized, the so called eating disorders not otherwise specified (EDNOS), which are incomplete forms of classical ED that are diagnosed when patients did not fulfill the classical ED diagnostic criteria. Type 1 diabetic patients have a high risk of suffering from ED due to these patients have to select the food they eat carefully in an early period of their development and because both entities, type 1 diabetes and ED, often affect adolescents and young adults. Furthermore, type 1 diabetic patients suffer from other eating behavior anomalies, which mainly appear in girls, that consist in spliting insulin doses or restricting food intake in order to reduce their body weight, but with the high price of the metabolic disturbance and subsequent chronic vascular complications if such behavior persists over time.
In this chapter we will review these psychological anomalies suffered by type 1 diabetic patients, especially problems with coping attitudes, disordered eating behaviors (DEB) and eating disorders (ED), and also discuss some aspects of their forms of presentation, management and prevention.

2. Search strategy for identification and selection of studies

We identified relevant studies published in English by searching MEDLINE from January 1990 to December 2010. We included randomised and quasi-randomised controlled studies, clinical series, reviews and systematic reviews on type 1 diabetic patients with inadequate coping attitudes, disordered eating behaviors and eating disorders, in which children, adolescents and young adults with type 1 diabetes were properly defined. As study strategy, relevant questions about type 1 diabetes and eating disorders were previously determined: coping with diabetes, epidemiology, clinical forms of eating disorders and specific behavioral anomalies in type 1 diabetic patients, metabolic consequences and vascular complications, management and prevention.

3. Inadequate coping attitudes in type 1 diabetic patients

People suffering from any type of chronic disease, need to make minor or major lifestyle adjustments. Diabetes, in particular, can eventually take its toll on the emotional, psychological, and physical well being of any person. These adjustments can lead to either successful adherence to medical regimens and control of the disease, or among other things, ineffective or maladaptive coping. The literature reveals that successfully adjusting to a chronic illness yields the following outcomes: successful performance of adaptive tests, absence of psychological disorders, low experience of negative affect, improved functional status, and appraisals of well-being in varying life domains (Stanton et al, 2001).

Coping can generally be defined as cognitive and/or behavioral attempts to manage and tolerate situations that are appraised as stressful to an individual. No single coping strategy or dimension can be considered maladaptive. The quality of the coping strategy and process is evaluated according to its impact on the outcome of interest. From the previous conceptual definition, Folkman and Lazarus (Folkman & Lazaruz, 1980; Folkman & Lazaruz, 1985; Folkman & Lazaruz, 1988) distinguished two primary dimensions of coping (or categories): emotion-focused (composed of individual coping strategies such as seeking emotional support) and problem-focused (composed of individual coping strategies such as making a plan of action). These coping categories described efforts to either alleviate the personal emotional stress induced by the stressor or alter the source of stress in the environment. Use of problem-focused coping has been found to be associated with better metabolic control, emotional status, and better adjustment overall in patients with diabetes (Lundman & Norberg, 1993); use of emotion-focused coping has been found to be associated with poor adjustment and adherence to health regimens in chronically ill samples (Bombardier et al, 1990).

Diabetic patients initially experience high levels of depression and anxiety (Lustman et al, 1997; Tuncay, 2008). Anderson et al. (Anderson et al, 2001) found that adults with diabetes have twice the odds of comorbid depression. It was also found that this prevalence was much higher in women than in men. Within their sample, one in every three individuals had a level of depression that impaired their ability to function on a daily basis which in turn affected quality of life, regimen adherence, and blood glucose control. Regarding to coping strategies, it has been shown that problem-focused coping was positively associated with glycaemia control and negatively associated with anxiety and depression (Maes et al, 1996). Smari and Valtysdottir (Smari & Valtysdottir, 1997) also found that problem-focused coping was associated with lower blood glucose levels—indicative of better adjustment. On the contrary, individuals who engaged in more emotion-focused types of coping experienced more anxiety, depression, and higher levels of glycaemia. It is obvious that any deviation from a normal routine or health status serves as a continual source of stress that leads to the individuals' inability to care for themselves (White et al, 1992). Therefore, management of this stress via coping strategies is crucial for psychological and physical health.

An author found that treating depression through therapy is effective for individuals with diabetes so they may regain confidence and abilities to control the disease, leading to improved quality of life and social and physiological functioning (Eisenberg, 1992). The treatment includes the development of coping skills through training programs (Grey & Berry, 2004) as well as patient empowerment (Anderson et al, 1995). DeRidder and Schreurs (DeRidder & Schreurs, 2001) observed that diabetic patients in particular are inclined to use coping strategies that are aimed at reducing the negative emotions surrounding the disease and its maintenance. If this suggestion was found to be empirically true across diabetes studies and patients, it may portend a particularly problematic issue since these strategies were generally viewed as less adaptive. It is apparent that stress permeates the management of diabetes and thus use of effective coping skills is imperative not only in illness management but general stress management as well. At present, there is no systematic quantitative review of the stress and coping literature in diabetes that links coping strategies to indices of adjustment. Thus, a summary statement of the adaptive versus maladaptive strategies identified for these coping-adjustment relations cannot be made with any degree of confidence.

4. Epidemiology of disordered eating behavior and eating disorders in type 1 diabetic patients

Disordered eating behavior (DEB) is common in young women living in westernized countries, where thinness is valued and dietary restraint is pursued (Attie & Brook-Gunn, 1989). Prevalence studies in North America indicate that full syndrome bulimia nervosa may be found in 1-3% of adolescents and young adult women and subthreshold disorders are even more common (American Psychiatric Association, 1994; Fairburn & Beglin, 1990; Jones et al, 2001). The rates of these disorders are lower but rising in less-westernized countries such as Asia and Africa as Western attitudes towards weight and shape become more pervasive (Hoek, 1993; Lee, 1993; Lee & Lee 1996). Differences in the prevalence of eating disorders varies according to different ethnic groups (Abrams et al, 1993; Kumanyika, 1993), however, a study found that ethnic differences in eating disorder symptoms disappeared when body mass index (BMI) was controlled (Arriaza & Mann, 2001). At present, there is no information on the effect of culture and race on eating disorders in people with diabetes.

The risk of eating disturbances has been postulated to be higher in type 1 diabetic patients than in the general population due to multiple interacting factors related to diabetes and its treatment (Colton et al, 1999; Rodin & Daneman, 1992). Diabetes management imposes some degree of perceived dietary restraint, particularly patients who eat according to a predetermined meal plan, rather than in response to internal cues for hunger and satiety. Such neglect of internal cues may contribute to dietary dysregulation in susceptible individuals (Polivy & Herman, 1985). The relationship between higher weight and DEB presents a management dilemma for clinicians, since both dietary restraint and higher weight are clear risk factors for the development of ED and their negative health consequences.

Although until recently it has been unclear whether there is a specific association of eating disorders with diabetes, some studies have suggested an increased incidence of eating disorders in young women with diabetes (Birk & Spencer, 1987; Engstrom et al, 1999; Hudson et al, Lloyd et al, 1987; 1985; Rodin et al, 1985; Rodin et al, 1986/1987; Rodin et al, 1991; Rosmark et al, 1986; Stancin et al, 1989; Steel et al, 1987; Vila, et al, 1993; Vila et al, 1995) whereas others did not find such an increase (Bryden et al, 1999; Fairburn et al, 1991; Friedman et al, 1995; Mannucci et al, 1995; Marcus et al, 1992; Meltzer et al, 2001; Peveler et al, 1992; Powers et al, 1990; Robertson & Rosenvinge, 1990; Striegel-Moore et al, 1992; Wing et al, 1986). However, the conclusions of these studies are limited by the small sample sizes of females in the age of the highest risk for eating disturbances, the absence of control groups, their low statistical power, and/or by the lack of structured diagnostic interviews for the assessment of eating disorders.

A study examined the association between ED and type 1 diabetic girls, aged 12-19, for at least 1 year. Subjects with diabetes were 2.4 times more likely than non diabetic controls to have a clinical ED and 1.9 times more likely to have a subthreshold ED (Affenito & Adams, 2001). In another investigation, the prevalence of ED in a population-based cohort of female adolescents with type 1 diabetes was compared with that found in aged-matched controls. DEB was found in 16.9% of adolescents with diabetes compared with 2.2% of the controls (Hoek, 1993). A longitudinal study of 87 patients with diabetes aged at baseline 11-25 years, in whom eating habits and attitudes were assessed by a semistructured research diagnostic

interview, showed that 14.9%, at baseline, and 26%, at the end of the follow-up period, had evidence of bingeing or purging while insulin misuse for weight control was reported by 35.6% of the patients (Peveler et al, 2005). A recent study from France (Ryan et al, 2008) concluded that abnormal eating behavior is present in French diabetic patients at higher levels than among the general population.
Thus, nowadays, there is clear evidence that EB and DEB are more prevalent in type 1 diabetic women than in the general population.

5. Clinical forms of eating disorders in type 1 diabetics

The three diagnostic forms of ED are AN, BN and EDNOS. Common to all three is a core problem in which the self-evaluation is unduly influenced by body weight or shape. This can be characterized by an extreme pursuit of thinness, in the case of AN, or recurrent episodes of binge eating and compensatory caloric purging behaviors, in the case of BN. EDNOS encompasses those ED that are clinically significant enough to compromise the patient health and the quality of life, but do not meet formal diagnostic criteria for AN or BN (American Psychiatric Association, 1994).
Eating disorders that meet Diagnostic and Statistical Manual of Mental Disorders four edition (DSM-IV) diagnostic criteria, mostly bulimia nervosa and EDNOS, are more than twice as common in girls with diabetes compared to their non-diabetic peers, furthermore, subthreshold eating disorders were also almost twice as common in girls with diabetes compared to controls (American Psychiatric Association, 1994). In line with these studies, it was found that the ED associated with bingeing and purging are the most common types of ED among girls with diabetes as they are in girls in the general population (American Psychiatric Association, 1994; Fairburn & Beglin, 1990; Jones et al, 2001). Restricting ED are much less common conditions (Jones et al, 2000), thus a specific association between anorexia nervosa and type 1 diabetes has not been demonstrated (Rodin et al, 2002).
In a longitudinal study by Colton et al, (Colton et al, 2007), at 5 years, 49% of a cohort of girls with type 1 diabetes reported current disordered eating behavior (DEB), 43.9% active dietary restraint, 6.1% binge-eating episodes, 3.1% self-induced vomiting, 3.1% insulin omission and 25.5% excessive exercise for weight control. Furthermore, 13.3% met criteria for an ED: three girls had bulimia nervosa, three had an eating disorder not otherwise specified and seven had a subthreshold ED.
Using the DSM-III-R or the DSM-IV for interview-based diagnosis, the prevalence of AN varies between 0.0-1.8% for diabetic patients, whereas 0.0-0.6% for controls. The prevalence of BN was 0.0-5.8% and 0.0-2.0%, respectively (Engström et al, 1999; Fairburn et al, 1991; Jones et al, 2000; Mannucci et al, 1995; Peveler et al, 1992; Robertson et al, 1990; Striegel-Moore et al, 1992; Vila et al 1995). In a study that aimed to determine the prevalence of ED in young adolescents, 98 type 1 diabetic patients and 575 age-matched controls were studied. The authors found neither AN nor BN case among diabetics and controls. However, the prevalence of EDNOS was significantly higher in adolescent diabetics than in controls both in boys (1.7% vs. 0.9% respectively) and girls (5.3% vs. 1.6% respectively). In addition, subthreshold ED were more common in male diabetic adolescents than in non-diabetic peers (García-Reyna et al, 2004). In a meta-analysis by Mannucci et al (Mannucci et al, 2005),

they found that the prevalence of AN in type 1 diabetes was not significantly different from that in controls, being 0.27 vs. 0.06 %, respectively, while the prevalence of BN was 1.23 vs. 0.69 %, respectively, $p < 0.05$, in line with previous studies (Affenito et al, 1997; Jones et al, 2000; Vila et al, 1995).
The cited data indicate that young type 1 diabetic patients have a higher prevalence of BN, EDNOS and subthreshold ED than their non-diabetic peers. Data are summarized in Table 1.

Clinical forms	Globally	Girls	Boys
AN	0.0-1.8 %	0.27 %	-
BN	0.0-5.8 %	1.23-13.3 %	-
EDNOS	7 %	5.3 %	1.7 %
DEB	16.9 %	14.9-49.4 %	-
Insulin misuse	-	3.1-35.6 %	-

Table 1. Estimated prevalence of ED and DEB in type 1 diabetic patients.

6. Specific behavioral anomalies in type 1 diabetics

It is well-known the association of chronic illness, such as type 1 diabetes, asthma, attention deficit disorder, physical disabilities and seizure disorders, with DEB (Neumark-Sztainer et al, 1995; Neumark-Sztainer et al, 1998). Adolescents with chronic illness present higher body dissatisfaction engaged in more high risk weight loss practices (Neumark-Sztainer et al, 1995). These data were confirmed by other studies (Neumark-Sztainer et al, 1998).
While adjusting to the changes of puberty, the adolescence is a period of rapid physical and psychological growth and development. During this time to control weight and to overcome body dissatisfaction, some adolescents commonly diet or exercise. Other may present more severe misbehaviors such as bingeing and purging, the use of laxatives or the adherence to an overly strict exercise regimen.
Before diagnosis and treatment, individuals with type 1 diabetes are likely to lose a large amount of weight. However, once the treatment begins the weight usually returns. By controlling diabetes with insulin injections many diabetics face a constant struggle with their weight (Collazo Clavell, 2010). As insulin encourages fat storage, many people with type 1 diabetes have discovered the relationship between reducing the amount of insulin they take and their corresponding weight loss (Mathur & Conrad, 2008; Mathur & Conrad, 2008). It is well-known that adolescents with type 1 diabetes tend to exhibit increased difficulty in maintaining optimal weight and also are more inclined to be concerned about their weight than their non-diabetic counterparts (Bryden et al, 1999).
Since weight management during this state of development can be especially difficult for those with type 1 diabetes, some diabetics may restrict or omit insulin, a condition known as diabulimia, as a form of weight control (Baginsky, 2009; Hasken et al, 2010; Ruth-Sahd et al, 2009). This is not a medically recognized condition yet, but describes the situation of a considerable number of type 1 diabetic patients.

Insulin restriction becomes a more significant problem in older adolescents, perhaps as parental supervision of insulin administration decreases. It becomes more common a potential worsening in severity and frequency throughout early adulthood. Once the pattern of frequent and habitual insulin restriction became entrenched, the cycle of negative feelings about body image, shape and weight; chronically elevated blood sugars; depression, anxiety and shame; and poor diabetes self-care can be complex and difficult to treat.

In a study that looked at 143 adolescents with type 1 diabetes who completed the Assessing Health and Eating among Adolescents with Diabetes survey; unhealthy weight control practice was observed in 37.9 % of females and 15.9% of males. Among the females, 10.3% reported skipping insulin and 7.4 % reported taking less insulin to control their weight (Neumark-Sztainer et al, 2002). Only one male reported doing either of these behaviors. In another 4 years follow-up study of 91 girls with diabetes aged 12 to 18, dieting was reported by 38% of the sample, binge eating by 45%, insulin omission by 14 % and self-induced vomiting by 8% at baseline, these behaviors were even more common at follow-up, when most of the girls were in the age of the highest risk for ED. At this time, more than half of the sample reported dieting for weight loss and binge eating, and one-third reported deliberate insulin omission to prevent weight gain (Rydall et al, 1997).

In general terms, it is estimated that between 30% and 40% of adolescents and young adults with diabetes skip or reduce insulin after meals to lose weight (Hasken 2010).

7. Metabolic consequences and vascular complications of disordered eating behaviors and eating disorders in type 1 diabetics

There is a spectrum of severity of disturbance of eating habits and attitudes, and subthreshold eating problems, seen as relatively mild in non diabetic patients, can give rise to clinically important disturbances of self-care and glycaemia control in diabetics. In general terms, glycosilated hemoglobin was higher in patients with diabetes who had ED compared with those with diabetes without ED (Affenito & Adams, 2001). A study by Rydall et al (Rydall et al, 1997), found that the mean HbA1c was significantly higher among girls with clinical DEB compared to those moderately disordered of eating habits or with no disordered behavior. Another 3-year longitudinal study by Figueroa Sobrero et al (Figueroa Sobrero et al, 2010) revealed that the presence and persistence of disordered eating behavior is associated with worse prognosis in type 1 diabetic children and adolescents.

The lack of proper insulin treatment in type 1 diabetics may lead to many harmful physical effects. Reducing insulin to lose weight increases the risk of dehydration, break down of muscle tissue, high risk of developed infections and fatigue. If this behavior continues, it may also result in kidney failure, eye disease leading to blindness, vascular disease and even death.

In particular, patients who misuse insulin to control body weight (Crow et al, 1998; Rodin et al, 1989), are thought to be at increased risk for microvascular complications (Rydall et al, 1997; Steel et al, 1987), but the extent of the risk has not been well characterized, as most studies have been cross-sectional. Clinical outcome in terms of physical and psychological health are not known with certainty. One longitudinal study of patients with diabetes and DEB over 9 years, found a low rate of microvascular complications (Pollock et al, 1995). On the contrary, another study, taking place over 4 years, found that insulin-dependent girls with DEB had an increased risk for retinopathy (Rydall et al, 1997). A more recent longitudinal study observed that diabetic patients aged 11 to 25 years with DEB or insulin misuse had a significant risk for the development of two or more serious complications, such as repeated episodes of diabetic ketoacidosis, increased rate of hospital admission and mortality (Peveler et al, 2005).

Therefore, ED in type 1 diabetics have clearly shown to be associated with impaired metabolic control (Jones et al, 2000; Vila et al, 1993; Friedman S et al, 1995; Affenito et al 1997; Affenito et al 1998; Rydall et al, 1997), more frequent episodes of ketoacidosis (Polonsky et al, 1994), and an earlier than expected onset of diabetes-related microvascular complications, particularly, retinopathy (Affenito et al, 1997; Colas et al, 1991; Rydall et al, 1997; Steel et al, 1987; Ward et al, 1995). In this sense, disordered eating status was more predictive of diabetic retinopathy than was the duration of diabetes, which is a well-established risk factor for microvascular complications (Diabetes Control and Complications Trial Research Group, 1993). Furthermore, ED in type 1 diabetic patients is associated with high mortality (Walker et al, 2002).

Regarding to mortality, an 11-year follow-up study reports that insulin restriction conveyed more than a three-fold increased risk of mortality in type 1 diabetic patients after controlling for age, body mass index and HbA1c values. Age of death was younger among insulin restrictors, with a mean age of death of 45 years, as compared to 58 years among those reporting appropriate insulin use (Goebel-Fabbri et al, 2007).

Insulin restriction becomes a more significant problem in older adolescents and in early adulthood. Once the pattern of frequent and habitual insulin restriction becomes entrenched, its consequent poor diabetes self-care can be complex and difficult to treat. Figure 1.

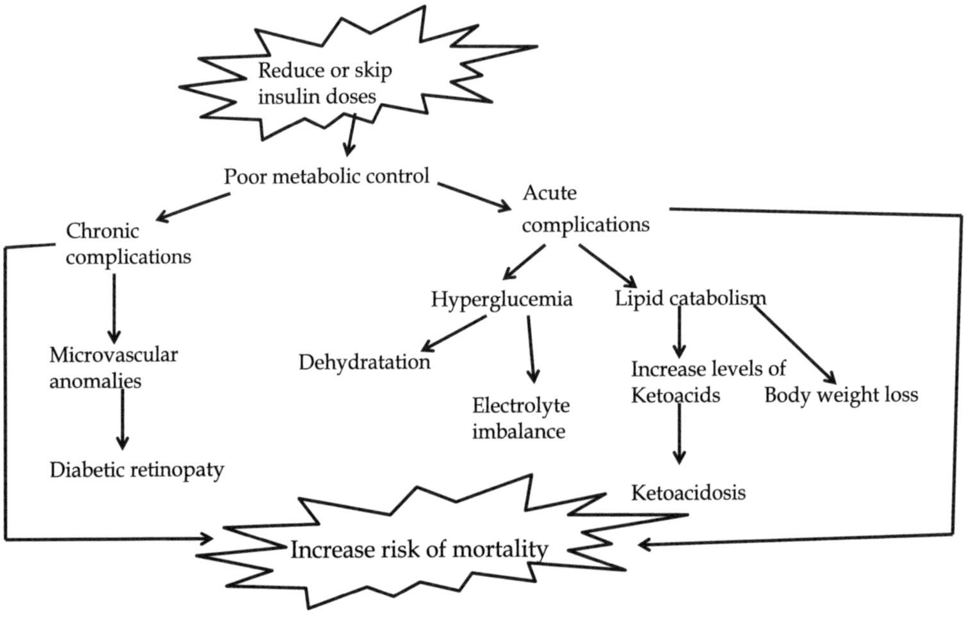

Fig. 1. Consequences of insulin misuse in type1 diabetic patients.

8. Management of inadequate coping attitudes in type 1 diabetic patients

Several major trial carried out in the past decades, have demonstrated that intensive diabetes management for type 1, as well as type 2 diabetes, can delay or prevent the onset and progression of many complications of the disease, especially microvascular complications (DCCT, 1993; UKPDS, 1998). Such studies also have demonstrated that achieving excellent glycaemia control requires complex self-management behaviors to be learned and maintained.

Traditionally, diabetes education has focused on increasing knowledge about diabetes and its care and increasing skills to perform self-care behaviors, such as blood glucose monitoring. However, it is clear that although knowledge and skills are important prerequisites to diabetes self-management, additional training in the application of this knowledge and skills in day-to-day living are necessary for longer-term maintenance and improved outcomes. Cognitive-behavioral interventions such as coping skills training focus primarily on improving behavioral skills are necessary to achieve better glycaemia and psychosocial outcomes in patients with diabetes and in their relative members (Grey & Berry, 2004).

8.1 Social problem solving

Social problem solving assists individuals when they are faced with peer or family pressures or any decision in which they are confronted with a dilemma. Social problem solving is a process by which an individual learns to think through the steps of having a problem and reaching a decision about how to handle the problem. The process assists individuals to look at all possible outcomes of situations and the possible consequences of their decisions (Duangdao & Roesch, 2008).

8.2 Conflict resolution

The basis of conflict resolution is the acquisition of skills necessary to resolve conflict in a positive manner that results in positive outcomes for all parties involved in the conflict (Deustsch & Brickman, 1994). The first step in this training is development of the understanding that in any conflict both parties can win and that every conflict should be approached in this manner. The individual is helped to focus on clear communication and problem-solving skills. Once the conflict is identified, all possible outcomes and the consequences to these outcomes are explored. Role-playing can then be set up to try out the communication of the decision. Role-play is used as both forms of practice and feedback on communication skills.

8.3 Communication skills training

This kind of training aims to help individuals express themselves in ways that are clear, appropriate, and constructive. Two main skills are identified under communication skills training: social skills training and assertiveness training. Models for social skills training include those by Carteledge & Milburn (Carteledge & Milburn, 1980) and Goldstein *et al.* (Goldstein et al, 1980). These models strive to teach individuals how to work with others in a way that will result in positive outcomes for all. Assertiveness training permits one to communicate in ways that are direct, honest, and appropriate. Working groups allow members to observe the behavior of others as well as practice and obtain feedback on how effectively they communicate with the other members of the group.

8.4 Coping skills training

Coping skills training has been utilized by Grey and Barry (Grey & Berry, 2004) in individuals with diabetes, particularly, in the area of problem solving. The framework is derived from Bandura's conceptualization of self-efficacy, where the individuals act as the catalyst for positive changes in their lives (Bandura, 1986). When a person can practice and rehearse a new behavior, such as learning how to cope successfully with a problem situation, self-efficacy or self-concept can be enhanced. Further, by enhancing self-efficacy, problems with psychosocial well-being may be decreased. When an individual cannot cope effectively with a problem situation, confidence is decreased for dealing with the next problem, and less successful coping patterns are employed (Marlatt & Gordon, 1985).

This kind of training was originally developed for work with youth to prevent drug and alcohol use, training in the use of coping skills can teach personal and social behaviors that can assist individuals in dealing with potential stressors they encounter in their daily lives and the stress reactions that may result from these situations (Forman et al, 1993). In children and youth, such interventions have been demonstrated to reduce substance abuse (Forman et al, 1993), improve social adjustment (Bierman & Furman, 1984), prevent smoking (DelGreco et al, 1986) and reduce responses to stressors (Elias et al, 1986). In adults, coping skills training has been used to address drug and alcohol use and weight reduction.

8.5 Cognitive-behavioural modification

The cognitive-behavioural modification process comprises three steps. The first is working with the individual to reflect on how they think and then respond to situations. The individual's thoughts are then examined to consider if the thoughts are based on fact or assumption. Once the thoughts are examined the next step is to solve the social problem. The last step consists in teaching the individual to use his or her thoughts to help follow through on the decision made in the previous step. The group members can list their negative thoughts and then the member and the group can formulate alternate positive thoughts to counter the negative thoughts.

8.6 Coping skills training with children and adolescents

The use of coping skills training for youth with diabetes was based on the hypothesis that improving coping skills would improve the ability of youth to cope with the problems faced on a day-to-day basis in managing diabetes. Initially, a number of studies were conducted in five to 10 years old school-children and preadolescents using coping skills training (Gross et al, 1982; Gross et al, 1983; Johnson et al, 1982). The results of these studies suggested that coping skills training increased appropriate verbal assertiveness and performance in social situation, but not glycaemia control. An experimental pilot study by Boardway et al (Boardway et al, 1993) also supported the potential of this intervention to assist adolescents to manage diabetes, the authors observed that diabetes-specific stress was found to decrease significantly after stress management training, but glycaemia control, coping styles, self-efficacy, and adherence to regimen remained unchanged.

Some controlled studies (Davidson et al, 1997; Grey et al, 1998; Grey et al, 2000) were conducted to determine whether coping skills training would improve glycaemia and psychosocial outcomes in adolescents with type 1 diabetes mellitus implementing intensive diabetes management. They showed that, at 3 months, adolescents who received coping skills training had lower hemoglobin A1c levels and less distress about coping with their diabetes than adolescents receiving intensive management alone. Furthermore, adolescents who received coping skills training found it easier to cope with their diabetes and experienced less negative impact from diabetes on their quality of life than those who did not receive the training. The authors also demonstrated that the effects on glycaemia control and quality of life associated with coping skills training combined with intensive diabetes management can be sustained over 1 year (Grey et al, 2000).

Hains et al, (Hains et al, 2001) examined the impact of a cognitive behavioral intervention for distressed adolescents with type 1 diabetes mellitus. They studied six youths who had increased levels of anxiety, diabetes stress, or anger who received eight individual sessions using cognitive restructuring with problem solving through a conceptualization phase, skill acquisition phase, and application phase. Four patients demonstrated improvement on anxiety, anger expression, or diabetes stress, compared with baseline.

The results of the aforementioned studies suggest that in children and adolescents with type 1 diabetes, coping skills training increases the repertoire of skills that youth have to self-manage diabetes. Thus, they can improve their metabolic control and their quality of life.

8.7 Coping skills training with parents and children or adolescents

Family environment has been found to play an important role in the adaptation of children with type 1 diabetes (McDougal, 2002). It has been shown that family interventions decrease parent-child conflicts about diabetes and improve metabolic control (Grey et al, 2003; Wysocki et al, 2000; Wysocki et al, 2001). One study that includes 119 families of adolescents with type 1 diabetes mellitus, assessed the effectiveness of an experimental group receiving Behavioral-Family Systems Therapy compared to both education and support groups in reducing parent-adolescent conflict in diabetes management. The Behavioral-Family Systems Therapy intervention targeted parent-adolescent conflict by focusing on family problem solving, communication skills training, cognitive restructuring, and aspects of functional and structural family therapy over 10 sessions. The results revealed that the experimental group showed significant improvement in parent-adolescent relationships, decreased diabetes-specific family conflicts, and increased treatment adherence when compared with education and support groups. At 6-month follow-up, parent-adolescent relationships remained significantly improved for the experimental group as compared to the control group. At 12 months, diabetes-specific family conflict was significantly improved compared to the control group. The experimental group showed improved treatment adherence compared with the control and education groups that both showed deteriorated adherence (Wysocki et al, 2000; Wysocki et al, 2001).

When parental involvement decreases, which is frequent in early adolescence, the metabolic control tends to deteriorate. Anderson et al. (Anderson et al, 1995) studied an office-based intervention to maintain parent adolescent teamwork in diabetes management. The study variables included parental involvement in diabetes care, family conflict, and subsequent metabolic control. Eighty-five patients aged 10 to 15 years were randomly assigned to one of three groups, which included teamwork, attention control, or standard control for 24 months. The teamwork families reported less conflict at 12 months. More adolescents in the teamwork group when compared to the comparison groups improved their HbA1c levels from the 12- to 24-month period. The results suggested the value of parent-adolescent partnership in diabetes management.

The results of the mentioned studies of coping skills training and problem-solving interventions in children, and adolescents with diabetes, as well as parents of children with diabetes, have demonstrated that these interventions are effective in assisting people to improve diabetes self management and to achieve better diabetes outcomes (Grey & Berry, 2004).

9. The management of eating behavioral anomalies in type 1 diabetics

No treatment outcome studies to date have examined treatment efficacy for DEB and ED in type1 diabetics, for this reason, many of the recommendations have not yet been empirically evaluated. ED have been shown to convey their own significant medical risk and also appear to persist and worsen over time. Treatment aimed at promoting family co-management of diabetes treatment tasks and decreasing diabetes-related family conflict have already been shown to promote improved diabetes outcomes in children and teens with type 1 diabetes (Nansel et al, 2008).

Despite the fact that little research has been done to determine the best treatment approaches for the problem of type 1 diabetic patients with ED or DEB, a multidisciplinary care team is considered the standard to treat these people. Such a team should include an endocrinologist/diabetologist, a nurse educator, a nutritionist with ED and/or diabetes training and a psychologist or social worker to provide weekly therapy. Depending on the severity of related psychiatric symptoms, such as depression and anxiety, a psychiatrist for psychopharmacologic evaluation and treatment should also be consulted. Team members must be allowed to frequently an openly communicate with each other to maintain congruent treatment approaches, messages and goals. Patients may require a medical or psychiatric inpatients hospitalization until they are medically stable and emotionally ready to engage in treatment as outpatients. Early in the treatment, monthly appointments with a team endocrinologist or nurse educator may be necessary to maintain medical stability, and monthly appointments with the nutritionists are also recommended. Laboratory tests, especially HbA1c and electrolytes, and weight checks should occur routinely at medical appointments. Unfortunately, such specialty services are rarely available to individuals with diabetes.

As a result, detection of insulin restriction may be unlikely until after the problem has become habitual and entrenched. Goebel-Fabbri et al (Goebel-Fabbri 2008) suggest that insulin restriction can be captured by a single screening item "I take less insulin than I should". The use of this question in routine clinical practice has the potential to identify at-risk subjects and, consequently, to make possible an early intervention. However, further studies are needed to assess the clinical utility of adopting such a question as a screening tool to identify insulin restrictors.

The overall goal of the treatment of patients with type 1 diabetes and DEB and ED is to return the patients to a state of premorbid physical and mental health. Treatment begins with emphasis on nutritional rehabilitation, weight restoration and adequate diabetes control (Anzai et al, 2002; Krakoff, 1991).

Psychotherapy should begin immediately for the patient and family, but it is not effective for the patient when is in a starvation mode (Walsh et al, 2000).

9.1 Diabetes treatment

The diabetes team has the important responsibility of monitoring insulin regimens and providing education about diabetes management and potential complications to patients and families (Krakoff, 1991). There are no studies looking at treatment of ED/DEB in youth with type 1 diabetes. The traditional approaches to poor blood glucose control involving a stricter and more intensive monitoring of the diabetic management may increase the risk for disordered eating (Colton et al, 1999). For this reason, it is recommended a less rigid approach in the insulin regimen and nutrition therapy to improve DEB. Lowering the amount of time spent on diabetes management during the day may help to lessen stress associated with the diabetes, which may in turn help alleviate DEB. Krokoff (Krokoff, 1991) suggested that self-destructive insulin manipulation within the context of an ED may also be an indirect call for help, signaling the need for more parental/adult intervention in patient's physical and mental health.

Trento et al, (Trento et al, 2009) suggest that offering a carbohydrate counting program within a group care management approach may help patients with type 1 diabetes acquire better self-efficacy and restructure their cognitive and lifestyle potential.

Technological advances can also be used to address specific treatment issues seen in these patients. For example, the first challenge that most patients face is weight gain associated with insulin restart. Patients need to be taught to indentify insulin edema, which may make them feel fat, bloated and uncomfortable, as temporary water retention that is different from the development of fatty tissue. Special tools designed to measure water-related weight versus lean muscle mass versus fat mass could help patients tolerate the temporary weight gain related to edema (Goebel-Fabbri 2008). Additionally, newer insulin analogs show evidence of improving weight profiles which could be of help (Goebel-Fabbri 2008; Russell-Jones & Khan, 2007).

9.2 Nutritional management

The dietician must balance the difficult tasks of providing diabetes education, ED education, writing meal plans and defining weight goals for patients and families (Anzai et al, 2002; Krakoff, 1991). The challenge presents when trying to balance the goal of slow weight gain and /or maintenance with diabetes meal planning. As the patient continues to increase calorie intake, insulin doses will need to be adjusted to match the amount of food eaten avoiding hyperglycemia. It is recommend a realistic goal of good blood glucose control instead of optimal blood glucose levels as the body readjusts to refeeding and the patient begins to benefit from psychotherapy. Multiple daily injections regimens that use insulin to carbohydrate ratios provide greater flexibility with meal times and amounts of food but do require increased blood glucose monitoring and insulin injections. Such intense diabetes management may increase the potential for disordered eating as the child or adolescent must think constantly about the effects of food, insulin and exercise on his or her blood glucose levels. This may not be an ideal approach to diabetes meal planning during the treatment and recovery from the ED. As the individual's physical and psychological health improves, the incorporation of more flexible meal-planning strategies may be useful. Care professionals, including nutrition therapists and diabetes educators, should be sensitive to weight-related changes and concerns in youth with type 1 diabetes. It is important for all health care professionals to be aware that weight loss may be related to glycaemia control.

9.3 Psychological therapy

Psychotherapy individual, group, and family therapy are the most common ways to treat ED. There are no studies showing the best psychotherapy modality for patients with type 1 diabetes and ED or DEB. Some authors propose individual therapy to help patients to recover from ED and diabetes mismanagement (Krokoff, 1991). Adolescents with type 1 diabetes often struggle with emotional issues related to having the illness and use an ED as a maladaptive coping mechanism. Individual therapy can help patients to develop more healthy coping strategies. Often families of patients with diabetes and ED have not adequately coped with the feelings of grief related to having a chronic illness in the family and thus they have not adequately supported the patient with diabetes. Dysfuntional family dynamics can exacerbate difficulties of adjusting to the illness and of resolving issues of grief and loss associated with the diagnosis. Family therapy is recommended to help the family in developing more functional ways of relating and in addressing issues of grief and loss that may be contributing to ED symptoms.

Psychoeducation is a useful method to aid the patient to develop skills that will help him or her to cope with a chronic disease. Therefore, it can be helpful in type 1 diabetic patients who have difficulties accepting the disease.

Psycho-pharmaceutical agents may be useful to treat comorbid mental health problems (Rosen, 2003). Table 2.

One uncontrolled study of cognitive behavior therapy (Peveler & Fairburn, 1992) and several case reports of other treatment approaches for ED associated with type1 diabetes have been reported (Nielsen et al, 1987; Peveler & Fairburn, 1989; Ramirez et al, 1990). Further research is needed to demonstrate whether more intensive, prolonged or alternative interventions may have a more significant impact on metabolic control and other diabetes-related outcomes.

Components	Recommendations
Diabetes therapy	Avoid intensive insulin regimens Avoid intensive glucose monitoring Use insulin analog with better weight gain profile Measure body weight with bioimpedance devices Involve family member in metabolic control
Nutrition	Less rigid diet recommendations Avoid excessive attention to the foods Meal planning based on family customs
Psychotherapy	Family therapy Psychoeducation Individual or group psychotherapy promote self-esteem Individual psychotherapy to promote adequate coping
Pharmacotherapy	Drugs to treat comorbidities associated with ED or DEB: depression, anxiety, etc.

Table 2. Components for the treatment of type 1 diabetic patients with ED or DEB.

10. Prevention

Since most type 1 diabetic patients do not admit to having an ED, this condition is commonly detected first by health care professionals (Walsh et al, 2000). The diabetes team may be the first to discover an ED and can play a crucial role in recommending proper treatment to the patient and family. It is unlikely that diabetes management will improve until appropriate treatment begins for the concurrent ED.

The results of studies on coping skills training and problem-solving interventions in children, adolescents, and adults with diabetes, as well as parents of children with diabetes, have demonstrated that these interventions are effective assisting people to improve diabetes self-management and to achieve better diabetes outcomes.

In childhood, the data suggest that interventions should include both children or adolescents and their parents within the first years after the diagnosis to improve self-management through learning problem-solving skills. Health care providers need to pay particular attention to adolescents with poorer glycaemia control and quality of life when they intensify their treatment, because they are less likely to reach treatment goals and may require additional support. Serious problems with self-management usually emerge during early adolescence and are difficult to correct [41,42]. The family management of diabetes should include a cooperative relationship between the patient, his or her family, and the diabetes health care provider team. The complexities of diabetes care demand a multifaceted approach that includes a strong foundation of diabetes education, medical supervision, reinforcement of positive self-care behaviors, and behavioral interventions that include problem solving and coping skills training. It is imperative to use problem solving strategies with psychological support that meet the developmental stage and level of adjustment for all family members involved in diabetes care.

Clinic-based group interventions for young women with diabetes and DEB may be the most practical and nonstigmatizing approach to prevention and early intervention for this problem. Rigid approaches to the dietary management of diabetes can contribute to the development of DEB. Rigid dieting has been shown to be a risk factor for ED in nonobese, nondiabetic women (Stewart et al, 2002). In type 1 diabetic patients feelings of deprivation associated with the perceived requirement for dietary restraint may trigger episodes of binge eating and subsequent insulin omission to prevent weight gain. Further, the weight gain associated with intensive diabetes management may amplify body dissatisfaction and the drive for thinness in susceptible girls (Daneman et al, 1998; Daneman & Rodin, 1999). For these reasons less intensive regimens are recommended in the initial stage of diabetes treatment, especially in young women.

It is recommended that the health care professional who treat young women with type 1 diabetes maintain a high index of suspicion for the presence of an eating disturbance, particularly among those patients with persistent poor metabolic control, repeated episodes of ketoacidosis and/or weight and shape concerns.

Screening for disordered eating behaviors in type 1 diabetics would be the best approach to get an early detection of behavioral abnormalities in these patients, however, a validated screening tool is not available yet (Dion Kelly et al, 2005). Clinicians working with adolescent and young adult women diabetes should be cognizant of patterns that might indicate the presence of DEB in their patients. They can include extreme concerns about weight and body shape, unusual patterns of intense exercise, sometimes accompanied or followed by frequent hypoglycemia, unusually low-calorie meal plans, unexplained elevations in HbA1c values, repeated problems with diabetic ketoacidosis and amenorrhea (Olmsted et al, 2008). Recently, Markowitz et al. (Markowitz et al, 2010) proposed a 16-items diabetes-specific self-reported measure of disordered eating for brief screening tool for disordered eating in diabetes. Table 3.

Individual or group intervention aimed to increase self-esteem, appearance and body acceptance, and family-based interventions with the objective of developing flexible approaches to food and meal planning may help to avoid the development of DEBs in type 1 diabetic patients.

CLUES
Adolescents or young women with type 1 diabetes
Patients with high concern on body weight or shape
Patients with not adequate coping with diabetes
Poor metabolic control including frequent episodes of ketoacidosis
Type 1 diabetic patients with amenorhea

Table 3. Clues to early diagnose ED or DEB in type 1 diabetics

11. Conclusions

Diabetes self-management is crucial to prevent early morbidity. Although more experimental research is needed, especially in minority populations and the non-adolescent age range, the addition of coping skills training and problem solving interventions to the clinical care of patients with diabetes appears warranted. Such interventions can be incorporated into routine diabetes education programs or the content included in regular diabetes care visits. Interventions using coping skills training and problem solving for children, adolescents, and adults with diabetes and their families should be individualized to their lifestyle, respect individual differences and routines, incorporate social support, and be reinforced and followed over time. Behavioral theory should be used in the design of future approaches.

Today is well-known that disordered eating behaviors and subthreshold disordered eating disorders are more prevalent in girls with type 1 diabetes than their peers without diabetes. DEB persists over time and its rates and symptoms severity increase with age. In type 1 diabetic women, the predominant ED are BN and EDNOS. Furthermore, these patients also develop specific DEB such as diet restriction, and insulin misuse in order to lose weight, with the consequent impairment of their metabolic control which is followed by acute diabetic complications such as diabetic ketoacidosis, dehydration or electrolyte anomalies, and chronic microvascular complications, mainly diabetic retinopathy, that even increase the risk of mortality.

Full established DEB and ED are difficult to manage. The management of these conditions requires a multidisciplinary team formed by an endocrinologist/diabetologist, nurse educator, nutritionist, psychologist and, frequently, a psychiatrist who should be consulted to evaluate and treat with psycho pharmaceutical products the possible psychiatric comorbidities of these patients. Unfortunately, the mentioned team is often not available for patients.

The best psychological methods to treat these anomalies are not determined yet. According to personal experience, patients tend to be treated individually or in group and, frequently, it is needed familiar therapy. Results of the treatment of these entities from experienced health professionals are waiting.

The key for the management of type 1 diabetic patients with ED or DEB is the early diagnosis and treatment. Unfortunately, validated questionnaires to screen type 1 diabetic population are not available so far. Therefore it is important that the staff of the diabetes team who treats these patients should know the relationship between poor diabetes metabolic control and intentional misuse of insulin, or the recommended diet to control weight gain. They also should know that strict diet and intensive insulin regimens are risk factors for the development of DEB or ED. Therefore, it would be important to be alert to detect excessive concern about body weight, shape or body dissatisfaction in these patients.

Eating disorders in type 1 diabetic patients represent some of the most complex patient problems to treat both medically and psychologically. Given the extent of the problem and the severe medical risk associated with it, more clinical and technological research aimed to improve its treatment is critical to the future health of this at-risk population.

12. References

Abrams, KK., Allen, L., & Gray, JJ. (1993). Disordered eating attitudes and behaviors, psychological adjustment, and ethnic identity: a comparison of black and white female college students. *Int J Eating Disord*, Vol.14, No. 1, (July 1993), pp. 49-57.

Affenito, SG., & Adams, CH. (2001). Are eating disorders more prevalent in females with type 1 diabetes mellitus when the impact of insulin omission is considered? *Nutr Rev*, Vol. 59, No. 6, (June 2001), pp. 179-182.

Affenito, SG., Backstrand, JR., Welch, GW., Lammi-Keefe, CJ., Rodriguez, NR., & Adams, CH. (1997). Subclinical and clinical eating disorders in IDDM negatively affect metabolic control. *Diabetes Care*, Vol. 20, pp. 182-184.

Affenito, SG., Rodriguez, NR., Backstrand, JR., Welch, GW., & Adams, CH. (1998) Insulin misuse by women with type 1 diabetes mellitus complicated by eating disorders does not favorably change body weight, body composition, or body fat distribution. *J AmDiet Assoc*, Vol.98, pp. 686-688.

American Psychiatric Association. Diagnostic and statistical manual of mental disorders. 4th ed. Washington (DC): American Psychiatric Association, 1994.

Anderson, RM., Funnel, MM., Butler, PM., Arnold, MS., Fitzgerald, JT., & Feste, CC. (1995). Patient empowerment. Results of a randomized controlled trial. *Diabetes Care*, Vol. 18, pp. 943-949.

Anzai, N., Lindsay-Dudley, K., & Bidwell, RJ. (2002). Impatient and partial hospital treatment for adolescent eating disorders. *Child Adolesc Psychiatr Clin North Am* , Vol. 11, pp. 279-309.

Arriaza, CA., & Mann, T. (2001). Ethnic differences in eating disorder symptoms among college students: the confounding role of body mass index. *J Am Coll Health*, vol. 49, pp. 309-315.

Attie, I., & Brooks-Gunn, J. (1989). Development of eating problems in adolescent girls: a longitudinal study. *Dev Psychol*, vol. 25, pp. 70-79.

Baginsky, P. (2009).A battle to overcome "Diabulimia". *Am Fam Physician*, vol. 79, pp. 263.

Bandura A. (1986). Social Foundations of Thought and Action: A SocialCognitive Theory. Prentice Hall. Englewood Cliffs, NJ.

Bierman, KL., & Furman, W. (1984). The effects of social skills training andpeer involvement on social adjustment of preadolescents. *Child Development*, Vol. 55, pp. 155–162.

Birk, R., & Spencer, ML. (1987).The prevalence of anorexia nervosa, bulimia and induced glycosuria in IDDM females. *Diabetes Educ*, vol. 15, pp. 336-341.

Boardway, RH., Delameter, AM., Tomakowsky, J., & Gutai, JP. (1993). management training for adolescents with diabetes. *Journal of Pediatric Psychology*, Vol. 18, pp. 183–195.

Bogner, HR., Morales, KH., Post, EP., & Bruce, ML. (2007). Diabetes, depression, and death. *Diabetes Care*, vol. 30, pp. 3005-3010.

Bombardier. CH., D'Amico, C., & Jordan, JS. (1990). The relationship of apprisal and coping to chronic illness adjustment. *Behavioral and Research Therapy*, Vol. 28, pp. 297-304.

Bryden, KS., Neil, A., Mayou, RA., Peveler, RC., Fairburn, CG., & Dunger, DB. (1999). Eating habits, body weight and insulin misuse: a longitudinal study of teenagers and young adults with type 1 diabetes. *Diabetes Care*, vol. 22, pp. 1956-1960.

Bryden, KS., Neil, A., Peveler, RC., Fairburn, CG., & Dundger, DB. (1999). Eating habits, body weight, and insulin misused. A longitudinal study of teenagers and young adults with type 1 diabetes. *Diabetes Care*, vol. 22, pp. 1956-1960.

Carteledge, MG., & Milburn, JF.(1980). eds: *Teaching Skills to Children: Innovative Approaches.* Pergamon, Elmsford, NY.

Colas, C., Mathieu, P., & Tehobroutsky, G. (1991). Eating disorders and retinal lesions in type 1 (insulin-dependent) diabetic women (letter). *Diabetología*, vol.34, pp.288.

Colton, PA., Olmsted, MP., Daneman, D., Rydall, AC., & Rodin, GM. (2007). Five-year prevalence and persistence of disturbed eating behavior and eating disorders in girls with type 1 diabetes. *Diabetes Care*, vol. 30 pp. 2861-2862.

Colton, PA., Rodin, GM., Olmsted, MP., & Daneman, D. (1999). Eating disturbances in young women with type 1 diabetes mellitus: mechanisms and consequences. *Psychiatr Ann*, vol. 40, pp. 193-201.

Cox, DJ., & Gonder-Frederick, L. (1992). Major developments in behavioural diabetes research. *J Consult Clin Psychol*, vol. 60, pp. 628-638.

Crow, SJ., Keel, PK., & Kendall, D. (1998). Eating disorders and insulin-dependent diabetes mellitus. *Psychosomatics*, vol. 39, pp. 233-243.

Daneman, D., Olmsted, M., Rydall, A., Maharaj, S., & Rodin, G. (1998). Eating disorders in young women with type 1 diabetes: prevalence problems and prevention. *Horm Res*, vol. 50, pp. 79-86.

Daneman, D., & Rodin, G. (1999). Eag disorders in young women with type 1 diabetes: a cause for concern? *Acta Paediatr*, vol. 88, pp. 117-119.

Davidson, M., Boland, EA., & Grey, M. (1997). Teaching teens to cope: coping skills training for adolescents with diabetes mellitus. *Journal Social Pediatric Nursery*, Vol. 2, pp.65–72.

DelGreco, L., Breitbach, L., Rumer, S, McCarthy, RH., & Suissa, S. (1986). Four-year results of a youth smoking prevention program using assertiveness training. *Adolescence*, Vol. 21, pp. 631–640.

De Mont-Marin, F., Hardy, P., Lepine, JP., Halfon, P., & Feline, A. (1995). Six-month and lifetime prevalences of psychiatric disorders in patients with diabetes mellitus. *European Psych*, vol.10, pp. 245-249.

DeRidder, D., & Schreus, K. (2001). Developing interventions for chronically ill patients: is coping a helpful concept?. *Clinical Psychology Review*, Vol. 2, pp. 205-240.

Deutsch, M., & Brickman, E. (1994). Conflict resolution. *Pediatric Review,* Vol. 15, pp. 16–22.

Diabetes Control and Complications Trial Research Group (DCCT) (1993). The effect of intensive treatment of diabetes on the development and progression of long-term complications in insulin-dependent diabetes mellitus. *N Engl J Med,* vol. 329, pp. 977-986.

Dion Kelly, S., Howe, CJ., Hendler, JP.,& Lipman, TH. (2005). Disordered eating behaviors in youth with type 1 diabetes. *The Diabetes Educator,* Vol. 31, pp. 572-583.

Duangdao, KM., & Roesch, SC. (2008). Coping with diabetes in adulthood: a meta-anlysis. *Journal of Behavior Medicine,* Vol. 31, pp. 291-300.

Eisenberg, L. (1991). Treating depression and anxiety in primary care. Closing the gap between knowledge and practice. *New England Journal of Medicine,* Vol. 326, pp. 1080-1084.

Engstrom, I., Kroon, M., Advirdsson, CG., Segnestam, K., Snellman, K., & Aman, J. (1999). Eating disorders in adolescent girls with insulin-dependent diabetes mellitus: a population- based case-control study. *Acta Paediatr,* vol. 88, pp. 117-119.

Fainburn, CG., & Beglin, SJ.(1990). Studies of the epidemiology of bulimia nervosa. *Am J Psychiatry,* vol. 147, pp. 401-408.

Fairburn, CG., Peveler, RC. (1991). Davies, B., Mann, JL., & Mayou, RA. Eating disorders in young adults with insulin dependent diabetes mellitus: a controlled study. *Br Med J,* vol. 303, pp. 17-20.

Fettahoglu, EC., Koparan, C., Özatalay, E., & Turkkahraman, D. (2007). The psychological difficulties in children and adolescents with insuline dependent diabetes mellitus. *Psych in Türkiye,* vol. 9, pp. 32-36.

Figueroa-Sobrero, A., Evangelista, P., Mazza, C., Basso, P., López, SM., Scaiola, E., Honfi, M., Ferraro, M., Eandi, ML., & Walz, F. (2010).Three-year follow up of metabolic control in adolescents with type 1 diabetes with and without eating disorders. *Arch Argent Pediatr,* vol. 108, pp. 130-135.

Folkman, S., & Lazarus, RS. (1980). An analysis of coping in a middle-aged community sample. *Journal of Health and Social Behavior,* Vol. 21, pp. 219-239.

Folkman, S., & Lazarus, RS. (1985). If it changes it must be a process: Study of emotion and coping during three stages of a college examination. *Journal of Personality and Social Psychology,* Vol. 48, pp. 150–170.

Folkman, S., & Lazarus, RS. (1988). Manual for the ways of coping questionnaire. Consulting Psychologist Press. Palo Alto (CA).

Forman, SG. (1993). Coping Skills Training for Children and Adolescents. Jossey-Bass. San Francisco, CA.

Friedman, S., Vila, G., Timsit, J., Boitard, C., & Mouren-Simeoni, MC. (1995). Troubles des conduits alimentaires et equilibre metabolique dans une population de jeunes adultes diabetiques insulino-dependants. *Ann Med-Psychol,* vol. 153, pp. 282-285.

García-Reyna, NI., Gussinyer, S., Raich, RM., Gussinyer, M., Tomás, J., & Carrascosa, A. (2004). Trastornos de la conducta alimentaria en adolescentes jóvenes con diabetes mellitas tipo 1. *Med Clin (Barc),* vol. 122, pp. 690-692.

Goebel-Fabbri, AE., Franko, DL., Pearson, K., Anderson, BJ., & Weinger, K. (2008). Insulin restriction and associated morbidity and mortality in women with type 1 diabetes. *Diabetes Care,* vol. 31, pp. 415-419.

Goebel-Fabbri, AE. (2008). Diabetes and eating disorders. *J Diabetes Sci Technol*,vol. 2, pp. 530-532.

Goldstein, AP., Sprafkin, RP., Gershaw, NJ., & Klein, P. (1980). Skillstreaming the Adolescent: A Structured Learning Approach to Teaching Prosocial Skills. Research Press. Champaign.

Goldston, DB., Kovacs, M., Obrosky, DS., & Iyenger, S. (1995). A longitudinal study of life events and metabolic control among youths with insulin-dependent diabetes mellitus. *Health Psychology*, Vol. 14, pp. 409-414.

Grey, M., Boland, EA., Davidson, M., Yu, C., Sullivan-Bolyai, S., & Tamborlane, WV. (1998). Short-term effects of coping skills training as an adjunct to intensive therapy in adolescents. *Diabetes Care*, Vol. 21, pp. 902–908.

Grey, M., Boland, EA., Davidson, M., Yu, C., & Tamborlane, WV. (2000). Coping skills training for youth with diabetes mellitus has long-lasting effects on metabolic control and quality of life. *Journal of Pediatrics*, Vol.137, pp. 107–113.

Grey, M., & Berry, D. (2004). Coping skills training and problem solving in diabetes. *Current Diabetes Reports*, Vol. 4, pp. 126-131.

Gross, AM., Johnson, WC., Wildman, H., Mullett, N. (1982). Coping skills training with insulin-dependent pre-adolescent diabetics. *Child Behavior Therapy*, Vol. 3, pp. 141–153.

Gross, AM., Heiman, L., Shapiro, R., & Schultz, RM. (1983). Children with diabetes: social skills training and hemoglobin A1c levels. *Behavior Modification*, Vol. 7, pp. 151–165.

Gülseren, L., Hekimsoy, Z., Gülseren, S., Bodur, Z., & Kültür, S. (2001). Depression-anxiety, quality of life and disability in patients with diabetes mellitus. *Turkish J Psych*, Vol. 12, pp. 89-98.

Hains, AA., Davies, WH., Parton, E., & Silverman, AH. (2001). Brief report: a cognitive behavioral intervention for distressed adolescents with type I diabetes. *Journal of Pediatric Psychology, Vol.* 26, pp. 61–66.

Hasken, J., Kresl, L., Nydegger, T., & Temme, M. Diabulimia and the role of school health personnel (2010). *Journal of School Health*, Vol. 80, pp. 465-469.

Hoek, HW. (1993). Review of the epidemiological studies of eating disorders. *Int Rev Psychiatry*, vol. 5, pp. 61-74.

Hudson, JL., Wentworth, SM., Hudson, MS., & Pope, HG. (1985). Prevalence of anorexia nervosa and bulimia among young diabetic women. *J Clin Psychiatry*, vol. 46, pp. 88-93.

Johnson, SB., Pollack, R., Silverstein, J., Rosenbloom AL., Spillar R., McCallum M., & Harkavy J. (1982). Cognitive and behavioral knowledge about insulin-dependent diabetes among children and parents. *Pediatrics*, Vol. 69, pp. 708–713.

Jones, JM., Bennett, S., Olmsted, MP., Lawson, ML., & Rodin, G. (2001). Disodered eating attitudes and behaviours in teenaged girls: an Ontario school-based study. *Can Med Assoc J*, vol. 165, pp. 547-552.

Jones, JM., Lawson, ML., Daneman, D., Olmsted, MP., & Rodin, G.(2000). Eating disorders in adolescent females with and without type 1 diabetes: cross sectional study. *Br Med J*,vol. 320, pp. 1563-1566.

King, H., Aubert, RE., & Herman, WH. (1998). Global burden of diabetes, 1995–2025 – Prevalence, numerical estimates, and projections. *Diabetes Care*, vol. 21, pp. 1414-1431.

King, H., Gruber, W., & Lander, T. (1995). Implementing National Diabetes Programmes.Report of a WHO Meeting Geneva: World Health Organization Division of Non-communicable Diseases.

Koopmanschap, M. (2002). Coping with Type II diabetes: the patient's perspective. *Diabetologia*, vol.45, pp. S18-S22.

Kovacs, M., Goldston D., Obrosky, DS., & Iyenger, S. (1992). Prevalence and predictors of pervasive noncompliance with medical treatment among youths with insulin-dependent diabetes mellitus. *Journal of American Academy Childs and Adolescent Psychiatry*, Vol. 31, pp. 1112-1119.

Krakoff, DB. (1991). Eating disorders as a special problem for persons with insulin-dependent diabetes mellitus. Nurs *Clin North Am*, vol. 26, pp. 707-714.

Kumanyika, SK., Wilson, JF., & Guilford-Davenport, M. (1993). Weight-related attitudes and behaviors of black women. *J Am Diet Assoc*, vol. 93, pp. 416-422.

Lee, S. (1993). How abnormal is the desire for slimness? A survey of eating attitudes and behaviour among Chinese undergraduates in Hong Kong. *Psychol Med*, vol. 23, pp. 437-451.

Lee, AM., & Lee, S. (1996). Disordered eating and its psychosocial correlates among Chinese adolescent females in Hong Kong. *Int J Eating Disord*, vol. 20, pp. 177-183.

Lundman, B., & Norberg, A. (1993). Coping strategies in people with insulin-dependent diabetes mellitus. *Diabetic Education*, Vol. 19, pp.198-204.

Lustman, PJ., Clouse, RE., Griffith, LS., & Carney, RM. (1997). Screening for depression in diabetes using the Beck Depression Inventory. *Psychosomatic Medicine*, Vol. 59, pp. 24-31.

Llorente, MD., & Urrutia, V. (2006). Diabetes, psychiatric disorders, and the metabolic effects of antipsychotic medications. *Clin Diabetes*, vol. 24, pp. 18-26.

Lloyd, GG., Steel, JM., & Young, RJ. (1987). Eating disorders and psychiatric morbidity in patients with diabetes mellitus. *Psychother Psychosom*, vol. 48, pp. 189-195.

Maes, S., Leventhal, H., & DeRidder, D. (1996). Coping with chronic diseases. Handbook of coping. Wiley. New York.

Mannucci, E., Ricca, V., Mezzani, B., Di Bernardo, M., Piani, F., Vannini, R., Cabras, PL., & Rotella, CM. (1995). Eating attitudes and behavior in IDDM patients: a case controlled study. *Diabetes Care*, vol.18, pp. 1503-1504.

Mannucci, E., Rotella, F., Ricca, V., Moretti, S., Placidi, GF., & Rotella, CM. (2005). Eating disorders in patients with type 1 diabetes: A meta-analysis. *J Endocrinol Invest*, vol. 28, pp. 417-419.

Marcus, MD., Wing, RR., Jawad, A.,& Orchard, TJ. (1992). Eating disorders symptomatology in a registry-based sample of women with insulin-dependent diabetes mellitus. *Int J Eatting Disord*, vol.12, pp. 425-430.

Markowitz, JT., Butler, DA., Volkening, LK., Anitisdel, JE., Anderson, B., & Laffel, LMB. (2010). Brief screening tool for disordered eating in diabetes. *Diabetes Care*, Vol. 33, pp. 495-500.

Marlatt, GA., & Gordon, JR. (1985). Relapse Prevention: Maintenance Strategies in Addictive Behavior Change. The Guilford Press. New York, NY.

McDougal, J. (2002). Promoting normalization in families with preschool children with type 1 diabetes. *Journal of Specialty Pediatric Nursering*, Vol. 7, pp. 113–120.

Meltzer, LJ., Bennett Johnson, S., Prine, JM., Banks, RA., Desrosiers, PM., & Silverstein, JH. (2001). Disordered eating, body mass and glycaemia control in adolescents with type 1 diabetes. *Diabetes Care*, vol. 24, pp.678-682.

Nansel, TR., Anderson, BJ., Laffel, LM., Simons-Morton, BG., Weissberg-Benchell, J., Wysocki, T., Iannotti, RJ., Holmbeck ,GN., Hood, KK., & Lochrie, AS. (2009). A multisite trial of a clinic-integrated intervention for promoting family management of pediatric type 1 diabetes: feasibility and design. *Pediatr Diabetes*, vol. 10, pp.105-115.

National Centre for Health Statistics. 2011. USA Government.

Neumark-Sztainer, D., Patterson, J., Mellin, A., Ackard, DM., Utter, J., Story, M., & Sockalosky, J. (2002). Weight control practices and disordered eating behaviors among adolescent females and males with type 1 diabetes: associations with sociodemographics, weight concerns, familial factors, and metabolic outcomes. *Diabetes Care*, vol.25, pp.1289-1296.

Neumark-Sztainer, D., Story, M., Falkner, NH., Beuhring, T., & Resnick, M. (1998). Disordered eating among adolescents with chronic illness and disability. *Arch Pediatr Adolesc Med*, vol. 152, pp.871-878.

Neumark-Sztainer, D., Story, M., Resnick, M., Garwick, A., & Blum, R. (1995). Body dissatisfaction and unhealthy weight-control practices among adolescents with and without chronic illness: a population-based study. *Arch Pediatr Adolesc Med*, vol. 149, pp.1330-1335.

Nielsen, S., Borner, H., & Kabal, M. (1987). Anorexia nervosa/ bulimia in diabetes mellitus: a review and presentation of 5 cases. *Acta Psychiatr Scand*, vol.75, pp.464-473.

Olmsted, MP., Coton, PA., Daneman, D., Rydall, AC., & Rodin, GM. (2008). Prediction of the onset of disturbed eating behavior in adolescent girls with type 1 diabetes. *Diabetes Care*, Vol. 31, pp. 1978-1982.

Peveler, RC., Bryden, KS., Neil, HAW., Fairburn, CG., Mayou, RA., Dunger, DB., & Turner, HM. (2005). The relationship of disordered eating habits and attitudes to clinical outcomes in young adult females with type 1 diabetes. *Diabetes Care*, vol. 28, pp.84-88.

Peveler, RC., & Fairburn, CG. (1999). Anorexia nervosa in association with diabetes mellitus: a cognitive-behavioural approach to treatment. *Behav Res Ther*, vol.27, pp.95-99.

Peveler, RC., & Fairburn, CG. (1992). The treatment of bulimia nervosa in patients with diabetes mellitus. *Int J Eating Disord*, vol.11, pp.45-53.

Peveler, RC., Fairburn, CG., Boller, I., & Dunger, DB. (1992). Eating disorders in adolescents with IDDM: a controlled study. *Diabetes Care*, vol. 15, pp.1356-1360.

Polivy, J., & Herman, CP. (1985). Dieting and binging: a casual analysis. *Am Psychol*, vol. 40, pp.193-201.

Polonsky, WH., Anderson, BJ., Lohrer, PA., Aponte, JE., Jacobson, AM., & Cole, CF. (1994). Insulin omission in women with IDDM. *Diabetes Care*, vol.17, pp.1178-1185.

Pollock, M., Kovacs, M., & Charron-Prochownik, D. (Eating disorders and maladaptive dietary/insulin management among youths with childhood-onset insulin-dependent diabetes mellitus

Powers, PS., Malone, JL., Coovert, DL., & Schulman, RG. (1990). Insulin-dependent diabetes mellitus and eating disorders: a prevalence study. *Compr Psychiatry*, vol.31, pp.205-210.

Robertson, P., & Rosenvinge, JH. (1990). Insulin-dependent diabetes mellitus: a risk factor in anorexia nervosa or bulimia nervosa? An empirical study of 116 women. *J Psychosom Res*, vol. 34, pp.535-541.

Ramirez, LC., Rosenstock, J., Strowig, S., Cercone, S., & Raskin P. (1990). Effective treatment of bulimia with fluoxetine, a serotonin reuptake inhibitor in patient with type 1 diabetes mellitus. *Am J Med*, vol. 88, pp. 540-541.

Rodin, G., Craven, J., Littlefield, C., Goldbloom, D., & Daneman, D. (1989). Insulin misuse through omission or reduction of dose. Psychosomatics, vol.30, pp.465-466.

Rodin, G., Craven, J., Littlefield, C., Murray, M., & Daneman, D. (1991). Eating disorders and intentional insulin undertreatment in adolescent females with diabetes. *Psychosomatics*, vol.32, pp.171-176.

Rodin, G., & Daneman, D. (1992). Eating disorders and IDDM: a problematic association. *Diabetes Care*, vol.15, pp.1402-1412.

Rodin, GM., Daneman, D., Johnson, LE., Kenshole, A., & Garfinkel, P. (1985). Anorexia nervosa and bulimia in female adolescents with insulin dependent diabetes mellitus: a systematic study. *J Psychiatr Res*, vol. 19, pp.381-384.

Rodin, GM., Johnson, LE., Garfinkel, P., Daneman, D., & Kenshole, A. (1986/1987). Eating disorders in female adolescents with insulin dependent diabetes mellitus. *Int J Psychiatry Med*, vol.16, pp. 49-57.

Rodin, GM., Olmsted, MP., Rydall, AC., Maharaj, SI., Colton, PA., Jones, JM., Biancucci, LA., & Daneman, D. (2002). Eating disorders in young women with type 1 diabetes mellitus. *J Psychosom Res*, vol. 53, pp.943-949.

Rosen, DS. (2003). Eating disorders in children and young adolescents: etiology, classification, clinical features and treatment. *Adolesc Med*, vol.14, pp. 49-59.

Rosmark, B., Berne, C., Holmgrem, S., Lago, C., Renholm, G., & Sohlberg, S. (1986). Eating disorders in patients with insulin-dependent diabetes mellitus. *J Clin Psychiatry*, vol. 47, pp.547-550.

Rubin. RR., & Payrot, M. (2001). Psychological Issues and Treatments for People with Diabetes. *Journal of Clinical Psychology*, vol. 57, pp.457-462.

Russell-Jones, D., & Khan, R. (2007). Insulin-assosociated weight gain in diabetes-causes, effects and coping strategies. *Diabetes Obesity & Metabolism*, Vol. 9, pp. 799-812.

Ruth-Sahd, LA., Schneider, M., & Haagen, B. (2009). Diabulimia: what it is and how to recognize it in critical care. *Dimens Crit Care Nurs*, vol. 28, pp. 147-153.

Ryan, M., Gallanagh, J., Livingstone, MB., Gaillard, C., & Ritz P. (2008). The prevalence of abnormal eating behaviour in a representative sample of the French diabetic population. *Diabetes & Metabolism*, vol. 34, pp.581-586.

Rydall, AC., Rodin, GM., Olmsted, MP., Devenyi, RG., & Daneman, D. (1997). Disordered eating behavior and microvascular complications in young women with insulin-dependent diabetes mellitus. *N Engl J Med*, vol.336, pp.1849-1854.

Smari, J., & Valtysdottir, H. (1997). Dispositional coping, psychological distress, and disease-control in diabetes. *Personality and Individual Differences*, Vol. 22, pp. 151–156.

Stancin, T., Link, DL., & Reuter, JM. (1989). Binge eating and purging in young women with IDDM. *Diabetes Care*, vol. 12, pp.601-603.

Stanton, AL., Collins, CA., & Sworowski, LA. (2001). Adjustment to chronic illness: Theory and research. In: *Handbook of health psychology*, Baum A, Revenon TA & Singer JS, pp. 387-403, Mahway NK, Erlbaum.

Steel, JM., Young, RJ., Lloyd, GG., & Clarke, BF. (1987). Clinically apparent eating disorders in young diabetic women: associations with painful neuropathy and other complications. *Br Med J*, vol. 294, pp.859-862.

Stewart, TM., Williamson, DA., & White, MA. (2002). Rigid vs. flexible dieting: association with eating disorder symptoms in nonobese women. *Appetite*, vol. 38, pp. 39-40.

Striegel-Moore, RH., Nicholson, TJ., & Tamborlane, WV. (1992). Prevalence of eating disorder symptoms in preadolescent and adolescent girls with IDDM. *Diabetes Care*, vol. 15, pp.1361-1368.

Trento, M., Borgo, E., Kucich, C., Passera, P., Trinetta, A., Charrier, L., Cavallo, F., & Porta, M. (2009). Quality of life , coping ability, and metabolic control in patients with type 1 diabetes managed by group care and a carbohydrate counting program. *Diabetes Care*, Vol. 32, pp. e134.

Tuncay, T., Musabak, I., Engin Gok, D., & Kutlu, M. (2008). The relationship between anxiety, coping strategies and characteristics of patients with diabetes. *Health and Quality of Life Outcomes*, Vol. 6, pp. 79-88.

UKPDS Group (1998). Intensive blood-glucose control with sulphonylureas or insulin compared with conventional treatment and risk of complications in patients with type 2 diabetes. *Lancet*, Vol. 352, pp. 837–843.

Vila, G., Nollet-Clemencon, C., Vera, L., Crosnier, H., Robert, JJ., & Mouren-Simeoni, MC. (1993). Etude des troubles des conduits alimentaires dans une population d`adolescents souffrant de diabete insulino-dependant. *Can J Psychiatry*, vol.38, pp. 606-610.

Vila, G., Robert, JJ., Nollet-Clemencon, C., Vera, L., Crosnier, H., Rault, G., Jos, J., & Mouren-Simeoni, MC. (1995). Eating and emotional disorders in adolescent obese girls with insulin-dependent diabetes mellitus. *Eur Child Adolesc Psychiatry*, vol. 4, pp. 270-279.

Walker, JD., Young, RJ., Little, J., & Steel, JM. (2002). Mortality in concurrent type 1 diabetes and anorexia nervosa. *Diabetes Care*, Vol. 25, pp. 1664-1665.

Walsh, JME., Wheat, ME., & Freund, K. (2000). Detection, evaluation and treatment of eating disorders: the role of the primary care physician. *J Gen Intern Med*, vol.15, pp.577-590.

Ward, A., Troop, N., Cachia, M., Watkins, P., & Treasure, J. (1995). Doubly disabled: diabetes in combination with an eating disorder. *Postgrad Med J*, vol. 71, pp.546-550.

Wing, RR., Nowalk, MP., Marcus, MD., Koeske, R., & Finegold, D. (1986). Subclinical eating disorders and glycaemia control in adolescents with type 1 diabetes. *Diabetes Care*, vol. 9, pp.162-167.

White, NE., Richter, JM., & Fry, C. (1992). Coping, social support and adaptation to chronic illness. *Western Journal of Nursing Research*, Vol. 14, pp. 211–224.

Wysocki, T., Greco, P., Harris, MA., Bubb, J., & White, NH. (2001). Behavior therapy for families of adolescents with diabetes: maintenance of treatment effects. *Diabetes Care*, Vol. 24, pp. 441–446.

Wysocki, T., Harris, MA., Greco, P., Bubb, J., Danda, CE., Harvey, LM., McDonell, K., Taylor, A., & White, NH. (2000). Randomized controlled trial of behavior therapy for families of adolescents with insulin-dependent diabetes mellitus. *Journal of Pediatric Psychology*, Vol. 25, pp. 23–33.

7

Predictors of Adherence, Metabolic Control and Quality of Life in Adolescents with Type 1 Diabetes

M. Graça Pereira[1], A. Cristina Almeida[2], Liliana Rocha[1] and Engrácia Leandro[2]
[1]*University of Minho, School of Psychology*
[2]*University of Minho, Social Sciences Institute*
Portugal

1. Introduction

Diabetes Mellitus Type I (DM1) is a diagnosed disease that appears before age 35 (Hanas, 2007) and is well known, in the pediatric population, as one of the most common diseases (Serafino, 1990). The diagnosis occurs mostly in childhood and adolescence, often between ages 5 and 11 (Eiser, 1990).
The definition of adolescence is a bit controversial but OMS (1965) establishes adolescence between 10 and 19 years old. The beginning of adolescence starts with the appearance of the first biological changes of puberty. According to Erikson's theory of psychosocial development (Erikson, 1968), the central task of adolescence is the development of autonomy, identity and self integration (Barros, 2003). In fact, identity formation, in adolescence, requires a reorganization of capacities, desires, needs and interests in the adolescent, as well as a quest for more independence towards parents. Nevertheless, the difficulties, even in the well succeeded resolution of the psychosocial tasks, may result in "identity confusion" (Erikson, 1968). In adolescents with diabetes, the disease can be an additional stressor functioning as another factor that requires acceptation and self integration. Diabetes exposes adolescents to potentially unpleasant experiences (having to explain others about the disease, medical exams, etc.) that can limit or prevent normal development and life experiences in adolescence (Close et al., 1986). On the other hand, physiological and hormonal changes that take place in adolescence may increase insulin resistance contributing to a weak control of diabetes (Duarte, 2002). In short, adolescence is a developmental phase, marked by changes and identity formation ,that requires a permanent and dynamic adaptation of the adolescent, ranging from feelings of acceptation to anger/anxiety and even depression (Leite, 2005) that can affect adherence to therapy and adaptation to illness. It is important to keep in mind that *being adolescent* is more important than *being diabetic* (Burroughs et al., 1997).

1.1 Adherence and metabolic control

Adherence to therapy in chronic disease is considered one of the main problems that may end in treatment failure (Leite, 2005). Kristeller and Rodin, in 1984, suggested that adherence to treatment was built on three dimensions: 1) Adherence (compliance) that refers to the degree of acceptance of the individual towards prescriptions and medical recommendation; 2) Adherence towards keeping and following the treatment that was agreed in the previous phase, and 3) Adherence (maintenance) to diabetes' self care tasks that have been integrated in the person's life style. Throughout these phases, the diabetic acquires control and develops the autonomy necessary in the maintenance phase.

Any detour from the treatment plan is defined as non adherence to therapy (Bishop, 1994) and can range from missing appointments, forgetting to take insulin (or take more or less than the prescribed amount) to not following the nutritional or the exercise plan. In DM1, adherence is often assessed through hemoglobin levels (HbA1c), (Sperling, 1996). The relationship between therapy adherence and metabolic control is complex and probably bidirectional i.e. low adherence to therapy is often preceded by a weak metabolic control and vice versa (Kakleas et al., 2009). However, there is some controversial regarding this issue. For some, HbA1c is the most valid indicator of adherence to therapy (DCCT, 1994) for others, there isn't a direct relationship between HbA1c and adherence (Silva et al., 2002).

The weak adherence to self-care in diabetes seems to result from a multifactor combination (Fagulha et al., 2004). Warren and Hixenbaugh, in 1998, found demographic variables to weakly predict adherence to self care in diabetes. Some studies have revealed that adolescents typically are less adherent to therapy than children, regarding insulin administration, exercise, nutrition and self monitoring of glucose (Hirschberg, 2001). Each adolescent apprehends and creates meanings about diabetes and its treatment's demands and how (s)he deals with them, in the social context, influences adherence to diabetes (Barros, 2003). Moreover, puberty changes, psychological dilemmas characteristic of adolescence (La Greca, 1992) and cognitive development may also contribute to an increase in non-adherence. Also, immaturity of thought, in adolescence, based on invulnerability may be one of the main causes of low adherence to diabetes treatment (Santos, 2001; Elkind, 1984), in adolescence.

In children and adolescents with diabetes, adherence is higher after diabetes diagnosis and deteriorates over time (Jacobson et al., 1987). On the other hand, non-adherence happens in average 3,5 years after the diagnosis and around age 15 (Anderson & Laffel, 1997). Compared to younger children and adults, adolescents exhibit poorer self-care behavior (Anderson et al., 1990) and poorer metabolic control (Kovacs et al., 1989).ADA (American Diabetes Association, 2003) recommends, as a therapeutic goal, that HbA1c stays below 7%.

Diabetics between 11 and 18 years old show a weak metabolic control (Mortensen et al., 1998; Fagulha et al., 2004). In the first years of diagnosis, lack of knowledge about the disease can affect metabolic control in children and adolescents (Butler et al., 2008) and, after this first phase, adolescents' compliance with treatment depends on adherence to self care tasks and to the degree of parenting supervision regarding disease management (Anderson et al., 1997). According to the authors, in an early phase, parents show more involvement in tasks related to treatment, particularly insulin administration, that best predicts metabolic control. However, throughout adolescence, parental involvement diminishes resulting in a decrease of adherence to therapy and, therefore, in a weak metabolic control.

Differences in adherence and metabolic control, in DM1, by gender, have been reported in the literature (Mortensenn & Hougaard, 1997). Girls tend to present a weaker adherence and poor metabolic control compared to boys. Girls enter puberty earlier than boys and a poor metabolic control is associated to normal physiological changes, in adolescence, such as increased levels of hormones responsible for insulin resistance (Carroll & Shade, 2005). However, other behavioral and psychosocial factors also tend to contribute to non-adherence in diabetes such as feeling reluctant in doing self monitoring of blood glucose, having irregular meals and not complying with the correct insulin doses.
Some studies show a relationship between bad metabolic control and family dysfunction, namely conflict in the family and low family cohesion, although this relationship has not been found in other studies. In fact, higher levels of cohesion and family stability have been related to better boundary definition between family subsystems and, as a result, more incentive to autonomy, more effective family communication and better metabolic control in diabetic adolescents (Fisher et al., 1982). Also, poor social support was found to predict bad metabolic control and low adherence to self care in diabetic adolescents (Fukunishi et al., 1998). In order to overcome the difficulties, related to adherence and metabolic control, it's important to concentrate on the adolescents' social competencies, family support and friends' support (Pereira & Almeida, 2008). There are several factors, that go beyond adherence to self care in diabetes, that can influence metabolic control. Therefore, a lack of a relationship between adherence and metabolic control may be due to insufficient rigorous efforts in adherence 's evaluation (McNabb, 1997).

1.2 Family functioning

The presence of a chronic disease, in a family's member, is a stressor for the entire family limiting the family's ability to go on with usual tasks and psychosocial roles requiring, as a result, flexibility in the family's system (Northam et al., 1996). Family functioning and a supportive parental style have been associated to better adherence to treatment (Manne et al., 1993). Conflict and family dysfunction predicted low adherence to self care in diabetes (Miller-Johnson et al., 1994) while higher levels of social support, cohesion and organization were associated to better metabolic control and adherence. Adolescents with better metabolic control seem to have parents that encourage independence, express feelings openly and communicate directly. On the other hand, adolescents with poor metabolic control have parents that are more critical, suspicious or indifferent to treatment (Anderson et al., 1981). However, the relationship between family functioning (cohesion, good communication, no conflict) and metabolic control is controversial since some studies found this association (Wysocki, 1993; Seiffge-krenke, 1998; La Greca & Thompson, 1998) but others have failed (Kovacs et al., 1989; Wysocki et al., 2001).

1.3 Family social support

Low adherence in diabetes has been associated to low family support and less parental supervision (Beveridge et al., 2006). In an initial phase, after diagnosis, adolescents receive more supervision from parents and adherence is stronger compared to late adolescence, when there is an increasing worry with body image, sexuality and independence from parental and authority figures (Jacbson et al., 1987). Relationships with others, at home or at school, play an important role in adolescence (Papalia et al., 2001). In an attempt to prove they belong and are like their peers, adolescents may abandon the therapeutic regimen (Fagulha et al., 2004). In fact, diabetes treatment does not help adherence i.e. daily insulin administration and the fact that diabetes treatment only avoids negative repercussions in the long term without bringing positive consequences, creates difficulties regarding adherence (Hanson et al., 1989).

Research has shown a relationship among social support, adolescents/family's characteristics and metabolic control in DM1 (Hanson et al., 1989; Wysocki, 1993). A family that provides warmth, advice, and adequate problem solving's strategies promotes adherence (Ellerton et al., 1996). From a developmental perspective, during childhood, parents assume the responsibility for the treatment regimen, however, in adolescence, the responsibility tends to be transferred to the adolescent and often, one or more treatment's components may not be followed. Family support is considered more important for younger adolescents or for those with a shorter duration of the disease (Stern & Zevon, 1990). Parents are the bigger suppliers of social support (more than friends) in diabetes treatment (Hanson et al., 1989) and, as a result, adolescents with parents less involved or with parents that provide poor support show less adherence to therapy and show a lower metabolic control. Nevertheless, in some studies, parental support has been positivity associated to adolescent's adherence but not to metabolic control (Hanson et al., 1989). The authors defend the hypothesis that family support may have a direct effect on adherence given parent's supervision over treatment's tasks. Due to the need for autonomy and independence, parents' support to deal with diabetes' psychosocial tasks may not always be desirable and adolescents may prefer to solve their problems alone or with friends' help.

1.4 Parental coping

There are few studies regarding parents' coping strategies towards diabetes. Some studies reveal that parents cope well with their children' diabetes (Macrodimitris & Endler, 2001) but others have problems adapting to the disease (e.g. Kovacs & Feinberg, 1982). Adequate coping strategies to deal with diabetes include family involvement and/or sharing tasks, participation of adolescent and family in support groups, knowledge about the disease, use of assertive behaviors in social environment and reorganization of meals. Recently, a study revealed differences between fathers and mothers regarding the use of coping strategies (Correia, 2010). Mothers show greater responsibility, in the daily care tasks of the diabetic adolescent, being responsible for blood glucose records, meals plan and insulin administration (Zanetti & Mendes, 2001). In fact, mothers often seek information regarding the onset and course of diabetes (Nunes & Dupas, 2004).

The strategies used by caregivers may create potential difficulties and obstacles to adherence and metabolic control in diabetes. Sometimes, when confronted with chronic disease, parents' response to stressful situations may lead to a family rupture influencing, as a result, the adolescent and family's adaptation to illness (Trindade, 2000). Some parents, after the diagnosis, cease participating in social parties and forbid the adolescent to eat sweets, transforming social interactions that involve food, in uncomfortable situations for the adolescent, particularly when related to peers (Nunes & Dupas, 2004). This type of coping strategies exacerbate dependency in the adolescent with diabetes increasing parent's stress since they feel they need to protect and control the adolescent in all situations and, as a result, family life needs to be organized and centered on the illness (Brito & Sadala, 2009).

1.5 Illness representations

The self regulation behavior model (Leventhal et al., 1992) emphasizes the importance of beliefs regarding adherence to treatment. In fact, illness representations play a role in personal decisions towards adherence to treatment, in diabetes' self care (Gonder-Frederick et al., 2002). In adults, recent research found that illness representations regarding diabetes accounted for the diversity in disease-related functioning (Petrie et al., 1996). Illness representations are concerned with those variables that patients themselves believe to be central to their experience of illness and its management. Edgar and Skinner, in 2003, described Leventhal's five dimensions of illness representations (Leventhal et al, 1980; Leventhal et al., 1984): *identity,* the label and symptoms associated with the illness (e.g., thirst); *cause,* beliefs about the factors responsible for the onset of illness; *timeline,* perceptions about the duration of illness; *consequences,* illness expected outcomes regarding physical, psychological, social, and economic functioning on a daily basis and in the long term; and *control/cure/treatment,* beliefs regarding the cure of the disease and patient's control over it. Later research, extended the original model adding more items by splitting the control dimension into personal control and treatment control; including also a cyclical timeline dimension; an overall comprehension of illness, and finally, an emotional representation of the illness (Moss-Morris et al., 2002).

In adolescents with diabetes, illness representations have been associated to medical and psychological outcomes. In particular, treatment effectiveness' beliefs have been associated to self-care (Griva et al., 2000; Skinner & Hampson, 2001; Skinner et al., 2002) and perceived consequences to lower levels of emotional well-being (Skinner et al., 2000; Skinner & Hampson, 2001). Illness representations, particularly consequences and emotional representations have been found to predict quality of life (Paddison et al., 2008). The belief that diabetes was a temporary disease, than a lifelong condition, and the perception that diabetes had serious consequences predicted poor metabolic control. Also a perception of control, over the course of illness, has been positively associated to quality of life (Paddison et al., 2008).

1.6 School support

Most of the research on DM1 focused on family support and its implications on adherence, as previously described and did not take in consideration school's support. However, managing a chronic illness in adolescents, who are trying to become independent from their families and integrate in their peer group, is not easy (Holmbeck et al., 2000). In fact, as the adolescent grows, peer relationships become paramount and an important source of emotional support (Wysocki & Greco, 2006). However, research on the implications of peers support on adherence, metabolic control and quality of life is scarce. Peer conflict has been associated to poor metabolic control in girls (Hegelson et al., 2009) and friend support has been related to adherence to blood glucose testing (Bearman & La Greca, 2002). Regardless of whether support from friends is associated to diabetes self-care and metabolic control, support from friends may always help adolescents to better adjust psychologically to diabetes (La Greca et al., 1995).

When faced with the choice of appropriate self-care behavior, older adolescents have better problem solving skills but are more vulnerable to non-adherence in the face of peer pressure (Thomas et al., 1997). Another study showed that adolescents, who perceive their friends reacting negatively to their diabetes' self-care behavior, report more stress which, in turn, is associated to poor metabolic control (Hains et al., 2007).

Research examining the positive and negative aspects of friends and peers, on diabetes outcomes and psychological well-being, is not clear. There seems to be more evidence that conflictual relationships are more harmful than supportive relations are beneficial, which is consistent with the literature on healthy adults (Helgson, 2006). Besides peers' support, teachers' support is also important. A study found that 9 % of parents had to change glucose monitoring and 16% changed treatment administration because of lack of support from teachers (Amillategui et al., 2007). In fact, teachers in general need to be knowledgeable of hyperglycemia and hypoglycemia's episodes in order to assist the adolescent if needed. Support from friends and peers are key factors that help the integration of the adolescent teenager in the school setting, facilitating adaptation to diabetes.

Although diabetes does not cause pain on adolescents, impacts nonetheless, the adolescent and family's daily living and, therefore, the quality of life of all involved (Hanas, 2007) at physical, emotional, social and family 's levels (Pereira et al., 2008).

1.7 Quality of Life (QOL)

Girls perceived lower levels of QOL compared to boys. Worries about metabolic control increase with age but, regardless of gender, as age increases QOL decreases (Hoey et al., 2001). Adolescents who monitor their glucose levels, several times a day, reported better quality of life (Novato, 2009). The monitoring of blood glucose levels allows the teenager to know the variation of blood sugar, over time, perceiving what behaviors impact metabolic control, resulting in better quality of life (Novato, 2009). Regarding the association between quality of life and adherence to self-care in diabetes, literature is contradictory. Diabetes treatment has adverse effects on quality of life (Watkins et al., 2000). In fact, adolescents with diabetes need to follow a set of requirements that can negatively impact the perception of their quality of life and interaction with others. However, other studies conclude that adherence to diabetes care is not related to quality of life (e.g. Snoek, 2000). Diabetics with good metabolic control (measured through glycated hemoglobin) show better quality of life (e.g Glasgow et al., 1997; Silva, 2003) however, in some studies, this relationships has not been found and, in other studies, this relationship is very weak or does not exist (e.g. Grey et al., 1998; Laffel et al., 2003). Family also plays an important role in the perception of adolescents' QOL because QOL is affected by how the family deals with the disease (Hanson, 2001). Family conflict predicts lower QOL in adolescents (Dickenson et al., 2003). Family environment was shown to influence QOL as well as adherence and metabolic control in adolescents with diabetes (Pereira et al., 2008).

While there is a growing interest in psychological issues in diabetes, it is important to identify which variables predict better outcomes. The present study aims to answer this question namely understanding the relationship between psychological variables and diabetes outcomes. The purpose is to find the best predictors of adherence, metabolic control and quality of life in adolescents with type 1 diabetes taking in consideration adolescent variables and family variables. Due to the fact that research on adolescents and chronic illness have failed to incorporate gender (Miller & La Greca, 2005), the present study considers gender in the regression models.

2. Methods

2.1 Sample characteristics

A convenient sample of 170 subjects participated in the study: 85 adolescents and 85 family members that accompanied the teenager to their routine medical appointments, in a diabetes pediatric unit in two central Hospitals, and in a Diabetics Association. All teens received treatment in the hospital and therefore no differences were present between the sample from the Diabetics Association versus Hospitals.

All participants (teenagers and family members) were volunteers. Adolescents' criteria for inclusion were: age between 12 and 19 years, fulfilling ISPAD (1995) criteria for the diagnosis of type 1 diabetes, having a diagnosis longer than a year, being in ambulatory treatment, absence of another chronic and/or mental disease, not being pregnant and having normal cognitive development.

2.2 Procedure

Questionnaires were answered separately by adolescents and family members after they had been informed of the study's goals and filled the informed consent. The value of glycated hemoglobin (HbA1c) was determined by a nurse who collected a drop of blood from the adolescent before the medical appointment. Criteria of good metabolic control was based on ISPAD (2009) i.e. smaller than 7,5% is considered optimal, 7,5% - 9,0% suboptimal and higher than 9%, high risk.

2.3 Instruments

2.3.1 Adolescents and parent

Clinical, Socio-Demographic Questionnaire (Pereira et al., 2010) that reports gender and age in adolescents and their family members as well as metabolic control (glycated hemoglobin) and duration of disease, in the adolescent.

Brief Illness Perception Questionnaire - Brief-IPQ - Broadbent et al. (2006), (Portuguese version of Figueiras & Alves, 2007). The Brief-IPQ is a 9 items questionnaire, measuring cognitive and emotional representations of illness, that includes nine dimensions of illness perceptions: consequences, timeline, personal control, treatment control, identity, concern, coherence, emotional representation and causal representations. Both adolescents and parents answered the questionnaire. *Higher results indicate a more threatening perception of illness.* Due to the fact that each subscale includes only one item, it is not possible to calculate an alpha. As a result, like in the original version, pearson correlations between dimensions were calculated. In adolescents, significant correlations were present between consequences and emotional representation (r=.635), personal control and coherence (r=.511) and personal control and treatment control (r=.371). In the family sample, significant correlations were obtained between consequences and emotional representation (r=.558), personal control and coherence (r=.522) and between concern and coherence (r=.324).

2.3.2 Adolescents

Self Care Inventory – SCI - La Greca, A. (1992), (Portuguese version of Almeida & Pereira, 2010). It´s a 14 items questionnaire assessing adherence to diabetes treatment's recommendations regarding self care that includes four subscales: blood glucose regulation, insulin and food regulation, exercise and emergency precautions. *Higher results indicate more adherence.* Only the full scale was considered in the present study. Internal consistency in the original version was .80 and in this sample was .73.

Diabetes Family Behaviour Scale - DFBS - McKelvey et al., (1993), (Portuguese version of Almeida & Pereira (in press). DFBS is a 47 items questionnaire that assesses family support given to the adolescent in diabetes self care. It is composed of two subscales: Guidance-Control (15 items) and Warmth-Caring (15 items). The remaining 17 items do not belong to any of the subscales. *High results indicate less social support.* Internal consistency, in the original version, was .86, .81 and .79 for the full scale, guidance-control and warmth-caring, respectively. The Portuguese version showed an alpha of .91 (total scale), .76 (guidance-control) and .81 (warmth-caring.). In this study only the full scale was considered (alpha of .75).

Diabetes Quality of Life - DQoL - Ingersoll & Marrero (1991), (Portuguese version of Almeida & Pereira (2008). DQol is a 52 items questionnaire that assesses quality of life in patients with diabetes that includes three subscales: impact of diabetes (23 items); worries towards diabetes (11 items) and satisfaction (towards treatment: 7 items; towards life in general: 10 items) and one item that assesses health and quality of life. Higher results indicate lower quality of life. In the original version, the alpha for the total subscale was .92, followed by .86 (satisfaction), .85 (impact of diabetes) and .82 (worries towards diabetes). In this sample alphas were .89 (total scale), .71 (impact on diabetes), .82 (worries towards diabetes) and .87 (satisfaction). All the subscales were considered in the hypothesis testing.

School Support (Pereira & Almeida, 2009). School Support is a 6 items questionnaire that measures school support (e.g. healthy snacks available in cafeteria) and peer support regarding daily diabetes' management (e.g. feeling supported by fiends regarding diabetes). *Higher results indicate more school support.* The alpha in this sample was .81.

2.3.3 Parent

Family Assessment Device - FAD - Epstein et al., (1983), (Portuguese version provided by Ryan et al., 2005). It´s a 60 items questionnaire distributed by seven subscales: Problems Solving, Communication, Roles, Affective Responsiveness; Affective Involvement; Behavior control and General Functioning. *Higher results indicate low family functioning.* In the original version, Epstein, Baldwin and Bishop (1983) found the following results: Problem solving: .74; Communication: .75; Roles: .72; Affective responsiveness: .83; Affective involvement: .78; Behavior Control: .72 and General Functioning: .92. Only the full scale was used in the present study and the alpha, in the present sample, was .93.

Coping Health Inventory for Parents - CHIP - McCubbin et al., (1983), (Portuguese version of Pereira & Almeida, 2001). CHIP is a 45 items questionnaire that measures parents' response to management of family life when they have a child who is seriously and/or chronically ill. It includes three subscales: 1) Maintaining family integration, cooperation and an optimist definition of the situation; 2) Maintaining social support, self-esteem and psychological stability; and 3) Understanding the medical situation through communication with other parents and consultation with medical staff. *Higher results indicate better coping*. In the original version, the alpha for the first and second subscale was .79 and .71 for the third. In this sample, alphas were: .65 for the first subscale, .79 for the second and .71 for the last subscale.

3. Data analysis

First, descriptive statistics were performed to find the rate of adherence to self-care, metabolic control and quality of life. Hierarchical regression analyses were later performed to identify the best predictors of adherence to self-care, metabolic control and quality of life. Due to the size of the sample, regression analysis were first performed taking in consideration all variables ,except illness perceptions, and later including only them in the regression equation. The first regression was performed using the method *enter* since the selection of variables was based on previous research. The second regression, due to its exploratory nature, was performed using the stepwise method.
For both regressions, the variables considered in the first step were socio-demographic and clinical variables i.e. gender of the adolescent, duration of disease and values of glycated hemoglobin. In the first regression analysis, the second step included adolescents' psychosocial variables i.e. family support, quality of life, adherence and school support. The third step included family variables i.e. family functioning and coping. In the second regression analysis, the second step included adolescents' illness perceptions and the third step included family member's illness perceptions.

4. Results

4.1 Sample caracteristics

The sample consisted of 85 adolescents, 51% males and 49% females. Their age ranged from 12 to 19 with an average of 15.13 (SD=1.97), 15.12 for males (SD=2.00) and 15.14 for females (SD=1.96). Glycated hemoglobin in the sample was, in average, 9.06 (SD=1.58) specifically 9.00 (SD=1.72) for boys and 9.13 (SD=1.44) for girls. Therefore, girls had a poor metabolic control than boys but they were all at high risk. Average of duration of diabetes was 6.61 years (SD=3.68) with boys being diagnosed longer (M=7.05 years; SD=4.10) than girls (M=6.17 years; SD=3.19). In our sample, girls reported better adherence to self-care, less social support, higher school support and family social support when compared to boys but differences were non-significant. Girls showed less quality of life than boys and this difference was significant (t(83)=-2.004; p=.048) (table 1).

Variables	Duration of Diabetes		Adherence		Metabolic Control		Quality of Life		Family Support		School Support	
	M	SD	M	SD	M	SD	M	SD	M	SD	M	SD
Male	7.05	4.10	4.00	0.59	9.00	1.72	75.91	16.96	106.63	13.15	27.93	6.34
Female	6.17	3.19	4.13	0.40	9.13	1.44	83.55	18.19	107.81	11.73	28.21	5.92

Statistics: M (mean), SD (standard deviation)

Table 1. Characteristics of the Adolescents' Sample by Clinical, Socio-demographic and Psychosocial variables

74% of adolescents lived with their nuclear families, 15% belonged to monoparental families, 9.4% to stepfamilies and, only, 1.2% lived in an extended family. 20% of family members, who participated in the study, were fathers and 80% mothers. Average age for fathers was 46 years (SD=4.55) and for mothers was 44 years (SD=6.19).

4.2 Predictors of adherence, metabolic control and quality of life in adolescents on gender, duration of disease, glycated hemoglobin, family support, school support and parental coping

When all variables were included in the model, adherence was predicted by gender of adolescent ($p<.05$), glycated hemoglobin ($p<.05$) and family support ($p<.001$), explaining 30% of the total variance. None of the family variables predicted adherence. Taking in consideration what a high score means, in each instrument, results showed that low perception of family support, gender (being male) and high glycated hemoglobin (bad metabolic control) predicted lower adherence to diabetes self-care.

Metabolic Control was predicted by family support (total) ($p<.05$), adherence (total) ($p<.05$), quality of life (total) ($p<.05$) and parental coping (understanding the medical situation) ($p<.05$), explaining 15.9% of total variance. As a result, higher adherence of adolescent to self-care and parental understanding of the medical situation predicted lower levels of glycated hemoglobin (better metabolic control). On the other hand, low quality of life and low perception of family support predicted high values of glycated hemoglobin (poor metabolic control).

Quality of life was predicted by gender ($p<.05$), glycated hemoglobin ($p<.05$) and school support (total) ($p<.01$) explaining 26.5% of the total variance. Higher values of glycated hemoglobin (poor metabolic control) predicted lower quality of life. On the other hand, higher adherence and a higher school support predicted better quality of life. Like in adherence, none of the family variables predicted quality of life, in adolescents. Table 2 shows the results.

4.3 Predictors of adherence, metabolic control and quality of life in adolescents on glycated hemoglobin and illness representations

Overall, adherence was predicted by personal control of adolescent's illness representations ($p<.001$) and family's representation of timeline ($p<.05$) explaining 20.3% of the total variance. Thus, lower adolescents' perception of personal control predicted lower adherence to self care and higher family perception of diabetes duration (timeline) predicted higher adherence to self care, in adolescents.

Metabolic control, in adolescents, was predicted by emotional representation of adolescents' illness perceptions ($p<.001$) and by family's perceptions of illness coherence ($p<.05$), explaining 16.6% of the total variance. Therefore, higher adolescents' perception of emotional representation (diabetes seen as a threatening disease) predicted higher values of glycated hemoglobin (poor metabolic control) and lower family's comprehension of diabetes predicted higher values of glycated hemoglobin.

Quality of life was predicted by glycated hemoglobin ($p<.05$), adolescent's perception of consequences ($p<.05$) and emotional representation ($p<.05$) explaining 31.6% of the total variance. Higher perception of the consequences of diabetes by adolescents and higher perception of emotional representation (diabetes seen as a threatening disease) predicted lower quality of life. None of the family variables predicted adolescent's quality of life. Table 3 shows the results.

Variables	Adherence				Hemoglobin (Metabolic Control)				Quality of Life			
	Δ R^2	B	SE B	β	Δ R^2	B	SE B	β	Δ R^2	B	SE B	β
Step 1	.071				-.023				.129			
Gender		-.133	.108	-.131		-.088	.350	-.028		-6.03	3.55	-.175
Duration of disease		-.011	.015	-.081		-.009	.048	-.020		-.369	.487	-.078
Glycated Hemoglobin		-.092	.034	**-.286****		----	----	----		3.745	1.12	**.340*****
Step 2	.312				.132				.258			
Gender		-.207	.096	**-.204***		-.123	.342	-.039		-7.91	3.36	**-.229***
Duration of disease		.001	.013	.005		.014	.046	.033		-.295	.464	-.062
Glycated Hemoglobin		-.077	.032	**-.239***		----	----	----		2.35	1.128	**.214***
Family Support		-.019	.004	**-.466*****		-.029	.015	-.232		-.104	.159	-.075
School Support		-.003	.009	-.030		-.018	.030	-.070		-.937	.287	**-.325****
Adherence		---	---	----		-.932	.381	**-.301***		-7.89	3.92	**-.232***
Quality of Life		-.006	.003	**-.215***		.023	.011	**.250***		-	-	-
Step 3	.300				.159				.265			
Gender		-.214	.097	**-.211***		-.160	.338	-.051		-6.97	3.389	**-.202***
Duration of disease		.001	.013	.006		.018	.045	.042		-.211	.465	-.045
Glycated Hemoglobin		-.085	.033	**-.262***		----	----	----		2.34	1.16	**.213***
Family Support		-.019	.004	**-.459*****		-.032	.015	**-.251***		-.146	.161	-.105
School Support		-.000	.009	-.008		-.015	.030	-.058		-.958	.292	**-.332****
Adherence		----	----	-----		-.976	.378	**-.315***		-6.865	3.976	-.202
Quality of Life		-.006	.003	-.192		.022	.011	**.244***		----	-----	-----
Family Functioning		-.099	.162	-.060		.146	.549	.029		9.008	5.554	.162
Coping -Medical Situation		-.019	.016	-.124		-.116	.052	**-.248***		.414	,547	.080
Coping - Social Support		.002	.007	.026		.018	.023	.086		-.274	.238	-.119

* $p < .05$; ** $p < .01$; *** $p < .001$

Table 2. Predictors of Adherence, Metabolic Control and Quality of Life in Adolescents on Gender, Duration of Disease, Glycated Hemoglobin, Family Support, School Support and Parental Coping (N=85 adolescents; N= 85 family members)

Variables	Adherence				Hemoglobin (Metabolic Control)				Quality of Life			
	Δ R^2	B	SE B	β	Δ R^2	B	SE B	β	Δ R2	B	SE B	β
Step 1	.070				n.s.				.121			
Glycated Hemoglobin		-.092	.034	**-.285****						4.117	1.160	**.363*****
Step 2	.169				.126				.288			
Glycated Hemoglobin										2.820	1.083	**.249***
Consequences - IPQ Adol.										2.762	.612	**.431*****
Personal Control - IPQ Adol.		-.081	.024	**-.350*****								
Emotional Representation - IPQ Adol.						.180	.050	**.369*****				
Step 3	.203				.166.				.316			
Glycated Hemoglobin										2.197	1.102	**.194***
Consequences - IPQ Adol.										1.822	.749	**.284***
Personal Control - IPQ Adol.		-.084	.024	**-.364*****								
Emotional Representation - IPQ Adol.						.173	.049	**.356*****		1.402	.670	**.254***
Timeline - IPQ Family		.046	.022	**.206***								
Coherence - IPQ Family						.154	.069.	**.224***				

* p < .05; ** p < .01; *** p < .001

Table 3. Predictors of Adherence, Metabolic Control and Quality of Life in Adolescents on Glycated Hemoglobin and Illness Representations (N=85 adolescents; N= 85 fam. members)

5. Discussion

In this study, adolescent's gender (i.e. being male) predicted lower adherence to diabetes self-care and higher quality of life. An association between gender and low adherence to diabetes, in adolescents girls, particularly regarding exercise, has been found in the literature (Patino et al., 2005). Girls with diabetes show lower quality of life than boys because they seemed to worry more regarding their illness (Grey et al., 1998; Rocha, 2010; Hoey et al., 2001). In fact, low quality of life, in girls, has been associated to more difficulties and worries regarding diabetes and less satisfaction with metabolic control. Girls enter puberty earlier than boys and a weak metabolic control may be associated to physiological changes, normal to adolescence, such as increased levels of hormones responsible for insulin resistance (Carroll & Shade, 2005).

In terms of predictors of adherence, taking in consideration the final model, higher values of glycated hemoglobin (poor metabolic control) predicted lower adherence to diabetes self-care and lower quality of life. These results are in accordance with the literature. Adolescents have more difficulties with metabolic control suggesting that hormonal changes, associated with puberty and the decline on adherence to self-care, were responsible for these results (Helgeson et al., 2009). In another study, glycated hemoglobin explained a small variance of quality of life in adolescents with diabetes suggesting that higher levels of glycated hemoglobin (poor metabolic control) had negative effects on the adolescent's perception of quality of life (Malik & Koot, 2009). In a study that addressed metabolic control and quality of life, good metabolic control (measured by glycated hemoglobin) was a predictor of better quality of life (Hoey et al.,2005).

Higher family support predicted higher adherence and better metabolic control (lower levels of glycated hemoglobin). These results are in accordance with the literature. Family support has been found to be a predictor of good metabolic control (Lewin et al., 2006). In fact, low family support was associated to low adherence to diabetes self-care and, indirectly, to a poor metabolic control. La Greca and Bearman, in 2002, suggested that family support predicts adolescents' adherence to diabetes self-care because family support is an important factor on the daily management of diabetes' self-care tasks in adolescents. Higher family support was found to be a predictor of higher adherence to self-care and good metabolic control suggesting the direct impact of parental support on diabetes' management tasks influencing , as a result, adherence and metabolic control, in the adolescent (Duke et al., 2008; Ellis et al., 2007). In a Portuguese sample of adolescents, family support was found to predict adherence in adolescents with type 1 diabetes (Pereira et al., 2008).

In the present study, a lower perception of personal control predicted lower adherence to diabetes self-care in adolescents. Beliefs in the effectiveness of treatment (control over the illness) were found to predict adherence to dietary self-care (Delamater, 2009). When the benefits, compared to costs of following the diabetes regimen were considered lower, diabetes was perceived as a less threatening disease and adherence to self care in diabetes , as a result, was poor (Patino et al., 2005).

Higher family perception of diabetes' duration, as an illness, predicted higher adherence of adolescents to diabetes self-care. In an attempt to understand if there were differences between illness representations in adults with type 2 diabetes and their partners, a relationship was found between partner's perceptions of the duration of diabetes (timeline) and treatment suggesting that partners' perceptions could influence positively patients' adherence to diabetes self-care (Searle et al., 2007). Based on these result, the same may be true for the dyads parent-adolescent. In fact, parent's perception as a long last condition in adolescent's life may be associated to more parental support regarding diabetes' management tasks in order to decrease future complications in the adolescent.

In terms of predictors of metabolic control, higher adherence to diabetes self-care predicted better metabolic control (lower levels of glycated hemoglobin). In fact, higher adherence to diabetes self-care has been found to predict good metabolic control in adolescents with type 1 diabetes, and lower quality of life, on the other hand, to predict poor metabolic control (Lewin et al., 2009). Higher levels of glycated hemoglobin have been associated to more worries regarding diabetes having, therefore, a negative impact on quality of life (Guttmann-Bauman et al., 1998).

Parents' understanding of the medical situation (coping with diabetes) predicted lower levels of glycated hemoglobin (better metabolic control) in the adolescent. This is a very interesting result. Family environment is important in the complex mechanism of adaptation to diabetes self-care having also an impact on metabolic control (Grey & Berry, 2004). In a study about behavioral therapy with families of adolescents with diabetes, when the relationship between parents and adolescents with diabetes improved, parents´ coping with their adolescents' diabetes got better producing also better outcomes, such as good metabolic control in the adolescent (Wysocki et al., 2000).

Adolescent's emotional representation of diabetes (as a threatening disease) predicted higher levels of glycated haemoglobin (poor metabolic control). In a study about health beliefs in adolescents with type 1 diabetes, negative illness perception, like illness severity and susceptibility were predictors of poor metabolic control. On the other hand, lower family's comprehension (illness coherence) of diabetes predicted bad metabolic control in the adolescent. This result emphasizes the importance of parents' understanding of the impact of diabetes on their child suggesting that those parents who understand less the disease may exercise less parental supervision and provide less family support regarding diabetes's management and, as a consequence, metabolic control decreases.

In terms of quality of life, higher school support predicted higher quality of life. This result is in accordance with the literature. Peers relationships are paramount on the psychological well-being of adolescents with diabetes (Helgeson et al., 2009). In fact, relationships with peers can positively or negatively (e.g. conflict experiences) influence quality of life of adolescents with type 1 diabetes. Adolescents who have more positive attitudes with their school experience tended to experience lower problems and worries with diabetes's management (Lehmkuhl & Nabors, 2007).

Lower quality of life was predicted by higher perceptions of diabetes consequences and higher perceptions of emotional representation (more threatening). This result is in accordance with the literature. In fact, using the same illness perceptions questionnaire, with adults with type 2 diabetes, lower quality of life was found to be related to stronger beliefs of diabetes consequences and negative emotional representations (Edgar et al., 2003). Also, in another study, illness beliefs predicted quality of life i.e. consequences and emotional representations of diabetes were found to predict low quality of life in adolescents (Paddison et al., 2008).

6. Conclusion

In this study, the importance of family factors (family support and parental coping) become evident on diabetes outcomes. As a result, it is important to include parents on intervention programs regarding diabetes in adolescence, School support is also an important factor and future studies should address how peers, teachers and school environment may help or hinder adherence, metabolic control and quality of life. According to results, psychological interventions should be included in the treatment protocol of adolescents receiving medical treatment.

Adolescents and parents' illness representations were predictors of adherence, metabolic control and quality of life, showing the importance of these constructs on diabetes outcomes and should, therefore, be included in intervention programs. Future studies should address how contradictory illness representations between parents and adolescents impact diabetes outcomes particularly if the adolescent perceives parents as intrusive trying to force their diabetes' representations on them.

It would be also interesting to assess family functioning from the adolescent point of view, besides parents' perspective (the only one addressed in the present study) and find out whether parents and adolescents' different perspectives, regarding family functioning, may impact diabetes outcomes.

7. References

Almeida, J. & Pereira, M. G. (no prelo). *Escala Comportamental de Suporte Social Familiar para Adolescentes com Diabetes* (DFBS).

Almeida, J. & Pereira, M.G. (2008). Questionário de Avaliação da Qualidade de Vida para Adolescentes com Diabetes: Estudo de validação do DQOL. *Análise Psicológica*, 2 (26), 295-307.

American Diabetes Association (2003). Test of Glycemia in Diabetes. Clinical Pratice Recommendations. *Diabetes Care*, 26 (1), 106-108.

Amillategui, B. , Calle, J. R. , Alvarez, M. A. Cardiel, M. A., & Barrio, R. (2007). Identifying the special needs of children with Type 1 diabetes in the school setting. An overview of parents' perceptions. *Diabetic Medicine*, 24(10), 1073-1079.

Amoros, M., Sanchez, J., & Carrillo, F. (2003). Adherencia al tratamiento. In Quiles, Sebastian & Carrillo (Eds.), *Manual de Psicología de la Salud con Niños, Adolescentes y Familia*, (pp. 73-94). Ediciones Pirâmide: Madrid.

Anderson, B. J., Auslander, W. F., Jung, K. C., Miller, J. P., & Santiago, J. V. (1990). Assessing family sharing of diabetes responsibilities. *Journal of Pediatric Psychology*, 15, 477-492.

Anderson, B., Brackett, J, Finkelstein, D., & Laffel, L. (1997). Parental Involvement in Diabetes Management Tasks: Relations to Blood Glucose Monitoring and Metabolic Control in Adolescents with Insulin-Dependent Diabetes-Mellitus. *The Journal of Pediatrics*, 130 (2), 257-265.

Anderson, B.J., & Laffel, L.M.B. (1997). Behavioral and psychology research with school aged children with type 1 diabetes. *Diabetes Spectrum*, 10 (4), 277-284.

Anderson, B.J., Miller, P., Auslander, W.F., & Santiago, J.V. (1981). Family Characteristics of Diabetic Adolescents: Relationship to Metabolic Control. *Diabetes Care*, 4, 586-594.

Barros, L. (2003). *Psicologia Pediátrica: perspectiva desenvolvimentista*. 2ªEdição. Climepsi Editores: Lisboa.

Bearman, K. J., & La Greca, A. M. (2002). Assessing friend support of adolescents' diabetes care: the diabetes social support questionnaire-friends version. *Journal of Pediatric Psychology*, 27(5), 417-428.

Beveridge, R.M., Berg, C.A., Wiebe, D.J., & Palmer, D.L. (2006). Mother and Adolescent representations of illness ownership and stressful events surrounding diabetes. *Journal of Pediatrics Psychology*, 31, 818-827.

Bishop, G. (1994). Interacting with the health care system. In Bishop (Ed.), *Health Psychology: Integrating mind and body* (pp. 220-227). Needham-Heights: Allyn and Bacon.

Brito, T.B., & Sadala, M.L.A. (2009). Diabetes mellitus juvenil: a experiência de familiares de adolescentes e pré-adolescentes. *Ciência & Saúde Coletiva*, 14 (3), 947-960.

Broadbent, E., Petrie, K. J., Main, J., & Weinman, J. (2006). The Brief Illness Perception Questionnaire. *Journal of Psychosomatic Research*, 60 631- 637.

Burroughs, T.E., Harris, M.A., Pontious, S.L., & Santiago, J.V. (1997). Research on social support in adolescents with IDDM: A critical review. *Diabetes Educator*, 23, 438-448.

Butler, D.A., Zuehlke, J.B., Tovar, A., Volkening, L.K., Anderson, B.J., & Laffel, L.M.B. (2008). The impact of modifiable family factors on glycemic control among youth with type 1 diabetes. *Pediatric Diabetes*, 9 (Part II), 373-381.

Cameron, F. J., Skinner, T. C., De Heaufort, C. E., Hoey, H., Swift, P. G. F., Aanstoot, H. et al., (2008). Are family factors universally related to metabolic outcomes in adolescents with type 1 Diabetes? *Diabetes Medicine*, 25 (4), 463-468.

Carroll M.F & Shade D.S. (2001). Ten pivotal questions about diabetic ketoacidosis. *Postgraduate Medicine*, 110, 89 -95.

Close H, Davies AG, Price DA, Goodyer IM. (1986). Emotional difficulties in diabetes mellitus. *Archives of Diseases Childhood.* 61(4), 337–340 .

Correia, A.C.R. (2010). *Coping e Auto-Eficácia em Pais de Crianças e Adolescentes com Diabetes tipo 1.* Tese de Mestrado em Psicologia Clínica e da Saúde não publicada. Faculdade de Ciências Humanas e Sociais. Porto. Portugal.

Delamater, A. M. (2009). Psychological care of children and adolescents with diabetes. *Pediatric Diabetes*, 10 (Suppl. 12), 175-184.

Diabetes Control and Complications Trial Research Group (DCCT) (1994). Effect of intensive diabetes treatment on the development and progression of long term complications in adolescents with insulin-dependent diabetes mellitus. *Journal of Pediatrics*, 12, 177-188.

Dickenson, L.M., Ye, X., Sack, J., & Hueston, W.(2003). General quality of life in youth with diabetes: Relationship to patient management and Diabetes - Specific Family and Conflict. *Diabetes Care*, 26, 3067-3073.

Duarte, R. (2002). *Epidemiologia da Diabetes.* In R. Duarte, J. Caldeira, J. Parreira, L. Sagreira, A. Odette & P. Lisboa (Eds). *Diabetologia Clínica*, Lidel - Edições Técnicas Lda. Lisboa.

Duke, D. C., Geffken, G. R., Lewin, A. B., Williams, L. B., Storch, E. A., & Silverstein, J. H. (2008). Glycemic Control in Youth with Type 1 Diabetes: Family Predictors and Mediators. *Journal of Pediatric Psychology*, 33 (7), 719-727.

Edgar, R. A. & Skinner, T. C. (2003). Illness Representation and Coping as Predictors of Emotional Well-being in Adolescents with Type 1 Diabetes. *Journal of Pediatric Psychology*, 28 (7), 485-493.

Eiser, C. 1990). *Chronic Childhood Disease.* New York: Cambridge University Press.

Elkind, D. (1984). *All grown up and no place to go: Teenagers in crisis.* Reading, MA: Add is on-Wesley.

Ellerton, M. L.; Stewart, M. J., Ritchie, J. A., & Hirth, A. M. (1996). Social support in children with a chronic condition. *Canadian Journal of Nursing Research*, 28 (4), 15-36.

Ellis, D. A., Podolski, C. L., Frey, M., Naar-King, S., Wang, B., & Moltz, K. (2007). The Role of Parental Monitoring in Adolescent Health Outcomes: Impact on Regimen Adherence in Youth with Type 1 Diabetes. *Journal of Pediatric Psychology*, 32(8), 907-917.

Epstein, N., Baldwin, L. & Bishop, D. (1983). The McMaster Family Assessment Device. *Journal of Marital and Family Therapy*, 9, 171-180.

Erikson, E. H. (1968) .*Identity, Youth and Crisis*. New York: Norton

Fagulha, A., Santos, I., & Grupo de Estudo da Diabetes (2004). Controlo glicémico e tratamento da Diabetes tipo 1 da Criança e Adolescente em Portugal. *Acta Médica Portuguesa*, 17, 173-179.

Figueiras, M.J. & Alves, N. C.(2007). Lay perceptions of serious illnesses: An adapted version of the Revised Illness Perception Questionnaire (IPQ-R) for healthy people. *Psychology and Health*, 22 (2), 143-158.

Fisher, E.B., Delamater, A.M., Bertelson, A.D., & Kirkley, B.G. (1982). Psychological factors in diabetes and its treatment. *Journal of Consulting and Clinical Psychology, 50*(6), 993-1003.

Fukunishi, I., Akimoto, M., Horikawa, N., Shirasaka, K., & Yamazaki, T. (1998). Stress and Social Support in glucose tolerance abnormality. *Journal of Psychosomatic Research,* 45 (4), 362-269.

Glasgow, R. E., Ruggiero, L., Eakin, E. G., Dryfoos, J., & Chobanian, L. (1997). Quality of life and associated characteristics in a large national sample of adults with diabetes. *Diabetes Care, 20* (4), 562-567.

Gonder-Frederick, L., Cox, D. J., & Ritterband, L. M. (2002). Diabetes and behavioral medicine: The second decade. *Journal of Consulting and Clinical Psychology,* 70(3), 611-625

Grey, M. & Berry, D. (2004). Coping Skills Training and Problem Solving in Diabetes. *Current Diabetes Reports*, 4, 126-131.

Grey, M., Boland, E., Yu, C., Sullivan-Bollyai, A., & Tamborlane, W.V. (1998). Personal and Family Factors Associated with Quality of Life in Adolescents with Diabetes. *Diabetes Care*, 212 (6), 909-914.

Griva, K., Myers, L. B., & Newman, S. (2000). Illness perceptions and self-efficacy beliefs in adolescents and young adults with insulin dependent diabetes mellitus. *Psychology and Health, 15,* 733–750.

Guttmann-Bauman, I., Flaherty, B. P., Strugger, M. & McEvoy, R. C. (1998). Metabolic Control and Quality-of-Life Self-Assessment in Adolescents With IDDM. *Diabetes Care*, 21 (6), 915-918.

Hanas, R. (2007). *Diabetes Tipo 1 em Crianças, Adolescentes e Jovens Adultos*. Abbott Diabetes Care. Lidel - Edições técnicas Lda: Lisboa.

Hanson, C. L., Cigrang, J. A., Harris, M. A., Carle, D. L., Relyea, G., & Burghen, G. A. (1989). Coping styles in youths with insulin-dependent diabetes mellitus. *Journal of Consulting and Clinical Psychology,* 57, 644–651.

Hanson, C.L. (2001). Quality of life in families of youths with chronic conditions. In H.M. Koot & J.L. Wallander (Eds.), *Quality of life in child and adolescent illness: Concepts, methods and findings* (pp. 182-209). New York: Brunner-Routledge.

Haynes, A., Bower, C., Bulsara, M. K., Finn, J., Jones, T. W. and Davis, E. A. (2007), Perinatal risk factors for childhood Type 1 diabetes in Western Australia—a population-based study (1980–2002). *Diabetic Medicine*, 24, 564–570.

Helgeson, V. S., Lopez, L. C., & Kamarck, T. (2009). Peer Relationships and Diabetes: Retrospective and Ecological Momentary Assessment Approaches. *Health Psychology*. 28(3), 273-282.

Helgeson, V. S., Siminerio, L., Escobar, O. & Becker, D. (2009). Predictors of Metabolic Control among Adolescents with Diabetes: A 4-Year Longitudinal Study. *Journal of Pediatric Psychology*, 34(3), 254–270.

Hirschberg, S.L. (2001). *The Self-regulation of health behaviour in children with insulin dependent diabetes mellitus*. Dissertation presented to the Faculty of Pacific Graduate School of Psychology. Palo Alto, California.

Hoey, H., Aanstoot, H. J., Chiarelli, F., Daneman, D., Danne, T., Dorchy, H. et al., (2001). Good Metabolic Control is Associated with Better Quality of Life in 2101 Adolescents with Type 1 Diabetes. *Diabetes Care*, 24 (11), 1923-1928.

Holmbeck, G. N., Colder, C., Shapera, W., Westhoven, V., Kenealy, L., & Updegrove, A. (2000). Working with adolescents: Guides from developmental psychology. In P. C. Kendall (Ed.), *Child and adolescent therapy: Cognitive behavioral procedures* (2nd ed.; pp. 334–385). New York: Guilford Press.

Ingersoll, G. & Marrero, D. (1991). A modified Quality of Life Measure for Youths: Psycometrics Properties. *The Diabetes Educator*, 17 (2), 114-118.

Jacobson A. M., Hauser, S. T., Wolfsdorf, J. I., Houlihan, J., Milley, J. E. & Watt, E. (1987). Psychological Predictors of Compliance in Children with Recent Onset of Diabetes Mellitus. *Journal of Pediatrics*, 805-811.

Kakleas, K., Kandyla, B., Karayianni, C., & Karavanaki, K. (2009). Psychosocial problems in adolescents with Type 1 diabetes mellitus. *Diabetes & Metabolism*. University of Athens.

Kovacs, M., & Feinberg, T. (1982). Coping with juvenile onset diabetes mellitus. In A. Baum & J. Singer (Eds), *Handbook of Psychology and Health*, 2,165-212. Erlbaum: Hillsdale, NJ.

Kovacs, M., Kass, R. E., Schnell, T. M., Goldston, D., & Marsh, J. (1989). Family functioning and metabolic control of school-aged children with IDDM. *Diabetes Care, 12,* 409-*414.*

Kristeller, J. l., & Rodin, J. (1984). A Three-stage model of treatment continuity: compliance, adherence and maintenance. In A. Baum, S. Taylor & J. Singer (Eds.), *Handbook of Psychology and Health.* (Vol. IV, pp. 85-112). New Jersey: Lawrence Erlbaum Associates.

La Greca, A. M. (1992). *Brief Manual for the Self Care Inventory*. University of Miami.USA.

La Greca, A. M. (1992). Peer Influences in Pediatric Chronic Illness: An Update. *Journal of Pediatric Psychology*; 17 (6), 775-784.

La Greca, A. M., & Bearman, K. J. (2002). The Diabetes Social Support Questionnaire-Family Version: Evaluating Adolescents' Diabetes-Specific Support From Family Members. *Journal of Pediatric Psycholog*, 27 (8), 665-676.

La Greca, A. M., & Thompson, K.M (1998). Family and friend Support for Adolescents with Diabetes. *Análise Psicológica*, 1 (XVI), 101-113.

La Greca, A. M., Auslander, W. F., Greco, P., Spetter, D., Fisher, E. B., Jr., & Santiago, J. V. (1995). I get by with a little help from my family and friends: Adolescents' support for diabetes care. *Journal of Pediatric Psychology, 20,* 449–476.

Laffel, L., Connell, A., Vangsness, L., Goebel-Fabri, A., Mansfield, A., & Anderson, B. (2003). General Quality of life in Youth with type 1 Diabetes. Relationship to patient management and diabetes-specific family conflit. *Diabetes Care,* 26, (11), 3067- 3073.

Lehmkuhl, H., & Nabors, L. (2007). Children with Diabetes: Satisfaction with School Support, Illness Perceptions and HbA1C Levels. *Journal of Developmental and Physical Disabilities,* 20, 101-114.

Leite (2005). Programa de promoção da adesão terapêutica em crianças diabéticas. In M. Guerra & L. Lima, (Eds.), *Intervenção Psicológica em Grupos em Contextos de Saúde.* Climepsi Editores: Lisboa.

Leventhal, H., Diefenbach, M.A., & Leventhal, E. A. (1992). Illness Cognition: Using common sense to understand treatment adherence and affect cognition interactions. *Cognitive Therapy and Research,* 16, 143-163.

Leventhal, H., Meyer, D., & Nerenz, D. (1980). The common-sense representation of illness danger. In S. Rachman (Ed.), *Contributions to Medical Psychology* (Vol. 2, pp. 7–30). New York: Pergamon Press.

Leventhal, H., Nerenz, D. R., & Steele, D. J. (1984). Illness representation and coping with health threats. In A. Baum, S. E. Taylor, & J. E. Singer (Eds.), *Handbook of Psychology and Health* (pp. 219 –252). Hillsdale, NJ: Lawrence Erlbaum Associates.

Lewin, A. B., Heidgerken, A. D., Geffken, G. R., Williams, L. B., Storch, E. A., Gelfand, K. M. & al., (2006). The Relation Between Family Factors and Metabolic Control: The Role of Diabetes Adherence. *Journal of Pediatric Psychology,* 31 (2), 174-183.

Lewin, A. B., La Greca, A. M., Geffken, G. R., Williams, L. B., Duke, D. C., Storch, E. A. & et al., (2009). Validity and Reliability of an Adolescent and Parent Rating Scale of Type 1 Diabetes Adherence Behaviors: The Self-Care Inventory (SCI). *Journal of Pediatric Psychology,* 34(9), 999-1007.

Macrodimitris S.D., & Endler N.S. (2001). Coping, control, and adjustment in Type 2 diabetes. Health Psychology, 20(3), 208-16.

Malik, J. A., & Koot, H. M. (2009). Explaining the Adjustment of Adolescents With Type 1 Diabetes. Role of diabetes-specific and psychosocial factors. *Diabetes Care,* 32, 774-779.

Manne, S.L., Jacobson, P.B.,Gorfinkle,K., Gerstein, F., & Redd, W.H. (1993).Treatment adherence diffilculties among children with cancer: the role of parenting style. *Journal of Pediatric Psychology,* 18 (1), 47-62.

McCubbin, H. I., McCubbin, M. A., Patterson, J. M., Cauble, A.E., Wilson, L. R., & Warwick, W. (1983). CHIP - Coping Health Inventory for Parents: An Assessment of Parental Coping Patterns in the Care of the Chronically Ill Child. *Journal of Marriage and Family,* 359-370.

McKelvey, J., Waller, D. A., North, A. J., Marks, J. F., Schreiner, B., Travis, L. B., & Murphy, J.N. Reliability and Validity of the Diabetes Family Behavior Scale (DFBS). *The Diabetes Educator,* 19, 125-132.

McNabb, W. L. (1997). Adherence in diabetes: can we define it an can we measure it? *Diabetes Care,* 20 (2), 215-218.

Miller, K. B., & La Greca, A. M. (2005). Adjustment to chronic illness in girls. In D. J. Bell, S. L. Foster, & E. J. Mash (Eds.), *Handbook of behavioral and emotional problems in girls* (pp. 489–522). New York: Kluwer Academic/Plenum Press Publishers.

Miller-Johnson, Emery, R, Marvin, R., Clarke, W., Loevinger, R., & Martin, M. (1994). Parent-Child Relationships And The Management Of Insulin-Dependent Diabetes Mellitus. *Journal of Consulting and Clinical Psychology*, 62 (3), 603-610.

Mortensen, H., Hougaard, P., & Hvidore Study Group (1997). Comparison of metabolic control in a cross-sectional study of 2873 children and adolescentts with IDDM from 18 countries. *Diabetes Care,* 20, 714-720.

Mortensen, H.B., Robertson, K.J., Aanstoot, H.J. Danne, T., Holl, R.H., Hougaard, P., et al., (1998). Insulin management and metabolic control of Type 1 diabetes mellitus in childhood and adolescence in 18 countries. Diabetic Medicine, 15, 752–759,

Moss-Morris, R., Weinman J., Petrie, K.J. Horn, R., Cameron, L. & Buick, D. (2002). The Revised Illness Perception Questionnaire (IPQ-R). Psychology and Health ,17 (1), 1-16.

Northam, E, Anderson, P, Adler, R., & Warne, M. (1996). Psychosocial and Family Functioning In Children with Insulin-Dependent Diabetes at Diagnosis and One Year Later. *Journal of Pediatric Psychology, 21,* 699-717.

Novato, T.S. (2009). *Factores preditivos de Qualidade de Vida Relacionada à Saúde em Adolescentes com Diabetes Mellitus tipo 1.* Tese não publicada de Pós-Graduação em Enfermagem na Saúde do Adulto. Brasil.

Nunes, M.D.R. & Dupas, G. (2004). Entregando-se à vivência da doença do filho: a experiência da mãe da criança/adolescente diabético. *Texto e Contexto de Enfermagem,* 13 (1), 83-91.

Olsen, B., Berg, C. A. and Wiebe, D. J. (2005). Dissimilarity in mother and adolescent illness representations of type 1 diabetes and negative emotional adjustment. *Psychology and Health,* 23 (1), 113-129.

Organización Mundial de la Salud (1965).Problemas de salud de la adolescência. Série de Informes técnicos, Geneva: OMS, 308,29p.

Paddison, C.A.M., Alpass, F.M., & Stephens, C.V. (2008). Psychological variables account for variation in metabolic control and quality of life among people with type 2 diabetes in New Zealand. *International Journal of Behavioural Medicine* 15: 180–186, 2008.

Papalia, D., Olds, S., & Feldman, R. (2001). *O Mundo da criança.* McGraw-Hill: Lisboa.

Patino, A. M., Sanchez, J., Eidson, M., & Delamater, A. M. (2005). Health Beliefs and Regimen Adherence in Minority Adolescents with Type 1 Diabetes. *Journal of Pediatric Psychology,* 30 (6), 503-512.

Pereira, M. G., & Almeida, J. P. (2001). CHIP - *Coping Health Inventory for Parents: An Assessment of Parental Coping Patterns in the Care of the Chronically Ill Child.* Research Version of University of Minho.Braga.Portugal.

Pereira, M.G., Berg-Cross, L., Almeida, P., & Machado, C. J. (2008). Impact of Family Environment and Support and Adherence, Metabolic Control, and Quality Life in Adolescents with Diabetes. *International Journal of Behavioral Medicine,* 15, 187-193.

Petrie, K. J., Weinman, J., Sharpe, N., & Buckley, J. (1996). Role of patients' view of their illness in predicting return to work and functioning after myocardial infarction: Longitudinal study. *British Medical Journal, 312,* 1191–1194..

Ray, C., Epstein N., Keitner, G., Miller, I., & Bishop, D. (2005). Evaluation and Treating Families: The McMaster Approach. *Routledge Taylor & Francis Group*. New York.

Rocha. L. (2010). *Variáveis familiares, adesão, controlo metabólico e qualidade de vida na diabetes tipo 1:* Um estudo com adolescentes e familiares Unpublished dissertation. University of Minho. Braga. Portugal.

Santos, R. J. (2001). *Adolescentes com Diabetes Mellitus Tipo 1: Seu cotidiano e enfrentamento da doença*. Dissertação apresentada ao Programa de Pós-Graduação em Psicologia da Universidade Federal do Espírito Santo. Brasil.

Sarafino, E. P. (1990). *Health psychology: Biopsychosocial Interactions*. New York: John Wiley & Sons.

Searle, A., Norman, P., Thompson, R., & Vedhara, R. (2007). Illness representations among patients with type 2 diabetes and their partners: Relationships with self-management behaviours. *Journal of Psychosomatic Research*, 63, 175-184.

Seiffe-Krenke, I.(1998). Psychological Adjustment of Adolescents with Diabetes: Functional or Dysfunctional for Metabolic Control? *Journal of Pediatric Psychology*, 23 (5), 313-322.

Silva, I. (2003). *Qualidade de vida e variáveis psicológicas associadas a sequelas de diabetes e sua evolução ao longo do tempo*. Tese de Doutoramento não publicada, Faculdade de Psicologia e de Ciências da Educação, Universidade do Porto.Portugal.

Silva, I., Pais Ribeiro, J., Cardoso, H., & Ramos, H. (2002). Questionário de Auto-cuidados na Diabetes - contributo para a criação de um instrumento de avaliação da adesão ao tratamento. *Psiquiatria Clínica*, 23 (3), 227-237.

Skinner T. C., Hampson S. E., & Fife-Schaw, C. (2002). Personality, personal model beliefs, and self-care in adolescents and young adults with Type 1 diabetes. *Health Psychology, 21*, 61–70.

Skinner, T. C., & Hampson, S. E. (2001). Personal models of diabetes in relation to self-care, well-being, and glycemic control: A prospective study in adolescence. *Diabetes Care, 24*, 828–833.

Skinner, T. C., John, M., & Hampson, S. E. (2000). Social support and personal models of diabetes as predictors of self-care and well-being: A longitudinal study of adolescents with diabetes. *Journal of Pediatric Psychology, 25*(4), 257–267.

Snoek F.J., Pouwer F., Welch G.W., & Polonsky WH.(2000). Diabetes-related emotional distress in Dutch and U.S. diabetic patients: cross-cultural validity of the problem areas in diabetes scale. *Diabetes Care*, 23(9), 1305-9.

Sperling, A. M. (1996). Diabetes Mellitus. In W. Nelson, R. Behrman, & A.Arvin (Ed.). *Nelson Textbook of Pediatrics*, 15ª Edição, WB Sanders & Company: Philadelphia.

Stern, M. & Zevon, M.A (1990). Stress, Coping and Family Environment: the Adolescent's Response to Naturally Occurring Stressors. *Journal of Adolescent Research*, 5, 290-305.

Thomas, A. M., Peterson, L., & Goldstein, D. (1997). Problem solving and diabetes regimen adherence by children and adolescents with IDDM in social pressure situations: A reflection of normal development. *Journal of Pediatric Psychology, 22*, 541–561.

Trindade, I. (2000). Abordagem Psicológica do doente crónico em centros de saúde. In I.Trindade, & J. Teixeira (Eds), Psicologia nos cuidados de saúde primários (pp. 47-53). Climepsi Editores: Lisboa.

Warren, L. & Hixenbaugh, P. (1998). Adherence and Diabetes. In L.B. Myers, & K. Midence (Eds), *Adherence to treatment in medical conditions* (pp.423-453). Harwood Academic Publishers: Netherlands

Watkins K.W., Klem L, Connell C.M., Hickey, T., Fitzgerald. J.T., Ingersoll-Dayton B. (2000) Effect of adults self-regulation of diabetes on quality of life. *Diabetes Care* 2000; 23, 1511–1515.

Wysocki et al. (2000). Randomized, Controlled Trial of Behavior Therapy for Families of Adolescents with Insulin-Dependent Diabetes Mellitus. *Journal of Pediatric Psychology*, 25 (1), 23-33.

Wysocki, T (1993). Associations Among Teen-Parent Relationships, Metabolic Control, and Adjustment to Diabetes in Adolescents. *Journal of Pediatric Psychology*, 18 (4), 441-452.

Wysocki, T., & Greco, P. (2006). Social support and diabetes management in childhood and adolescence: Influence of parents and friends. *Current Diabetes Reports, 6,* 117–122.

Wysocki, *T.*, Greco, P., Harris, M. A., Bubb, J., & White, N. H. (2001). Behavior therapy for families of adolescents with IDDM: Maintenance of treatment effects. *Diabetes Care, 24, 441–446.*

Zanetti, M.L. & Mendes, I.A.C. (2001). Análise das actividades relacionadas às actividades diárias de crianças e adolescentes com diabetes mellitus tipo1: depoimento de mães. *Revista Latino-Americana de Enfermagem*, 9 (6), 25-30.

8

Contributing Factors to Poor Adherence and Glycemic Control in Pediatric Type 1 Diabetes: Facilitating a Move Toward Telehealth

Joseph P. H. McNamara[1], Adam M. Reid[2], Alana R. Freedland[3], Sarah E. Righi[1] and Gary R. Geffken[1]
[1]*University of Florida, Department of Psychiatry*
[2]*University of Florida, Department of Clinical and Health Psychology*
[3]*University of Florida, Department of Counselor Education*
USA

1. Introduction

The study of family's with children with T1D and their regimens has led to a burgeoning literature by psychologist's with an interest in the relationship between adherence and glycemic control. Research in pediatric or child health psychology may be described as focusing on studying behavioral health, or psychological factors including learning, development, psychopathology, and culture as they interact with biological and physiological factors involved with illness, and in many cases, chronic illnesses. T1D is a chronic illness where an increasingly complex medical regimen for the child's illness interacts with the child's family, their school, their peers, and their culture. T1D is a chronic illness where the research of child health psychologists and other health care professionals can be seen as providing a prototype or model of other chronic illness of childhood that have a lower prevalence, and hence have a literature that is comparatively less developed than that of T1D.

2. The challenges of type 1 diabetes

Type 1 Diabetes (T1D) is a complex and challenging disease for children and adolescents due to the necessary integration of daily medical tasks (e.g., blood glucose monitoring) and lifestyle modifications. Evidence suggests that a substantial percentage of children are non-adherent to these demands.[1,2] Although some of those who are non-adherent experience few negative consequences, a large number of non-adherent children are at risk for significant medical complications including diabetic ketoacidosis (DKA), neuropathy, nephropathy, retinopathy, and cardiovascular disease.[3] Despite improvements in fluid and insulin therapy, fatality rates are still estimated at 1 to 2% of youth who experience a DKA episode. Non-adherence can also negatively impact clinical decisions made by health care providers such as prescribing incorrect insulin doses. Further, poor adherence results in increased morbidity and mortality, as well as problematic medication use and excessive use of health care services.[4,5] Numerous factors have a significant impact on adherence and glycemic control.

3. Family and psychological factors influencing adherence and glycemic control

Research suggests that family factors have a large impact on adherence and glycemic control in populations with pediatric T1D. Young children's management of T1D is highly dependent on family factors due to their high reliance on parental care. Parenting style is an important variable to examine when measuring adherence and glycemic control. Davis and colleagues[6] found parental warmth was associated with better adherence among preschool through elementary aged children with T1D. Parental restrictiveness was associated with low glycemic control. Establishing good self-care habits at an early age is critical in the maintenance of T1D since young children diagnosed with T1D are more likely to experience longer disease duration.[7] Healthy habits, such as engagement in physical activity, are crucial for the management of T1D. Mackey and Streisand[8] found parental support of exercise activity to be related to higher rates of physical activity in youth with T1D. Support included encouragement and parent participation in the exercise activity. Healthy eating behaviors are also essential to the management of T1D. In a qualitative study examining the effects of family meals on youth with T1D, the authors found that family meals were important to the participants.[9] The participants found it easier to maintain healthy eating habits when they shared meals with their families. In contrast parental conflict, characterized by criticism of exercise activity, was negatively associated to rates of physical activity. This study implicates the importance of including family-focused strategies in nutritional interventions.

While diet and exercise are important for the management of T1D, new technologies such as continuous subcutaneous insulin infusion (CSII) or the insulin pump have made their way into diabetic management. Evidence supports use of the insulin pump to improve quality of life and patients using the pump exhibit higher levels of glycemic control compared to patients on daily injections.[10] While the pump allows patients to achieve improved glycemic control, maintaining these results is difficult and often deteriorates over time.[11] According to Wiebe and colleagues,[12] low parental involvement was associated with lower pump duration. Parent involvement was lowest among older adolescents. The authors concluded that older adolescents' desire for independence might have affected parental involvement. Therefore it is important for clinicians to promote shared responsibility for pump management. Assessment of parental support prior to implementation of the insulin pump can provide clinicians with valuable information pertaining to the appropriateness of its use. The Diabetes Family Behavior Checklist (DFBC) is a common instrument used for the assessment of parental support for pediatric T1D.[13] Lewin and colleagues[14] found the measure to display high internal consistency and moderate to high convergent validity with other instruments measuring family behaviors related to diabetes, adherence, and glycemic control. The authors concluded that using both parent and child forms of the DFBC as well as administering these forms separately were important for the validity of the assessments.

In addition to parental support, authoritative parenting, classified by parental demand and responsiveness, has been associated with higher metabolic control and self-care in adolescents with T1D.[15] Authoritative mothering displayed the closest relationship to improved glycemic control and self-care. This could be explained by the mothers' higher involvement in care than the fathers in the study. Both maternal permissiveness and authoritarian parenting styles were associated with poorer diet adherence.[15] Similar to these findings, Lloyd and colleagues[16] found maternal empathy to be positively correlated with adherence and glycemic control in a sample of T1D adolescents. It is common for mothers to be more involved in the care giving process than their male counterparts, which can often lead to high levels of stress among mothers with children with T1D. In a study by Lewin, Storch, Silverstein, Baumeister, Strawser, and Geffken[17] illness-related stressors linked with a mother's caretaking role were highly correlated to a mother's stress and state anxiety. Parenting stress was positively correlated to child behavior problems. Similarly, Hilliard, Monaghan, Cogen, and Streisand[18] found that general anxiety and parenting stress were associated with parents' perceptions of their children's problematic behavior in children with T1D.

In addition to the management of T1D and behavioral problems, parenting stress has been related to initial diagnosis of the disorder. Streisand and colleagues[19] found that parents exhibited the highest levels of anxiety and depressive symptoms at the time of their child's diagnosis. These results implicate the importance of providing additional support and education to parents of newly diagnosed children as well as assessing for anxious and depressive symptoms. Parents are also at risk for developing chronic sorrow pertaining to the diagnosis of pediatric T1D. Results of a study examining chronic sorrow showed that parents exhibited a grief reaction upon initial diagnosis and continued to experience intermittent emotional distress.[20] The mothers in the study sample were more comfortable talking about their grief than fathers, however, both mothers and fathers displayed evidence of chronic sorrow. With growing evidence supporting the positive association between parenting stress and other issues related to T1D, recent interventions have been created to focus specifically on these issues among parents of children with the disorder. In a study by Monaghan, Hilliard, Cogen, and Streisand,[21] the authors assessed the efficacy and practicality of a telephone-based intervention designed for parents of children with T1D. The intervention aimed to improve parental quality of life by decreasing parenting stress, increasing social support and improving the management of pediatric T1D. The subjects scored lower on parenting stress and higher on social supportpost-intervention. This evidence suggests the utility of interventions with families coping with T1D. The Pediatric Inventory for Parents has been proven to be an effective instrument for measuring parenting stress in mothers of children with T1D.[14] The instrument displayed internal consistency reliability and validity for this population.

Current research suggests that family conflict may also have a negative impact on the management of pediatric T1D. In a study examining youth and adolescents with T1D, perception of family conflict was the highest predictor of medical adherence.[22] Perception of family cohesion predicted improved adherence. Parent-child conflict has also been linked to poor adherence as well as poor metabolic control in children with T1D.[23] Similarly, Williams, Laffel, and Hood[24] found a positive relationship between psychological distress and diabetes-specific conflict in pediatric T1D. The results of these studies indicate the importance of family cohesion for better management of pediatric T1D. According to the findings of Harris, Freeman, and Beers[25] Behavioral Family Systems Therapy (BFST) produced an improvement in mother-adolescent conflict related to diabetes specific issues as well as an improvement in general parent-adolescent conflict.

Given the impact of family cohesion on diabetes management, it is no surprise that spousal support is also an important factor in the examination of adherence and glycemic control in children with T1D. Marital conflict has been shown to influence the link between mother-adolescent relationships and adherence. Lewandowski and Drotar[26] found that higher levels of perceived spousal support were associated with lower mother-adolescent conflict and higher medical adherence of adolescents with T1D. Single-parent households have been associated with lower adherence.[27] In a study on family dynamics in adolescents with T1D, the authors found that divorced, separated and single-parent families appeared to pose the highest risk to poor glycemic control among this population.[28] The study also showed that parent-child agreement on blood glucose monitoring responsibility was related to more frequent monitoring. The results from this study provide support for interventions aimed at facilitating the transition from parental responsibility to adolescent responsibility of metabolic management. Clinicians should be aware of these implications when assessing for diabetes management. The Diabetes Family Conflict Scale is a clinical tool that is used to measure negative emotions surrounding blood glucose monitoring, quality of life and perceived parental burden caused by the management of diabetes.[29] This measure is the most commonly used assessment for measuring diabetes-related family conflict. Hood, Butler, Anderson, and Laffel[30] revised the scale to include updated technology and language pertaining to diabetes management. The revised scale has high construct validity, predictive validity and internal consistency.

Similar to the aforementioned family factors, several child behavioral patterns also contribute to poor adherence and glycemic control. How a child behaves is one of the most important predictors of a multitude of important outcomes, including academic success,[31] social acceptance,[32] and development of psychological problems.[33] Two of these psychological problems are externalizing and internalizing behaviors, which are two of the biggest broad spectrum behavioral classification terms used in psychological literature since its popularization with the work of Achenbach.[34] Externalizing problems, problems that are manifested in outward behavior and reflect a child's negative reactions to his or her environment, and internalizing problems, behaviors in which youth direct feelings and emotions inward, are predictive of numerous behavioral outcomes, especially adherence and glycemic control within the pediatric diabetes literature.[35][36]

Externalizing symptoms have been found to relate to a poorer prognosis for youth with diabetes.[37] This likely can be explained by the poor adherence and glycemic control in these youth with diabetes.[38][39][40] Children with externalizing problems, such as oppositional or aggressive behaviors, likely fail to listen to their parents when told to take their insulin injection or maintain an appropriate diet regimen, as evidenced by Duke & colleagues[41] who conducted a study on 120 youth with diabetes and found that adherence mediated the relationship between externalizing behaviors and low HbA_{1c} levels. Attention deficit-hyperactivity disorder, a common externalizing disorder, has received little attention in the pediatric diabetes literature. One case study of two children with co-morbid ADHD and diabetes found that standard behavioral treatment for ADHD significantly reduce problems with adherence to the diabetes treatment regimen.[41][42] Emerging research investigating improvements in adherence and glycemic control as the result of treatments tailored solely toward addressing co-morbid internalizing disorders, such as depression or generalized anxiety disorder, reveal similar results.[42][43] Keeping in mind the clear inhibiting role of externalizing and internalizing problems (highlighted below) on adherence, and the importance of adherence in glycemic regulation, future treatment plans for youth with T1D should incorporate concurrent psychological therapy.

Parent reported internalizing disorders are believed to be present in approximately 28% of individuals with diabetes[44][45] and, similar to externalizing disorders, co-morbid presenting internalizing disorders have been associated with a worse prognosis in youth with T1D.[46] As suggested by empirical findings both cross sectionally and longitudinally,[47][36][35][46] one reason for this worse prognosis likely stems from poorer adherence and glycemic control as a result of the internalizing symptoms. For example, a youth with depression may struggle to adhere to the recommendations of their primary care physician due to a lack of motivation, feelings of helplessness, and decreased energy. Indeed, research has shown that depressed individuals do often engage in less self-care and health promoting activities.[48] It has been proposed that a bidirectional relationship may exist between depression and glycemic control, implying that lower glycemic control may lead to increased dysphoria while dysphoria may in turn lead to worse adherence which causes poorer glycemic management.[49]

These children who struggle to adhere to their doctor's recommendations and manage their diabetes properly will continue to experience the multiple health-related issues associated with diabetes, as well as put themselves at risk for more serious health problems as they get older, such as coronary heart disease.[50] Clearly, externalizing and internalizing disorders can have a crippling effect on adherence and glycemic control in diabetic youth, yet, the standard approach to treatment fails to address these internalizing and externalizing problems. A new approach which could circumvent some of the barriers to treatment caused by these internalizing and externalizing symptoms, such as poor self-care, lack of motivation, and avoidance behaviors would likely improve the poor prognosis of these youth with type 1 diabetes. An example of addressing these treatment barriers would be incorporating motivational interviewing, a therapeutic approach aimed at increasing motivation and self-esteem, that has been found to improve glycemic control in youth with diabetes.[51]

The role of depression in causing poorer adherence and glycemic control can be explained further when examining the role of peer victimization in this relationship. Peer victimization, as used in the psychological literature, can be overt forms (such as physical and verbal assault) and/or relational forms (social ostracism),[52] and both kinds of peer victimization are higher in several clinical pediatric populations, such as in youth with learning disorders,[53] obesity,[54] endocrine disorders,[55] inflammatory bowel disease,[56] etc. While little research has been conducted on peer victimization in a population of youth with diabetes, some recent studies have replicated the previous results with other chronic health conditions, finding that youth with diabetes have higher rates of relational peer victimization than their peers without diabetes.[57] Further, the importance of investigating the impact of victimization in diabetes is highlighted by Storch & colleagues[57] further findings that, within the sample of youth with diabetes, children who had higher rates of peer victimization were more likely to be depressed, lonely, and socially anxious. As discussed earlier, research in the past few years has began to identify depression as a driving mechanism of the link between peer victimization and poor adherence and glycemic control. Research by Storch & colleagues[58] found that depression partially mediated the relationship between peer victimization and diabetes self-management, or simply put that peer victimized, youth with diabetes manage their diabetes worse as they endorse higher levels of depression. Specifically related to their self-management, this study found that the more the youth were victimized by their peers, the worse HbA1c, adherence to glucose testing, and dietary management. While these findings are certainly preliminary, they do have important clinical implications. Forth most, clinicians treating pediatric diabetes need to be aware that they are working with an at risk population for peer victimization. Assessment procedures for peer victimization should be implemented in order to develop a better understanding of a probable cause for any presenting depression related issues with the child or adolescent.

Higher cognitive functions that underlie problem solving abilities, specifically executive functioning, has been found to be more developed in youth who are better at forseeing long term consequences.[59] Thus it is no surprise that higher executive functioning is associated with adherence to the diabetes regimen.[60] In other words, children who are better at measuring the risks of not monitoring there glucose intake, carrying around snacks or other recommendations of their doctor are more likely to adhere to their diabetes regimen. Recent research has identified that children with higher executive functioning are better at problem solving, planning, organization, and working memory and that all of these derivatives of executive functioning have been associated with adherence, which in turn was associated with higher glycemic control.[61][62] It is important for clinicians to be aware of youth's deficits in executive functioning and understand the value in discussing problem solving techniques with the children, which likely could improve overall diabetes management.[63] Future research in pediatric diabetes should investigate possible paradigms that could improve aspects of a child's problem solving abilities related to diabetes in a clinically feasible manner.

Other research has suggested that executive functioning may relate less to adherence in younger youth with diabetes,[63] but this may result from the increased involvement from parents in younger children, which improves glycemic control,[64][65] and therefore future research should investigate the relationship between parental executive functioning and younger children's glycemic control. Parents do play an obviously beneficial role in how a youth manages their diabetes, such as monitoring their adherence to treatment recommendations,[66] however, parents can also negatively impact their child's prognosis as the result of parental accommodation. Parental accommodation relates to parents giving in to their youth's resistance to beneficial treatment recommendations or treatment procedures in order to lower their child's anxiety, increase mood, or just as a result of the parent's poor insight into the necessity of the procedure.

Parental accommodation has received little attention in the diabetes literature, but is well researched in other pediatric populations, specifically related to the treatment of anxiety disorders.[67] This literature discusses how parents can create a barrier to the treatment of pediatric anxiety disorders by facilitating avoidance of anxiety provoking stimuli, such as a spider or germs, so that their child does not become anxious, even though this serves to reinforce the maladaptive anxiety. Research on parental accommodation is beginning to identify a similar predicament in pediatric diabetes populations. Simply put, parents are the frontline caregivers for their youth with diabetes.[68] They generally are responsible for preparing insulin injections or controlling the blood glucose levels consumed in their youth's diet. All too often however, parents are poorly educated on their child's diabetes regimen, which leads to poor HbA_{1C} levels,[69] or the youth may be resistant to their parents enforcement of the treatment recommendations. If the latter is the case, parents who accommodate to their youths resistance (e.g. allowing youth to not adhere to their diet, not routinely check their urine for ketones, etc.) and utilize permissive parenting styles are more likely to have youth with worse glycemic control than parents who are more strict and encourage mature decision making in relation to diabetes management (authoritative parenting style).[70] Thus, emerging research on diabetes underlines the importance of educating parents on the management of their child's diabetes and suggests that certain parenting approaches, specifically ones which allow for youth to take charge of their diabetes management but also sets strict boundaries about what is expected (such as mandatory daily checking of glucose levels, maintaining dietary restrictions, etc.) results in better adherence and improved glycemic control in youth with type 1 diabetes. Additionally, a child's adherence to their diabetes regimen is a product of the tools they use to monitor glucose and administer insulin.

4. New technology influencing adherence and glycemic control

Many aspects of medical care are undergoing a technological revolution; diabetes management is no exception. The advent of portable insulin pumps has had positive implications for youth with T1D mellitus in that this new technology simplifies diabetes management and allow for a more flexible lifestyle. Insulin pumps allow users to follow a less strict diet than non-pump users. Moreover, insulin pumps administer insulin more accurately than by hand thereby rendering individual insulin injections unnecessary and decreasing the incidence of severe hypoglycemia[71][72]

Compared to those administering multiple daily injections (MDI), youth using a continuous subcutaneous insulin infusion (CSII), more simply known as an insulin pump, have significantly lower A1C levels[73][73] and reduced daily insulin requirements.[74] Compared to MDI regimens, children using CSII experienced a significant reduction in their glycosylated hemoglobin level.[74] In addition to the positive effects of using a CSII, pumps are safe and well tolerated even among young children.[75][76]

The sensor-augmented insulin pump (SAP), a sophisticated tool, is an advancement in CSII technology that facilities the administration of insulin and monitors blood glucose. These insulin pumps represent a new era of diabetes management that simplifies the daily treatment regimens youth and their parents must follow. For instance, among youth using either a conventional insulin pump or SAP for a duration of six months to 3 years, SAP users' glycosylated hemoglobin level improved significantly more than that of conventional insulin pump users'.[77] In a study by Hirsch and colleagues,[78] SAP users had significantly decreased hypoglycemia and improved A1C levels as compared with conventional insulin pump users. As diabetes management becomes easier due to technological developments in insulin pump design, children and adolescents will become more likely to adhere to their diabetes regimens.

Technological devices in diabetes management are not the only promising tools for youth with Type 1 Diabetes. Carbohydrate counting is a simple and effective strategy that helps youth and their parents decide how much insulin to administer and can lead to an improvement in glycemic control. In a study by Mehta, Quinn, Volening, and Laffel[79] with children aged 4 through 12 found a relationship between parents who precisely counted the amount of carbohydrates consumed each day and lower A1C levels. Furthermore researchers found that it is feasible for children and their caregivers to accurately estimate the amount carbohydrates in food. In a study with 2530 children and children with diabetes, 73 percent were within 10-15 grams of the actual carbohydrate amount.[80] However, a study by Bishop and colleagues[81] found that in their sample of 48 adolescents aged 12 to 18, most youth could not accurately count carbohydrates. However they found that children who did successfully count carbohydrates had significantly lower A1C levels. As evidenced by the aforementioned studies, knowing how to accurately count carbohydrates is strongly associated with adherence to diabetes treatment.

Assessment of diabetes related knowledge is a means of understanding a patient's level of illness-specific knowledge as a necessary prerequisite of a youth's adherence to their diabetes regimen. The Diabetes Awareness and Reasoning Test (DART) is composed of 122 questions that effectively measures general diabetes knowledge, nutrition, diabetes care at school, hyperglycemia/hypoglycemia, insulin pump, problem solving, blood glucose testing, and sick days diabetes care. The DART was given to both children and their caregivers and A1C levels of each child were provided. It was shown that the children's insulin pump sub-score and children's parents total DART score significantly predicted A1C levels in that higher test scores predicted lower A1C levels.[82] The PedCarbQuiz is another questionnaire that was completed by adolescents or their caregivers and measures carbohydrate and insulin-dosing knowledge. Similar to the results of the study by Heidgerken and colleagues,[82] higher scores achieved by adolescent and their caregivers on the PedCarbQuiz[83] significantly correlated with lower A1C levels. The relationship between diabetes knowledge and A1C levels underlines the importance of diabetes management education in treatment adherence. New interventions are being developed to help enhance adherence and glycemic control.

5. Role of new interventions

Woolston and colleagues[84] stated the principles for new interventions should be family-focused with services provided in the home to enhance effectiveness. The team providing these services should be multidisciplinary in nature, in order to identify concerns from different perspectives that might benefit the family. This type of intervention should help the child and family achieve self-sufficiency and ultimately no longer require the in-home services.

An innovative approach to home-based intervention is through telehealth. Telehealth interventions permit diabetes educators and mental health providers trained in behavioral treatment of diabetes adherence to assist their patients in their home environment without contending with logistical challenges of scheduling face-to-face contact.[85][86] Telemedicine provides an immediate and efficient way for health care providers and their patients to communicate. This improved communication increases the timeliness of feedback, which makes treatment more efficient and responsive.[87]

In a review of how telehealth could be integrated into mental health care, Stamm[88] noted that one of the great strengths of telehealth is that it can overcome significant barriers to treatment, including economics and geography. These barriers are often identified in mental health, as patients report that they cannot keep their appointments because they cannot afford transportation, or because they do not have the flexibility in their job to leave work to attend sessions. Additionally, telehealth allows providers to increase their availability over a wider geographical area, since patients will no longer have to travel long distances to receive appropriate services.[89]

Two of the ways in which telehealth can be used has been used with patients with diabetes are home telemonitoring and telephone support.[90] Home telemonitoring can be further divided based on a timing distinction: real-time interaction or delayed.[92] Phone calls and videoconferencing fall into this category. Delayed telemonitoring involves data or information that is accessed by a provider after the patient initially sends the information. Telephone support is provided by the clinician but does not necessarily require electronic transmission of patient data.[92]

Video teleconferencing has been examined as a means of maintaining face-to-face contact between provider and patient. Stamm[89] noted that advances in technology are fueling improvements in the utility of these services. A review of the literature provided support for telehealth services in increasing the likelihood of therapy attendance with no loss in treatment benefits. Preliminary data suggests that this approach may be effective in increasing adherence to medical regimens, and can be used as a tool to support ongoing therapy. Piette and colleagues[91] designed an intervention where adult patients with diabetes received biweekly telephone calls from diabetes educators to discuss diabetes care. The educators were allowed to individualize the information provided to the specific needs of each patient. They found that their intervention improved glycemic control, and reduced diabetes-related symptoms.[90] Additionally, they found that this intervention reduced patient-reported depressive symptoms, improved self-efficacy with regard to diabetes care, and reduced the number of days spent in bed. These patients also reported greater satisfaction with the level of health care provided.[91]

Polisena and colleagues[92] metaanalysis on telehealth for diabetes found that telehealth had a positive impact on both the utilization of health services as well as glycemic control. In the 26 studies they examined, they consistently found significant benefits of home telemonitoring on glycemic control, reduced hospital visits, and shorter hospital stays. The results on telephone support in the metaanalysis by Polisena and colleagues[92] were less clear although some studies found increased patient satisfaction and reported improved quality of life. A possible reason for the inconsistent findings within the telephone support was the significant variability in the strategies used.[92]

A possible strategy to address this problem in youth with T1D would be implementing Behavioral Family Systems Therapy (BFST) through telehealth. BSFT has shown to improve family relationships and communication in families with children who have diabetes.[92][93] In addition, Wysocki and colleagues[95] found that BSFT led to improved treatment adherence and metabolic control.

BSFT includes numerous strategies to improve adherence.[95][96] More specifically, BSFT has 4 treatment strategies including problem solving, communication skills training, structural family therapy for role clarification, and cognitive restructuring. The first strategy is a structured approach to problem solving. As adolescence can be a period of increased conflict between parents and teens, the use conflict resolution skills to reduce family tension can be very therapeutic. The steps in the problem solving technique are: a) define the problem, b) set a goal, c) brainstorm ways to accomplish the chosen goal, d) evaluate the ideas, e) implement the plan, and f) revise the goal.[95][96]

The second strategy in BFST is communication skills training that focuses on improving communication between parents and adolescents around diabetes related tasks and adherence. Often parents and adolescents engage in negative communication patterns, particularly during times of conflict or when negotiating adherence strategies. The communication skills training component is designed to remediate negative communication patterns within the family. This can be an idiosyncratic component, which allows the therapist to tailor interventions to the specific needs of the families. The steps in communication skills are: a) feedback, b) instruction, c) modeling, and d) behavioral rehearsal.[95][96]

The third strategy in BSFT that is useful in improving adherence and glycemic control in families with youth with T1D is the use of structural family therapy to focus on defining roles within the family. Individuals may have ideas about the roles of each family member that have not been shared with other family members. Role confusion within the family can contribute to increased communication problems and conflict. Role clarification and explicit role negotiation within the family, as explicated in structural family therapy, can be used to reduce problems in the family that adversely impact adherence and glycemic control.[95][96]

The fourth strategy in BFST that can be used therapeutically to improve adherence and glycemic control in families with youth with T1D is cognitive restructuring. Cognitive restructing can used to address cognitive distortions and irrational thinking that can impair problem solving ability within the family. Cognitive distortion can contribute to the maintenance of maladaptive communication patterns and conflict between parents and adolescents, and thereby adversely impacting regimen adherence. Helping parents and adolescents to restructure or "soften" their strong unproductive belief patterns can facilitate more effective communication.[95][96]

Several studies conducted within the research program of Geffken and colleagues provide evidence for the effectiveness of telehealth family psychotherapy for youth with T1D. A case study[94] and case series[95] demonstrated decreased HbA1c in participants as well as improved family dynamics surrounding the diabetes regimen. An open trial of 27 adolescents[96] demonstrated a 0.7% reduction in HbA1c and no diabetes related hospitalizations in an at-risk sample of youth. Additionally, results from a controlled trial show improved metabolic control and family interactions.[97][98] Specifically, relative to those in the wait-list, families in immediate treatment had an average decrease in HbA1c of 1.32% and fewer disagreements around the diabetes regimen between parents and children ($p<.05$). Participants also showed improved adherence to their regimen at end of treatment ($p<.05$). After a one-month follow-up period, however, many participants did not maintain their treatment gains. Over one third had an increase of 0.6% or greater in HbA1c, suggesting that additional sessions would likely aid in maintaining treatment gains. Of the remaining youth, approximately one third maintained gains, while the remaining youth were unable to be reached for follow-up assessments. Although not systematically assessed, our non-study related interactions with these youth (i.e., consultations during their scheduled endocrinology visits) suggest that the overwhelming majority of these youth experienced partial or full relapses. Taken together, these studies demonstrate that intensive telehealth family psychological treatment using a BSFT model improves adherence to the medical regimen, glycemic control, and family dynamics.

According to Azar and Gabbay[87], telemedicine interventions have a wide range of variability. Some systems are more basic and focus phone, email or short message services to faciliatate communication between patients and their providers. In contrast other systems use complex web interfaces that can include home meter information as well as logs for diet and activitiy levels.[99] For example, Carelink, an insulin-pump monitoring system accessed online, significantly improved glycemic control equally among children in both rural and urban areas even though children in rural areas visited clinics less frequently. The Carelink system allowed children and their parents to upload and access information about their glucose levels, amount of insulin required each day, and informed patients of where their blood sugar levels were in comparison to their goal daily sugar level. If dose adjustments were necessary, the diabetes care provider emailed or called their patient to alert them of the change.[100]

6. Conclusions

This review of the literature demonstrates a wide variety of psychological variables may mediate the relationship between regimen adherence and glycemic control in the families of youth with T1D. These psychological variables range from parental warmth and support to coerciveness and conflict in the parent-child relationship. It was also demonstrated that a wide variety of childhood behavioral patterns such as internalizing and externalizing, behavioral self-regulation and executive functioning, and peer-victimization may have similar relationships with regimen adherence and glycemic control in youth with T1D. The role of diabetes knowledge and the importance of it's measurement are suggested. Finally the development of new technology in diabetes care and management have been reviewed. The value of newer telehealth technologies are highlighted towards the latter sections of the review. The review demonstrates that Telehealth, used via the telephone or internet, is a cost-effective, convenient way for patients and their healthcare providers to manage and communicate about their diabetes regimen. The work by Geffken and colleagues demonstrates that telehealth can particularly useful for service delivery with families with youth with T1D. Telehealth allows treatment for families with youth with T1D with considerable barriers to their diabetes management such as those who require complex treatments and more frequent consultation with their diabetes care provider than distance or funding will allow. This review provides evidence on the value and critical inclusion of behavioral health services and research for the treatment of families youth with T1D.

7. References

[1] M.A. Rapoff, & M.U. Barnard, "Compliance with pediatric medical regimens", *Patient compliance in medical practice and clinical trials.* New York: Raven Press, 73-98. 1991.

[2] M. Kovacs, D. Goldston, S. Obrosky, & S. Iyengar, "Prevalence and predictors of pervasive noncompliance with medical treatment among youths with insulin-dependent diabetes mellitus" *Journal of the American Academy of Child and Adolescent Psychiatry,* Vol. 31, pp. 1112-1119. 1992.

[3] Diabetes Control and Complications Research Group, "The effect of intensive treatment of diabetes on the development and progression of long-term complications in insulin-dependent diabetes mellitus", *New England Journal of Medicine,* Vol. 329, pp.977-986.1993.

[4] K.L. Lemanek, J. Kamps, & N.B. Chung, "Empirically supported treatments in pediatric psychology: Regimen adherence", *Journal of Pediatric Psychology,* Vol. 26, pp. 253-275. 2001.

[5] A.L.Quittner, D.L. Espelage, C. Ievers-Landis, & D. Drotar, "Measuring adherence to medical treatment in childhood chronic illness: Considering multiple methods and sources of information", *Journal of Clinical Psychology in Medical Settings,* Vol. 7, pp. 41-54. 2002.

[6] C. L. Davis, A. M. Delamater, K. H. Shaw, A.M. La Greca, M. S. Eidson, J. Perez-Rodriguez, & R. Nemery, "Parenting styles, regimen adherence, and glycemic control in 4- to 10-year-old children with diabetes", *Journal of Pediatric Psychology,* Vol. 26(2), pp. 123-129. 2001.

[7] Diabetes Control and Complications Trial Research Group, "Effect of intensive diabetes treatment on the development and progression of long-term complications in adolescents with insulin-dependent diabetes mellitus: Diabetes control and complications trial", *The Journal of Pediatrics,* Vol. 125(2), pp. 177-188. 1994.

[8] E. R. Mackey, & R. Streisand, "Brief report: The relationship of parental support and conflictto physical activity in preadolescents with type 1 diabetes", *Journal of Pediatric Psychology,*Vol. 33(10), pp. 1137-1141. 2008.

[9] A. J. Rovner, S. N. Mehta, D. L. Haynie, E. M. Robinson, H. J. Pound, D. A.Butler et al., "Perceived benefits, barriers, and strategies of family meals among children with type 1 diabetes mellitus and their parents: Focus-group findings", *Journal of the American Dietetic Association*, Vol. 110(9), pp. 1302-1306. 2010.

[10] J. R. Wood, E. C. Moreland, L. K. Volkening, B. M. Svoren, D. A. Butler, & L. M. B. Laffel, "Durability of insulin pump use in pediatric patients with type 1 diabetes", *Diabetes Care*, Vol. 29(11), pp. 2355-2360. 2006.

[11] I. Rabbone, A. Bobbio, K. Berger, M. Trada, C. Sacchetti, & F. Cerutti, "Age-related differences in metabolic response to continuous subcutaneous insulin infusion in pre-pubertal and pubertal children with type 1 diabetes mellitus", *Journal of Endocrinological Investigation*, Vol. 30(6), pp. 477-483. 2007.

[12] D. J. Wiebe, A. Croom, K. T. Fortenberry, J. Butner, J. Butler, M. T. Swinyard, et al., "Parental involvement buffers associations between pump duration and metabolic control among adolescents with type 1 diabetes", *Journal of Pediatric Psychology*, Vol. 35(10), pp.1152-1160. 2010.

[13] L. C. Schafer, K. D. McCaul, & R. E. Glasgow, "Supportive and nonsupportive family behaviors: Relationships to adherence and metabolic control in persons with type I diabetes", *Diabetes Care*, Vol. 9(2), pp. 179-185. 1986.

[14] A. B. Lewin, E. A. Storch, J. H. Silverstein, A. L. Baumeister, M. S. Strawser, & G. R. Geffken, "Validation of the pediatric inventory for parents in mothers of children with type 1 diabetes: An examination of parenting stress, anxiety, and childhood psychopathology", *Families, Systems, & Health*, Vol., 23(1), pp. 56-65. 2005.

[15] M. S., Greene, B., Mandleco, S. O. Roper, E. S. Marshall, & T. Dyches, "Metabolic control, self-care behaviors, and parenting in adolescents with type 1 diabetes: A correlational study", *The Diabetes Educator*, Vol. 36(2), pp. 326-336. (2010).

[16] S. M. Lloyd, M. Cantell, D. Pacaud, S. Crawford, & D. Dewey, "Brief report: Hope, perceived maternal empathy, medical regimen adherence, and glycemic control in adolescents with type 1 diabetes", *Journal of Pediatric Psychology*, Vol.34(9), pp. 1025-1029. 2009.

[17] A. B. Lewin, G. R. Geffken, A. D. Heidgerken, D. Duke, W. Novoa, L. B. Williams, & E.A. Storch, "The diabetes family behavior checklist: A psychometric evaluation", *Journal of Clinical Psychology in Medical Settings*, Vol. 12(4), pp. 315-322. 2005.

[18] M. E. Hilliard, M. Monaghan, F. R. Cogen, & R. Streisand, "Parent stress and child behaviour among young children with type 1 diabetes", *Child: Care, Health & Development*, Vol. 37(2), pp. 224-232. 2011.

[19] R. Streisand, E. R. Mackey, B. M. Elliot, L. Mednick, I. M. Slaughter, J. Turek, & A. Austin, "Parental anxiety and depression associated with caring for a child newly diagnosed with type 1 diabetes: Opportunities for education and counseling", *Patient Education & Counseling*, Vol. 73(2), pp. 333-338. 2008.

[20] S. Bowes, L. Lowes, J. Warner, & J. W. Gregory, "Chronic sorrow in parents of children with type 1 diabetes", *Journal of Advanced Nursing*,Vol. 65(5), 992-1000. 2009.

[21] M. Monaghan, M. E. Hilliard, F. R. Cogen, & R. Streisand, "Supporting parents of very young children with type 1 diabetes: Results from a pilot study", *Patient Education & Counseling*, Vol. 82(2), pp. 271-274. 2011.

[22] S. T. Hauser, A. M. Jacobson, P. Lavori, J. I. Wolfsdorf, R. D. Herskowitz, J. E. Milley, et al., "Adherence among children and adolescents with insulin-dependent diabetes

mellitus over a four-year longitudinal follow-up: II. immediate and long-term linkages with the family milieu", *Journal of Pediatric Psychology*, Vol. 15(4), pp. 527-542. 1990.

[23] S. Miller-Johnson, R. E. Emery, R. S. Marvin, W. Clarke, R. Lovinger, & M. Martin, "Parent-child relationships and the management of insulin-dependent diabetes mellitus", *Journal of Consulting and Clinical Psychology*, (1994). Vol. 62(3), pp. 603-610. 1994.

[24] L. B. Williams, L. M. B. Laffel, & K. K. Hood," Diabetes-specific family conflict and psychological distress in paediatric type 1 diabetes", *Diabetic Medicine*, Vol. 26(9), pp. 908-914. 2009.

[25] M. A. Harris, K. A. Freeman, & M. Beers, "Family therapy for adolescents with poorly controlled diabetes: Initial test of clinical significance", *Journal of Pediatric Psychology*, Vol. 34(10), pp. 1097-1107. 2009.

[26] A. Lewandowski, & D. Drotar, "The relationship between parent-reported social support and adherence to medical treatment in families of adolescents with type 1 diabetes", *Journal of Pediatric Psychology*, Vol. 32(4), pp. 427-436. 2007.

[27] K. M. Grabill, G. R. Geffken, D. Duke, A. Lewin, L. Williams, E. Storch, & J. Silverstein, "Family functioning and adherence in youth with type 1 diabetes: A latent growth model of glycemic control", *Children's Health Care*, Vol. 39(4), 279-295. 2010.

[28] F. J. Cameron, T. C. Skinner, C. E. de Beaufort, H. Hoey, P. G. F. Swift, H. Aanstoot, et al., "Are family factors universally related to metabolic outcomes in adolescents with Type 1 diabetes?", *Diabetic Medicine*, Vol. 25(4), pp. 463-468. 2008.

[29] D. Rubin Young-Hyman, & M. Peyrot "Parent-child responsibility and conflict in diabetes care", *Diabetes*, Vol.38:28. 1989.

[30] K. K. Hood, D. A. Butler, B. J. Anderson, & L. Laffel, "Updated and revised diabetes family conflict scale", *Diabetes Care*, Vol. 30(7), pp.1764-1769. 2007.

[31] D. Arnold, "Co-occurrence of externalizing behavior problems and emergent academic difficulties in young high-risk boys: A preliminary evaluation of patterns and mechanisms," *Journal of Applied Developmental Psychology*, Vol. 18, pp. 317-330, 1997.

[32] D. Schwartz, K.A. Dodge, G.S. Pettit, J.E. Bates, & The Conduct Problems Prevention Research Group, "Friendship as a moderating factor in the pathway between early harsh home environment and later victimization in the peer group," *Developmental Psychology*, Vol. 36, pp. 646-662, 1999.

[33] C.R. Petty, J.F. Rosenbaum, D.R. Hirshfeld-Becker, A. Henin, S. Hubley, S., LaCasse, et al., "The Child Behavior Checklist broad-band scales predict subsequent psychopathology: a 5-year follow-up," *Journal of Anxiety Disorders*, Vol. 22, pp. 532–539, 2008.

[34] T.M. Achenbach, "Integrative guide for the 1991 CBCL/4-18,YSR, and TRF profiles," Burlington: University of Vermont, Department of Psychiatry, 1991.

[35] D. M. Cohen, M. A., Lumley, S. Naar-King, T. Partridge, & N. Cakan, "Child behavior problems and family functioning as predictors of adherence and glycemic control in economically disadvantaged children with type 1 diabetes: A prospective study," *Journal of Pediatric Psychology*, Vol. 29, pp. 171–284, 2008.

[36] L. Greening, L. Stoppelbein, C. Konishi, S.S. Jordan, & G. Moll, "Child routines and youths' adherence to treatment for type 1 diabetes," Vol. 32, pp. 437-447, 2007.

[37] M. Kovacs, D. Charron-Prochownik, & D. S. Obrosky, " A longitudinal study of biomedical and psychosocial predictors of multiple hospitalizations among young people with insulin-dependent diabetes mellitus," *Diabetic Medicine*, Vol. 12, pp. 142-148, 1995.

[38] C.M. McDonnell, E.A. Northam, S.M. Donath, G.A. Werther, & F.J. Cameron, "Hyperglycemia and externalizing behavior in children with type 1 diabetes," *Diabetes Care, 30*, pp. 2211–2215, 2007.

[39] S. Naar-King, A. Idalski, D. Ellis, M. Frey, T. Templin, P.B. Cunningham, et al."Gender differences in adherence and metabolic control in urban youth with poorly controlled type 1 diabetes: The mediating role of mental health symptom," *Journal of Pediatric Psychology,* 31, pp. 793-802, 2005.

[40] D.K. Duke, G.R. Geffken, A.B. Lewin, L.B. Williams, E.A. Storch, & J.H. Silverstein, "Glycemic control in youth with type 1 diabetes: Family predictors and mediators," *Journal of Pediatric Psychology,* Vol. 33, 719-727, 2008.

[41] K. Gelfand, G. Geffken, A. Lewin, A. Heidgerken, M. Grove, T. Malasanos, et al, "An initial evaluation of the design of pediatric psychology consultation service with children with diabetes," *Journal of Child Health Care,* Vol. 8, pp.113-123, 2004.

[42] L. M. Sancheza, A.M. Chronisa & S.J. Hunter, "Improving Compliance With Diabetes Management in Young Adolescents With Attention-Deficit/Hyperactivity Disorder Using Behavior Therapy," *Cognitive and Behavioral Practice,* Vol. 13, pp. 134-145, 2006.

[43] S.M. Markowitz, J.S. Gonzalez, J.L. Wilkinson, & S.A. Safren, "A Review of Treating Depression in Diabetes: Emerging Findings," *Psychosomatics,* Vol. 15, pp. 1-18, 2011.

[44] R.M. Ghandour, M.D. Kogan, S.J. Blumberg, & D.F. Perry, "Prevalence and correlates of internalizing mental health symptoms among CSHCN," *Pediatrics,* Vol. 125, pp. e269-e277, 2010.

[45] P.J. Lustman & R. E. Clouse, "Depression in diabetic patients: the relationship between mood and glycemic control," *Journal of Diabetes Complications,* Vol. 19, pp. 113–122, 2005.

[46] M.M. Garrison, W.J. Katon, & L.P. Richardson. "The impact of psychiatric comorbidities on readmissions for diabetes in youth." *Diabetes Care,* Vol. 28, pp. 2150-2154, 2005.

[47] V. S. Helgeson, K. A. Reynolds, L. Siminerio, O. Escobar, & D. Becker, "Parent and adolescent distribution of responsibility for self-care: Links to health outcome." Journal of Pediatric Psychology, Vol. 33, pp. 497-508, 2008.

[48] A.M. La Greca & J.S. Skyler, "Psychological issues in IDDM; A multivariate framework," in *Stress, Coping, and Disease,* Erlbaum, 1991, pp. 169-109.

[49] P. J. Lustman, R.J. Anderson, K.E. Freedland, M. de Groot, R.M. Caney, & R.E. Clouse, "Depression and poor glycemic control: a meta-analytic review of the literature. *Diabetes Care,* Vol. 23, pp. 934-942, 2000.

[50] S. He, H. Cao, C.G.M. Magnusson, M. Eriksson-Berg, M. Mehrnaz, K. Schenck-Gustafsson, & M. Blombäck, "Are increased levels of von Willebrand factor in chronic coronary heart disease caused by decrease in von Willebrand factor cleaving protease activity? A study by immunoassay with antibody against intact bond," *Thrombosis Research,* Vol. 103, pp. 241–248, 2001.

[51] Channon, S. J., Huws-Thomas, M. V., Rollnick, S., Hood, K., Cannings-John, R. L., Rogers, C. et al., "A multicenter randomized controlled trial of motivational interviewing in teenagers with diabetes." *Diabetes Care,* Vol. 30, 1390–1395, 2007.

[52] N. R. Crick, & M. A. Bigbee, "Relational and overt forms of peer victimization: A multiinformant approach," *Journal of Consulting and Clinical Psychology,* Vol. 66, 337-347, 1998.

[53] A. Baumeister, E.A. Storch, & G.R. Geffken, "Peer victimization in children with learning disabilities," *Child and Adolescent Social Work Journal,* Vol. 25, pp.11-23, 2008.

[54] C.S. Lim, P.A. Graziano, D.M. Janicke, W.N. Gray, L.M. Ingerski, & J.H. Silverstein,"Peer Victimization and Depressive Symptoms in Obese Youth: The Role of Perceived Social Support Children's Health Care," *Children's Heath Care,* Vol. 40, pp. 1-15, 2011.

[55] E.A. Storch, A. Lewin, J.H. Silverstein, A.D. Heidgerken, M.S. Strawser, A. Baumeister, et al., "Social-psychological correlates of peer victimization in children with endocrine disorders," *The Journal of Pediatrics,* Vol. 145, pp. 784-789, 2004.

[56] D.M. Janicke, W.N. Gray, N.A. Kahhan, K.W. Follansbee Junger, K.K. Marciel, et al., "Brief Report: The Association Between Peer Victimization, Prosocial Support, and Treatment Adherence in Children and Adolescents with Inflammatory Bowel Disease," *Journal of Pediatric Psychology,* Vol. 34, pp. 769-773, 2009.

[57] E.A. Storch, A. Lewin, J. Silverstein, A. Heidgerken, M. Strawser, A. Baumeister, et al., "Peer victimization, and psychosocial adjustment in children with type 1 diabetes," *Clinical Pediatrics,* Vol. 43, pp. 467-471, 2004

[58] E.A. Storch, A. Heidgerken, G.R. Geffken, A. Lewin, V. Ohleyer, M. Freddo, et al., "Bullying, regimen self-management, and metabolic control in youth with type 1Diabetes," *Journal of Pediatrics,* Vol. 148, pp. 784-787, 2006.

[59] A. Bechara, A.R. Damasio, H. Damasio, & S.W. Anderson, "Insensitivity to future consequences following damage to human prefrontal cortex," *Cognition,* Vol. 50, pp. 7–15, 1994.

[60] D.M. Bagner, L.B. Williams, G.R. Geffken, J.H. Silverstein, & E.A. Storch, "Type 1 diabetes in youth: The relationship between adherence and executive functioning," *Children's Healthcare,* Vol. 36, pp.169-179, 2007.

[61] K. McNally, J. Rohan, J. Pendley, A. Delamater, & D. Drotar, "Executive functioning, treatment adherence, and glycemic control in children with Type 1 Diabetes," *Diabetes Care,* Vol. 33, pp. 1159–1162, 2010.

[62] L.B. Williams, "Executive functioning, parenting stress, and family factors as predictors of diabetes management in pediatric patients with type 1 diabetes using intensive insulin regimens," *University of Florida, 2008.*

[63] T. Wysocki, R. Iannotti, J. Weissberg-Benchell, K. Hood, L. Laffel, B.J. Anderson, et al., "Diabetes problem solving by youths with type 1 diabetes and their caregivers: Measurement, validation and longitudinal associations with glycemic control," *Journal of Pediatric Psychology,* Vol. 33, pp. 875-884, 2008.

[64] O. Hsin, A.M. La Greca, J.M. Valenzuela, C.T. Moine, & A.M. Delamater, "Adherence and glycemic control among Hispanic youth with type 1 diabetes: role of family involvement and acculturation," *Journal of Pediatric Psycholology,* Vol. 26, 2009.

[65] M. Grey, E. Boland, C. Yu, S. Sullivan-Bolyai, & W. Tamborlane, "Personal and family factors associated with quality of life in adolescents with diabetes." *Diabetes Care,* Vol. 21, pp. 909-914, 1998.

[66] D.A. Ellis, C.L. Podolski, M. Frey, S. Naar-King, B. Wang, & K. Moltz, "The role of parental monitoring in adolescent health outcomes: Impact on regimen adherence in youth with type 1 diabetes." *Journal of Pediatric Psychology,* Vol. 32, pp. 907-917, *2007.*

[67] C. Suveg, T.L. Roblek, J. Robin, A. Krain, S. Schendbrand, & G.S. Ginsburg, "Parental involvement when conducting cognitive-behavioral therapy for children with anxiety disorders," *Journal of Cognitive Psychotherapy,* Vol. 20, pp. 287–301, 2006.

[68] M., Kovacs, T. L. Feinberg, S. Paulauskas, R. Finkelstein, M. Pollack, & M. Crouse-Novak, "Initial psychological responses of parents to the diagnosis of insulin-dependent diabetes mellitus in their children," *Diabetes Care,* Vol. 8. pp. 568–575, 1985.

[69] H. Tahirovic & A. Toromanovic, "Glycemic control in diabetic children: role of mother's knowledge and socioeconomic status," *European Journal of Pediatrics,* Vol. 169, pp. 961-964, 2010.

[70] M.S. Greene, B. Mandleco, S.O. Roper, E.S. Marshall & T. Dyches, "Metabolic control, self-care behaviors, and parenting in adolescents with type 1 diabetes: a correlational study," *Diabetes Education,* Vol. 36, pp. 326–336, 2010.

[71] American Diabetes Association, *Living with diabetes: Advantages of using an insulin Pump,* 2010.

[72] J. C. Pickup, & A. J. Sutton, "Severe hypoglycaemia and hypocaemic control in type 1 diabetes: Meta-analysis of multiple daily insulin injections compared with continuous subcutaneous insulin infusion", *Diabetic Medicine,* Vol. 25(7), pp. 765-774. 2008.

[73] C. A. Paris, G. Imperatore, G. Klingensmith, D. Petitti, B. Rodriguez, A. M. Anderson, et al., "Predictors of insulin regimens and impact on outcomes in youth with type 1 diabetes: The search for diabetes in youth study", *Journal of Pediatrics,* Vol. 155(2), pp. 183-189. 2009.

[74] E. Pankowska, M. Blazik, P. Dziechciarz, A. Szypowska, & H. Szajewska, "Continuous subcutaneous insulin infusion vs. multiple daily injections in children with type 1 diabetes: A systematic review and meta-analysis of randomized control trials", *Pediatric Diabetes,* Vol. 10(1), pp. 52-58. (2008).

[75] L. A. Fox, L. M. Buckloh, S. D. Smith, T. Wysocki, & N. Mauras, "A randomized controlled trial of insulin pump therapy in young children with type 1 diabetes", *Diabetes Care,* Vol. 28(6), pp. 1277-1281. 2005.

[76] J. N. Churchill, R. L. Ruppe, & A. Smaldone, "Use of continuous insulin infusion pumps in young children with type 1 diabetes: A systematic review", *Journal of Pediatric Health Care,* Vol. 23(3), pp.173-179. 2008.

[77] A. E. Scaramuzza, D. Iafusco, I. Rabbone, R. Bonfanti, F. Lombardo, R. Schiaffini, et al., "Use of integrated real-time continuous glucose monitoring/insulin pump system in children and adolescents with type 1 diabetes: A 3-year follow-up study", *Diabetes Technology & Therapeutics,* Vol. 13(2), pp. 99-103. 2011.

[78] I. B. Hirsch, J. Abelseth, B. W. Bode, J. S. Fischer, F. R. Kaufman, J.Mastrototaro, et al., "Sensor-augmented insulin pump therapy: Results of the first randomized treat-to-target study", *Diabetes Technology & Therapeutics*, Vol. 10(5), pp. 377-383. 2008.

[79] S. N. Mehta, N. Quinn, L. K. Volkening, & M. B. Laffel, "Impact of carbohydrate counting on glycemic control in children with type 1 diabetes", *Diabetes Care*, Vol. 32(6), 1014-1016. 2009.

[80] C. E. Smart, K. Ross, J. A. Edge, B. R. King, P. McElduff, & C. E. Collins, "Can children with type 1 diabetes and their caregivers estimate the carbohydrate content of meals and snacks?", *Diabetic Medicine*, (2010). (2010). Vol. 27(3), pp. 348-353. 2010.

[81] F. K. Bishop, D. M. Maahs, G. Spiegel, D. Owen, G. J. Klingensmith, A. Bortsov, et al., "The carbohydrate counting in adolescents with type 1 diabetes (CCAT) study", *Diabetes Spectrum*, Vol. 22(1), pp. 56-62. 2009.

[82] A. D. Heidgerken, L. Merlo, L. B. Williams, A. B. Lewin, K. Gelfand, T. Malasanos, et al., "Diabetes awareness and reasoning test: A preliminary analysis of development and psychometrics", *Children's Health Care*, Vol. 36(2), pp. 117-136. 2007.

[83] M. B. Koontz, L. Cuttler, M. R. Palmert, M. O'Riordan, E. A. Borawski, J. McConnell, & E. O. Kern, "Development of validation of a questionnaire to assess carbohydrate and insulin-dosing knowledge in youth with type 1 diabetes", *Diabetes Care*, Vol. 33(3), pp. 457-462. 2010.

[84] J.L. Woolston, S.J. Berkowitz, M.C. Schaefer, & , J.A. Adnopoz, "Intensive, integrated, in-home psychiatric services: The catalyst to enhancing outpatient intervention", *Child and Adolescent Psychiatric Clinics of North America*, Vol. 7, 615-633. 1998.

[85] E. A. Balas, F. Jaffrey, G. J. Kuperman, S. A. Boren, G. D. Brown, F. Pinciroli, & J. A. Mitchell, "Electronic communication with patients: Evaluation of distance medicine technology", *Journal of the American Medical Association*, Vol. 278, pp. 152-159. 1997.

[86] D. C. Klonoff, "Diabetes and telemedicine: Is the technology sound, effective, cost effective,and practical?", *Diabetes Care*,Vol. 26, pp. 1626-1628. 2003.

[87] M. Azar, & R. Gabbay, "Web-based management of diabetes through glucose uploads: Has the time come for telemedicine?" *Diabetes Research and Clinical Practice, Vol. 83*, pp. 9-17. 2009.

[88] B. H. Stamm, "Integrating telehealth into mental health care", *In T. L. Jackson (Ed.), Innovations in clinical practice: A source book*, Vol. 18. pp. 385-400.2000.

[89] N. Holt, & M.A. Crawford, "Medical information service via telephone: The pioneer of physician consultation services", *Annals of the New York Academy of Science*, Vol. 670. pp. 155-162. 1992.

[90] J. Polisena, K. Tran, K. Cimon, B. Hutton, S. McGill, & K. Palmer, "Home telehealth for diabetes management: A systematic review and meta-analysis", *Diabetes, Obesity & Metabolism*, Vol. 11(10). pp. 913-930. 2009.

[91] J.D. Piette,M. Weinberger M, S. J. McPhee, C.A. Mah, F.B. Kraemer, L.M., Crapo, "Do automated calls with nurse follow-up improve self-care and glycemic control among vulnerable patients with diabetes?" *Am J Med*, Vol. 108, pp. 20-27. 2000.

[92] T. Wysocki, M. A. Harris, L. M. Buckloh, D. Mertlich, A. S. Lochrie, A. Taylor, et al., "Effects of behavioral family systems therapy for diabetes on adolescents' family relationships, treatment adherence, and metabolic control", *Journal of Pediatric Psychology*, Vol. 31, pp. 928-938. 2006.

[93] T. Wysocki, M. A. Harris, P. Greco, J. Bubb, C.E. Danda, L.M. Harvey, et al., "Randomized, controlled trial of behavior therapy for families of adolescents with insulin-dependent diabetes mellitus", *Journal of Pediatric* Psychology, Vol. 25, pp. 23–33. 2000.

[94] J.W. Adkins, E.A. Storch, A.B. Lewin, L. Williams, J.H. Silverstein, T. Malasanos, et al., "Home-based behavioral health intervention: Use of a telehealth model to address poor adherence to type-I diabetes medical regimens", *Journal of Telehealth and Telemedicine,* Vol. 12, pp. 370-372. 2006.

[95] K. Gelfand, G. Geffken, M. Halsey-Lyda, A. Muir, & T. Malasanos, "Intensive telehealth management of five at risk adolescents with diabetes", *Journal of Telehealth and Telecare,*Vol. 9, pp. 117-121. 2003.

[96] A. Heidgerken, E.A. Storch, L. Williams, A. Lewin, J.H. Silverstein, J. Adkins, et al., "Telehealth intervention for adolescents with type 1 diabetes", *Journal of Pediatrics,* Vol. 148, pp. 707-708. 2006.

[97] H.D. Lehmkuhl, E.A. Storch, C. Cammarata, K. Meyer, O. Rahman, J. Silverstein, et al., "Telehealth Behavior Therapy for the Management of Type I Diabetes in Adolescent", *Journal of Diabetes and Science Technology,* Vol. 4(1), pp. 199-208. 2010.

[98] E.A. Storch, G. Geffken, J. Adkins, D. Duke, K. Kiker, T. Malasanos, & J. Silverstein,"Wait-list controlled trial of telehealth behavior therapy: Preliminary results", *Scientific Proceedings of Therapeutic Patient Education,* Vol. 68. 2006.

[99] R. Bellazzi, M. Arcelloni, G. Bensa, H. Blankenfeld, E. Brugués, E. Carson,. . . M. Stefanelli, "Design, methods, and evaluation directions of a multi-access service for the management of diabetes mellitus patients", *Diabetes Technology & Therapeutics,* Vol. 5(4), pp. 621-629. 2003.

[100] E. A. Corriveau, P. J. Durso, E. D. Kaufman, B. J. Skipper, L. A. Laskaratos, & K. B. Heintzman, "Effect of carelink, an internet-based insulin pump monitoring system, on glycemic control in rural and urban children with type 1 diabetes mellitus", *Pediatric Diabetes,*Vol. 9(4), pp. 360-366. 2008.

Part 3

Perspectives of Diabetes Pathogenesis

9

Fulminant Type 1 Diabetes Mellitus in IRS-2 Deficient Mice

Toshiro Arai, Nobuko Mori and Haruo Hashimoto
Nippon Veterinary and Life Science University
Japan

1. Introduction

Type 1 diabetes mellitus (T1DM), one of two major forms of diabetes, results from nearly complete destruction of pancreatic beta (β) cells. According to the classification of diabetes made by the American Diabetes Association, T1DM is divided into two subtypes: immune-mediated (type 1A) and idiopathic (type 1B) (American Diabetes Association, 2008). Fulminant type 1 diabetes mellitus (FT1DM), which was first reported by Imagawa et al. in 2000, is thought to be a unique subtype of type 1B diabetes. The initial reports of FT1DM were exclusively in Japanese population and accounted for about 20% of their T1DM (Imagawa et al., 2000; 2003). Outside Japan, Cho et al. (2007) reported prevalence for FT1DM of 7.1% in the newly diagnosed Korean T1DM patients. However, epidemiological study of FT1DM is lacking in other Asian populations and its incidence and pathogenesis remain to be elucidated. While a search for FT1DM was reported to be negative in the Caucasian population, case reports on FT1DM had surfaced in different ethnic groups, predominantly from Asian origins (Jung et al., 2004; Taniyama et al., 2004; Moreau et al., 2008). However, the causative mechanism of FT1DM is currently unknown. On the other hand, insulin receptor substrate (IRS) disorders are associated with onset of insulin resistance and diabetes mellitus (Withers et al., 1998; Kido et al., 2000). A small population of male IRS-2 deficient mice showed hyperglycemia associated with markedly diminished pancreatic islet size, and these extremely hyperglycemic IRS-2 deficient mice exhibited 1) abrupt onset of diabetes and 2) very short duration of diabetic symptoms, such as polyuria, thirst, and body weight loss. These symptoms resembled the features of human nonautoimmune FT1DM (Hashimoto et al., 2006). Characteristics of abrupt onset of hyperglycemia associated with marked diminished islet mass in IRS-2 deficient mice were investigated to analyze the onset mechanism of FT1DM.

2. Characteristics of fulminant type 1 diabetes mellitus

2.1 Onset of fulminant type 1 diabetes mellitus

Fulminant type 1 diabetes mellitus (FT1DM) is a novel clinical entirely within diabetes mellitus and accounts for 20% of T1DM in Japan. Since its initial description by Imagawa et al. (2000), many cases have been reported predominately in Japan and Korea. FT1DM shows clinical characteristics of (1) remarkably abrupt onset of disease; (2) very short (< 1 week) duration of diabetic symptoms, such as polyuria, thirst and body weight loss; (3) acidosis at diagnosis; (4) negative status of islet-related antibodies, islet cell antibodies (ICA), anti-glutamic acid decarboxylase antibodies (GADAb), insulin autoantibodies (IAA) or anti-islet antigen 2 antibodies (IA-2); (5) virtually no C-peptide secretion (< 10 μg/day in urine); and (6) elevated serum pancreatic enzyme level. Fas and Fas ligand expression are lacking and the mechanism of β cell destruction differs from that in autoimmune T1DM. However the degradation mechanism of β cell in FT1DM of humans is unknown. Recently, it has been reported that the onset of FT1DM may be attributed to certain HLA subtype, to viral infection, or to pregnancy (Imagawa et al., 2003; Imagawa et al., 2005; Shimizu et al., 2006; Kawabata et al., 2009). In recent study, macrophages and T cells - but not natural killer cells – had infiltrated the islets and the exocrine pancreas and Toll-like receptor (TLR) 3, a sensor of viral components, was detected in most of macrophages and T cells in FT1DM patients (Shibasaki et al., 2010). Their study showed remarkably decreased numbers of pancreatic beta and alpha cells, macrophage-dominated insulitis and the expression of TLRs, a signature of viral infection, in FT1DM soon after the disease onset. These results suggest a new mechanism of virus-induced macrophage-dominated inflammatory process, rather than autoimmune T cell response, plays a major role in β cell destruction in FT1DM.

2.2 FT1DM associated with viral infection

Causative mechanism for accelerated β cell destruction in FT1DM is unclear. To date, viral infection has been the most popular speculated cause of acute destruction of the pancreatic β cell as many patients reported flu-like symptoms prior to the disease onset (Zheng et al., 2011). Tanaka et al (2009) investigated islet cell status, including the presence of enterovirus and chemokine/cytokline/major histocompatibility complex (MHC) expression in the pancreata using immunohistochemical analyses in three subjects with FT1DM. Immunohistochemical analyses revealed the presence of enterovirus-capsid protein in all three affected pancreata. Extensive infiltration of CXCR3 receptor-bearing T-cells and macrophages into islets was observed. Dendritic cells were stained in and around the islets. Interferon-γ and CXC chemokine ligand 10 (CXCL10) were strongly coexpressed in all subtypes of islet cells, including β cell and α cells. No CXCL10 was expressed in exocrine pancreas. Serum levels of CXCL10 were increased. Expression of MHC class II and hyper-expression of MHC class I was observed in some islet cells. These observations strongly suggest the presence of a circuit for destruction of β cells in FT1DM. Enterovirus infection of the pancreata initiates coexpression of interferon-γ and CXCL10 in β cells. CXCL10 secreted from β cells activates and attracts autoreactive T-cells and macrophages to the islets via CXCR3. These infiltrating autoreactive T-cells and macrophages release inflammatory cytokines including interferon-γ in the islets, not only damaging β cells but also accelerating CXCL10 generation in residual β cells and thus further activating cell-mediated autoimmunity until all β cells have been destroyed. On the other hand, Shibasaki et al (2010) investigated pathogenesis of FT1DM with special reference to insulitis and viral infection using pancreatic autopsy samples from three patients. Both β and α cell area were significantly decreased in comparison with those of normal controls. Macrophages and T cells – but not natural killer cells – had infiltrated the islets and the exocrine pancreas. Toll-like receptor (TLR) 3, a sensor of viral components, was detected in 84.7% of macrophages and 62.7% of T cells in all three patients. TLR7 and TLR9 were also detected in the pancreas of all three patients. Enterovirus RNA was detected in β cells positive islets in one of the three patients by *in situ* hybridization. These results suggest that macrophage-dominated inflammatory process, rather than autoimmune T cell response, plays a major role in β cell destruction in FT1DM.

2.3 FT1DM associated with pregnancy

FT1DM associated with pregnancy is very rare. However if it occurs, the rapid onset is associated with an extremely high risk of fetal death. Therefore, it is important for physicians to make an appropriate diagnosis as early as possible and to begin immediate treatment of both the mother and the fetus (Murabayashi et al., 2009). Shimizu et al. (2006) characterized the clinical and immunogenetic features of Japanese pregnancy-associated FT1DM (PF). A group of patients with PF was compared with a group of patients of child-bearing age with FT1DM that was not associated with pregnancy (NPF) in a nationwide survey conducted from 2000-2004. The criteria used for inclusion of FT1DM were 1) ketosis or ketoacidosis within 1 week after the onset of hyperglycemic symptoms; 2) urinary C peptide excretion less than 10 μg/day, fasting serum C peptide levels less than 0.3ng/ml, or serum C peptide levels less than 0.5 ng/ml after glucagon injection or a meal load soon after the onset of the disease; and 3) hemoglobin A_{1c} levels less than 8.5% on the first visit. Twenty two PF patients showed increased plasma amylase values and negative for GADab except one with transient increase in GADab (12U/ml). In 22 PF patients, 18 developed disease during pregnancy, whereas four cases occurred immediately after delivery. Twelve cases that developed during pregnancy resulted in stillbirty, and five of the six fetal cases that survived were delivered by cesarean section. The haplotype frequency of HLA DRB1*0901-DQB1*0303 in PF was significantly higher than those in NPF and controls, whereas that of DRB1*0405-DQB1*0401 in NPF was significantly higher than those in PF. The type 1 diabetes-susceptible HLA class II haplotype is distinct in PF and NPF patients, suggesting that different HLA haplotypes underlie the presentation of PF or NPF. Moreau et al. (2008) reported three cases of FT1DM in Caucasian French women. HLA phenotyping of these Caucasian patients did not find the specific HLA haplotype (DRB1*0405-DQB1*0401) found to be linked to FT1DM in Japanese patients. Two cases of FT1DM associated with pregnancy was reported from Malaysia (Tan & Loh, 2010), and FT1DM as subtype of type1B diabetes with severe and persistent β cell failure may be an important subtype in the young adult Asian populations. More international collaborative epidemiological studies are warranted in order to better understand and characterize FT1DM associated with pregnancy.

3. Metabolic disorders in IRS-2 deficient mice

3.1 IRS-2 deficient mouse

Insulin receptor substrate (IRS) disorders are associated with onset of insulin resistance and diabetes mellitus. IRS-1 deficient mice are growth-retarded and show skeletal muscle insulin resistance but do not develop diabetes because the hyperinsulinemia associated with the β cell hyperplasia in these mice efficiently compensates for the insulin resistance (Withers et al., 1998; Kido et al., 2000). IRS-2 deficient mice develop diabetes, presumably due to inadequate β cell proliferation combined with insulin resistance, and the insulin resistance in IRS-2 deficient mice is ameliorated by reduction of adiposity. IRS-2 deficient mice are widely used for analysis of pathophysiology of human type 2 diabetes mellitus (T2DM). In male IRS-2 deficient mice (C57BL/6 x CBA hybrid background) generated by Kubota et al. (2000) with C57BL/6J:Jcl mice established an inbred line of IRS-2 deficient mice, serious T1DM accompanied by abrupt and marked increase of their plasma glucose concentrations and ketonuria was sometimes observed (Hashimoto et al., 2006). The symptoms observed in IRS-2 deficient mice with serious T1DM with insulin-deficient hyperglycemia resembled those of human nonautoimmune FT1DM reported by Imagawa et al. (2000). Analyses of plasma metabolite, insulin, C-peptide, hepatic enzyme activities related to energy metabolism and histopathological changes in pancreas and islet-related antibodies may clarify the mechanism of β cell destruction and onset of FT1DM in animals.

3.2 Metabolic characteristics in IRS-2 deficient mice

We established an inbred line of mice deficient in insulin receptor substrate-2 (IRS-2) that have a C57BL/6J genetic background (B6J-IRS2$^{-/-}$ mice). At 6 week of age, there was no difference in body weight between wild-type (control) and IRS-2 deficient mice, but IRS-2 deficient mice showed remarkable impaired glucose tolerance and insulin resistance (Hashimoto et al., 2006). IRS-2 deficient mice showed significant increases in plasma glucose, free fatty acid (FFA), triglyceride (TG), total cholesterol (TC) and insulin concentrations compared to wild-type (control) mice at 6-week-old. In the livers of male IRS-2 deficient mice, the activities of cytosolic pyruvate kinase (PK), glucose-6-phosphate dehydrogenase (G6PD), ATP citrate lyase (ACL), fatty acid synthase (FAS) and malic enzyme (ME) were significantly higher than those of control mice (Table 1). Increase in activities of G6PD, ACL, FAS and ME, which are crucial enzymes for fatty acid synthesis, means activation of lipid synthesis in liver of IRS-2 deficient mice. Insulin resistance observed in IRS-2 deficient mice tends to deteriorate with aging. On the other hand, two of eight male IRS-2 deficient mice each at the ages of 14 and 24 week suddenly showed extreme hyperglycemia, similar to that in case of FT1DM. Another 2 male IRS-2 deficient mice developed extreme hyperglycemia at the age of 11 and 12 week and died. Plasma glucose and FFA concentrations in the extremely hyperglycemic IRS-2 deficient mice showed abnormal increases compared with moderately hyperglycemic IRS-2 deficient mice. Plasma insulin concentrations in extremely hyperglycemic IRS-2 deficient mice were below the detection limit. On histopathologic examination, the pancreatic islets of extremely hyperglycemic IRS-2 deficient mice were either absent or decreased in size and number compared with those of moderately hyperglycemic IRS-2 deficient mice. The islets of extremely hyperglycemic IRS-2 deficient mice showed karyorrhexis, cytoplasmic swelling, and partial necrosis. In addition, the liver of one extremely hyperglycemic IRS-2 deficient mouse showed collagen fibrinoid degeneration and macrophages.

In conclusion, at 6 week of age, IRS-2 deficient mice showed profiles compatible with several features of metabolic syndrome, including hyperglycemia, hyperinsulinemia, insulin resistance, hypertriglyceridemia, and high FFA concentrations. Therefore even young IRS-2 deficient mice are useful animal models for studying T2DM. Moreover, hyperglycemia and insulin resistance in these mice progressed to their highest levels when the animals were 14 week of age. A small population of male IRS-2 deficient mice developed abrupt onset of hyperglycemia associated with markedly diminished islet mass, resembling the features of human nonautoimmune FT1DM. The IRS-2 deficient mice may also serve as an animal model for studying FT1DM.

			Wild-type (n=8)	IRS-2 deficient (n=8)
Plasma	Glucose (mg/dl)		152 (8)	223 (23)*
	Free fatty acid (mEq/l)		0.26 (0.03)	0.49 (0.09)*
	Triglyceride (mg/dl)		55.4 (2.5)	75.8 (8.4)*
	Total cholesterol (mg/dl)		54.8 (2.6)	88.0 (8.1)*
	Insulin (ng/ml)		0.74 (0.10)	2.01 (0.35)*
Liver	Cytosol	HK	5.6 (0.3)	6.0 (0.6)
		GK	1.4 (0.1)	1.6 (0.2)
		PK	11.1 (1.5)	14.8 (1.4)*
		G6PD	6.0 (0.7)	8.5 (0.8)*
		LDH	1658 (75)	1633 (83)
		MDH	4340 (211)	4342 (162)
		AST	546 (60)	577 (57)
		ACL	4.4 (0.4)	5.9 (0.4)*
		FAS	7.7 (0.6)	10.8 (1.1)*
		ME	10.1 (1.2)	20.1 (2.0)*
		PEPCK	20.9 (2.2)	22.3 (2.8)
	Microsomes	G6Pase	424 (11)	440 (22)
	Mitochondria	GLDH	1264 (96)	1462 (78)
		MDH	3985 (216)	4247 (349)
		AST	1008 (110)	981 (55)

Data are presented as mean (SE).
*P<0.05 (Student's *t* test) versus value for wild-type mice.
Hepatic enzyme activities are presented as nmol/min/mg protein.
HK, hexokinase; GK, glucokinase; PK, pyruvate kinase; G6PD, glucose-6-phosphate dehydrogenase; LDH, lactate dehydrogenase; MDH, malate dehydrogenase; AST, aspartate aminotransferase; ACL, ATP citrate lyase; FAS, fatty acid synthase; ME, malic enzyme; PEPCK, phosphoenolpyruvate carboxykinase; G6Pase, glucose-6-phosphatase; GLDH, glutamate dehydrogenase

Table 1. Plasma metabolite concentrations and hepatic enzyme activities in 6-week-old male wild-type and IRS-2 deficient mice

3.3 Obesity with insulin resistance in IRS-2 deficient mice with high-fat diet feeding

Type 2 diabetes mellitus (T2DM) appears to be increasing mainly in the United States, Africa and Asia. In 2000 there were one hundred and fifty million T2DM patients, but they are predicted to increase substantially to two hundred and twenty million world-wide in 2010. Since World War II (WWII), T2DM patients have increased markedly with dramatic changes of lifestyle in Japan. Typical changes of the lifestyle include the increases in high fat diets, sedentary habit and driving. Especially, the level of fat in modern Japanese diets increased from 20.0 g/day in 1953 to 59.9 g/day in 1995 according to the nation-wide nutrition monitoring survey in Japan. Japanese population is predisposed to develop T2DM due to insufficient insulin secretion in spite of no predisposition to obesity. IRS-2 deficient mice show at 6 weeks of age showed profiles compatible with several features of the metabolic syndrome, including hyperglycemia, hyperinsulinemia, insulin resistance, hypertriglyceridemia, and high FFA. To investigate the characteristics in energy metabolism in IRS-2 deficient, three kinds of diets with different lipid concentrations were supplied to IRS-2 deficient mice (4 weeks old) for 2weeks. Total calories of diets were calculated as 395.1

kcal/100g for Modern American diet, 365.0 kcal/100g for Modern Japanese diet and 328.9 kcal/100g for Japanese diet after WWII. Each diet contained 15.5% (American diet, Ad), 10.1% (Japanese diet, Jd) and 3.9% (WWII diet) as crude fat, respectively. Regular diet (Rd) for laboratory animals (390kcal/100g) contained 5.0% as crude fat were based on human Japanese diet after WWII. Male IRS-2 deficient mice (4 weeks old) were provided with

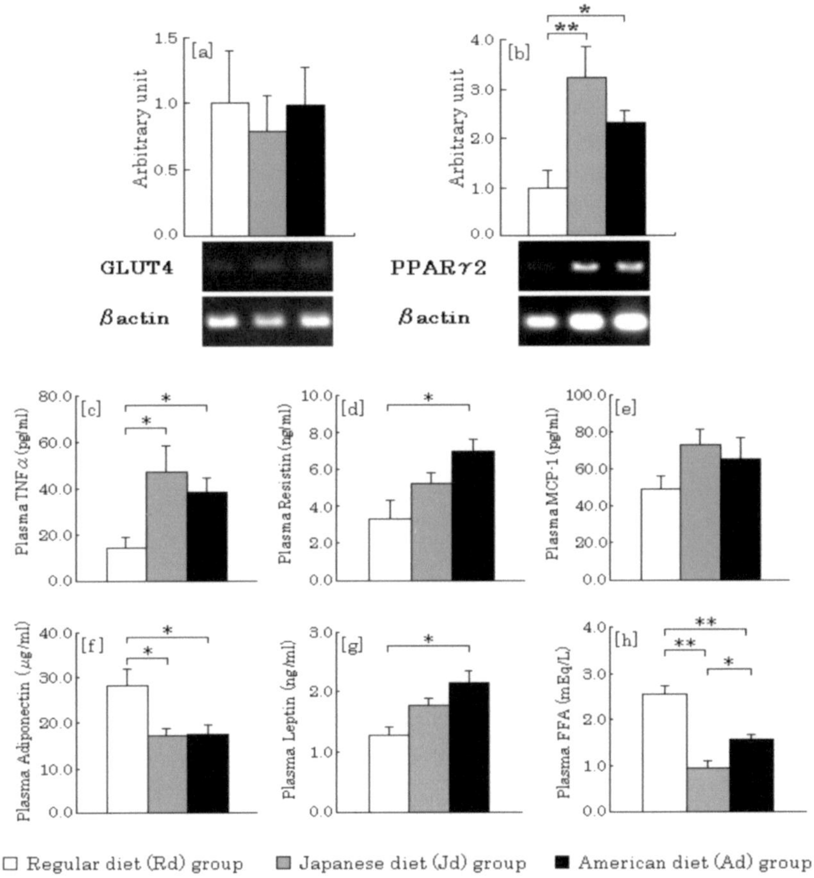

Fig. 1. Effects of modern Japanese and American diets on RNA expression of GLUT4 and PPARγ2 of adipose tissues and plasma adipocytokines concentrations in IRS-2 deficient mice fed with three kinds of diets with different lipid levels.

regular and Japanese and American diets as well as tap water *ad libitum* for 2 weeks, and used for glucose tolerance test, insulin tolerance test, and harvests of blood, liver, femoral muscles, white adipose tissue (WAT), and pancreas for chemical analysis at the age of 6 weeks (Hashimoto et al., 2009). Average body weight of Rd, Jd and Ad group at 6 week of age were 20.8, 22.7 and 22.9g each. Japanese and American diet increased significantly the body weight of IRS-2 deficient mice when compared with regular diet. Ad group showed severely impaired glucose tolerance, and Jd and Ad group showed deterioration of insulin resistance. Expression of SREBP-1c mRNA in the livers of Ad group was increased with Rd group ($p<0.05$). In addition, expression of PPARγ2 mRNA and GLUT2 mRNA in the Ad group were higher than in other groups ($p<0.05$). Cytosolic ACL and ME activities in the

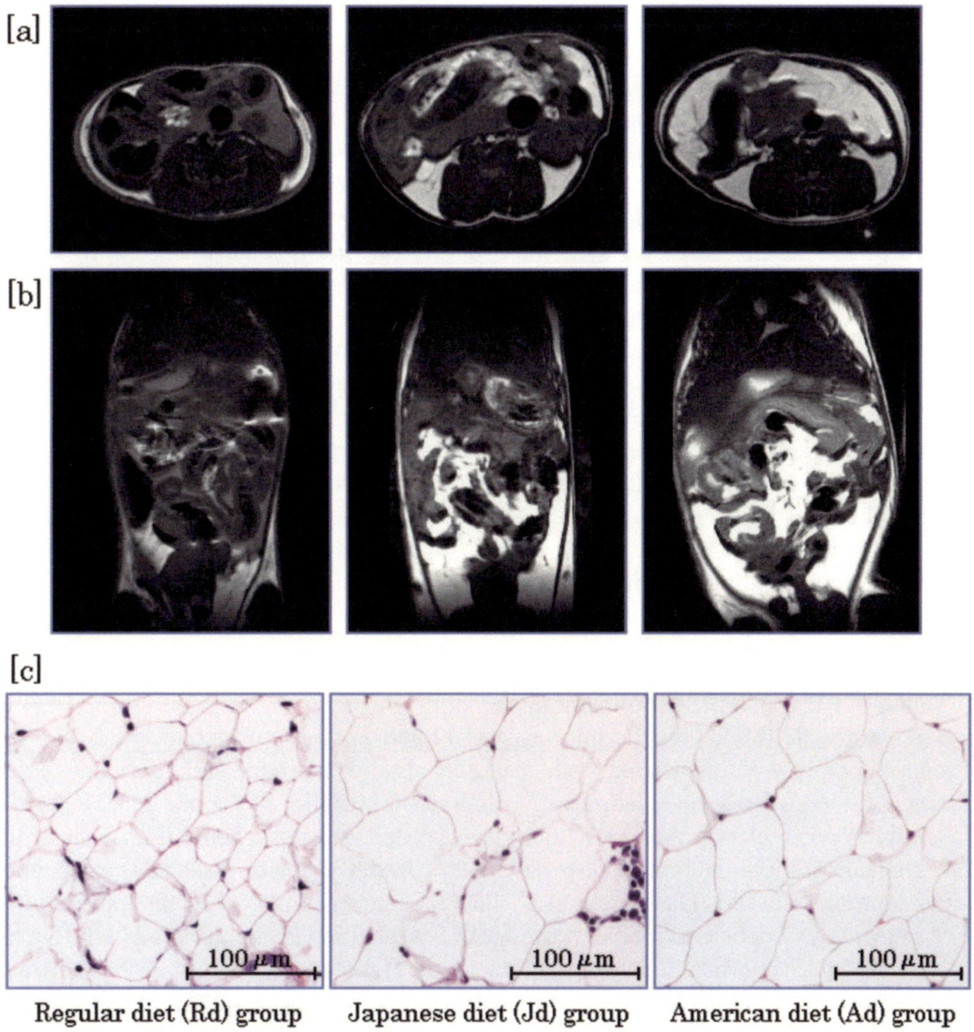

Fig. 2. Effects of modern Japanese and American diets on intraperitoneal white adipose tissues, (a) Axial views, (b) Coronal views of MRI, and (c) Adipocytes in white adipose tissues of IRS-2 deficient mice with three kinds of diets with different lipid levels.

livers of the Jd and Ad groups increased when compared with the Rd group ($p<0.05$). Expression of GLUT4 mRNA in the skeletal muscle of the Jd and Ad groups were lower than that in the Rd group ($p<0.01$). Figure 1 shows expression of mRNA in WAT and plasma cytokine concentrations in IRS-2 deficient mice. Expression of GLUT4 mRNA was not changed in WAT of each group. Expression of PPARγ2 mRNA in the Jd and Ad groups was higher than that in the Rd group ($p<0.05$). Both the Jd and Ad groups showed increased plasma TNF-α concentrations compared with the Rd group ($p<0.05$). In addition, the Ad group showed increased plasma resistin concentrations compared with other groups ($p<0.05$). However, plasma MCP-1 concentrations were not altered. On the other hand, both of Jd and Ad groups showed decreased plasma adiponectin concentrations compared with the Rd group ($p<0.05$). The Ad group showed increased plasma leptin concentrations compared with the Rd group ($p<0.05$). Both the Jd and Ad groups showed decreased plasma FFA concentrations compared with the Rd group ($p<0.05$). MRI showed the effects of Japanese and American diets on intraperitoneal WAT in IRS-2 deficient mice. Peritoneal WAT was accumulated in mice fed on Japanese and American diets. WAT around the kidney and testes in the Jd and Ad groups increased in proportion to fat concentrations of diets when compared with the Rd group. In addition, adipocytes of the Jd and Ad groups were corpulent when compared with those of the Rd group (Figure 2c). Expression of GLUT2 mRNA in pancreas of the Ad group was the lowest among all groups ($p<0.05$). The Jd and Ad groups showed hyperinsulinemia when compared with Rd group ($p<0.05$). On histopathologic examination of islets, insulin secretion was observed in all three groups.

In conclusion, high-fat diet feeding induced rapid accumulation of fat intraperitoneal cavity of IRS-2 deficient mice. Obese IRS-2 deficient mice showed higher activities of lipid synthesis in their livers and the increase in TNF-α of corpulent adipocyte origin further aggravated insulin resistance and the increase in resistin also aggravated the impaired glucose tolerance, leading to aggravation of T2DM. Plasma adiponectin concentrations decreased significantly in obese IRS-2 deficient mice fed on high-fat diet, and decreased adiponectin concentrations might worsen T2DM to severe diabetic condition.

4. Fulminant type 1 diabetes mellitus (FT1DM) in IRS-2 deficient mice

4.1 Onset of FT1DM in IRS-2 deficient mice

Two of eight male IRS-2 deficient mice each at 14 and 24 weeks of age suddenly showed extreme hyperglycemia associated with markedly diminished pancreatic islet size. These extremely hyperglycemic mice had greatly diminished activities of hepatic ACL, FAS, and ME. In these mice, plasma ALT activities were elevated and histochemical analysis of the liver confirmed inflammation. These cases of extreme diabetes resemble the human nonautoimmune FT1DM (Hashimoto et al., 2006). Occurrence rate of FT1D appears to be ~20% in male IRS-2 deficient mice after the age of 8 weeks, and is not observed in the female mice. FT1DM mice showed clinical characteristics of (1) remarkably abrupt onset of disease; (2) very short (< 1 week) duration of diabetic symptoms; (3) acidosis at diagnosis; (4) negative status of islet-related antibodies, ICA, GADAb, IAA or IA-2; (5) virtually no C-peptide secretion; and (6) elevated serum pancreatic enzyme level.

4.2 Characteristics of plasma metabolite and hormones in IRS-2 deficient mice with FT1DM

Because over 50% of male IRS-2 deficient mice after 10 weeks of age tended to show glycosuria with obesity, male IRS-2 deficient mice (8 weeks old) without glycosuria according to Diasticks (Bayer Medical Ltd., Tokyo, Japan) were used as the control. Eight IRS-2 deficient mice (8-20 weeks old) with abrupt increase of blood glucose concentrations over 450 mg/dl (25 mmol/l) within a week and ketonuria with ketosticks (Bayer Medical Ltd.) were determined as FT1DM. Plasma glucose, FFA, TG, TC, insulin and C-peptide concentrations and hepatic enzyme activities were compared between control and diabetic mice. The body weights of the diabetic mice were 26.0 ± 4.6 g (mean ± SD), smaller than those of the control mice (29.6 ± 3.8 g). As the diabetic mice (8-24 weeks old) were older than the control mice (8 weeks old), the reduction of body weights in the diabetic mice was significant. All the diabetic mice showed ketonuria. In the diabetic mice, the plasma glucose and TC concentrations were significantly higher than those in the controls, whereas plasma insulin and C-peptide concentrations decreased significantly under one third of the control values. There were no significant differences in FFA and TG concentrations between the diabetic and control mice (Table 2).

4.3 Activities of hepatic enzymes related to glucose and lipid metabolism

Activities of HK and GK as rate-limiting enzymes in glycolysis, G6PD as rate-limiting in pentose-phosphate pathway, LDH as cytosol marker enzyme, MDH and AST as crucial enzymes in the malate-aspartate shuttle, PEPCK and FBPase as rate-limiting enzymes in gluconeogenesis, ACL, ME and FAS as rate-limiting enzymes in fatty acid synthesis, PC as oxaloacetate-supplying enzyme to the tricarboxylic acid (TCA) cycle, GLDH as mitochondrial marker enzyme and 3HBD as rate-limiting enzyme in ketone body synthesis were measured. Removed pancreas from the control and the diabetic mice (12 weeks old, plasma glucose 560 mg/dl, plasma insulin <0.2 ng/ml) were examined histopathologically. Existence of the islet-related antibodies was investigated immunohistochemically in sera of NOD mice as autoimmune type 1 diabetic model and IRS2-deficient mice using pancreatic sections prepared from mice before (control mice) and after (diabetic mice) onset of FT1DM.
Activities of HK and GK in glycolysis and MDH in the malate-aspartate shuttle in cytosolic fraction of liver in the diabetic mice were significantly lower than those of the control mice. Activities of FBPase in gluconeogenesis and ME in fatty acid synthesis in liver of the diabetic mice were significantly higher than those of the controls. In the mitochondrial fraction of liver of the diabetic mice, activities of 3-HBD were significantly higher than the controls, whereas activities of AST and PC were significantly lower than those of the controls. In the liver of the diabetic mice, activities of cytosolic LDH, G6PD, AST and mitochondrial GLDH were lower than those of the control mice. The clinical symptoms of FT1DM observed in male IRS-2 deficient mice are significant increase in plasma glucose and cholesterol concentrations and a significant decrease in plasma insulin and C-peptide concentrations. All diabetic mice showed reduction of body weight, glycosuria and ketonuria and they were considered to fall into complete insulin deficiency. In the diabetic mice with insulin deficiency, their plasma TG and FFA concentrations were expected to increase generally, however those concentrations were not changed in IRS-2 deficient diabetic mice. In our previous report (Hashimoto et al., 2006), plasma TG and FFA concentrations decreased significantly notwithstanding plasma glucose and cholesterol concentrations increased significantly in the diabetic IRS-2 deficient mice at 14 weeks old. Liver-specific insulin receptor knockout (LIR-KO) mice with remarkable insulin resistance showed a significant decrease in their plasma TG and FFA concentrations. As IRS-2 deficient mice seemed to have unique regulation mechanism of plasma TG and FFA concentrations, their characteristics in lipid metabolism should be further studied in more IRS-2 deficient mice.
In livers of the diabetic IRS-2 deficient mice, activities of enzymes in glycolysis and the malate-aspartate shuttle were significantly decreased, whereas those in gluconeogenesis and ketone body synthesis were significantly elevated. Decreased activities of pyruvate carboxylase, supplying oxaloacetate to the TCA cycle, suggested depression of citrate synthesis, the rate limiting reaction of TCA cycle, and activation of ketone body synthesis. Moreover, depression in the malate-aspartate shuttle means decreased ATP production. Decrease in glycolysis or increase in gluconeogenesis and ketone body synthesis may be

typical metabolic changes induced by complete insulin deficiency. Decreased activities of LDH, MDH, AST and GLDH in the diabetic IRS-2 deficient mice reflected depression of liver function frequently observed in the diabetic animals.

			Control (n=8)	Diabetic (n=8)
Plasma	Glucose (mg/dl)		223 (20)	569 (77)*
	Free fatty acid (mEq/l)		0.60 (0.02)	1.20 (0.30)*
	Triglyceride (mg/dl)		79.7 (8.9)	97.5 (17.7)
	Total cholesterol (mg/dl)		88.9 (7.7)	162.3 (27.1)*
	Insulin (ng/ml)		1.32 (0.16)	0.28 (0.05)*
	C-peptide (ng/ml)		3.4 (0.4)	1.1 (0.3)*
Liver	Cytosol	HK	6.9 (0.5)	4.7 (0.4)*
		GK	4.2 (0.6)	1.3 (0.3)*
		G6PD	5.1 (0.5)	4.6 (0.3)
		LDH	1294 (86)	1108 (163)
		MDH	4288 (160)	3499 (250)*
		AST	653 (75)	615 (40)
		PEPCK	26 (3)	31 (3)
		FBPase	68 (8)	101 (6)*
		ACL	3.5 (0.4)	3.5 (0.3)
		FAS	4.7 (0.5)	4.9 (0.8)
		ME	17 (2)	30 (2)*
	Mitochondria	GLDH	1834 (116)	1635 (124)
		MDH	2480 (101)	2524 (334)
		AST	1684 (62)	1354 (52)*
		3-HBD	4.1 (0.2)	8.6 (1.4)*
		PC	153 (8)	66 (6)*

Data are presented as mean (SE).
Control means 8-week-old male IRS-2 deficient mice without glycosuria according to Diasticks.
*$p<0.05$ vs. controls
Hepatic enzyme activities are presented as nmol/min/mg protein.
FBPase, fructose-1,6-bisphophatase; 3-HBD, 3-hydroxybutyrate dehydrogenase; PC, pyruvate carboxylase

Table 2. Plasma metabolite concentrations and hepatic enzyme activities in control and diabetic IRS-2 deficient mice

4.4 Pathology and islet antibodies in IRS-2 deficient mice with FT1DM

On histopathological examination, the pancreatic islets of the diabetic mice were significantly decreased in size and number compared to those of the control mice. In particular, size and number of insulin secreted β cells in the diabetic mice decreased significantly compared to those in the controls, whereas number of glucagon secreted α cells decreased a little. Remarkable insulitis by autoimmunity was not observed in pancreatic sections in the diabetic mice (Figure 3). In the sera of the diabetic NOD mice, the islet-related antibodies reacted with their own islets (Figure 4, B1) and IRS2-deficient mouse islets before (Figure 4, B2) and after (Figure 4, B3) onset of FT1DM. In the serum of the control NOD mouse without glycosuria, the islet-related antibodies were not observed (Figure 4, A1-3). In sera of control and diabetic IRS2-deficient mice, the islet-related antibodies were not observed (Figure 4, C1-3 and D1-3). We also noted observed fatty degeneration in the liver of FT1DM mice. The cause of this degeneration might be increased adiposity due to increased activities of lipogenic enzymes (such as ACL, FAS, and ME) before the change of glucose tolerance in IRS-2 deficient mice. We consider that macrophages noted on histopathologic examination likely appeared to phagocytize the degraded collagen fibrinoid induced by fatty degeneration.

In the diabetic IRS-2 deficient mice, hepatic steatosis is frequently observed. The finding of severe, selective destruction of pancreatic β cells was considered to be one of the characteristics in FT1DM in IRS-2 deficient mice. The diabetic IRS-2 deficient mice did not show the islet-related antibodies observed in the diabetic NOD mice as autoimmune T1DM model. The destruction mechanism of pancreatic islet cells in IRS-2 deficient mice may differ clearly from that in the diabetic NOD mice. IRS-2 deficient mice develop diabetes because of insulin resistance in the liver and failure to undergo β cells hyperplasia. Progress of changes in islet mass should be further studied to investigate pancreatic β cells destruction. At the moment abrupt increase in plasma concentrations and appearance of ketonuria are available indicators to decide complete insulin deficiency caused by pancreatic β cells destruction in diabetic mice. In IRS-2 deficient mice, the sterol regulatory element binding protein (SREBP)-1 downstream genes, such as ATP citrate lyase and fatty acid synthase genes, are significantly increased and an excess amount of lipid is accumulated in their tissues. Accumulated lipid is also considered to be one of the causes of injury to their pancreatic islets. As FT1DM in IRS-2 deficient resembles human FT1DM, IRS-2 deficient mice are a good animal model for T2DM of human and some IRS-2 deficient mice with FT1DM may be a useful animal model for studying the destruction mechanism of pancreatic β cells in progressing to FT1DM.

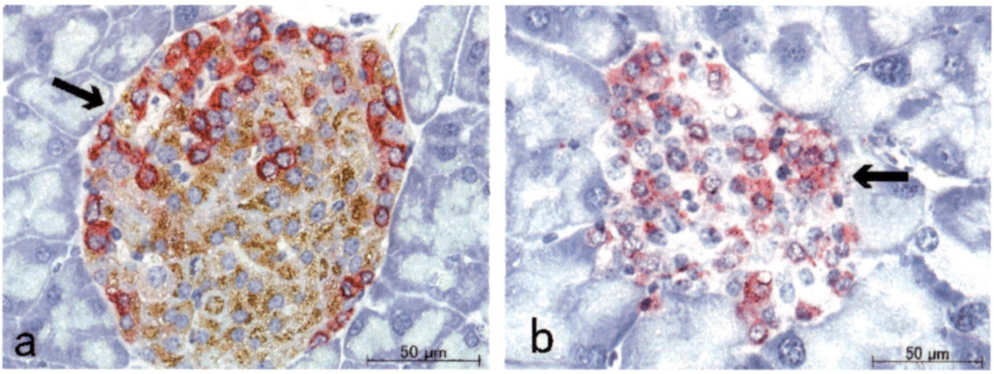

Fig. 3. Histopathological examinations of pancreatic islet cells of IRS-2 deficient mice. Pancreatic islets (arrowheads) in a control mouse (a) and a diabetic mouse (b). Pancreas sections were pretreated with 0.03% H_2O_2 in methanol to block endogenous peroxidase activity, and incubated for 60 min at room temperature with guinea pig anti-swine insulin (Dako Cytomation), followed by 30 min incubation with peroxidase-conjugate rabbit anti-guinea pig immunoglobulin. Then, the sections were incubated for 60 min at room temperature with rabbit anti-human glucagon (Dako Cytomation), followed by 30 min incubation with alkaline phosphatase-labelled polymer conjugated goat anti-rabbit antibody (Nichirei). For double staining, peroxidase (brown, DAB) and alkaline phosphatase (red, New Fuchsin) were used, respectively. Magnification, x 200

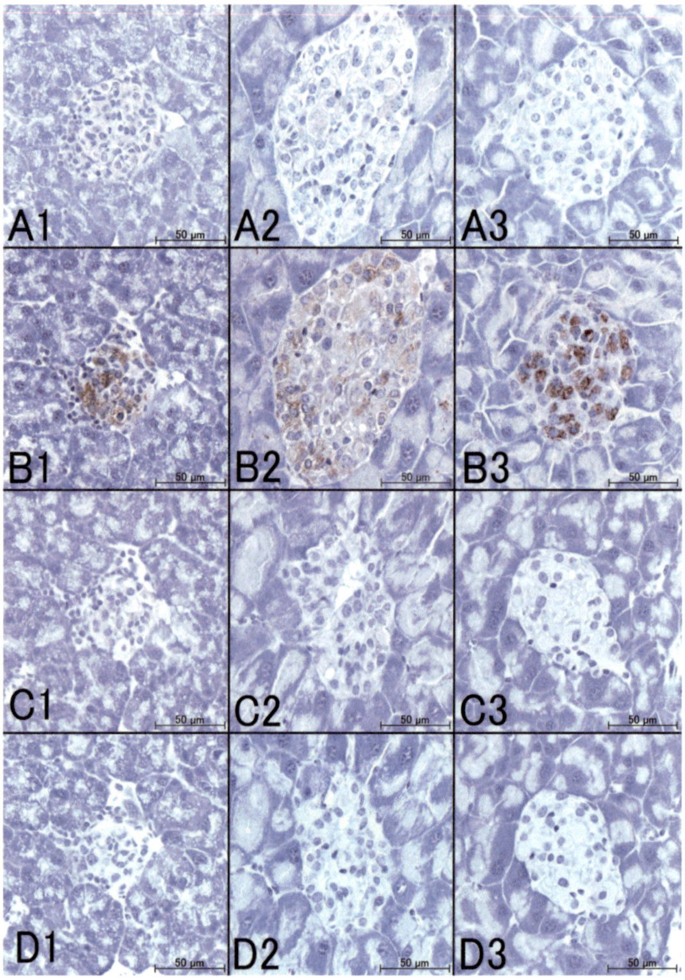

Fig. 4. Observation of islet-associated autoantibodies in serum of NOD and IRS-2 deficient mice. All pancreas specimens were fixed in 10% buffered formalin and embedded paraffin, mounted on amino-silane coated glass slide and stained using the indirect immunoperoxidase method. For each mouse, sera were treated with 0.03% H_2O_2 in methanol to measure the endogenous peroxidase activity. After pre-incubation with the 10% normal rabbit serum (Dako Cytomation) for 10 min at room temperature, sections were then incubated with preclinical NOD/shi mice sera, diabetic NOD/shi mice sera, control IRS-2 mice sera and diabetic IRS-2 mice sera, followed by incubation overnight at 4℃. Sections were serially incubated with polyclonal rabbit anti-mouse IgG/HRP antibodies (Dako Cytomation) for 60 min at room temperature. The peroxidase activity was visualized by incubation in a 0.05M Tris-HCl buffer (pH 7.6) containing 0.02% 3,3′-diaminobenzidine (DAB) and 0.006% H_2O_2 solution for 5 min. Immunostained sections were counterstained with hematoxylin for visualization of nuclei. Column 1, 2 and 3 present diabetic NOD, control IRS-2 deficient and diabetic IRS-2 deficient mouse pancreatic sections, respectively. Control NOD mouse serum (A) reacted with diabetic NOD (A1), control IRS-2 deficient (A2) and diabetic IRS-2 deficient mouse (A3) pancreatic sections. Diabetic NOD (B1-3), control IRS-2 (C1-3) and diabetic IRS-2 (D1-3) mouse sera reacted with pancreatic sections, respectively.

5. Onset mechanism of obesity and diabetes in IRS-2 deficient mice

5.1 Onset mechanism of FT1DM in IRS-2 deficient mice

Figure 5 summarizes onset mechanism of obesity and diabetes in IRS-2 deficient mice. IRS-2 deficient mice tend to fall in insulin resistance. Excess calorie and physical inactivity induce hyperglycemia followed by increased insulin secretion, which accelerates fatty acid synthesis via activation of transcriptional factor, SREBP-1c etc. Acceleration of fatty acid synthesis induces heterotopic accumulation of lipid, and visceral fat accumulation is increased. This situation is defined as obesity. Adiponectin exerts antidiabetic effects on muscles and the liver through AMP-activated protein kinase (AMPK) activation (Yamauchi et al., 2002) and antiatherosclerotic effects by inhibiting monocyte adhesion to endotherial cells and lipid accumulation into macrophages (Ouchi et al., 2001). Thus adiponectin increases glucose uptake and fatty acid oxidation in muscles via the type 1 adiponectin receptor (Yamauchi et al., 2003), and hepatic gluconeogensis via type 2 adiponectin receptor. Moreover adiponectin protects against oxidative stress in skeletal muscle by activating nuclear factor (NF)-κB target genes, manganese superoxide dismutase and inducible nitric oxide synthase (Ikegami et al., 2009). Decreased adiponectin secretion and increased inflammatory cytokines secretion from swelling adipose tissue deteriorate insulin resistance in obese animals (1st stage). Decreased adiponectin causes depression of activity of AMPK which increases glucose utilization and fatty acid β-oxidation in skeletal muscle and adipose tissues (Whitehead et al., 2006). Then hyperglycemia, hyperinsulinemia and accelerated lipid synthesis are maintained and hyper-secretion of insulin force excessively heavy work on pancreatic β cells. In over functional pancreatic islets, β-oxidation of fatty acid is accelerated resulting in excess amount of reactive oxygen species (ROS) production, which induces ROS stress leading to mitochondrial dysfunction and apoptosis of β-cells with low scavenging activity of ROS (2nd stage). It has been reported that adiponectin inhibits fatty acid-induced apoptosis by suppression of ROS generation via both the cAMP/PKA and AMPK pathway in endothelial cells (Kim et al, 2010). Macrophages (but not T cells) infiltration is observed frequently in FT1DM (Shibasaki et al., 2010). In IRS-2 deficient mice with FT1DM macrophage infiltration induced by MCP-1 was observed. Infiltrated macrophages may participate in destruction process of pancreatic islets leading to T1DM. The β cell deficit is believed to be due to autoimmune induced β cell apoptosis mediated by the release of inflammatory cytokines, such as IL-1β and TNF-α, from T lymphocytes and macrophages (Donath et al., 2003). Cytokine-induced β cell death preferentially affects newly forming beta cells, which implies that replicating beta cells might be more vulnerable to cytokine destruction. Efforts to expand beta cell mass in type 1 diabetes by fostering β cell replication are likely to fail unless cytokine-induced apoptosis is concurrently suppressed (Meier et al., 2006). Inflammatory cytokines from corpulent adipocytes appear to participate in destruction of islets β cells leading to T1DM. In autoimmune T1DM, β cells are assumed to be destroyed through a long-standing autoimmune process, whereas in FT1DM, β cells seem to be destroyed very rapidly, probably by a destructive process triggered by viral infection (Hanafusa & Imagawa, 2008). Since IRS-2 deficient mice were maintained under specific pathogen free conditions (Hashimoto et al., 2006), viral infection was deleted from the causes of β cell destruction. Adipocyte-secreted factors associate the pancreatic β cells destructions. Chronic exposure of human islets to leptin leads to β cell apoptosis (Donath et al., 2003). TNFα, in combination with other cytokines, accelerates dysfunction and destruction of the β cell (Eizirik & Mandrup-Poulsen, 2001). IL-6 released by adipocytes may be responsible for the increases in plasma IL-6 concentrations observed in obesity and at least in combination with other cytokines, IL-6 has cytotoxic effects on β cell (Eizirik et al., 1994). Increased FFA levels are known to be toxic for β cell, leading to the concept of lipotoxicity (McGarry & Dobbins, 1999). The toxic effect of FFA is mediated via formation of ceramide, increased nitric oxide production and activation of the apoptotic mitochondrial pathway (Maedler et al., 2001). Elevated glucose concentrations induced β cell apoptosis at higher concentration in rodent islet (Efanova et al., 1998). In human islets glucose-induced β cell apoptosis and dysfunction are mediated by β cell production and secretion of IL-1β. Chronic hyperglycemia increases production of ROS, which may cause oxidative damage in β cell (Matsuoka et al., 1997; Laybutt et al., 2002). IL-1β and ROS activate the transcription factor nuclear transcription factor (NF) κB, which plays a critical role in mediating inflammatory responses. A series of inflammatory reaction appear to have important roles in the β cell destruction process in IRS-2 deficient mice with insulin resistance.

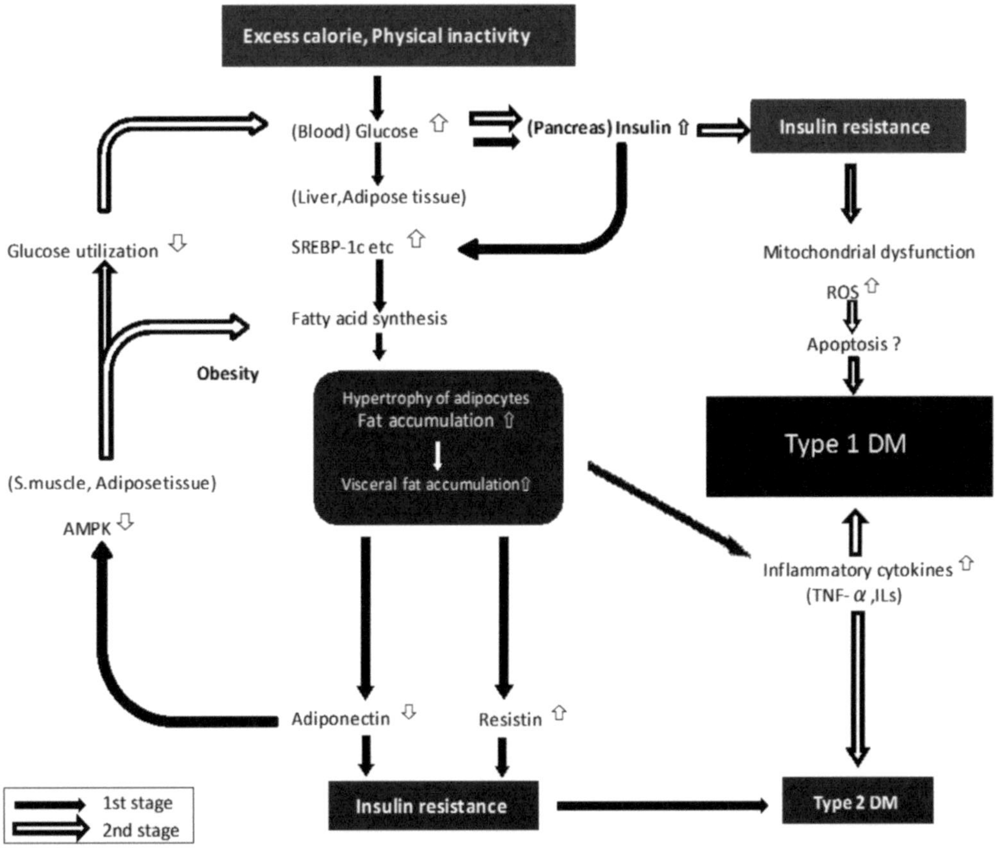

SREBP, sterol regulatory element binding protein; AMPK, AMP-activated protein kinase; ROS, reactive oxygen species;
TNF, tumor necrosis factor; IL, interleukins

Fig. 5. Onset mechanism of obesity and diabetes in IRS-2 deficient mice

5.2 Comparison of pathology of FT1DM between IRS-2 deficient mice and human patients

IRS-2 deficient mice with FT1DM show remarkable body weight loss, polydipsia, polyuria, glycosuria and ketonuria as typical symptoms of T1DM as reported in human FT1DM patients. Laboratory data in IRS-2 deficient mice with FT1DM reveal hyperglycemia, hyperlipidemia and remarkable decrease in insulin secretion as in human FT1DM patients (Table 3). The above symptoms of T1DM were onset abruptly after hyperglycemia was observed in IRS-2 deficient mice. Insulitis with macrophage dominant infiltration was observed in IRS-2 deficient mice and human FT1DM. Destruction mechanism of β cells associated HLA, viral infection and pregnancy were investigated in detail in human FT1DM patients (Kawabata et al., 2009; Murabayashi et al., 2009; Tan & Loh, 2010), whereas association with MHC was not investigated in IRS-2 deficient mice. Since FT1DM was observed in only male IRS-2 deficient mice, pregnancy is not associated with onset of FT1DM. Inflammatory cytokines play a major role in destruction process of pancreatic β cell in both IRS-2 mice and human FT1DM patients. Trigger of the β cell destruction process is different between IRS-2 mice and human. Insulin resistance by increase in inflammatory cytokines seemed to be main cause to lead β cell destruction in IRS-2 deficient mice, whereas viral infection may be a trigger for destruction mechanism in human FT1DM patients.

	IRS-2 deficient mice	Human patients	References
Clinical characteristics			
Body weight loss	Remarkable	Remarkable	Imagawa et al. (2003)
Polydipsia	Positive	Positive	Imagawa et al. (2003)
Polyuria	Positive	Positive	Imagawa et al. (2003)
Glycosuria	Positive	Positive	Imagawa et al. (2003)
Ketonuria	Positive	Positive	Imagawa et al. (2003)
Laboratory data			
Fasting plasma glucose (mg/dl)	570 (480 – 640)	711 (300 – 1293)	Shimizu et a. (2006)
Fasting plasma C peptide (ng/ml)	1.1 ± 0.3*	< 0.5	Shibasaki et al. (2010)
Serum triglyceride (mmol/l)	1.1 ± 0.2*	2.0 ± 1.8**	Imagawa et al. (2003)
Serum total cholesterol (mmol/l)	4.2 ± 0.7*	5.1 ± 1.6**	Imagawa et al. (2003)
Insulitis	Macrophages dominant infiltration	Macrophages as the main cell type in insulitis lesion, followed by T lymphocytes	Hanafusa & Imagawa (2008)
Islet related autoantibodies	Negative	Negative	Imagawa et al. (2003)

*Mean ± SE, **Mean ± SD

Table 3. Characteristics of FT1D in IRS-2 deficient mice and human patients

Type 1 diabetes is a polygenic disease. Approximately 50% of the genetic susceptibility can be explained by allele in HLA class II region, in particular certain DQ alleles. More than 95%

of type 1 diabetic patients carry these predisposing alleles, but the occurrence of these alleles in the background population is high, approximately 50%. It is believed that the diabetes predisposing DQ antigens have a shape of the antigen presenting groove of the molecule that leads to more efficient presentation of β cell associated autoantigens (Donath et al., 2003). HLA comment should be in the text. In FT1DM patients, the haplotype frequency of HLA DRB1*0901-DQB1*0303 was significantly higher than those in controls (Moreau et al., 2008). HLA phenotyping of these Caucasian patients did not find the specific HLA haplotype (DRB1*0405-DQB1*0401) found to be linked to FT1D in Japanese patients. More investigation about haplotype frequency of MHC was necessary for IRS-2 mice in the destruction process of pancreatic β cells.

6. Conclusion

IRS-2 mice tend to become obese accompanying insulin resistance after 8 weeks of age. IRS-2 deficient mice develop diabetes, presumably due to inadequate β cell proliferation combined with insulin resistance compared to IRS-1 deficient mice with the β cell hyperplasia to compensate for the insulin resistance. Heterotopic accumulation of lipid observed frequently in obese IRS-2 mice, and corpulent adipocytes secrete various inflammatory cytokines, such as TNF-α and ILs, whereas production of adiponectin as antidiabetic agent is decreased significantly. About 20% of male IRS-2 deficient mice showed clinical characteristics of (1) remarkably abrupt onset of disease; (2) very short (< 1 week) duration of diabetic symptoms; (3) acidosis at diagnosis; (4) negative status of islet-related antibodies; (5) virtually no C-peptide secretion; and (6) elevated serum pancreatic enzyme level. These symptoms resembled the features of human nonautoimmune FT1DM. In IRS-2 deficient mice with FT1DM, insulitis with macrophage dominated infiltration to islet β cell area was observed frequently as in human FT1DM patients. Inflammatory cytokines appear to have important roles in the process of β cell destruction leading to FT1DM. IRS-2 deficient mice are considered to be useful animal model for studying the mechanism of β cell destruction leading to FT1DM.

7. References

American Diabetes Association. (2008). Diagnosis and classification of diabetes. *Diabetes Care* Vol. 31 (Suppl. 1): S55-S60. ISSN 0149-5992

Cho, Y.M., Kim, J.T., Ko, K.S., Koo, B.K., Yang, S.W., Park, M.H., Lee, H.K. & Park, K.S. (2007). Fulminant type 1 diabetes in Korea: highprevalence among patients with adult-onset type 1 diabetes. *Diabetologia* Vol. 50 (No. 11): 2276-2279. ISSN 0012-186x

Donath, M.Y., Storling, J., Maedler, K. & Mandrup-Poulsen, T. (2003). Inflammatory mediators and islet β-cell failure: a link between type 1and type 2 diabetes. *Journal of Molecular Medicine* Vol. 81 (No. 8): 455-470. ISSN 0946-2716

Efanova, I.B., Zaitsev, S.V., Zhivotovsky, B., Kohler, M., Efendic, S., Orrenius, S & Berggren, P.O. (1998). Glucose and tolbutamide induce apoptosis in pancreatic beta-cells. A process dependent on intracellular Ca2+ concentration. *Journal of Biological Chemistry* Vol.273 (No. 50): 33501-33507. ISSN 0021-9258

Eizirik, D.L., Sandler, S., Welsh, N., Cetkovic-Cvrlje, M., Nieman, A., Geller, D.A., Pipeleers, D.G., Bendtzen, K. & Hellerstrom, C. (1994).Cytokines suppress human islet function irrespective of their effects on nitric oxide generation. *Journal of Clinical Investigation* Vol. 93 (No. 5): 1968-1974. ISSN 0021-9738

Eizirik, D.L. & Mandrup-Poulsen, T. (2001). A choice of death-the signal-transduction of immune-mediated beta-cell apoptosis. *Diabetologia* Vol. 44 (No. 12): 2115-2133. ISSN 0021-186x

Hanafusa, T. & Imagawa, A. (2008). Insulitis in human type 1 diabetes. *Annals of the New York Academy of Science* Vol. 1150: 297-299. ISSN 0077-8923

Hashimoto, H., Arai, T., Takeguchi, A., Hioki, K., Ohnishi, Y., Kawai, K., Ito, M., Suzuki, R., Yamauchi, T., Ohsugi, M., Saito, M., Ueyama, Y., Tobe, K., Kadowaki, T., Tamaoki, N. & Kosaka, K. (2006). Ontogenetic characteristics of enzyme activities and plasma metabolites in C57BL/6J:Jcl mice deficient in insulin receptor substrate 2. *Comparative Medicine* Vol. 56 (No. 3): 176-187. ISSN 1532-0820

Hashimoto, H., Arai, T., Mori, A., Kawai, K., Hikishima, K., Ohnishi, Y., Eto, T., Ito, M., Hioki, K., Suzuki, R., Ohsugi, M., Saito, M., Ueyama, Y., Okano, H., Yamauchi, T., Kubota, N., Ueki, K., Tobe, K., Tamaoki, N., Kadowaki, T. & Kosaka, K. (2009). Reconsideration of insulin signals induced by improved laboratory animal diets, Japanese and American diets, in IRS-2 deficient mice. *Experimental and Clinical Endocrinology & Diabetes* Vol. 117(No. 2): 577-586. ISSN 0947-7349

Ikegami, Y., Inukai, K., Imai, K., Sakamoto, Y., Katagiri, H., Kurihara, S., Awata, T. & Katayama, S. (2009). Adiponectin upregulates ferritin heavy chain in skeletal muscle cell. *Diabetes* Vol. 58 (No. 1): 61-70. ISSN 0012-1797

Imagawa, A., Hanafusa, T., Miyagawa, J. & Matsuzawa, Y. (2000). A novel subtype of type 1 diabetes mellitus characterized by a rapid onset and an absence of diabetes-related antibodies. *The New England Journal of Medicine* Vol. 342 (No. 5): 301-307. ISSN 0028-4793

Imagawa, A., Hanafusa, T., Uchigata, Y., Kanatsuka, A., Kawasaki, E., Kobayashi, T., Shimaka, A., Shimizu, I., Toyoda, T., Maruyama, T. & Makino, H. (2003). Fulminant type 1 diabetes. A nationwide survey in Japan. *Diabetes Care* Vol. 26 (No. 8): 2345-2352. ISSN 0149-5992

Imagawa, A., Hanafusa, T., Uchigata, Y., Kanatsuka, A., Kawasaki, E., Kobayashi, T., Shimada, A., Shimizu, I., Maruyama, T. & Makino, H. (2005). Different contribution of class II HLA in fulminant and typical autoimmune type 1 diabetes mellitus. *Diabetologia* Vol. 48 (No. 2): 294-300. ISSN 0012-186x

Jung, T.S., Chung, S.I., Kim, S.J., Park, M.H., Kim, D.R., Kang, M.Y. & Hahm, J.R. (2004). A Korean patient with fulminant autoantibody-negative type 1 diabetes. *Diabetes Care* Vol. 27 (No. 12): 3023-3024. ISSN 0149-5992

Kawabata, Y., Ikegami, H., Awata, T., Imagawa, A., Maruyama, T., Kawasaki, E., Tanaka, S., Shimada, A., Osawa, H., Kobayasahi, T.,Hanafusa, T., Tokunaga, K., Makino, H. & the Committee on Type 1 Diabetes, Japan Diabetes Society. (2009).Differential association of HLA with three subtypes of type 1 diabetes: fulminant, slowly progressive and acute-onset.*Diabetologia* Vol. 52 (No. 12): 2513-2521. ISSN 0021-186x

Kido, Y., Burks, D.J., Withers, D., Bruning, J.C., Kahn, C.R., White, M.E. & Accili, D. (2000). Tissue-specific insulin resistance in mice withmutations in the insulin receptor, IRS-1, and IRS-2. *Journal of Clinical Investigation* Vol. 105 (No. 2): 199-205. ISSN 0021-9738

Kim, J-E., Song, S.E., Kim, T-W., Kim, J-Y., Park, S-C., Park, Y-K., Baek, S-H., Lee, I.K. & Park, S-Y. (2010). Adiponectin inhibits palmitate-induced apoptosis through suppression of reactive oxygen species in endothelial cells: involvement of cAMP/protein kinase A and AMP-activated protein kinase. *Journal of Endocrinology* Vol. 207(No. 1): 35-44. ISSN 0022-0795

Kubota, N., Tobe, K., Terauchi, Y., Eto, K., Yamauchi, T., Suzuki, R., Tsubamoto, Y., Komeda, K., Nakano, R., Miki, H., Satoh, S., Sekihara, H., Sciacchitano, S., Lesniak, M., Aizawa, S., Nagai, R., Kimura, S., Akanuma, Y., Taylor, S.I. & Kadowaki, T. (2000). Disruption of insulin receptor substrate 2 causes type 2 diabetes because of liver insulin resistance and lack of compensatory beta-cell hyperplasia. *Diabetes* Vol. 49 (No. 11): 1880-1889. ISSN 0012-1797

Laybutt, D.R., Kaneto, H., Hasenkamp, W., Grey, S., Jonas, J.C., Sgroi, D.C., Groff, A., Ferran, C., Bonner-Weir, S., Sharma, A. & Weir, G.C. (2002). Increased expression of antioxidant and antiapoptotic genes in islets that may contribute to beta-cell survival during chronic hyperglycemia. *Diabetes* Vol. 51 (No. 2): 413-423. ISSN 0012-1797

Maedler, K., Spinas, G.A., Dyntar, D., Moritz, W., Kaiser, N. & Donath, M.Y. (2001). Distict effects of saturated and monosaturated fatty acids on beta-cell turnover and function. *Diabetes* Vol. 50 (No. 1): 69-76. ISSN 0012-1797

Matsuoka, T., Kajimoto, Y., Watada, H., Kaneto, H., Kishimoto, M., Umayahara, Y., Fujitani, Y., Kamada, T., Kawamori, R. & Yamasaki, Y. (1997). Glycation-dependent, reactive oxygen species-mediated suppression of the insulin gene promoter activity in HIT cell. *Journal of Clinical Investigation* Vol. 99 (No. 1): 144-150. ISSN 0012-9738

McGarry, J.D. & Dobbins, R.L. (1999). Fatty acid, lipotoxicity and insulin secretion. *Diabetologia* Vol. 42 (No. 1): 128-138. ISSN 0012-186x

Meier, J.J., Ritzel, R.A., Maedler, K., Gurlo, T. & Butler, P.C. (2006). Increased vulnerability of newly forming beta cells to cytokine-induced cell death. *Diabetologia* Vol. 49 (No. 1): 83-89. ISSN 0012-186x

Moreau, C., Drui, D., Arnault-Ouary, G., Charbonnel, B., Chaillous, L. & Cariou, B. (2008). Fulminant type 1 diabetes in Caucasians: a report of three cases. *Diabetes and Metabolism* Vol. 34 (No. 5): 529-532. ISSN 1262-3636

Murabayashi, N., Sugiyama, T., Kihara, C., Kusaka, H., Sugihara, T. & Sagawa, N. (2009). A case of fulminant type 1 diabetes mellitus associated with pregnancy. *Journal of Obstetrics and Gynaecology Research* Vol. 35 (No. 6): 1121-1124. ISSN 1341-8076

Ouchi, N., Kihara, S., Arita, Y., Nishida, M., Matsuyama, A., Okamoto, Y., Ishigami, M., Kurihara, H., Kishida, K., Nishizawa, H., Hotta, K., Muraguchi, M., Ohmoto, Y.,

Yamashita, S., Funahashi, T. & Matsuzawa, Y. (2001). Adipocyte-derived plasma protein, adiponectin,suppresses lipid accumulation and class A scavenger receptor expression in human monocyte-derived macrophages. *Circulation* Vol. 103 (No. 8): 1057-1063. ISSN 0009-7322

Shibasaki, S., Imagawa, A., Tauriainen, S., Iino, M., Oikarinen, M., Abiru, H., Tamaki, K., Seino, H., Nishi, K., Takase, I., Okada, Y., Uno, S., Murase-Mishiba, Y., Terasaki, J., Makino, H., Shimomura, I., Hyoty, H. & Hanafusa, T. (2010). Expression of Toll-like receptors in the pancreas of recent-onset fulminant type 1 diabetes. *Endocrine Journal* Vol. 57 (No. 1): 211-219. ISSN 0918-8959

Shimizu, I., Makino, H., Imagawa, A., Iwahashi, H., Uchigata, Y., Kanatsuka, A., Kawasaki, E., Kobayashi, T., Shimada, A., Maruyama, T.& Hanafusa, T. (2006). Clinical and immunogenetic characteristics of fulminant type 1 diabetes associated with pregnancy.*Journal of Clinical Endocrinology & Metabolism* Vol. 91 (No. 2): 471-476. ISSN 0021-972x

Tanaka, S., Nishida, Y., Aida, K., Maruyama, T., Shimada, A., Suzuki, M., Shimura, H., Takizawa, S., Takahashi, M., Akiyama, D., Arai-Yamashita, S., Furuya, F., Kawaguchi, A., Kaneshige, M., Katoh, R., Endo, T. & Kobayashi, T. (2009). Enterovirus infection, CXC chemokine ligand 10 (CXCL10), and CXCR3 circuit. A mechanism of accelerated β cell failure in fulminant type 1 diabetes.*Diabetes* Vol. 58 (No. 10): 2285-2291. ISSN 0012-1797

Tan, F. & Loh, K. (2010). Fulminant type 1 diabetes associated with pregnancy: A report of 2 cases from Malaysia. *Diabetes Research and Clinical Practice* Vol. 90: e30-e32. ISSN 0168-8227

Taniyama, M., Katsumata, R., Aoki, K., Suzuki, S. (2004). A Filipino patient with fulminant type 1 diabetes. *Diabetes Care,* Vol. 27(No. 3): 842-843, ISSN 0149-5992

Whitehead, I.P., Richards, A.A., Hickman, I.J., Macdonald, G.A. & Prins, J.B. (2006). Adiponectin - a key adipokine in the metabolic syndrome. *Diabetes, Obesity and Metabolism* Vol. 8 (No. 2): 264-280, ISSN 1462-8902

Withers, D.J., Gutierrez, J.S., Towery, H., Burks, D.J., Ren, J.M., Previs, S., Zhang, Y., Bernal, D., Pons, S., Shulman, G.I., Bonner-Weir, S., & White, M.E. (1998). Disruption of IRS-2 causes type 2 diabetes in mice. *Nature* Vol. 391: 900-904. ISSN 0028-0836

Yamauchi, T., Kamon, J., Minokoshi, Y., Ito, Y., Waki, H., Uchida, S., Yamashita, S., Noda, M., Kita, S., Ueki, K., Eto, K., Akanuma, Y., Froguel, P., Foufelle, F., Ferre, P., Carlin, D., Kimura, S., Nagai, R., Kahn, B.B. & Kadowaki, T. (2002). Adiponectin stimulates glucose utilization and fatty-acid oxidation by activating AMP-activated protein kinase. *Nature Medicine* Vol. 8: 1288-1295. ISSN 1078-8956

Yamauchi, T., Kamon, J., Ito, Y., Tsuchida, A., Yokomizo, T., Kita, S., Sugiyama, T., Miyagishi, M., Hara, K., Tsunoda, M., Murakami, K., Ohzeki, T., Uchida, S., Takekawa, S., Waki, H., Tsuno, N.H., Shibata, Y., Terauchi, Y., Froguel, P., Tobe, K., Koyasu, S., Taira, K., Kitamura, T., Shimizu, T., Nagai, R. & Kadowaki, T. (2003). Cloning of adiponectin receptors that mediate antidiabetic metabolic effects. *Nature* Vol. 423: 762-769. ISSN 0028-0836

Zheng, C., Zhou, Z., Yang, L., Huang, G., Li, X., Zhou, W., Wang, X. & Liu, Z. (2011). Fulminant type 1 diabetes mellitus exhibits distinct clinical and autoimmunity features from classical type 1 diabetes mellitus in Chinese. *Diabetes Metabolism Research and Reviews* Vol. 27 (No. 1): 70-78. ISSN 1520-7552

10

Obesity in the Natural History of Type 1 Diabetes Mellitus: Causes and Consequences

Fernando Valente[1], Marília Brito Gomes[2] and Sérgio Atala Dib[1]
[1]*São Paulo Federal University, São Paulo*
[2]*State University of Rio de Janeiro, Rio de Janeiro*
Brazil

1. Introduction

There has been a worldwide epidemic increasing in the prevalence of sedentary, overweight and obesity that comes with modernity and urbanization (Wang et al., 2002). The consequence is the development of insulin resistance (IR) and type 2 diabetes (T2D). This is classically defined as a metabolic disease that occurs due to a higher IR that leads to a slow setting of lower insulin production (more relative than absolute), in general in adult age. T2D is associated also with a genetic predisposition. The majority of T2D individuals are overweight or obese and the ones who do not, at least present increased abdominal adipose mass (ADA, 1997). The rising prevalence of overweight and obesity is happening also in children and adolescents (Pinhas-Hamiel et al., 1996; Willi & Egede, 2000; Rosenbloom et al., 1999). The metabolic syndrome (MS), which physiopathology is based on IR, shows the same trend in children and adolescents (Jago et al., 2008), as well as isolated pre-diabetes (Li et al., 2009).

In parallel, it has been seen an elevation in the number of type 1 diabetes (T1D) cases and its establishment at a younger age (EURODIAB ACE Study Group, 2000). T1D is characterized primarily by a pancreatic beta cell destruction, which may lead to ketosis. It can be classified as autoimmune (with positive anti-islet, anti-insulin, anti-GAD, anti-IA2 and/or anti-IA2 beta antibodies) or idiopathic, in which no autoantibodies can be detected, and occurs more frequently in individuals of African-American or Asian origin. Multiple genetic predisposition and environmental factors are involved with T1D (ADA, 1997). At least one of those autoantibodies is present in 85-90% of T1D on diagnosis. The treatment for T1D consists of multiple insulin injections, known as intensive treatment, to obtain adequate glycemic control and therefore prevent micro (The DCCT Research Group, 1993) and macrovascular (Nathan et al., 2005 and 2003) chronic complications. However, it can be followed by weight gain most of the times (Arai et al., 2008), which can amplify the risk of cardiovascular disease (CVD) in spite of good glycemic control. This weight gain can start on puberty and persist along adulthood (Särnblad et al., 2007). Therefore, some of these patients present clinical features of both T1D and T2D, confounding its classification. This phenotype was initially called double diabetes (DD) (Libman & Becker, 2003; Becker et al.,

2001), and is characterized by positive pancreatic autoantibodies in patients with clinical features of T2D, as IR and overweight and/or obesity (Pozzilli & Buzzetti, 2007; Gilliam et al., 2005; Reinehr et al., 2006), as shown in Table 1 (Pozzilli & Buzzetti, 2007) and in Figure 1.

	T1D	DD	T2D
Age at disease onset	Childhood +++ Adolescence +++ Adult +	Childhood ++ Adolescence ++ Adult (LADA) +	Childhood + Adolescence ++ Adult +++
Major genetics predisposition	MHC class I and II, *InsVNTR, CTLA-4, PTPN22*	?	*APM1, PPARγ 2, PtdCho-1, TCF7L2*
Environmental factors	Diet, viruses Cow´s milk in infancy	Life style (diet, sedentary life)	Life style (diet, sedentary life)
Circulating antibodies to β cells	+++	+	-
T cell-mediated immunity to β cells	+++	++	-
C-peptide secretion	-	+	+++
IR	-/+	++	+++
Inflammatory markers (cytokines, adipokines)	+	++	+++
Macrovascular complications	+	++	+++

Table 1. Clinical and pathogenic features of DD compared to T1D and T2D (Pozzilli & Buzzetti, 2007).

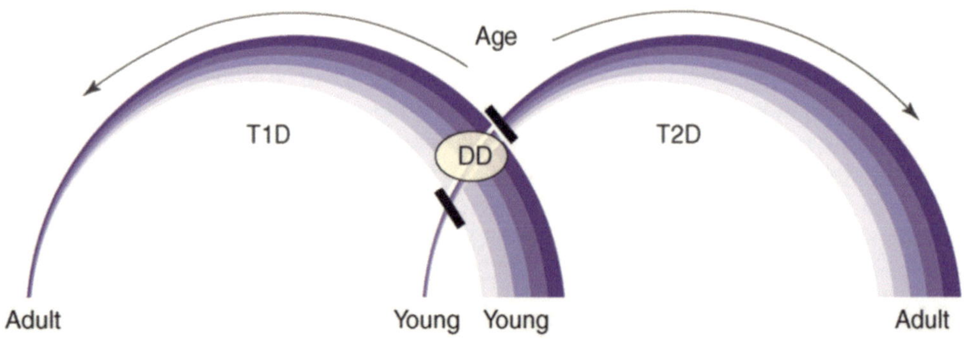

Fig. 1. Schematic representation showing where DD lies in respect to age and the two types of diabetes, as illustrated by two 'rainbows' (Pozzilli & Buzzetti, 2007).

2. Obesity as a accelerate factor to type 1 diabetes mellitus development

Studies with streptozotocin-induced diabetic baboons showed that to have an abnormal glucose tolerance it is necessary an isolated huge loss of beta-cell mass or a moderate loss of these cells associated to an IR (McCulloch et al., 1991), that could be in humans the physiologically IR of adolescence (Acerini et al., 2000) or gestation (Buschard et al., 1987), periods with higher incidence of T1D, or pathological situations like infection (usually one of the triggering factors of T1D) or weight gain.

Others studies suggest that the increase in the body mass index (BMI) and the consequent IR may accelerate the β cell destruction process in individuals predisposed to T1D, due to the release of obesity-related cytokines that show inflammatory and/or immunomodulatory properties (Aldhahi & Hamdy, 2003), triggering diabetes. This hypothesis may be reinforced by one study that correlated high anti-GAD levels with high BMI (Rolandsson et al., 1999). Two interesting data from studies with non-obese diabetic (NOD) mice are that hyperinsulinemia, an IR marker, precede clinical T1D (Armani et al., 1998) and that T1D incidence falls after treatment with rosiglitazone, an insulin sensitizer drug (Beales & Pozzili, 2002).

The IR, autoimmunity and apoptosis of the β cells constitutes the three factors of the called "accelerator hypothesis", proposed by Wilkin (Wilkin, 2001), that contemplate the factors presented in both more common types of diabetes, that is, T2D and T1D. There is a constitucional (intrinsic) high speed of apoptosis of β cells that is necessary to the development of diabetes, but rarely enough. The other two factors, extrinsic, that can speed the apoptosis of beta-cells are IR (result of weight gain and/or physical inactivity) and autoimmunity against beta-cells.

It is known that obese individuals have elevated serum levels of leptin, a cytokine secreted by adipocytes in proportion to adipose tissue mass and that is responsible, among other functions, for regulating food intake and thus BMI. Moreover, leptin controls the cellular immune response and is involved in the pathogenesis of autoimmune diseases (Lord, 2002). Studies have shown that administration of leptin in NOD mice promoted an early inflammatory infiltrate in the pancreatic islets, increased production of interferon gamma (IFN-gamma) by T lymphocytes, which accelerated the establishment of a T1D (Matarese, 2002 e 2005).

On the other hand, adiponectin, another important cytokine produced by adipose tissue, inversely proportional to its fat mass, can decrease the systemic and pancreatic islets inflammatory process, acting as a protective factor in the development of T1D, in addition to reducing IR (Kadowaki et al., 2006; Wellen & Hotamisligil, 2005).

However, development report (OECD, 2009) from 16 countries does not show any obvious relationship between national estimates of childhood obesity prevalence and incidence rates of T1D (Table 2). Therefore, obesity does not account for the wide between-country differences in T1D incidence, which range from 0.57 per 100 000 person-years in China to more than 48 per 100 000 person-years in Sardinia and Finland in the 0- to 14-year age group (Daneman, 2006).

On the other hand, in a meta-analysis of nine studies (eight case-control studies and one cohort study) comprising a total of 2658 cases (Verbeeten et al., 2011), seven reported a significant association between childhood obesity, BMI or %weight-for-height and increased risk for T1D. Four of these studies reported childhood obesity as a categorical exposure and produced a pooled odds ratio of 2.03 (95% CI 1.46–2.80) for subsequent T1D, but with age at obesity assessment varying from age 1 to 12 years (Figure 2). A dose-response relationship was supported by a continuous association between childhood BMI and subsequent T1D in a meta-analysis of five studies (pooled odds ratio 1.25 (95%CI 1.04–1.51) per 1 SD higher BMI) (Figure 3).

Country	T1D incidence rate in children aged 0-14 years (per 100.000 person-years)	% of children aged 11-15 years overweight or obese
Finland	57,4	15,8
Sweden	41	10,5
Norway	27,9	10
UK	24,5	12
Denmark	22,2	9,7
Canada	21,7	21,3
USA	20,8	29,8
Netherlands	18,8	8
Germany	18	12
Ireland	16,3	14,2
Iceland	14,7	14,5
Spain	13	16,7
Poland	12,9	11,2
France	12,2	10,5
Greece	9,9	18,8
Italy	8,4	18,3

Table 2. Relationship between Type 1 diabetes incidence and prevalence of childhood overweight or obesity in 16 Organization for Economic Co-Operation and Development (OECD) countries, from Health at a Glance 2009: OECD Indicators (OECD, 2009).

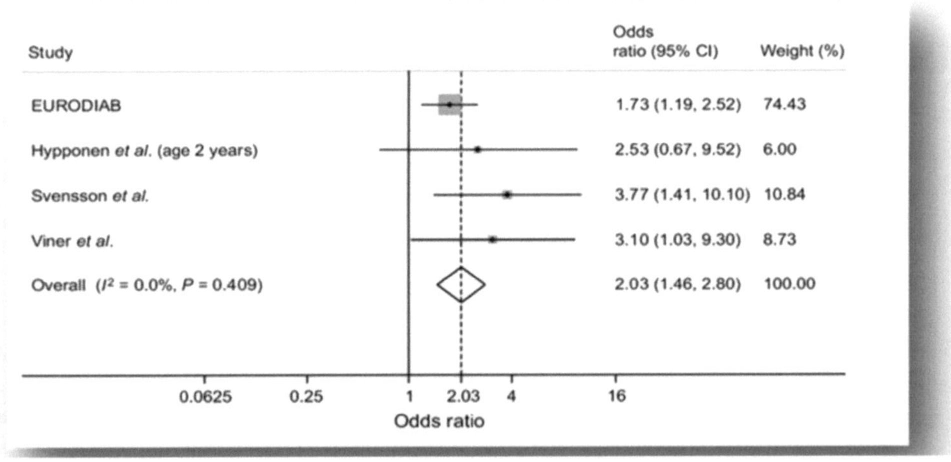

Fig. 2. Meta-analysis (fixed-effects inverse variance model) of studies of childhood obesity as a risk factor for subsequent T1D (Verbeeten et al., 2011).

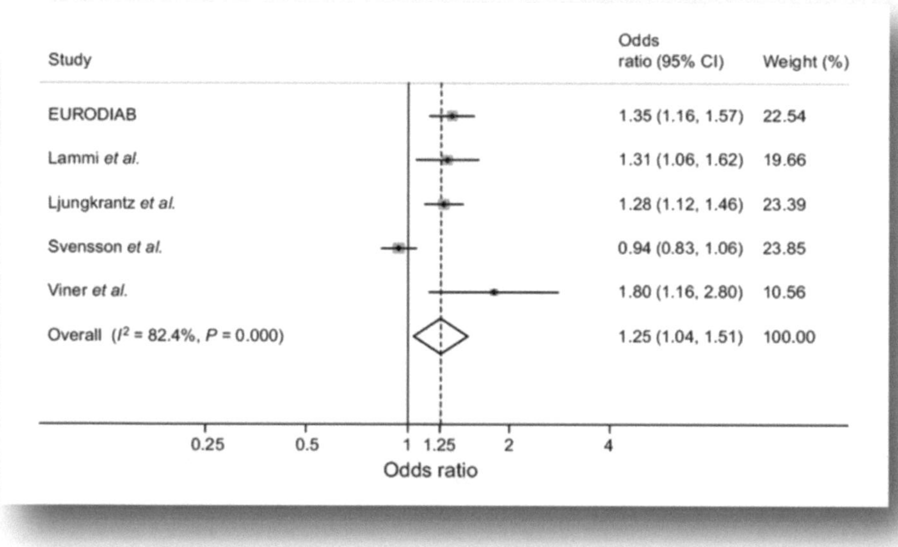

Fig. 3. Meta-analysis (random-effects inverse variance model) of studies of childhood BMI as a risk factor for subsequent T1D. Odds ratios correspond to a 1-unit increase in BMI standard deviation score (SDS)(Verbeeten et al., 2011).

3. Obesity after clinical Type 1 diabetes diagnostic

If on one hand intensive insulin prevents microvascular and macrovascular complications associated with poor glycemic control, the other brings an increased risk of severe hypoglycemia and weight gain, traditionally viewed as a normalization of weight, i.e. the correction of glycosuria, diuresis, and wasting with the initiation of insulin therapy. Insulin stimulates lipogenesis, inhibits protein catabolism, and slows basal metabolism. Other important aspect is the abnormal physiological route of insulin via its peripheral administration in those with T1D, which is also associated with reduced energy metabolism (Charlton & Nair, 1998). Classically normal or underweight, the phenotype of the T1D individuals is thus changing. A follow-up of 18 years of 589 individuals from the Pittsburgh Epidemiology of Diabetes Complications Study (EDC), a cohort of childhood-onset T1D, showed an increase in the prevalence of overweight by 47% (from 28.6% at baseline to 42%) and of obesity by sevenfold (from 3.4% at baseline to 22.7%), concomitantly with the highest prevalence of intensive insulin therapy - 7% and 82% were on intensive insulin therapy (≥ 3 insulin injections per day or on insulin pump) at baseline and 18 years after, respectively (Conway et al., 2010). Although injection frequency increased, total daily insulin dose decreased from 0.76 to 0.62 U/kg/day. Figure 4 shows the temporal patterns in the prevalence of being overweight and obese and the use of intensive insulin treatment, and these data was not influenced by the aging of the cohort and survivorship, as can be seen on Table 3. (age-group-specific prevalence for the 40–49-year-old age group by time period): overweight or obesity were present in 25% of the T1D individuals in 1986–1988 and in 68.2% in 2004–2007 (Conway et al., 2010).

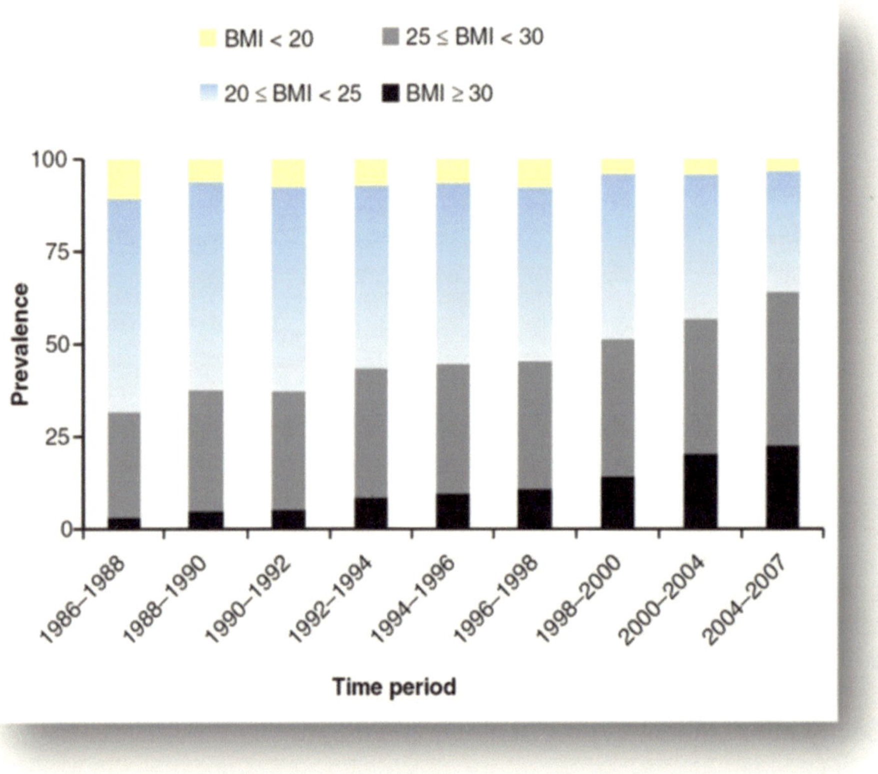

Fig. 4. Temporal patterns in overweight and obesity in Type 1 diabetes (Conway et al., 2010).

	BMI < 20 kg/m² (underweight)	20 ≤ BMI < 25 kg/m² (normal weight)	25 ≤ BMI < 30 kg/m² (overweight)	BMI ≥ 30 kg/m² (obese)
1986–1988	4 (9.1)	29 (65.9)	10 (22.7)	1 (2.3)
1988–1990	3 (5.8)	29 (55.8)	17 (32.7)	3 (5.8)
1990–1992	6 (8.5)	43 (60.6)	18 (25.4)	4 (5.6)
1992–1994	10 (12.2)	39 (47.6)	27 (32.9)	6 (7.3)
1994–1996	14 (11.9)	58 (49.2)	35 (29.7)	11 (9.3)
2004–2007	5 (2.9)	50 (28.9)	79 (45.7)	39 (22.5)

Table 3. Age-specific prevalence of underweight, normal weight, overweight, and obese for those aged 40-49 years in each time period, n (%)(Conway et al., 2010)

The prevalence of overweight/obesity in this T1D population was lower at baseline than general population (31.9 vs. 55.9%), although the incidence in both was similar after a mean of 7 years' follow-up (12%), and after 18 years' follow-up the prevalence of overweight in T1D people appear to have increased at a faster pace than in the general population.
Predictors of weight change were a higher baseline HbA1c, symptomatic autonomic neuropathy (inversely), overt nephropathy (inversely), and going onto intensive insulin therapy during follow-up. By the end of this study, 24% of the T1D people had died. Thus, as overt nephropathy and symptomatic autonomic neuropathy are associated with weight loss, the survivors are biased toward weight gain. The EDC Study also showed that, in T1D with a higher baseline HbA1c, moderate weight gain did not adversely affect the cardiovascular risk profile and favorably influenced the lipid profile in the setting of ameliorated glycemic control, but increased LDL cholesterol levels in the absence of a major improvement in glycemic control (Williams et al., 1999). Subjects who gained the least weight had the lowest LDL cholesterol levels at the follow-up period regardless of changes in HbA1 category. But when the weight gain after insulin was great, case of part of the patients who received intensive treatment in the Diabetes control and complications trial (DCCT) study and placed in the highest quartile of change in BMI, there was unmasking of central obesity or even MS in T1D (Purnell et al, 1998). These patients gained an average of 14 kg during the course of the study, about twice the weight gain equivalent to the third quartile of intensive care and the last quartile of patients on conventional treatment. Patients with the highest weight gain had the highest values of waist-hip ratio, blood pressure and insulin requirements when compared to the group with the same degree of glycemic control and also in intensive care, but who did not gain much weight. These youngsters also had a relatively atherogenic lipid profile, with elevations to levels of triglyceride, LDL cholesterol and apolipoprotein B (apoB) compared to their peers, also intensively treated, but without similar weight gain. The DCCT study (Purnell et al., 2003) also showed that the presence of family history of T2D was one of the strongest predictors for the weight gain in individuals with T1D who underwent intensive insulin therapy in the DCCT. In individuals with a family history of T2D, the weight gain, the final weight, the central fat distribution assessed by waist circumference, the insulin dose (units/kg/day) and degree of dyslipidemia were higher than in those without history familial T2D. Dyslipidemia included increases in triglycerides (TG) in VLDL particles and IDL (intermediate-density lipoprotein), which changes are common in individuals with central adiposity (Terry et al., 1989) and T2D (Brunzell & Chait, 1997). This could correspond to the expression of genes predisposing to T2D in this population. The findings of this study support the hypothesis that insulin treatment allows the expression of various components of MS in individuals with T1D who have family history of T2D, but also suggests that this group should be monitored more closely and earlier in relation to their potential of developing macrovascular complications, which is responsible for most of the increase in mortality found in patients with T1D (Laing et al., 1999), more than three times the general population.

4. Type 1 diabetes and Metabolic Syndrome

The insulin resistance is a soil to MS development and it is present during T1D evolution, even because of weight gain or because of the glucotoxicity – there was shown a proportion between fasting glycemic and IR, and improvement of glycemic control is linked to better insulin sensitivity, for example contributing to the so-called period of "honeymoon", the remission phase of diabetes, well known by clinicians, and may occur in up to 50% of patients during the first year of disease (DCCT Research Group, 1987). Yki-Jarvinen et al. (1986), studied insulin sensitivity using the hyperinsulinemic euglycemic clamp in 15 adult patients with T1D and normal BMI during the first 2 weeks, 3 months and 1 year after clinical diagnosis. In the first two weeks of diagnosis, they had a decrease in insulin sensitivity when compared to controls. However, three months after diagnosis, there was an improvement in insulin sensitivity in these patients, and it became similar to that of controls. Importantly, this improvement in insulin sensitivity coincided with the period of "honeymoon" in these patients, and showed a good correlation with HbA1c values and insulin doses in the treatment. Insulin sensitivity of patients who entered clinical remission was 40% greater than those who did not have this condition. Recently, our group performed a cohort and multicenter study (Gabbay et al, 2005; Dib, 2006) to determine the prevalence of MS in a group of patients with T1D and assessing their relation with the time of diagnosis. The study included 524 (276 females) T1D (according to the criteria of the Brazilian Diabetes Society and American Diabetes Association) with an average age of 20 ± 9 years and divided according to the time of T1D in 4 groups: GI, ≤ 5 years (n = 264), G-II, 6-10 years (n = 108), G III, 11-15 years (n = 96) and G IV,> 15 years (n = 56). In these groups were analyzed BMI (kg/m^2), total daily doses of insulin for treatment (U/kg/day), HbA1c values and the prevalence of MS. The criterion used for characterization of MS was the one of the World Health Organization, that is, diabetes mellitus and 2 or more of the following: increase in waist circumference (criterion set for youth) (Freedman et al., 1999), TG ≥ 150 mg/dL or HDL-C < 40 mg/dL (males) and < 50 mg/dL (females), urinary albumin excretion (≥ 20 µg/min) and hypertension (according to criteria adjusted for age and sex) (Brazilian Hypertension, Heart and Nephrology , Societies 2002). The daily insulin dose and HbA1c values were significantly lower in G-I than in other groups (G-I: 0.7 ± 0.3, G-II: 1.1 ± 0.3, G-III: 1.0 ± 0.3 and G-IV: 0.8 ± 0.2 U/kg/day, p = 0.000) and (G-I: 8.7 ± 2.6, G-II: 9.5 ± 2.2, G-III, 9.5 ± 2.3 and G-IV: 9.4 ± 2.8%, p = 0.000), respectively. There was a significant increase in the values of waist circumference (G-I: 71.9 ± 2.2, G-II: 75.7 ± 11.1, G-III: 76.5 ± 8.4 and G-IV: 80.2 ± 7.5 cm, p = 0.000) and BMI (G-I: 20.6 ± 3.8, G-II: 22.4 ± 3.6, G-III: 22.5 ± 3.1 and G- IV: 23.1 ± 4.1 kg/m2, p = 0.000) after 5 years of diagnosis of T1D. However, it is important to note that the BMI values were not superior to classical criteria of obesity or even overweight. The prevalence of MS (G-I: 5.1, G-II: 11.2, G-III: 18.9 and G-IV, 31.5%, p = 0.000) increased with time of diagnosis (Figure 5). The odds ratio (OR) for the development of MS in the other groups in relation to G-I was significant G-III onwards, being equal to 3.59 and 7.18 for this for G-IV in relation to G-I, both with p = 0.001. That is, the odds for the development of MS in patients with T1D and over 15 years of diagnosis is 618% higher than under 5 years of disease. Similarly, the odds for the development of MS for patients with T1D between 11 and 15 years duration is 259% higher than those with less than 5 disease in this group of patients. Other factors related to insulin resistance, such as visceral fat, BMI and TG, even when considered separately, also increased with the duration of the disease.

In another study (Giuffrida et al., 2005), 500 T1D patients [age 19.7 ± 8.9 years (mean ± SD), 52% female], we observe that, also analyzed separately, the prevalence of microalbuminuria (GI: 24.1%, G-II, 25.0%, G-III: 31.0% and G-IV: 55.6%, p <0.05) and hypertension (GI, 8.3%;

G-II: 13.6%, G-III: 28.6% and G-IV: 44.4%, p = 0.000) increased with duration of disease. Data from these studies suggest that chronic glucotoxicity (elevated HbA1c) and factors involved in diabetic nephropathy (microalbuminuria and hypertension) may be one of the mechanisms for the development of MS in T1D, among many others.

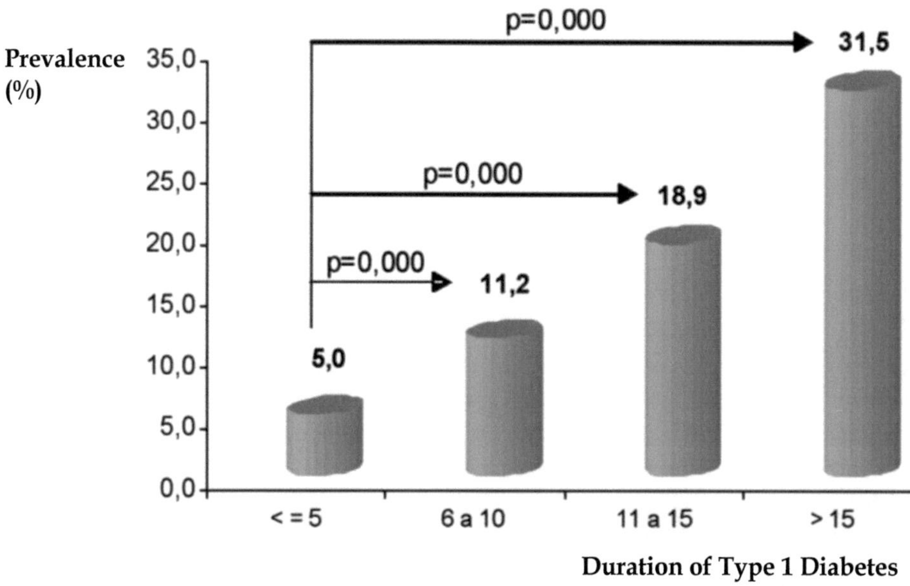

Fig. 5. Prevalence of MS in patients with T1D, according to disease duration. (Dib, 2006)

Aiming to compare the prevalence of MS using the ATP III criteria modified for age in our group of T1D, we studied 521 (51.2% female, age 20 ± 9 years; time of diagnosis of diabetes: 7.7 ± 6.9 years and HbA1c: 9.0 ± 2.4%) and found that this was equal to 12% (unpublished data).

The lowest concentration in the insulin in the liver causes a decrease in the synthesis of GHBP levels (Growth Hormone Binding Protein) (Bereket et al., 1999) that leads to a decrease in GH action, in the values of IGF-1 and in the inhibitory counter-regulation of this hormone, resulting in an exaggerated secretion of GH and increased insulin resistance.

The realization of a strict glycemic control in T1D, according to current guidelines, many often leads to use of supraphysiological doses of insulin, which could result in a stimulation of androgen synthesis, mediated by insulin, as occurs in cases of insulin resistance. Accordingly, the prevalence of Polycystic Ovary Syndrome (PCOS) and other symptoms and signs of hyperandrogenism were evaluated in a group of 85 patients with T1D (Escobar-Morreale et al., 2000). PCOS was defined by the presence of menstrual changes and clinical or laboratory evidence of hyperandrogenism. Other causes of elevated androgen hormones were excluded. Eighteen normal eumenorrheic women served as controls. Thirty-three patients (38%) presented with T1D changes associated with an androgen excess (16 with PCOS and 17 with hirsutism without menstrual abnormalities). The patients with T1D and PCOS had elevated total and free testosterone and androstenedione but normal levels of sex-hormone binding globulin (SHBG) and dehydroepiandrosterone sulfate (DHEAS). However, despite the finding of a high prevalence of hyperandrogenism (including PCOS and hirsutism), there was no difference between clinical variables such as duration of diabetes, age at diagnosis, conventional or intensive insulin treatment, average daily dose of insulin or glucose control between the T1D patients with and without hyperandrogenism in study.

The gold-standard method for evaluating IR is the hyperinsulinemic euglycemic clamp that directly measures the relationship between blood glucose and insulin levels, but it is difficult to be executed on a large scale since it is an invasive and expensive procedure. For this reason, HOMA-IR is used as a surrogate method to indirectly measure IR, calculated through fasting glycemia and insulinemia relationship. On the other hand, this calculation cannot be used for T1D as these patients do not produce endogenous insulin. So to evaluate the insulin sensitivity in these patients eGDR calculation (Equation 1) was developed that shown a good correlation with hyperinsulinemic euglycemic clamp (Chillarón et al., 2008):

$$\text{eGDR (mg.kg-1.min-1)} = 24{,}4 - 12{,}97\,(\text{W/H}) - 3{,}39\,(\text{Hypertension}) - 0{,}60\,(\text{HbA1c}) \quad \text{(E1)}$$

In which W/H is the waist-hip ratio(cm), hypertension is the presence or absence of hypertension (0 = no and 1 = yes) and the value of HbA1c is represented in %. It is also a good predictor of mortality, coronary arterial disease (CAD), microalbuminuria - a precocious hallmark of endothelial dysfunction (Pambianco et al., 2007) - and MS for T1D individuals, according to IDF (International Diabetes Federation), WHO (World Health Organization) and NCEP/ATPIII modified by AHA (American Heart Association).

As we know the insulin resistance is linked to an ectopic store of fat in insulin sensitive tissues like liver and muscle, but it is not clear if this fat accumulation leads to a hyperinsulinemic state or if it is its consequence. In a study with T2D patients, the glycemic control obtained after 67 hours of insulin treatment caused an accrual in intramyocellular and intrahepatic lipid content measured by nuclear magnetic resonance (NMR) spectroscopy, without compromising insulin sensitivity (Anderwald et al., 2002). Like T2D individuals, the intramyocellular lipid content in T1D ones was increased compared to controls and there was a direct relation with the glycemic control (Sibley et al., 2003).

There has been also noted a clear association between IR and visceral fat store, that can take its content extended in consequence of intensive insulin treatment independently of the type of diabetes, aggravating the CVD risk. In the DCCT study, the subgroup of T1D individuals that received intensive insulin treatment had a higher growth in BMI compared to the ones who were treated conventionally and it was noted a stronger correlation of this BMI variation with visceral fat deposit than with subcutaneous fat (Sibley et al., 2003). In this study, there are also demonstrations of direct association between visceral fat content and hepatic lipase, which favors the emergence of atherogenic dyslipidemia in these intensive treated individuals that put on more weight, reaching lipid levels similar to those of the conventionally treated group, suggesting loss of the benefits of intensive insulin therapy on lipids in this group of patients who had an excessive weight gain.

In other study (Nadeau et al., 2010), lean T1D adolescents with short time of disease (average of 7.5 years) without any inflammatory, clinical or lipid abnormalities had a IR - measured by hyperinsulinemic euglycemic clamp - similar to non diabetic obese adolescents and a superior IR than control subjects matched for age, pubertal stage, physical activity level and BMI, despite normal waist and intramyocellular lipid content.

There was also a demonstrated association between fat mass and blood pressure levels in T1D children and adolescents - high fat content, identified by the bioimpedance (BIA), and BMI were related to higher systolic and diastolic blood pressure (Pietrzak et al., 2009). The BIA is an easy, noninvasive, portable, no risk, relatively inexpensive method to measure the percentage of fat and provides results comparable to dual energy X-ray absorptiometry (DXA) (Elberg et al., 2004; Völgyi et al., 2008), that is reliable but expensive, requiring trained operators, individuals exposed to ionizing radiation and is not portable (Thomson et al., 2007).

There are data indicating good correlation between BIA and DXA, including Brazilian (Braulio et al., 2010) and T1D subjects (Leiter et al., 1994). Although overestimating the percentage of fat in lean individuals and underestimate it in obese (Sun et al., 2005), proves useful for predicting metabolic risk (including IR) as well as BMI and waist circumference (Lee et al., 2008). Through the BIA, it is possible to calculate the CDI (central fat distribution index), which assesses the impact of subcutaneous fat in the central fat distribution, and can be measured by dividing the area of abdominal subcutaneous fat mass by total fat (Silva et al., 2009). This measure seems to be relevant in that, according to some studies (Silva et al., 2009; Van Harmelen et al., 1998), the main source of leptin is the abdominal subcutaneous adipose tissue, either by mass effect - the subcutaneous adipose tissue is the major fat depot - as to produce more leptin (larger cell size and leptin gene expression) that omental adipose tissue. However, depending on the impedance (eg the trunk), the results may vary according to position changes, skin temperature, variation in electrode impedance and errors in their placement (Scharfetter et al., 2001).

A new adipokine identified visfatin, increases in proportion to visceral fat mass (Fukuhara et al., 2005) and decreases after gastric band placement (Haider et al., 2006). It is high in individuals with T2D (Chen et al., 2006) and even more in T1D (López-Bermejo et al., 2006), suggesting that its rising is linked to deterioration of pancreatic β cells. In vitro, visfatin activates the insulin receptor regardless of fasting state, increasing glucose uptake in muscle and adipose tissue and reducing hepatic glucose production independently of insulin levels (Fukuhara et al., 2005).

Hyperhomocysteinemia, known risk factor for coronary atherosclerosis (Okada et al., 1999), has also been shown to be detrimental to pancreatic insulin secretion (Patterson et al., 2006). The C-reactive protein (CRP), an inflammatory marker that confers increased risk for atherosclerosis (Hayaishi-Okano et al., 2002), is increased in T2D patients (Nabipour et al., 2008) and obese subjects (Richardson et al., 2009), and also relates to the control of diabetes (King et al., 2003), i.e. may increase due to the weight gain caused by intensive control of diabetes (Schaumberg et al., 2005).

Ferritin is another acute phase inflammatory marker, correlate positively with CRP and BMI (Richardson et al., 2009), and also more specifically with visceral adiposity and insulin resistance (Iwasaki et al., 2005), leading to increased ferritin levels in T2D patients, concurrent with an augmentation of visfatin (Fernandez-Real et al., 2007).

Recently, several studies have indicated that the gene associated with fat mass and BMI (FTO) has an important genetic effect on BMI and risk of obesity through the rs9939609 polymorphism. This polymorphism is linked to an impaired responsiveness to satiety, ie have an effect on appetite (Wardle et al., 2008). The homozygous AA genotype results in an average gain of 3 kg or 1 unit of BMI over the TT genotype. There is evidence that this polymorphism is linked to BMI gain in subjects with T1D (Gu et al., 2010) and higher levels of leptin and CRP (Welsh et al., 2010).

5. Conclusion

Obesity may both contribute to the onset of T1D as being a consequence of intensive treatment with insulin, that is, good glycemic control in T1D can lead to excessive weight gain in predisposed individuals (eg relatives of T2D), IR and consequently MS. Thus, the current approach of patients T1D should happen as it is done in T2D, multifactorial with an early and intensive monitoring of lifestyle, blood glucose, blood pressure and lipids, with the aim of identifying, correcting these factors and potentially reduce the high risk for cardiovascular disease in these patients. So gain weight can accelerate the presentation and modify the initial TID phenotype as increase the cardiovascular risk factors during evolution do the disease .

6. References

Acerini CL, Vheetham TD, Ege JA, Dunger DB. Both insulin sensitivity and insulin clearance in children and young adults with type 1 (insulin-dependent) diabetes vary with growth hormone concentrations and with age. *Diabetologia* 2000; 43: 61-8.

Aldhahi, W. and Hamdy, O. Adipokines, inflammation and the endothelium in diabetes. *Curr. Diab. Rep.*2003, 3, 293-298.

American Diabetes Association. Report of the Expert Committee on the Diagnosis and Classification of Diabetes Mellitus. *Diabetes Care* 1997; 20: 1183-97.

Anderwald C, Bernroider E, Krsšák M, Stingl H, Brehm A, Bischof MG, Nowotny P, Roden M and Waldhäusl W. Effects of Insulin Treatment in Type 2 Diabetic Patients on Intracellular Lipid Content in Liver and Skeletal Muscle. *Diabetes* 2002, 51: 3025–3032.

Arai K, Yokoyama H, Okuguchi F et al. Association between Body Mass Index and Core Components of Metabolic Syndrome in 1486 Patients with Type 1 Diabetes Mellitus in Japan (JDDM 13). *Endocrine Journal*, 2008, vol 55 (6), 1025-1032.

Armani A, Durant S, Throsby M, Coulad J, Dardenne M, Homo-Delarche F. Glucose homeostasis in the nonobese diabetic mouse at the pre-diabetic stage. *Endocrinology* 1998; 139: 1115-24.

Beales PE, Pozzili P. Thiazolidinediones for the prevention of diabetes in the non-obese diabetic (NOD) mouse: implications for human type 1 diabetes. *Diabetes Metab Res Rev* 2002; 18: 114-7.

Becker DJ, Libman I, Pietropaolo M, Dosch M, Arslanian S, LaPorte R. Changing phenotype of IDDM: is it type 1 or type 2? *Pediatr. Res.* 2001, 49, 93A.

Bereket A, Lang CH, Wilson TA. Alterations in the growth hormone-insulin-like growth factor axis in insulin dependent diabetes mellitus. *Horm Metab Res* 1999; 31: 172-81.

Braulio VB, Furtado VC, Silveira MG, Fonseca MH, Oliveira JE. Comparison of body composition methods in overweight and obese Brazilian women. *Arq Bras Endocrinol Metab.* 2010; 54/4.

Brunzell JD, Chait A. Diabetic dyslipidemia: pathology and treatment. In: Porte D, Sherwin J (eds.). *Ellenberg and Rifkin's Diabetes Mellitus*. 5th ed. Norwalk: Appleton and Lange; 1997. p.1077-98.

Buschard K, Buch I, Molsted-Pedersen L, Hougaard P, Kuhl C. Increased incidence of true type I diabetes acquired during pregnancy. *Br Med J (Clin Res Ed)* 1987; 294 (6567): 275-9.

Charlton M, Nair K. Role of hyperglucagonemia in catabolism associated with type 1 diabetes. Effects of leucine metabolism and the resting metabolic rate. *Diabetes* 1998; 47: 1748–1756.

Chen M-P, Chung F-M, Chang D-M, Tsai JC-R, Huang H-F, Shin S-J and Le Y-J. Elevated plasma level of visfatin/PBEF in patients with type 2 diabetes. *JCEM*, 2006, 91: 295-299.

Chillarón JJ, Goday A, Pedro-Botet J. Síndrome metabólico, diabetes mellitus tipo 1 y resistencia a la insulina. *Med Clin (Barc)* 2008, 130(12): 466-71.

Conway B, Miller RG, Costacou T, Fried L, Kelsey S, Evans RW and Orchard TJ. Temporal patterns in overweight and obesity in Type 1 diabetes. *Diabet. Med.* 27, 398–404 (2010).

Daneman D. Type 1 diabetes. Lancet 2006; 367: 847–858.

Dib, SA. Insulin Resistance and metabolic syndrome in Type 1 Diabetes Mellitus. *Arq Bras Endocrinol Metab* vol 50 nº 2 Abril 2006

Elberg J, McDuffie JR, Sebring NG, Salaita C, Keil M, Robotham D, Reynolds JC and Yanovski JA. Comparison of methods to assess change in children's body composition. *Am J Clin Nutr*. 2004 July; 80 (1): 64–69.

Escobar-Morreale HF, Roldan B, Barrio R, Alonso M, Sancho J, de Calle H, et al. High prevalence of the polycystic ovary syndrome and hirsutism in women with type 1 diabetes mellitus. *J Clin Endocrinol Metab* 2000; 85: 4182-7.

EURODIAB ACE Study Group. Variation and trends in incidence of childhood diabetes in Europe. EURODIAB ACE Study Group. *Lancet* 2000, 355, 873-876.

Fernandez-Real JM, Moreno JM, Chico B, López-Bermejo A and Ricart W (2007). Circulating Visfatin Is Associated With Parameters of Iron Metabolism in Subjects With Altered Glucose Tolerance. *Diabetes Care* 30: 616–621, 2007.

Freedman D, Serdula MK, Srinivasan SR, Berenson GS. Relation of circumference and skin fold thicknesses to lipid and insulin concentrations in children and adolescents: the Bogalusa Heart Study. *Am J Clin Nutr* 1999; 69: 308-17.

Fukuhara A, Matsuda M, Nishizawa M, Segawa K, Tanaka M, Kishimoto K, Matsuki Y, Murakami M, Ichisaka T, Murakami H, Watanabe E, Takagi T, Akiyoshi M, Ohtsubo T, Kihara S, Yamashita S, Makishima M, Funahashi T, Yamanaka S, Hiramatsu R, Matsuzawa Y, Shimomura I.Visfatin: a protein secreted by visceral fat that mimics the effects of insulin. *Science* 2005, 307, 426-430.

Gabbay MAL, Gomes MB, Pires AC, Dib SA. Prevalence and trends of metabolic syndrome in type 1 diabetes according to duration of the disease. *Diabetes* 2005; 54 (suppl.1): A176.

Gilliam LK, Brooks-Worrell BM, Palmer JP, Greenbaum CJ, Pihoker C. Autoimmunity and clinical course in children with type 1, type 2 and type 1.5 diabetes. *J Autoimmun.* 2005, 25, 244-250.

Giuffrida FMA, Gabbay MAL, Pires AC, Brito M, Dib SA. Desenvolvimento dos sinais da síndrome metabólica em pacientes com diabetes mellitus tipo 1 de acordo com o tempo de duração da doença. *Arq Bras Endocrinol Metab* 2005; 49: S96.

Gu HF, Alvarsson A and Brismar K. The Common FTO Genetic Polymorphism rs9939609 is Associated with Increased BMI in Type 1 Diabetes but not with Diabetic Nephropathy. *Biomarker Insights* 2010:5 29–32.

Haider DG, Schindler K, Schaller G, Prager G, Wolzt M and Ludvik B. Increased plasma visfatin concentration in morbidly obese subjects are reduced after gastric banding. *JCEM*, 2006, 91: 1578-1581.

Hayaishi-Okano R, Yamasaki Y, Katakami N, Ohtoshi K, Gorogawa S-I, Kuroda A, Matsuhisa M, Kosugi K, Nishikawa N, Kajimoto Y, Hori M. Elevated C-reactive protein associates with early-stage carotid atherosclerosis in young subjects with type 1 diabetes. *Diabetes Care* 2002, 25: 1432–1438.

Iwasaki T, Nakajima A, Yoneda M, Yamada Y, Mukasa K, Fujita K, Fujisawa N, Wada K and Terauch Y (2005). Serum Ferritin Is Associated With Visceral Fat Area and Subcutaneous Fat Area. *Diabetes Care* 28: 2486–2491, 2005.

Jago, R. et al. Studies to Treat or Prevent Pediatric Type 2 Diabetes (STOPP-T2D) Prevention Study Group * Prevalence of the metabolic syndrome Among a Racially/Ethnically Diverse Group of U.S. Eighth-Grade Adolescents and Associations With Fasting Insulin and Homeostasis Model Assessment of Insulin Resistance Levels. *Diabetes Care* 2008, 31(10): 2020-2025.

Kadowaki T, Yamauchi T, Kubota N, Hara K, Ueki K, Tobe K. Adiponectin and adiponectin receptors in insulin resistance, diabetes, and the metabolic syndrome. J. *Clin. Invest.* 2006, 116: 1784–1792.

King DE, Mainous AG, Buchanan TA and Pearson WS. C-reactive protein and glycemic control in adults with diabetes. *Diabetes Care* 2003, 26: 1535–1539.

Laing SP, Swerdlow AJ, Slater SD, Botha JL, Burden AC, Waugh NR, et al. The British Diabetic Association Cohort Study II: cause-specific mortality in patients with insulin treated diabetes mellitus. *Diabet Med* 1999;16:466-71.

Lee K, Song Y-M and Sung J. Which Obesity Indicators Are Better Predictors of Metabolic Risk? Healthy Twin Study. *Obesity* (2008) 16, 834–840.

Leiter LA, Lukaski HC, Kenny DJ. The use of bioelectrical impedance analysis (BIA) to estimate body composition in the diabetes control and complications trial (DCCT). *Int J Obesity* 1994; 18: 829–835.

Li C., Ford ES, Zhao G, Mokdad AH. Prevalence of Pre-Diabetes and Its Association With Clustering of Cardiometabolic Risk Factors and Hyperinsulinemia Among U.S. Adolescents National Health and Nutrition Examination Survey 2005–2006. *Diabetes Care* 2009, 32: 342–347.

Libman, I.M. and Becker, D.J. (2003). Coexistence of type 1 and type 2 diabetes mellitus: 'double' diabetes? *Pediatr. Diabetes* 2003, 4, 110-113.

López-Bermejo A, Chico-Julià B, Fernàndez-Balsells M, Recasens M, Esteve E, Casamitjana R, Ricart W, Fernández-Real JM Serum visfatin increases with progressive beta cell-deterioration. *Diabetes* 2006, 55, 2861-2875.

Lord, G. Role of leptin in immunology. *Nutr. Rev.* 2002, 60, S35-S38.

Matarese G, Moschos S, Mantzoros CS. Leptin in immunology. *J. Immunol.* 2005, 174, 3137-3142.

Matarese G, Sanna V, Lechler RI, Sarvetnick N, Fontana S, Zappacosta S, La Cava A. Leptin accelerates autoimmune diabetes in female NOD mice. *Diabetes* 2002, 51, 1356-1361.

McCulloch DK, Kahn SE, Schwartz MW, Koerker DJ, Palmer JP. Effect of nicotinic acid-induced insulin resistance on pancreatic B cell function in normal and streptozotocin treated baboons. *J Clin Invest* 1991; 40: 166-80.

Nabipour I, Vahdat K, Jafari SM, Beigi S, Assadi M, Azizi F, Sanjdideh Z. Elevated High Sensitivity C-Reactive Protein Is Associated with Type 2 Diabetes Mellitus: The Persian Gulf Healthy Heart Study. *Endocrine Journal*, 2008, vol 55 (4), 717-722.

Nadeau KJ, Regensteiner JG, Bauer TA, Brown MS, Dorosz JL, Hull A, Zeitler P, Draznin B. and Reusch JEB. Insulin Resistance in Adolescents with Type 1 Diabetes and Its Relationship to Cardiovascular Function. *Clin Endocrinol Metab*, February 2010, 95 (2): 513–521.

Nathan DM, Lachin JM, Cleary P., Pomar T., Brillon DJ, Backlund JY, O'Leary DH, Genuth SM. Diabetes Control and Complications Trial / Epidemiology of Diabetes Interventions and Complications Study Research Group. Intensive Diabetes therapy and carotid intima-media thickness in type 1 diabetes mellitus. *NEJM* 2003, 348: 2294-2303.

Nathan DM et al. Diabetes Control and Complications Trial / Epidemiology of Diabetes Interventions and Complications Study Research Group. Intensive Diabetes treatment and cardiovascular disease in patients with type 1 diabetes. *NEJM* 2005, 353: 2643-2653.

OECD. Health at a Glance 2009: OECD Indicators. Paris: Organization for Economic Co-Operation and Development Press, 2009: 38–51.

Okada E, Oida K, Tada H, Asazuma K, Eguchi K, Tohda G, Kosaka S, Takahashi S and Miyamori I. Hyperhomocysteinemia Is a Risk Factor for Coronary Arteriosclerosis in Japanese Patients With Type 2 Diabetes. *Diabetes Care* 1999, 22: 484–490.

Pambianco G, Costacou T, Orchard TJ. The Prediction of Major Outcomes of Type 1 Diabetes: a 12-Year Prospective Evaluation of Three Separate Definitions of the metabolic syndrome and Their Components and Estimated Glucose Disposal Rate - The Pittsburgh Epidemiology of Diabetes Complications Study experience. *Diabetes Care* 2007, 30: 1248–1254.

Patterson S, Flatt PR, Brennan L, Newsholme P, McClenaghan NH. Detrimental actions of metabolic syndrome risk factor, homocysteine, on pancreatic B-cell glucose metabolism and insulin secretion. Journal of Endocrinology 2006, 189: 301-10.

Pietrzak I, Mianowska B, Gadzicka A, Młynarski W, Szadkowska A. Blood pressure in children and adolescents with type 1 diabetes mellitus – the influence of body mass index and fat mass. *Pediatric Endocrinology, Diabetes and Metabolism* 2009, 15 (4): 240-5.

Pinhas-Hamiel O, Dolan LM, Daniels SR, Standiford D, Khoury PR, Zeitler P. Increased incidence of non-insulin-dependent diabetes mellitus among adolescents. *J Pediatr* 1996, 128, 608-15.

Pozzilli,P. and Buzzetti, R. A new expression of diabetes: double diabetes. *TRENDS in Endocrinology and Metabolism* 2007, 18 (2), 52-57.

Purnell JQ, Hokanson JE, Marcovina SM, Steffes MW, Cleary PA, Brunzell JD. Effect of excessive weight-gain with intensive therapy of type 1 diabetes on lipid levels and blood pressure: results from the DCCT. Diabetes Control and Complications Trial. *JAMA* 1998; 280: 140-6.

Purnell JQ, Dev RK, Steffes MW, Cleary PA, Palmer JP, Hirsch IB, et al. Relationship of family history of type 2 diabetes, hypoglycemia, and auto antibodies to weight gain and lipids with intensive and conventional therapy in the Diabetes Control and Complications Trial. *Diabetes* 2003; 52: 2623.

Reinehr T, Schober E, Wiegand S, Thon A, Holl R. DPV-Wiss Study Group. B-Cell autoantibodies in children with type 2 diabetes mellitus: subgroup or misclassification? *Arch. Dis. Child.* 2006, 91, 473-477.

Richardson MW, Richardson MW, Ang L, Visintainer PF, Wittcopp CA.The abnormal measures of iron homeostasis in pediatric obesity are associated with the inflammation of obesity. *Int J Pediatr Endocrinol.*; 2009:713269. Epub 2009 Oct 8.

Rolandsson O, Hägg E, Hampe C, Sullivan EP, Nilsson M, Jansson G, Hallmans G, Lernmark A. Glutamate decarboxylase (GAD65) and tyrosine phosphatase-like protein (IA-2) autoantibodies index in a regional population is related to glucose intolerance and body mass index. *Diabetologia* 1999, 42, 555-559.

Rosenbloom A, Joe JR, Young RS, Winter WE. Emerging Epidemic of Type 2 Diabetes in Youth. Diabetes Care 1999, 22: 345–354.

Särnblad S., Ingberg CM, Åman J, Schvarcz E. Body composition in young female adults with Type 1 diabetes mellitus. A prospective case-control study. *DIABETIC Medicine,* DOI: 10.1111/j.1464-5491.2007.02144.x

Scharfetter H, Schlager T, Stollberger R, Felsberger R, Hutten H and Hinghofer-Szalkay H. Assessing abdominal fatness with local bioimpedance analysis: basics and experimental findings. *International Journal of Obesity* (2001) 25, 502 ± 511.

Schaumberg DA, Glynn RJ, Jenkins AJ, Lyons TJ, Rifai N, Manson JE, Ridker PM, Nathan DM (2005). Effect of Intensive Glycemic Control on Levels of Markers of Inflammation in Type 1 Diabetes Mellitus in the Diabetes Control and Complications Trial. *Circulation* 2005; 111; 2446-2453.

Sibley SD, Palmer JP, Hirsch IB and Brunzell JD. Visceral Obesity, Hepatic Lipase Activity, and Dyslipidemia in Type 1 Diabetes. *J Clin Endocrinol Metab,* July 2003, 88 (7): 3379–3384.

Silva EA, Flexa F, Zanella MT. Impact of abdominal fat and insulin resistance on arterial hypertension in non-obese women. *Arq Bras Endocrinol Metab.* 2009; 53/3.

Sociedade Brasileira de Hipertensão. Sociedade Brasileira de Cardiologia e Sociedade Brasileira de Nefrologia 2002 IV. Diretrizes Brasileiras de hipertensão arterial. p.5-7.

Sun G, French CR, Martin GR, Younghusband B, Green RC, Xie Y, Mathews M, Barron JR, Fitzpatrick DG, Gulliver W and Zhang H. Comparison of multifrequency bioelectrical impedance analysis with dual-energy X-ray absorptiometry for assessment of percentage body fat in a large, healthy population. *Am J Clin Nutr* 2005; 81: 74–8.

Terry RB, Wood PDS, Haskell WL, Stefanick ML, Krauss RM. Regional adiposity patterns in relation to lipids, lipoprotein cholesterol, and lipoprotein subfraction mass in men. *J Clin Endocrinol Metab* 1989; 68: 191-9.

The Diabetes Control and Complications Trial (DCCT) Research Group. Effects of age, duration and treatment of insulin-dependent diabetes mellitus on residual betacell function: observations during eligibility testing for the Diabetes control and Complications Trial (DCCT). *J Clin Endocrinol Metab* 1987; 65: 30-6.

The Diabetes Control and Complications Trial Research Group. The effect of intensive treatment of diabetes on the development and progression of long-term complications in insulin-dependent diabetes mellitus. *NEJM*, 1993, 329 (14): 977-986.

Thomson R, Brinkworth GD, Buckley JD, Noakes M and Clifton PM. Good agreement between bioelectrical impedance and dual-energy X-ray absorptiometry for estimating changes in body composition during weight loss in overweight young women. *Clinical Nutrition* (2007) 26, 771–777.

Van Harmelen V, Reynisdottir S, Eriksson P, Thörne A, Hoffstedt J, Lönnqvist F and Arner P. Leptin Secretion From Subcutaneous and Visceral Adipose Tissue in Women. *Diabetes*, Vol. 47, June 1998.

Verbeeten KC, Elks CE, Daneman D, Ong KK. Association between childhood obesity and subsequent Type 1 diabetes: a systematic review and meta-analysis. *Diabetic Medicine* 2011 Jan: 28 (1): 10-8.

Völgyi E, Tylavsky FA, Lyytikäinen A, Suominen H, Alén M and Cheng S. Assessing Body Composition With DXA and Bioimpedance: Effects of Obesity, Physical Activity, and Age. *Obesity* (2008) 16, 700–705.

Wang, Y., Monteiro C., Popkin B.M. Trends of obesity and underweight in older children and adolescents in the United States, Brazil, China, and Russia1–3. *Am J Clin Nutr*; 75:971–7, 2002.

Wardle J, Carnell S, Haworth CMA, Farooqi IS, O'Rahilly S and Plomin R. Obesity Associated Genetic Variation in *FTO* Is Associated with Diminished Satiety. *J Clin Endocrinol Metab* 93: 3640–3643, 2008.

Wellen K., Hotamisligil G. Inflammation, stress, and diabetes. *J. Clin. Invest.* 2005, 115:1111–1119.

Welsh P, Polisecki E, Robertson M, Jahn S, Buckley BM, Craen AJM, Ford I, Jukema JW, Macfarlane PW, Packard CJ, Stott DJ, Westendorp RGJ, Shepherd J, Hingorani AD, Smith GD, Schaefer E and Sattar N. Unraveling the Directional Link between Adiposity and Inflammation: A Bidirectional Mendelian Randomization Approach. *J Clin Endocrinol Metab* 95: 93–99, 2010.

Wilkin TJ. The accelerator hypothesis: weight gain as the missing link between Type I and Type II diabetes. *Diabetologia* 2001;44:914-22.

Willi SM, Egede LE. Type 2 diabetes mellitus in adolescents. *Current Opinion in Endocrinology & Diabetes*, 2000, 7:71–76.

Williams KV, Erbey JR, Becker D, Orchard TJ. Improved glycemic control reduces the impact of weight gain on cardiovascular risk factors in type 1 diabetes. The Epidemiology of Diabetes Complications Study. *Diabetes Care* 1999; 22: 1084–1091.

Yki-Jarvinen H, Koivisto VA. Natural course of insulin resistance in type 1 diabetes. *N Engl J Med* 1986; 315: 224-30.

11

Meta-Analysis of Genome-Wide Association Studies to Understand Disease Relatedness

Stephanie N. Lewis, Elaine O. Nsoesie, Charles Weeks,
Dan Qiao and Liqing Zhang
Virginia Tech, Blacksburg, VA
USA

1. Introduction

Genome-wide association studies (GWAS) have become a popular method of surveying haplotype variations within populations. The recent explosion and success of these studies has allowed for identification of multiple gene variations and non-genetic risk factors that are often involved in pathogenesis of many diseases (Xavier&Rioux, 2008). Efforts to archive these single nucleotide polymorphisms (SNPs) and make the information publicly available have been made possible by the International Haplotype Map Project (HapMap) (The International HapMap Consortium, 2005; The International HapMap Consortium, 2007) and development of GWAS databases (Johnson&O'Donnell, 2009) such as Genomes.gov (Hindorff et al., 2009). The HapMap database of genetic variants and the ever progressing technology involved in identifying genetic disease susceptibility markers has allowed for identification of shared genetic associations that were undetectable with previous methods for identifying deleterious mutations effects for individual genes (Xavier&Rioux, 2008). We are now capable of detecting common susceptibility markers between previously unassociated diseases with the ability to assess combined association signals shared by biological pathways (Wang et al., 2011).

Research of immune-mediated disease susceptibility has benefited from the discovery of shared haplotypes. GWAS with a focus on autoimmune diseases, which included celiac disease, Crohn's disease, multiple sclerosis, rheumatoid arthritis, systemic lupus erythematosus, and type 1 diabetes (Lettre&Rioux, 2008), have shed light on shared genetic markers. Such markers can be exploited to identify biomedical traits that translate to improved diagnostic and treatment techniques (McCarthy et al., 2008). Under the common disease/common variant hypothesis (Wang et al., 2005), one would assume that shared variants result in shared disease phenotypes, and this commonality could serve as a global target for effective treatment options. It is under this assumption that many disease association studies are conducted. The Wellcome Trust Case Control Consortium (WTCCC) conducted a study in which nearly 2000 individuals were examined for coronary artery disease (CAD), hypertension, type II diabetes (T2D), rheumatoid arthritis (RA), Crohn's disease (CD), type I diabetes (T1D) and bipolar disorder (BD) susceptibility against a shared set of about 3000 controls (The Wellcome Trust Case Control Consortium, 2007). The study revealed several association loci for the seven diseases, with some of these indicating risk for more than one of the studied diseases (The Wellcome Trust Case Control Consortium, 2007).

Huang et al. used the data from the WTCCC study to see if associations could be made between the seven diseases given the loci and collections of other data regarding disease susceptibility (Huang et al., 2009). Huang et al. performed analyses at four levels (nucleotide, gene, protein, and phenotype) to determine the existence of overlap across SNPs associated with the seven diseases and constructed protein-protein interaction networks to visualize similarities between diseases (Huang et al., 2009). The group found strong associations across all four levels of analysis for the autoimmune group (CD, RA, and T1D), while no genetic associations were found at any level within the metabolic/cardiovascular group (CAD, hypertension and T2D) (Huang et al., 2009). These results reasserted some expectations derived from clinical literature in the case of the autoimmune group, and suggested inappropriate disease grouping in the case of the metabolic/cardiovascular group (Huang et al., 2009).

For this study, we proposed a large-scale disease and phenotype comparison based on the WTCCC and Huang et al. studies. To this end, we have combined data from GWAS with expression pattern data to determine if genetic and expression similarities exist between diseases. A total of 61 human diseases and phenotypes were assessed. Disease relatedness networks (DRNs) were constructed to visually assess associations on a larger scale. We also took advantage of high-throughput molecular assay technologies to incorporate mRNA expression profiles of diseases, and thus added another dimension of analysis toward assessing disease relationships. Gene expression is an indicator of cellular state, and gene expression profiles can be considered as quantitative traits that are highly heritable. The link between organismal complex traits, such as disease-related phenotype, and gene expression variation has been theoretically accepted (Goring et al., 2007; Moffatt et al., 2007; Chen et al., 2008; Emilsson et al., 2008). With the declining per-sample costs of high-throughput microarray experiments, the amount of gene expression data in international repositories has grown exponentially. The availability of these datasets for many different diseases provides an opportunity to use data-driven approaches to improve our understanding of disease relationships. Hu and Agarwal (Hu&P., 2009) determined disease-disease and disease-drug networks using large-scale gene expression data. Very recently, Suthram et al. (Suthram et al., 2010) presented a quantitative framework to compare and contrast diseases by combining both disease-related mRNA expression data and human protein interaction data. Although GWAS provide comprehensive views of disease interrelationships at the DNA level, the insights from the gene expression aspect, which reflects cellular phenotype, will further advance and strengthen the understanding of this issue. A large-scale disease comparison study such as this has the potential to uncover relationships between diseases and phenotypes that are often overlooked in single disease SNP data analysis.

2. Methods

2.1 SNP-based genetic analysis

Five populations were considered for this expansion study: Han Chinese (CHB), Japanese (JPT), a combined CHB and JPT population (CHB+JPT), Yoruba (YRI), and U.S. residents with northern and western European ancestry (CEU). SNP dataset 2009-02_rel24 (The International HapMap Consortium, 2005; The International HapMap Consortium, 2007) was downloaded from the HapMap site and the SNP set was expanded by means of linkage disequilibrium (LD). SNPs with an r^2 greater than or equal to 0.5 were included. SNPs were divided by associated disease or phenotype (listed in Table 1) and the divisions were maintained for each succeeding level of analysis. SNPs were divided into blocks based on an r^2 greater than or equal to 0.1. Gene names from Ensembl (Birney et al., 2004) were assigned to blocks if the genetic location was within 2 kilobases up- or downstream of the gene of interest or within the start and end bases for the gene. Gene data were cross-referenced against pathway-specific gene lists generated from the KEGG database (Kanehisa&Goto, 2000; Kanehisa et al., 2006; Kanehisa et al., 2010) in order to assign genes to identified pathways. Pairwise comparisons for each level were conducted to see if diseases and phenotpyes shared SNPs, blocks, genes, or pathway designations. Jaccard index values were calculated for each comparison at each level to assess similarity. Using the Jaccard indexes, DRNs were constructed to visualize the strength of relatedness between diseases. DRNs were visually inspected to identify the strongest relationships. Suggested associations were verified by principal components analysis (PCA) and minor data mining for clinical relevance. Complete details of these methods were previously described by Lewis et al (Lewis et al., 2011).

2.2 Gene expression dataset

The gene expression data used in this analysis was obtained from the NCBI Gene Expression Omnibus (GEO) (Barrett et al., 2009). Not all of the 61 diseases were represented by expression data on the GEO site. Data for a subset of diseases was found by scanning the experimental context of a collection of GEO data (or GEO Series, GSE) for microarrays that were assigned to human disease conditions. Only those microarrays that were curated and reported in the GEO Datasets (or GDS) were used in our analysis. The data set was also restricted to those GSEs in which both the disease and the corresponding control condition (from healthy tissue samples) were measured in the same tissue. For consistency, we further restricted the GSEs to only those datasets which used Affymetrix Gene Chip Human Genome U133 Array Set HG-U133A (GPL96), HG-U133B (GPL97) and HG-U133plus2 (GPL570), which are among the most commonly used platforms. Probes for these platforms were mapped to the current gene identifiers (Chen et al., 2007). This process yielded nineteen diseases for the final GEO analysis.

2.3 Expression measurement

To quantitatively compare expression data, we first normalized the data in each microarray sample using the Z-score transformation to make the expression values across various microarray samples and diseases comparable. Next, we performed an unpaired two-sample Student t-test to compute the t-test statistic and p-value of each gene between the disease and control groups. We only used the most appropriate Affymetrix probe set in which a single probe was representative of each gene. The most appropriate Affymetrix probe set was adopted from the work of Hu et al. (Hu&Agarwal, 2009) as many genes were represented by multiple probe sets in Affymetrix U133 microarray chips. This modification avoided correlation and scoring biases brought on by over-representation of those genes. 18,600 most appropriate probes/genes for each of nineteen diseases were identified. The genes were grouped with statistically significant high t-test statistics ($p<0.05$) as "up-regulated genes" and statistically significant low t-test statistics ($p<0.05$) as "down-regulated genes". Instead of using a p-value threshold as a cutoff to identify significantly changed genes, the 200 and 1000 most changed genes were designated as the disease-associated significantly changed genes for each disease state. The lowest p-values in each category

Abbre-viation	Disease/ Phenotype	Abbre-viation	Disease/ Phenotype	Abbre-viation	Disease/ Phenotype	Abbre-viation	Disease/ Phenotype
AD	Alzheimer's disease	EO	Early onset extreme obesity	LM	Lipid measurements	QT	Cardiac repolarization (QT interval)
AF	Atrial Fibrillation/At-rial Flutter	GCA	General cognitive ability	LOAD	Late-onset Alzheimer's disease	RA	Rheumatoid Arthritis
ALS	Amyotrophic Lateral Sclerosis	GD	Gallstone disease	LONG	Longevity and age-related phenotypes	RLS	Restless Leg Syndrome
BA	Brain aging	GLA	Glaucoma	MHA	Minor histocompat-ibility antigenicity	SA	Subclinical atherosclerosis
BC	Breast cancer	HAE	Hepatic adverse events with thrombin inhibitor ximelagatran	MI	Myocardial infarction	SALS	Sporadic Amyotrophic lateral Sclerosis
BD	Bipolar disorder	HBF	Adult fetal hemoglobin levels (HbF) by F cell levels	MS	Multiple sclerosis	SCP	Sleep and circadian phenotypes
BL	Blood lipids	HEI	Height	ND	Nicotine dependence	SLCL	Serum LDL cholesterol levels
BMG	Bone mass and geometry	HEM	Human episodic memory	NEU	Neuroticism	SLE	Systemic Lupus Erythematosus
BPAS	Blood pressure and arterial stiffness	HIV1	HIV-1 disease progression	OBE	Obesity-related traits	SP	Schizophrenia
CA	Childhood asthma	HT	Haematological (blood) traits	PA	Polysubstance addiction	SPBC	Sporadic post-menopausal breast cancer
CAD	Coronary Artery Disease	HYP	Hypertension	PC	Prostate cancer	SPM	Skin pigmentation
CC	Colorectal cancer	IC	Iris color	PD	Parkinson's disease	STR	Stroke
CD	Crohn's disease	IMAN	Immunoglo-bulin A nephropathy	PF	Pulmonary function phenotypes	T1D	Type I Diabetes
CDI	Celiac disease	IS	Ischemic stroke	PR	Psoriasis	T2D	Type II Diabetes
CS	Coronary spasm	KFET	Kidney function and endocrine traits	PSP	Progressive Supranuclear Palsy	TG	Triglycerides
CVD	Cardiovascular Disease outcomes						

Table 1. List of diseases and phenotypes considered for this study and the previous study (Lewis et al., 2011) with corresponding abbreviations.

(up-regulated, down-regulated, and combined) for the top 200 or 1000 genes were pooled for each disease. All of the genes with significant expression changes were grouped together and Jaccard index values were calculated. Gene lists for each disease were compared pair-wise for each of the three expression categories. Here, a high Jaccard index implied a high degree of commonality between diseases/phenotypes. The Jaccard indexes were normalized to produce Z-scores, which were then used as a measure of disease relatedness. The significantly changed genes shared by two diseases were also subjected to Gene Ontology (GO) term enrichment analysis using the web-based Gene Ontology enrichment analysis and visualization (GOrilla) tool (Eden et al., 2007; Eden et al., 2009).

2.4 Medical subject headings (MeSH) term mapping

MeSH is the National Library of Medicine's controlled vocabulary thesaurus (Bodenreider et al., 1998). It consists of sets of terms associated with descriptors in a hierarchical structure. For the nineteen GEO validation diseases (Table 2), the MeSH trees were downloaded and the first level of each tree was used as the disease category. The category that could best indicate the cause of the disease was taken as the disease category.

3. Results

3.1 Summary of significant disease associations for screening of 61 diseases and phenotypes

Jaccard index values were used to assess similarity between diseases and phenotypes within each level of analysis. Correlation between the levels was also assessed using the Spearman correlation method. High correlation was seen between the SNP and block data sets, while low correlation was seen between the pathway data and the other three levels of analysis. The progression from SNP to block, block to gene, and gene to pathway levels resulted in a grouping of susceptibility markers. Visualization of the associations by means of DRNs suggested the grouping translated to an increase in the strength of associations between diseases. This was also reflected in the distribution of Jaccard indexes for each level. Figure 1 shows a slight distribution shift to the right from SNP level to pathway level.

The DRNs suggested consistent association between several diseases for the SNP, block, and gene levels. The strongest associations seen for all populations were observed between (multiple sclerosis [MS], T1D, and RA), with noticeable association between (haematological traits [HT] and adult fetal hemoglobin levels [HBF]) and (serum low-density lipopolysaccharide cholesterol levels [SLCL] and lipid measurements [LM]). Several other less significant associations were suggested by the DRNs as well, but these associations were not consistent in significance for all populations. The qualitative assessments made by examining the DRNs were verified using PCA, which allowed for quantitative isolation of the strongest relationships. The PCA results matched the visual assessment for all levels, and suggested additional strong associations unique to specific populations were present. For example, an association between (LM and triglyceride levels [TG]) that was unique to the JPT population was suggested that was not outwardly apparent by visual inspection of the DRNs. This association was found in the CHB+JPT populations, but not the CHB population. JPT was also missing the (HBF and HT) association that was observed in the other populations. Further details regarding the results of this portion of the study were previously submitted for publication (Lewis et al., 2011).

Disease	platform	GEO record	Sample Size		MeSH category
			Disease	Control	
AD	GPL96	GSE1297	22	9	Nervous System Diseases [C10] Mental Disorders [F03]
ALS	GPL96 and 97	GSE3307	9	16	Nervous System Diseases [C10] Nutritional and Metabolic Diseases [C18]
BD	GPL96	GSE5388	30	31	Mental Disorders [F03]
BC	GPL96 and 97	GSE6883	6	3	Neoplasms [C04] Skin and Connective Tissue Diseases [C17]
CD	GPL96	GSE3365	59	42	Digestive System Diseases [C06]
IS	GPL96	GSE1869	6	10	Cardiovascular Diseases [C14]
OBE	GPL96	GSE474	16	8	Nutritional and Metabolic Diseases [C18]
PD	GPL96	GSE6613	50	22	Nervous System Diseases [C10]
PR	GPL96	GSE6710	13	13	Skin and Connective Tissue Diseases [C17]
SLE	GPL96 and 97	GSE11909	103	12	Skin and Connective Tissue Diseases [C17] Immune System Diseases [C20]
CAD	GPL96	GSE12288	110	120	Cardiovascular Diseases [C14]
T1D	GPL570	GSE10586	12	15	Nutritional and Metabolic Diseases [C18] Endocrine System Diseases [C19] Immune System Diseases [C20]
T2D	GPL96 and 97	GSE9006	12	24	Nutritional and Metabolic Diseases [C18] Endocrine System Diseases [C19]
CA	GPL570	GSE8052	268	136	Respiratory Tract Diseases [C08] Immune System Diseases [C20]
CC	GPL570	GSE9348	70	12	Neoplasms [C04] Digestive System Diseases [C06]
ND	GPL570	GSE11208	6	5	Disorders of Environmental Origin [C21] Mental Disorders [F03]
SP	GPL570	GSE4036	14	14	Mental Disorders [F03]
AF	GPL96 and 97	GSE2240	10	5	Cardiovascular Diseases [C14]
PSP	GPL96	GSE6613	6	22	Nervous System Diseases [C10] Eye Diseases [C11]

Table 2. List of nineteen diseases in gene expression analysis and their MeSH classification.

3.2 Clustering of genetic associations

Based on the observations made using the DRNs, agglomerative hierarchical clustering was used to find groups of diseases. At each level, the 61 diseases/phenotypes were clustered into ten groups. The number of clusters was set to ten based on visual inspection of the

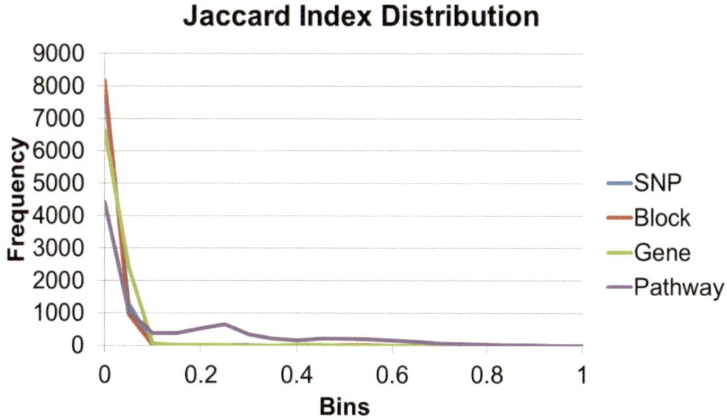

Fig. 1. Graphical representation of histogram data showing distribution of all Jaccard indexes for all populations at each level of analysis. Index values were grouped and then divided into twenty bins across the range zero to one. (N = 9150 for each analysis level)

hierarchical branching of the trees. Representative clustering results are shown for the CHB+JPT population in Figure 2. The CHB+JPT population showed a high correlation to most populations at all levels of analysis based on the Rand Index for similarity. The Rand Index for similarity was used to compare the clustering across populations at each level. The diseases within each cluster were least similar at the SNP level for all populations and most similar at the gene level across most of the populations. At the SNP level groupings, associations between (MS, RA, and T1D), (HBF and HT), and (breast cancer [BC] and sporadic post-menopausal breast cancer [SPBC]) were found for all populations (Figure 2A). The grouping of (RA and T1D), (BC and SPBC), (HBF and HT), (Amyotrophic Lateral Sclerosis [ALS] and Parkinson's disease [PD]) and (colorectal cancer [CC] and prostate cancer [PC]) were consistent at the block level for all populations (Figure 2B). At the gene level, the number of diseases/phenotypes included in each cluster increased with consistent groups again observed for all populations. These groups included (MS, RA, and T1D), (ALS, PD, CAD, Alzheimer's disease [AD] and T2D), and (neuroticism [NEU], brain aging [BA], and sleep and circadian phenotypes [SCP]) (Figure 2C). Clusters at the pathway level were also much larger than at the other levels. No consistent relationships were seen for the clusters containing a larger number of diseases, but the smaller groupings consistently showed relationships between (longevity and age-related phenotypes [LONG] and early onset extreme obesity [EO]), (cardiovascular disease outcomes [CVD], CD, and NEU) and (blood lipids [BL], LM, and Restless Leg Syndrome [RLS]) (Figure 2D). Four populations suggested clustering of (LONG, EO, and T1D), while one, YRI, showed a relationship between (LONG, EO, and SLCL).

3.3 Gene expression analysis

The gene expression profiles showed some patterns for the three expression categories (up-regulated, down-regulated, and combined), with the number of strong associations increasing with cutoff type (top 200 most changed genes, top 1000 most changed genes, and changes with a p-value less than 0.05). Jaccard indexes for each disease/phenotype pair were calculated and used to construct DRNs, which are shown in Figure 3. Strong associations between (PD, Progressive Supranuclear Palsy [PSP], and nicotine dependence

[ND]), (ischemic stroke [IS], CC, and CD), and (CAD and childhood asthma [CA]) were observed under all three cutoff scenarios for all three expression categories of analysis. Of these, the (CAD and CA) pair showed the most variation in association strength for all the variables considered.

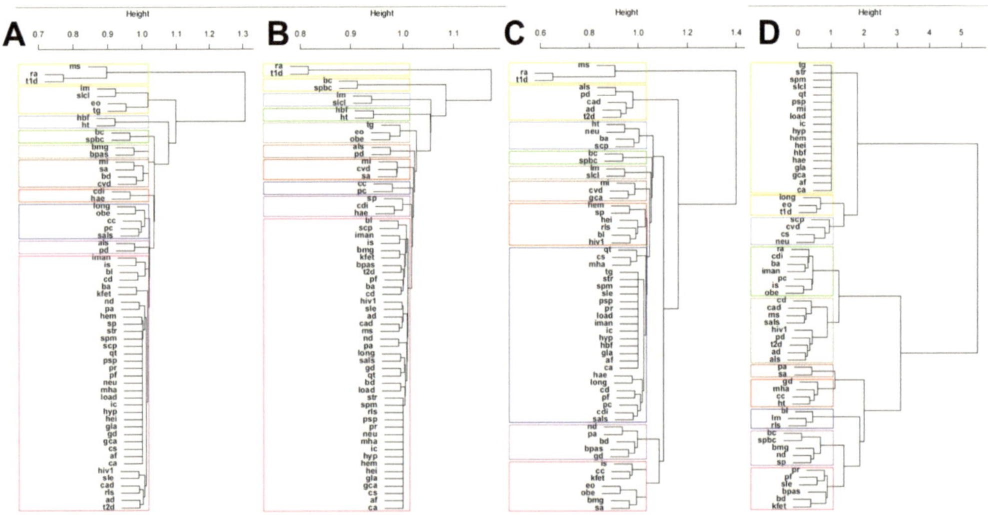

Fig. 2. Clustering dendrogram for 61 disease/phenotype comparisons at the (A) SNP, (B) block, (C) gene, and (D) pathway levels. Colored boxes indicate the clusters derived from Rand Index analysis. Results for the CHB+JPT population are shown as a representative data set for all populations.

Links between disease classifications were also seen. Connections between nervous system diseases and disorders of environmental origin (i.e., (PSP and ND) and (PD and ND)) were seen in all three expression categories and cutoff types. Associations between nervous system and mental disorders (e.g., AD and BD) were seen for the top 200 and top 1000 groups, but this association was masked in the *p*-value-derived group. For the p-value group, predominate associations between metabolic, cardiovascular, digestive, and immune system diseases were found. One unexpected classification association was the nervous system-metabolic disease link exemplified by (PSP and OBE) and (PD and OBE) for the down-regulation and subsequently combined expression groups with the top 1000 and p-value cutoffs.

As expected, the number of significant associations increased as the threshold criteria increased given that the quantity of data available for comparison was greater. Seemingly strong associations observed at the top 200 cutoff, such as the (AD and BD) and (BD and SP) associations were masked in the *p*-value cutoff data as other stronger associations were present. The increase in maximum Jaccard index for the combined expression data set from 0.44 to 0.81 agreed with this observation. Though we saw an increase in relationship strength with less stringent cutoff thresholds, the additional comparison data resulted in reduction in significant associations. Therefore, the expression categories for the *p*-value cutoff group were used to compare with the SNP-based data in order to avoid assigning an arbitrary cutoff for the expression data and to ensure enough data was available for the nineteen-disease comparison.

3.4 Comparison of the SNP and expression data for nineteen diseases

Correlation between data sets may have been influenced by the data sources. Both the SNP and block levels encompassed data from the HapMap site. The gene level data was obtained by cross referencing the HapMap data against the Ensembl database of gene names. The pathway data was obtained by cross referencing the Ensembl-derived data against the KEGG database. Given that the amount of data available through each of these sources is not consistent, there was loss of data in the transition from blocks to genes and genes to pathways. Of the reduced set of nineteen diseases and phenotypes compared, only atrial fibrillation/atrial flutter (AF) did not contain gene data for the SNP-based comparisons. The number of missing diseases/phenotypes increased to four at the pathway level (i.e., AF, CA, psoriasis [PR], and PSP). Despite the missing disease associations for AF, the gene level of analysis was used for comparison to the expression data. The range of Z-scores for this dataset was closest to the range seen for the expression data, and intuitively, the gene data should show some correlation to gene expression.

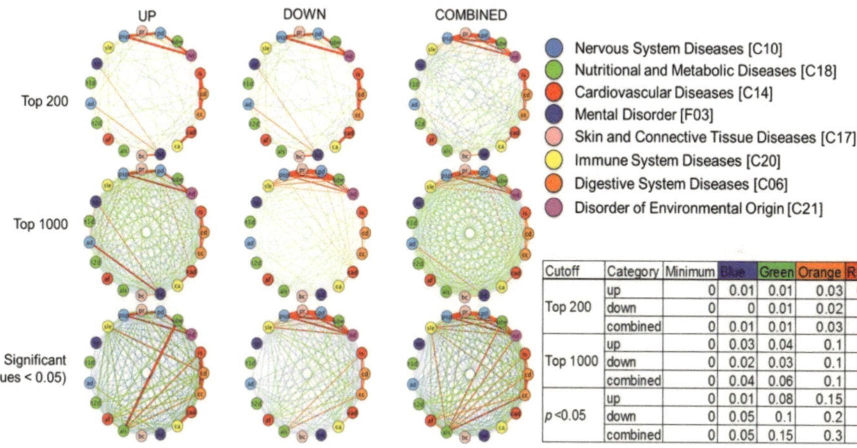

Cutoff	Category	Minimum	Blue	Green	Orange	Red	Maximum
Top 200	up	0	0.01	0.01	0.03	0.15	0.2
	down	0	0	0.01	0.02	0.1	0.87
	combined	0	0.01	0.01	0.03	0.2	0.44
Top 1000	up	0	0.03	0.04	0.1	0.2	0.38
	down	0	0.02	0.03	0.1	0.5	0.91
	combined	0	0.04	0.06	0.1	0.3	0.6
p <0.05	up	0	0.01	0.08	0.15	0.2	0.33
	down	0	0.05	0.1	0.2	0.5	0.74
	combined	0	0.05	0.15	0.3	0.5	0.81

Fig. 3. DRNs for expression data for the three cutoff levels (top 200, top 1000, and significance with p-value < 0.05) and three expression categories (up-regulated, down-regulated, and combined). Disease nodes are color coded to show grouping of diseases based on MeSH classification. Edges are color coded according to increasing strength of disease association. Values for the color scale are listed in the inserted table.

DRNs comparing the gene level of analysis for the CEU, CHB+JPT, and YRI populations to the expression data are shown in Figure 4. The JPT and CHB populations are not shown since the CHB+JPT population is highly representative of the individual populations. A Spearman correlation was calculated between each population for the SNP-based data set and the expression data (Table 3). A weak negative correlation was observed between the genetic and expression data, suggesting no significant relationships were shared between the two data sets. A qualitative analysis of the networks and clustering from the SNP-based data analysis suggested a high degree of similarity between the predicted associations for all population. However, the strong associations observed in the genetic analysis were not seen in the expression data. Rather, a seemingly reciprocal relationship appeared between the genetic and expression DRNs. The strongest expression-based association was between ALS and obesity-related traits (OBE), which was in the weakest associations group for the SNP-based associations. An examination of the genetic DRNs suggested the strongest associations between (ALS and PD), (AD and T2D), and (T1D and SLE). These associations were weak for the expression data. Some associations near the middle of the Z-score range appeared more common between the data sets, such as the (IS and CC), (AD and BD), and (OBE and CC) pairs.

61 diseases	CEU	CHB	JPT	CHB+JPT	YRI
CEU	1	0.9599	0.9595	0.9574	0.9447
CHB		1	0.9779	0.9925	0.9726
JPT			1	0.9858	0.9556
CHB+JPT				1	0.9686
YRI					1
19 diseases					
GEO	-0.1367	-0.1228	-0.1278	-0.1254	-0.1176

Table 3. Spearman correlation coefficients between populations and between each population and the GEO data. The Spearman correlation is a comparison of the ranked Z-scores for each data set.

Despite the overall lack of correlation between the genetic and expression analyses, several unexpected links between neurological and cardiovascular/metabolic diseases were observed in both data sets (i.e., (AD and T2D) and (PD and OBE)). These potentially novel disease relationships may primarily rely on genetic similarity or genomic expression similarity instead of phenotypic classification, but this idea would need to be further explored.

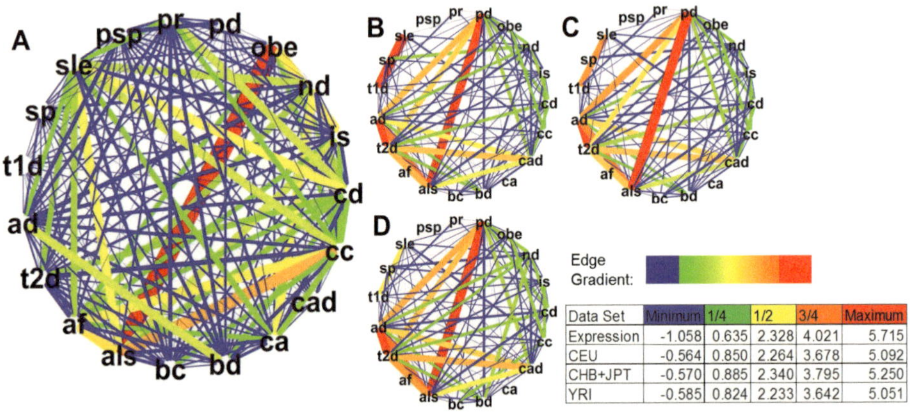

Fig. 4. DRNs based on Z-scores for three populations and expression data. DRNs for (A) combined expression data for significantly changed genes (p<0.05), (B) CEU gene level, (C) CHB+JPT gene level, and (D) YRI gene level are shown. Edge live color and width correspond to strength of association between disease pairs. The gradient and corresponding values are listed in the inserted table.

4. Discussion

The results from this study suggested it is possible to elucidate genetic similarities that can be overlooked during single disease GWAS. Several expected associations supported by literature were found (e.g. association between (SLE and RA) and (EO and SLCL)) while some unexpected associations were also observed. The unexpected neurological-cardiovascular/metabolic disease associations were observed for both the genetic analysis and the expression profile analysis. Though the origin and symptoms associated with diseases in each category may be different, the results suggest genetic similarities. Possible explanations for these associations cannot be elucidated solely from this study given the broad nature of the comparison. A detailed SNP-by-SNP and gene-by-gene examination may indicate the reason behind the neurological-cardiovascular/metabolic relatedness. Those relationships are particularly interesting and may indicate some common underlying molecular mechanism among these disease groups that has not yet been widely studied.

Clinical evidence supports the strongest relationships identified from the expression data. PSP and PD share some common symptoms such as stiffness, and movement difficulties which could explain the common expression pattern indicating some degree of relatedness between the two. On the other hand, explaining the relationship between PSP and ND is more difficult. Several studies have shown that smokers have a lower risk of developing Parkinson's disease (Soto-Otero et al., 1998; Hernan et al., 2001; Quik, 2004). One recently published paper showed that smoking for a greater number of years may reduce the risk of the disease (Chen et al., 2010). An earlier study suggested that younger patients with CD might be under an increased risk of IS (Andersohn et al., 2010). Extensive studies have demonstrated a strong association between CD and CC (Gillen et al., 1994). The relationship between (IS and CC) and (CAD and CA) is also unclear, but shared immune-dependent responses may be the common link.

Similarities and differences were observed between the three categories (up-regulated, down-regulated and combined) of gene expression analysis (see Figure 3). The different association patterns may be due to the use of a single rule to identify disease associated genes for all kinds of diseases, which over simplifies the problem. Theoretically, variance of gene expression can be considered as a quantitative trait inherited from genetic variation. It is possible that a combined DNA variant and expression phenotype can better explain genetic architecture with reduced environmental and biological noise (Dermitzakis, 2008). However, the precise and reliable estimation of molecular link between functional genomic effects and complex organism phenotypes depends on a large number of pooled variant and gene expression data from corresponding tissues or cell types, since tissue-specific differences can be found widely (Dermitzakis, 2008). A combined genetic and gene expression profile study, as presented here, can shed light on disease relatedness from different perspectives. Parikh et al. performed a more direct comparison of GWAS and expression data in an effort to prioritize T2D susceptibility genes (Parikh et al., 2009). The group isolated SNPs from GWAS, searched for associated genes, and then found corresponding tissue-specific expression profiles for a subset of all the SNP-associated genes (Parikh et al., 2009). Parikh et al. were able to identify five genes common to individuals with T2D and twelve genes with differentiating expression patterns in individuals with versus without the disease (Parikh et al., 2009). Rather than focusing on a single disease to identify targets, we strove for a more global comparison of genetic and expression data.

Even though discrepancies between our data sets were observed, it is possible that the reduction in data between the gene and pathway level could have excluded some genes common to multiple diseases. With the increased density of GWAS and gene expression studies, the discrepancies and anomalies observed in this study might be better understood. We set out to support the idea that diseases potentially share phenotype similarity as a result of genetic factors, pathway associations, expression regulation, or some combination of these three ideas. Within the autoimmune disease group, we observed diseases that possessed some genetic similarity. We saw expected strong associations between T1D, MS, and RA, as well as less expected associations between AD and T2D. It would appear that systemic inflammation responses may be the key to shared susceptibility among many of the diseases and phenotypes for which we observed relatedness. Clinical studies suggested individuals with one immune-mediated disease, such as T1D, may be more susceptible to pathogenesis of another (Dorman et al., 2003; Nielson et al., 2006; Toussirot et al., 2006; Doran, 2007). It has also been clinically suggested that inflammation plays a role in neurological diseases like AD (Akiyama et al., 2000; Perry, 2004) and PD (Perry, 2004). We also know that cardiovascular and metabolic diseases, such as atherosclerosis, T2D, and OBE have links to chronic inflammatory responses (Stienstra et al., 2006; Tontonoz&Spiegelman, 2008). In all of these cases, our results suggest the clinical manifestations may have genetic relevance and the unexpected cardiovascular/neurological links may be important. Given the broad scope of this study, the conclusions made here are suggestions for where genetic commonality could be found without specific identification of the related targets. A more detailed disease-by-disease analysis similar to the study conducted by Parikh et al. (Parikh et al., 2009) would need to be conducted to identify specific genes of interest shared by diseases. The methods used in the Parikh et al. study can be specifically applied to the study of T1D by performing a detailed step-by-step comparison between this disease and other possibly related diseases in order to elucidate genetic commonalities to T1D. The results from our study and from one tailored specifically for T1D could influence current treatment options and suggest new approaches for managing and treating the disease. We feel our study is a strong example of how GWAS and expression data can be used conjunctively to predict significant disease associations relevant to improving and unifying diagnoses and treatment options for multiple immune-mediated diseases.

5. Acknowledgements

The authors would like to acknowledge the faculty and students of the Spring 2010 Genetics, Bioinformatics, and Computational Biology Problem Solving course for feedback regarding the progress of this study.

6. References

Akiyama, H., S. Barger, et al. (2000). "Inflammation and Alzheimer's." Neurobiology of Aging 21(3): 383-421.

Andersohn, F., M. Waring, et al. (2010). "Risk of ischemic stroke in patients with Crohn's disease: A population-based nested case-control study." Inflammatory Bowel Disease 16(8): 1387-1392.

Barrett, T., D. Troup, et al. (2009). "NCBI GEO: archive for high-throughput functional genomic data." Nucleic Acids Research 37: D885-D890.

Birney, E., T. D. Andrews, et al. (2004). "An overview of Ensembl." Genome Research 14(5): 925-928.

Bodenreider, O., S. Nelson, et al. (1998). Beyond synonymy: exploiting the UMLS semantics in mapping vocabularies. Annual Symposium of the American Medical Informatics Association, Orlando, FL, Hanley & Belfus, Inc.

Chen, H., X. Huang, et al. (2010). "Smoking, duration, intensity, and risk of Parkinson disease." Neurology 74(11): 878-884.

Chen, R., L. Li, et al. (2007). "AILUN: reannotating gene expression data automatically." Nature Methods 4(11): 879.

Chen, Y., J. Zhu, et al. (2008). "Variations in DNA elucidate molecular networks that cause disease." Nature 452(7186): 429-435.

Dermitzakis, E. T. (2008). "From gene expression to disease risk." Nature genetics 40(5): 492-493.

Doran, M. (2007). "Rheumatoid arthritis and diabetes mellitus: evidence for an association?" The Journal of Rhematology 34(3): 460-462.

Dorman, J. S., A. R. Steenkiste, et al. (2003). "Type 1 Diabetes and Multiple Sclerosis." Diabetes Care 26(11): 3192-3193.

Eden, E., D. Lipson, et al. (2007). "Discovering Motifs in Ranked Lists of DNA Sequences." PLoS Computational Biology 3(3): e39.

Eden, E., R. Navon, et al. (2009). "GOrilla: A Tool for Discovery and Visualization of Enriched GO Terms in Ranked Gene Lists." BMC Bioinformatics 10: 48.

Emilsson, V., G. Thorleifsson, et al. (2008). "Genetics of gene expression and its effect on disease." Nature 452(7186): 423-428.

Gillen, C. D., H. A. Andrews, et al. (1994). "Crohn's disease and colorectal cancer." Gut 35(5): 651-655.

Goring, H. H. H., J. E. Curran, et al. (2007). "Discovery of expression QTLs using large-scale transcriptional profiling in human lymphocytes." Nature Genetics 39: 1208-1216.

Hernan, M. A., S. M. Zhang, et al. (2001). "Cigarette Smoking and the Incidence of Parkinson's Disease in Two Prospective Studies." Annals of Neurology 50(6): 780-786.

Hindorff, L. A., P. Sethupathy, et al. (2009). "Potential etiologic and functional implications of genome-wide association loci for human diseases and traits." PNAS 106(23): 9362-9367.

Hu, G. and P. Agarwal. (2009). "Human disease-drug network based on genomic expression profiles." PLoS One 4(8): e6536.

Huang, W., P. Wang, et al. (2009). "Indentifying disease associations via genome-wide association studies." BMC Bioinformatics 10: 1-11.

Johnson, A. D. and C. J. O'Donnell (2009). "An Open Access Database of Genome-wide Association Results." BMC Medical Genetics 10: 1-6.

Kanehisa, M. and S. Goto (2000). "KEGG: Kyoto Encyclopedia of Genes and Genomes." Nucleic Acids Research 28(27-30).

Kanehisa, M., S. Goto, et al. (2010). "KEGG for representation and analysis of molecular networks involving diseases and drugs." Nucleic Acids Research 38: D355-D360.

Kanehisa, M., S. Goto, et al. (2006). "From genomics to chemical genomics: new developments in KEGG." Nucleic Acids Research 34: D354-D357.

Lettre, G. and J. D. Rioux (2008). "Autoimmune diseases: insights from genome-wide assocation studies." Human Molecular Genetics 17(2): R116-R121.

Lewis, S. N., E. Nsoesie, et al. (2011). "Prediction of Disease and Phenotype Associations from Genome-Wide Association Studies." PLoS One Submitted for Review.

McCarthy, M. I., G. R. Abecasis, et al. (2008). "Genome-wide Association Studies for Complex Traits: Consensus, Uncertainty and Challenges." Nature 9: 356-369.

Moffatt, M. F., M. Kabesch, et al. (2007). "Genetic variants regulating ORMDL3 expression contribute to the risk of childhood asthma." Nature 448(7152): 470-473.

Nielson, N. M., T. Westergaard, et al. (2006). "Type 1 Diabetes and Multiple Sclerosis: A Danish Population-Based Cohort Study." Archives of Neurology 63(7): 1001-1004.

Parikh, H., V. Lyssenko, et al. (2009). "Prioritizing genes for follow-up from genome wise assocation studies using information on gene expression in tissues relevant for type 2 diabetes mellitus." BMC Medical Genetics 2(72).

Perry, V. H. (2004). "The influence of systemic inflammation on inflammation in the brain: implications for chronic neurodegenerative disease." Brain, Behavior, and Immunity 18(5): 407-413.

Quik, M. (2004). "Smoking, nicotine and Parkinson's disease." Trends in Neurosciences 27(9): 561-568.

Soto-Otero, R., E. Mendez-Alvarez, et al. (1998). "Studies on the interaction between 1,2,3,4-tetrahydro-B-carboline and cigarette smoke: a potential mechanism of neuroprotection for Parkinson's disease." Brain Research 802(1-2): 155-162.

Stienstra, R., C. Duval, et al. (2006). "PPARs, Obesity, and Inflammation." PPAR Research 2007: 1-10.

Suthram, S., J. T. Dudley, et al. (2010). "Network-Based Elucidation of Human Disease Similarities Reveals Common Functional Modules Enriched for Pluripotent Drug Targets." PLoS Computational Biology 6(2): 1-10.

The International HapMap Consortium (2005). "A Haplotype Map of the Human Genome." Nature 437(7063): 1299-1320.

The International HapMap Consortium (2007). "A second generation human haplotype map of over 3.1 million SNPs." Nature 449: 851-861.

The Wellcome Trust Case Control Consortium (2007). "Genome-wide association study of 14,000 cases of seven common diseases and 3,000 shared controls." Nature 447: 661-678.

Tontonoz, P. and B. M. Spiegelman (2008). "Fat and Beyond: The Diverse Biology of PPARγ." Annual Review of Biochemistry 77: 289-312.

Toussirot, E., E. Pertuiset, et al. (2006). "Association of Rheumatoid Arthritis with Multiple Sclerosis: Report of 14 Cases and Discussion of Its Significance." The Journal of Rhematology: Correspondence 33(5): 1027-1028.

Wang, L., P. Jia, et al. (2011). "An efficient hierarchical generalized linear mixed model for pathway analysis of genome-wide assocation studies." Bioinformatics 27(5): 686-692.

Wang, W. Y. S., B. J. Barratt, et al. (2005). "Genome-Wide Association Studies: Theoretical and Practical Concerns." Nature Reviews Genetics 6: 109-118.

Xavier, R. J. and J. D. Rioux (2008). "Genome-wide association studies: a new window into immune-mediated diseases." Nature Reviews Immunology 8: 631-643.

12

Cytokine-Induced β-Cell Stress and Death in Type 1 Diabetes Mellitus

Lisa Vincenz[1], Eva Szegezdi[1], Richard Jäger[1],
Caitriona Holohan[1], Timothy O'Brien[2] and Afshin Samali[1]
[1]*Apoptosis Research Centre*
[2]*Regenerative Medicine Institute,*
National University of Ireland Galway
Ireland

1. Introduction

1.1 Pathophysiology of type I diabetes mellitus: Role of pro-inflammatory cytokines

Type 1 diabetes mellitus (T1DM) is an autoimmune disease characterised by the destruction of insulin-producing β-cells in the pancreatic islets of Langerhans (Fig.1), which is mediated by autoreactive T cells, macrophages and pro-inflammatory cytokines (Fig.2). This leads to an inability to produce sufficient insulin resulting in elevated blood glucose levels and pathological effects (Eizirik & Mandrup-Poulsen, 2001).

T1DM is believed to be initiated by physiological β-cell death or islet injury triggering the homing of macrophages and dendritic cells that in turn launch an inflammatory reaction. The infiltrating macrophages secrete pro-inflammatory cytokines, namely interleukin-1β (IL-1β) and tumour necrosis factor α (TNFα) as well as various chemokines that attract immune cells such as dendritic cells, macrophages and T lymphocytes. T cells recognising β-cell-specific antigens become activated, infiltrate the inflamed islets and attack the β-cells (Baekkeskov et al., 1990, Elias et al., 1995, Lieberman et al., 2003, Nakayama et al., 2005). In a normally functioning immune system, T cells with a high affinity for self-antigens are eliminated during their differentiation resulting in immune 'tolerance'. Autoreactive cells that have escaped these mechanisms are subject to 'peripheral immune regulation' that blocks their activation and clonal expansion, preventing development of an autoimmune disease (Mathis & Benoist, 2004). For reasons we do not fully understand, these immune regulatory mechanisms either fail to launch, or are ineffective in stopping the immune attack against the β-cells in T1DM, and a positive feedback cycle is established (Mathis & Benoist, 2004). This forward-feeding process of T cell- and cytokine-mediated β-cell killing can be ongoing for years progressively destroying the β-cells. When over 80 % of the β-cells are deleted by this continuous T lymphocyte and inflammatory cytokine-driven attack the insulin secretory capacity falls below a certain threshold and the disease manifests itself.

Activated T cells induce death of a target cell by (1) secreting perforin and granzymes, (2) releasing pro-inflammatory cytokines including interferon-γ (IFNγ) and TNFα or (3) activation of Fas receptors on the surface of target cells. All these factors have also been described to contribute to β-cell killing in T1DM (Kägi et al., 1997, D. Liu et al., 2000, Petrovsky et al., 2002, Suk et al., 2001). In particular, recent evidence suggests that the

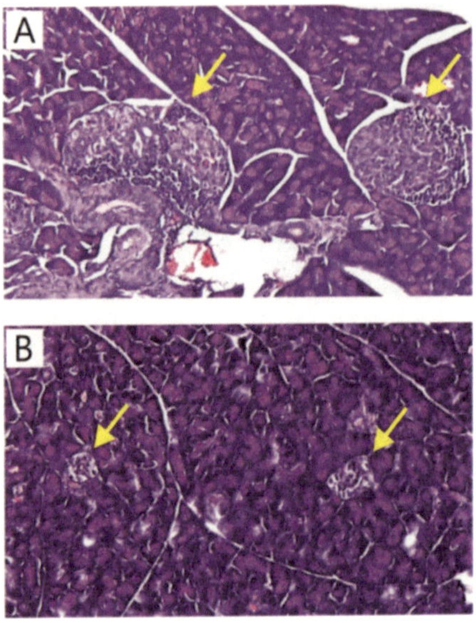

Fig. 1. β-cell islets in the pancreas of (A) pre-diabetic and (B) diabetic NOD mice. The yellow arrows indicate the islets in the haematoxylin-eosin stained tissue section (original magnification 200X).

cytokines IL-1β, TNFα and IFNγ that are secreted by macrophages and T cells have a broader role in the development of T1DM than previously thought. They are the main inducers of β-cell stress responsible for significant levels of β-cell death in both rodent (Iwahashi et al., 1996, Rabinovitch et al., 1994) and human (Delaney et al., 1997) experimental models of T1DM.

Underlining the importance of the cytokines, it has been shown that neutralisation of the pro-inflammatory cytokines by antibodies and/or soluble cytokine receptors against IL-1β, IFNγ, IL-6 and TNFα can inhibit the development of T1DM in NOD mice or BB rats (Mandrup-Poulsen, 1996). Transgenic mice expressing IFNγ in β-cells develop severe insulitis (pre-diabetes) and destruction of β-cells. Treatment of these mice with anti-IFNγ antibody prevents the development of T1DM. IFNγ-deficient mice as well as mice injected with neutralising anti-IFNγ receptor antibodies were resistant to development of experimentally-induced T1DM (Cailleau et al., 1997, Seewaldt et al., 2000, B. Wang et al., 1997). Similar to IFNγ, genetic or pharmacological abrogation of IL-1β action also reduces disease development in animal models of T1DM (Mandrup-Poulsen et al., 2010).

Although many factors contribute to β–cell destruction during T1DM, in this book chapter we review current knowledge regarding the role of cytokines mediating β–cell stress and death in T1DM.

1.2 Signal transduction of pro-inflammatory cytokines in β-cells

IL-1β, IFNγ and TNFα exert a variety of effects on β-cells. They sensitise β-cells to apoptosis by increasing the expression of pro-apoptotic proteins, such as the Fas receptor (Stassi et al., 1997). They drive and stabilise the autoimmune response by triggering the secretion of chemokines (e.g. CXCL9 and CXCL10) by β-cells (Frigerio et al., 2002), which results in constant recruitment of autoreactive T cells. Finally, pro-inflammatory cytokines directly

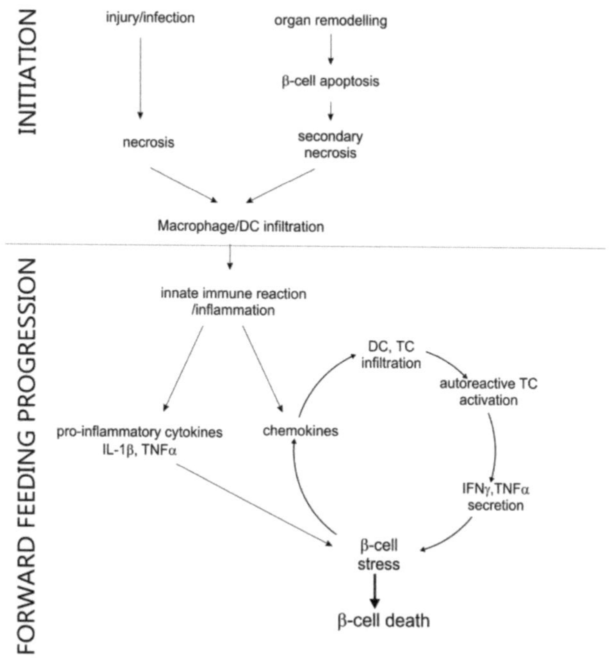

Fig. 2. Cytokine-induced β-cell death. Initial β-cell death caused by injury, infection or physiologically during development can activate an autoimmune response that leads to activation and infiltration of cytokine-secreting macrophages, dendritic cells (DC) and T cells (TC). Pro-inflammatory cytokines IL-1β, TNFα and IFNγ secreted by macrophages and TCs cause β-cell stress and death and secretion of chemokines that further stimulate autoimmune cell infiltration.

cause stress in β-cells which eventually activates the cell's death machinery. The signal transduction pathways activated by these pro-inflammatory cytokines leading to chemokine secretion, β-cell stress and death are detailed below (also see Fig. 3).

It is very important to note that any of the above pro-inflammatory cytokines alone has limited effects in terms of cell stress or death, on β-cells. However, combinations of IL-1β/IFNγ or TNFα/IFNγ have very strong, synergistic effects that trigger serious levels of stress culminating in cell death.

1.2.1 IL-1β signalling

The main mediator of IL-1β signalling is the transcription factor nuclear factor kappa B (NF-κB) (Flodström et al., 1996, Kwon et al., 1995). The pathway by which IL-1β activates NF-κB has been delineated in a number of cell types and experimental models (Fig.3). It is thought that the same mechanisms are involved in pancreatic β-cells. IL-1β, secreted by activated macrophages and T cells, binds to the IL-1 receptor 1 (IL-1R1) on the surface of target cells. IL-1R1 then recruits IL-1 receptor accessory protein (IL-1RAcP) (Dinarello, 1997). This allows binding of the adaptor protein myeloid differentiation factor 88 (MyD88) and recruitment of IL-1R1 activated kinase 1 (IRAK1) and/or IRAK2 (Burns et al., 1998, Muzio et al., 1997, Wesche et al., 1997). IRAK proteins are in complex with a protein named Tollip prior to recruitment to the receptor (Burns et al., 2000). Tollip associates with IL-1RacP when the IRAK/Tollip complex is recruited to the activated receptor. TNF-receptor-associated

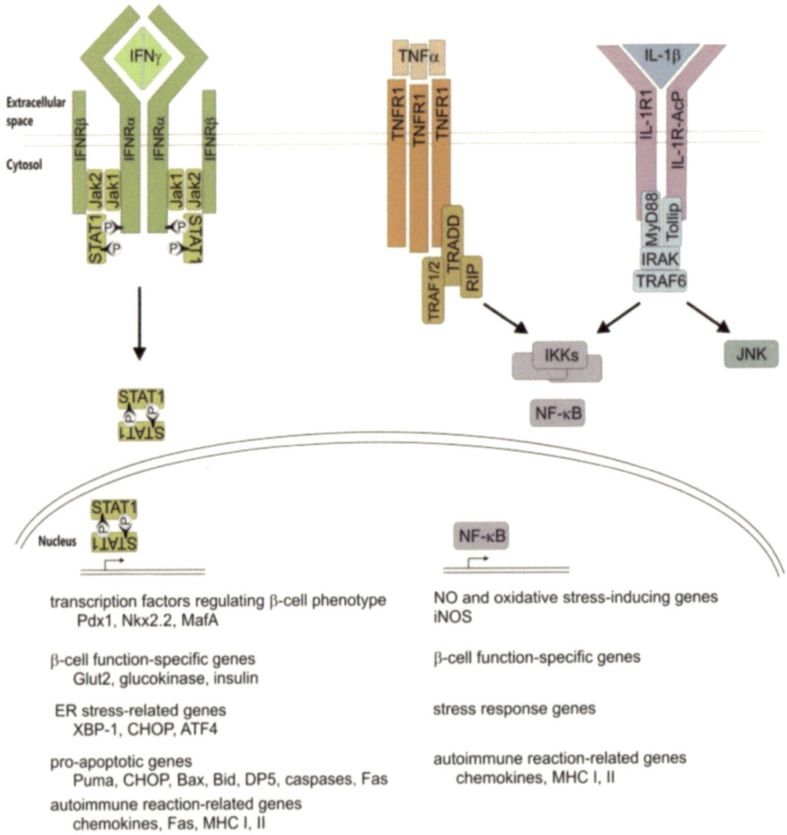

Fig. 3. Cytokine-signalling in pancreatic β-cells. IL-1β, TNFα and IFNγ activate receptors on the surface of β-cells inducing a signalling cascade leading to the activation of transcription factors STAT1 and NF-κB that control numerous genes involved in β-cell function, inflammation, stress responses and apoptosis.

factor-6 (TRAF6) is recruited to IRAK1 and IRAK2 (Muzio et al., 1997, Yamin & Miller, 1997) leading to the activation of inhibitor of NF-κB (IκB) kinase (IKK) *via* NF-κB inducing kinase (NIK). IKK then phosphorylates IκB which triggers its degradation and the release of the transcription factor NF-κB from the inhibitory interaction.

In addition, phosphatidyl inositol-3 kinase (PI3K) is recruited to the activated IL1-R1 complex where it becomes activated (Reddy et al., 1997, Reddy et al., 2004). PI3K activity is required, but not sufficient for NF-κB activation (Reddy et al., 1997).

NF-κB can regulate the transcription of numerous target genes (for review see (Pahl, 1999)). The target genes include cytokines (e.g. IL-1β, TNFα, IFNγ), chemokines, immunoreceptors, proteins involved in antigen presentation, cell adhesion molecules, stress response genes, regulators of apoptosis (both pro- and anti-apoptotic), growth factors and other transcription factors. The effects of NF-κB signalling are highly cell type-specific. In most cell types the net effect of NF-κB activation is to promote cell survival. In contrast, in β-cells NF-κB activation has a pro-apoptotic effect (Eldor et al., 2006, Ortis et al., 2008). These studies demonstrate that inhibition of NF-κB protects rodent pancreatic β-cells from the damaging effects of cytokine-exposure *in vitro* and prevents streptozocin-induced diabetes *in vivo*.

A large number of NF-κB target genes were identified using DNA microarray technology in cytokine-treated primary rat β-cells (Cardozo et al., 2001a). Cytokines induced NF-κB-dependent up-regulation of genes involved in stress responses (including CHOP, C/EBPβ and δ, Hsp27 and MnSOD), immune responses (e.g. MHC-II-associated invariant chain γ and MHC-I) and down-regulation of genes involved in β-cell function (glucose transporter-2 (Glut-2)), insulin production (Isl-1), insulin processing (PC-1), insulin release (PLD-1, CCKA-receptor) and Ca^{2+} homeostasis (SERCA2, IP 3-kinase) (Cardozo et al., 2001a).
Inducible nitric oxide synthase (iNOS) is strongly induced and is the best characterised NF-κB target in both rat β-cells (Cardozo et al., 2001a, Kutlu et al., 2003) and human pancreatic islets (Flodström et al., 1996). Induction of iNOS increases nitric oxide (NO) production in β-cells, resulting in the generation of reactive oxygen species (ROS) and oxidative stress. The cellular stress triggered by NO in rodent and human cells will be discussed later in this chapter (under section 2.2).
In addition to NF-κB, IL-1β signalling also activates the mitogen activated protein kinase (MAPK) extracellular signal-regulated kinase (ERK) 1/2 and induces suppressor of cytokine signalling-3 (SOCS-3) (Emanuelli et al., 2004). Signal transduction pathways induced by MAPKs and SOCS-3 are interlinked with the NF-κB-regulated pathways; MAPK activation potentiates IL-1β-dependent NF-κB activation and subsequent iNOS induction, and (ERK)1/2 activation was shown to contribute to cytokine-induced apoptosis in rat pancreatic β-cells (Pavlovic et al., 2000). While MAPKs positively affect NF-κB signalling and enhance β-cell death, SOCS-3 has a negative effect. SOCS-3 belongs to a family of proteins that provide a negative feedback for cytokine-induced signalling. It was also identified as an inhibitor of insulin signalling (Emanuelli et al., 2000) as SOCS-3 can bind to the insulin receptor and block its insulin-induced autophosphorylation and activation (Emanuelli et al., 2004). SOCS-3 inhibits IL-1β signalling upstream and thus negatively regulates nearly all effects of IL-1β. SOCS-3 suppresses the expression of several IL-1β-induced pro-apoptotic genes, many of them known to be NF-κB-dependent (Karlsen et al., 2004) and protects rat β-cells from IL-1β- and TNFα-induced cell death (Bruun et al., 2009).
As mentioned above, over 200 genes have been identified to be NF-κB-regulated in β-cells treated with pro-inflammatory cytokines. However, which of these genes are targets of IL-1β signalling, or to what extent their expression is regulated by IL-1β alone is currently unknown. Determining the individual targets of the cytokines would lead to a better understanding of how the cytokines synergise to cause β-cell stress and death.

1.2.2 TNFα signalling

TNFα was also shown to lead to activation of NF-κB in pancreatic β-cells (Ortis et al., 2006). TNFα binds to and activates the TNF receptor (TNFR1), which is present on the surface of β-cells (Kägi et al., 1999). TNFα binding to TNFR1 leads to the latter's trimerisation and activation (Fig. 3). Upon activation, the cytosolic death domain of TNFR1 recruits TNF receptor-associated death domain (TRADD) (Hsu et al., 1995), TRAF2 (Hsu et al., 1996b) and the death domain kinase receptor interacting protein (RIP) (Hsu et al., 1996a). TRAF2, in turn, recruits IκB kinase (IKK) and induces its activation in a RIP-dependent manner via activation of an IKK kinase (e.g. NIK) (Devin et al., 2000). Activated IKK phosphorylates IκB proteins leading to their proteasomal degradation and release of NF-κB. The activation of NF-κB by both TNFα and IL-1β has a pro-apoptotic effect in rat pancreatic β-cells (Ortis et al., 2008). This effect was more pronounced in response to IL-1β than TNFα.

TNFα signalling can lead to RIP-dependent activation of three MAPKs (c-Jun N-terminal kinase JNK, p38 and ERK) in a cell type-specific manner (Devin et al., 2003). In rat pancreatic β-cells, TNFα treatment induced activation of JNK and p38 which has been suggested to contribute to an inhibitory effect of TNFα on glucose-stimulated insulin secretion (H.-E. Kim et al., 2008) and hence β-cell dysfunction in response to TNFα.

1.2.3 IFNγ signalling

IFNγ is a homodimeric cytokine. It binds to two IFNγ receptor α (IFNγRα) chains (Fig. 3). A third unit of IFNγRα and two molecules of IFNγ receptor β (IFNγRβ, also termed accessory factor 1, AF-1) bind to the IFNγRα (Thiel et al., 2000). This leads to the activation and transphosphorylation of Janus tyrosine kinase 1 and 2 (JAK1 and JAK2) which are associated with IFNγRα and IFNγRβ, respectively, and are brought together upon receptor oligomerisation (Igarashi et al., 1994, Kotenko et al., 1995). JAK1 and JAK2 phosphorylate IFNγR leading to the recruitment of two molecules of the transcription factor, signal transducer and activator of transcription-1 (STAT-1). After phosphorylation and activation by JAK2, STAT-1 homodimerises and translocates to the nucleus where it stimulates the expression of target genes (Takeda & Akira, 2000). Islet cells isolated from STAT-1$^{-/-}$ non-obese diabetic (NOD) mice were resistant to apoptosis induced by combined treatment with IFNγ and TNFα or IFNγ and IL-1β (S. Kim et al., 2007). In support of this, blockade of STAT-1 protected against diabetes induced by injection of multiple low doses of streptozotocin in mice (Callewaert et al., 2007, C.A. Gysemans et al., 2005). A recent gene expression analysis showed that nearly two thousand genes are regulated by STAT-1 in response to cytokine exposure (IL-1β and IFNγ) in β-cells (Moore et al., 2011). STAT-1 was found to regulate the IL-1β/IFNγ-mediated induction of chemokines, including CXCL9, CXCL10, CXCL11 and CCL20 (Moore et al., 2011) and islets from STAT-1$^{-/-}$ mice have decreased production of CXCL10 upon cytokine exposure both *in vitro* and *in vivo* (C.A. Gysemans et al., 2005).

STAT-1 also down-regulates several genes specific to β-cell functions, such as insulin, glucokinase, Glut2, prohormone convertases, as well as many transcription factors involved in the differentiation and maintenance of β-cell phenotype (e.g. Pdx1, MafA, Nkx2.2) (Moore et al., 2011, Perez-Arana et al., 2010).

Finally, STAT-1 is an important regulator of genes mediating intracellular stress and apoptotic pathways. Several apoptosis-related genes such as Puma, CHOP, Bax, Bid, caspase-3, -4, -7, DP5/Hrk and endoplasmic reticulum stress-transducing genes (XBP1, ATF4) are regulated by STAT-1 (Eizirik & Darville, 2001, Moore et al., 2011, Anastasis Stephanou et al., 2000). IFNγ has been found to profoundly accelerate IL-1β-mediated iNOS induction and thus cause oxidative stress. We have demonstrated that treatment of a rat insulinoma cell line (RIN-r) with a combination of IL-1β and IFNγ induces the mitochondrial apoptotic pathway in an iNOS-dependent manner (Holohan et al., 2008). This is in line with reports from other groups (Gurzov et al., 2009).

The inflammatory effects of IFNγ are controlled by negative feedback regulation, exerted by interferon regulated factor-1 (IRF-1) (Moore et al., 2011) and SOCS-1 and -3 (Alexander, 2002). IRF-1 is likely to exert its STAT-1 regulatory role by up-regulation of SOCS-1 (Moore et al., 2011). IRF-1 expression reduces chemokine expression in β-cells and resulting T cell infiltration in Langerhans islets (C. Gysemans et al., 2008, Moore et al., 2011), however the effect of IRF-1 on STAT-1-mediated β-cell de-differentiation (loss of β-cell function) and β-cell stress is minor (Moore et al., 2011). In line with this, transgenic expression of SOCS-1 in β-cells reduced diabetes development in non-obese diabetic (NOD) mice (Flodström-

Tullberg et al., 2003) and protected β-cells against infiltrating autoreactive T cells (Chong et al., 2004). In summary, the effect of IFNγ in β-cells is primarily mediated by STAT-1 through which IFNγ controls key processes culminating in loss of β-cell function, stress and finally death. IFNγ regulates a number of genes that increase the sensitivity of β-cells to apoptotic stimuli and intracellular stress.

2. Cytokine-induced β-cell death

2.1 Mechanisms of cytokine-induced β-cell death

During the development of T1DM, there are two waves of β-cell death. It is believed that β-cell death is the initial trigger for the autoimmune attack. While autoimmune attack was thought to be initiated by cytolytic activity or immune-stimulation of viruses (Jun & Yoon, 2003), it is also possible that physiological β-cell death might be a trigger. Instead of an exogenous impact, or environmental effect, induction of diabetes might be initiated during physiological tissue remodelling of the pancreas peaking at age 2-3 weeks in rodents. At this time, an increased level of β-cell death occurs in the islets and might be the primary trigger of the autoimmune attack (Turley et al., 2003). Programmed cell death associated with normal tissue remodelling does not induce inflammation. However, if the dead cells are not removed promptly by phagocytosis they can disintegrate and release cellular contents in a manner similar to pathological tissue damage which can trigger inflammation. In fact, accumulation of dead cells has been noticed in NOD mice and similarly, disintegrating, so called secondary necrotic cells were sufficient to induce inflammation, macrophage infiltration and pre-diabetic insulitis in NOD mice (H.S. Kim et al., 2007).

The second wave of β-cell death is driven by the autoimmune reaction. This is an ongoing process gradually killing the β-cells and culminating in the disease phenotype. The mechanism of β-cell death induced by the autoreactive leukocytes has been extensively examined with consensus that the major form of β-cell death is apoptosis, however, under certain conditions and especially in rodent experimental models of T1DM, necrotic β-cell death can also contribute to β-cell loss.

Apoptosis is a physiological form of cell death involved in the elimination of cells that have served their function, are no longer needed or are damaged. It is an active, highly ordered and rapid process characterised by the detachment of the dying cell from its neighbours, cell shrinkage, condensation of chromatin, fragmentation of the nucleus and finally fragmentation of the cell into membrane bound particles, called apoptotic bodies which are engulfed by neighbouring cells or professional phagocytic cells (Samali et al., 1996). By this means, cells are eliminated without leakage of otherwise inflammatory cellular material.

The morphological changes typical of apoptosis are orchestrated by the caspase family of proteases (Samali et al., 1999). Caspases are activated by two distinct mechanisms. The extrinsic pathway is triggered by an extracellular pro-apoptotic stimulus, usually a cytokine that belongs to the death ligand subfamily of the TNF superfamily. Upon engagement of the death ligand with its cognate death receptor on the cell surface of the target cell, the receptors trimerise and induce the formation of a protein complex, called the death-inducing signalling complex (DISC). The DISC is an activation platform for caspases-8 and/or -10 (Peter & Krammer, 2003). Once these initiator caspases are activated they activate downstream effector caspases, which leads to a burst of caspase activity and subsequent proteolysis that dismantles the cells.

The second, so called intrinsic pathway is initiated at the level of mitochondria. Upon intracellular stress these organelles release cytochrome *c* that associates with the adaptor protein APAF-1 to build a multimeric cytoplasmic protein complex termed the apoptosome, which functions to activate another initiator caspase, caspase-9 (Riedl & Salvesen, 2007). Mitochondrial release of cytochrome *c*, and thus activation of the intrinsic apoptosis pathway, is controlled by members of the Bcl-2 family of proteins (see section 2.3). Once cytochrome *c* is released and caspase-9 is activated, the same caspase cascade is triggered as during the extrinsic apoptotic pathway that leads to the final demise of the cell.

Interestingly, TNFα was shown to induce expression of an endogenous caspase inhibitor in β-cells that prevents apoptosis, the X-linked inhibitor of apoptosis protein (XIAP). This NF-kB-mediated induction of XIAP is inhibited by IFNγ signalling, providing a mechanism for synergistic cytoxicity of TNFα and IFNγ in β-cells (H.S. Kim et al., 2005).

Apoptosis is distinguished from **necrosis**, a pathological, mostly uncontrolled mode of cell death. During necrosis cells swell, their membranes disintegrate and their content is released, inducing inflammation. Recently, an active mode of necrosis, termed necroptosis, has been described that can be induced upon activation of TNFR1 when caspase-8 activation is blocked (Vandenabeele et al., 2010). A possible role of necroptosis in initiation of diabetes seems worthy of further investigation in light of the known involvement of TNFR1 signalling in diabetes and of a recent study that provided evidence of necrotic β-cell death playing a role in initiating autoimmune-type diabetes (Steer et al., 2006).

2.2 The role of nitric oxide in cytokine-mediated β-cell loss

It is thought that cytokine-induced β-cell stress and death is partly caused by intracellular production of ROS and NO. NO is a gaseous hydrophobic signalling molecule that readily diffuses through membranes and plays an essential role in various neurological, immunological and cardiovascular processes. The biosynthesis of NO is catalysed by nitric oxide synthases (NOS). In β-cells IL-1β signals up-regulation of iNOS and subsequent generation of NO. The main physiological effect of NO is mediated via the direct activation of guanylyl cyclase by NO leading to production of cyclic GMP (cGMP) and activation of cGMP-dependent signal transduction pathways. However, if present for a prolonged period or in high quantities, NO can nitrosylate specific cysteine residues of various proteins (S-nitrosylation) forming nitrosothiols and thereby affect the protein's activity, stability and localisation (Hess et al., 2005). In most cases this leads to rapid degradation of the nitrosylated proteins but a small subgroup of proteins have been shown to gain stability after nitrosylation (Paige et al., 2008). NO can have anti-apoptotic and cytoprotective effects in some cell types (McCabe et al., 2006), but can become toxic if present at high levels due to formation of ROS and protein nitrosylation which, amongst other things, also causes mitochondrial damage.

It has been shown that NO can induce both necrotic and apoptotic cell death (Bonfoco et al., 1995). With respect to β-cell destruction, it has been shown that endogenous levels of NO are sufficient to induce β-cell injury in rodent models of T1DM (Thomas et al., 2002) and increased levels of NO caused by cytokine-mediated iNOS induction cause cell death by both necrosis (Hoorens et al., 2001, Welsh et al., 1994) and apoptosis (Holohan et al., 2008). The relative involvement of NO in the destruction of β-cells in human and rodent islets is not fully elucidated. Several studies have shown that a combination of IL-1β with IFNγ or TNFα induces cell death in rodent pancreatic islet cells, predominantly by induction of apoptosis but also partly by necrosis (D. Liu et al., 2000, Saldeen, 2000). In rodent β-cells the cytokine-induced induction of necrosis seems to be dependent on iNOS-induced production of NO as the level of necrotic cell death was greatly reduced in purified β-cells from iNOS-deficient mice (D. Liu et al., 2000). Another study found that inhibition of iNOS in rat islets reduced both necrosis and apoptosis induction (Saldeen, 2000). In any case, the cytokine-induced production of NO seems to play a major role in mediating β-cell death in rodent experimental models of T1DM. Additionally, we recently demonstrated that a combination of IL-1β and IFNγ induces the intrinsic apoptosis pathway in a synergistic manner in a rat insulinoma cell line (RIN-r) and showed that iNOS-mediated production of NO was both required and sufficient for apoptosis induction (Holohan et al., 2008). This is in agreement with previous findings that showed that apoptosis induced by a combination of IL-1β and IFNγ is NO-dependent in a rat insulinoma cell line (Storling et al., 2005).

Human islets have been shown to be less sensitive to NO-induced damage compared to rodent cells. As such, inhibition of iNOS could not protect human islets from cytokine-induced cell death suggesting a NO-independent cytotoxicity. (Delaney et al., 1997, Eizirik & Mandrup-Poulsen, 2001, Hoorens et al., 2001). The resistance of human islets towards NO compared to rodent islets is speculated to be due to higher levels of heat shock protein 70 (Hsp70) in human β-cells (Burkart et al., 2000) which protects cells from the oxidative stress inflicted by NO (Welsh et al., 1994).

2.3 Role of the Bcl-2 family proteins

Cytokines can modulate the expression and/or activity of several members of the Bcl-2 family (Gowda et al., 2008, A. Stephanou et al., 2000, P. Wang et al., 2009, L. Zhang et al., 2008). The various interactions between the pro- and anti-apoptotic members of this family of proteins lie at the heart of the intrinsic pathway of apoptosis (Youle & Strasser, 2008). Bcl-2 family members are characterised by up to four conserved regions termed Bcl-2 homology (BH) domains. The pro-apoptotic multidomain family members Bax and Bak contain three BH domains and can be activated to form oligomeric structures in the outer mitochondrial membrane that trigger cytochrome *c* release, which then initiates the intrinsic pathway of caspase activation. Activation proceeds through interaction with BH3-only family members (harbouring only the third BH domain) that are induced or activated by cellular stress signals. Activation of Bax or Bak is counteracted by anti-apoptotic multidomain Bcl-2 family members (such as Bcl-2, Bcl-xL, or Mcl-1), which bind and sequester the BH3-only proteins.

Viral transduction of Bcl-2, the prototype member of the family, was shown to protect human islet cells from cytokine-induced apoptosis, giving a first indication that regulation of Bcl-2 family proteins by cytokines might contribute to β-cell apoptosis (Rabinovitch et al., 1999). Likewise, adenoviral transduction of Bcl-X_L prevented cytokine-mediated apoptosis of RIN-r cells (Holohan et al., 2008).

Several recent studies have addressed the involvement of Bcl-2 family proteins in cytokine-induced β-cell death in more detail. Treatment of human or rat islets with inflammatory cytokines resulted in activation of the intrinsic pathway of apoptosis and involved activation of the pro-apoptotic BH3-only protein Bad by dephosphorylation (Grunnet et al., 2009). Dephosphorylation of Bad was also found in a second study analysing cytokine-treated rat islets, and in addition up-regulation of pro-apoptotic BH3-only proteins Bim and Bid was also detected (Mehmeti et al., 2011). In a different study it was shown that in primary rat β-cells cytokines as well as ER stress lead to increased expression of the pro-apoptotic BH3-only protein DP5/Hrk in a JNK-dependent manner (Gurzov et al., 2009). Up-regulation of DP5 in β-cells is mediated by the transcription factor STAT-1 which is regulated by IFNγ (Moore et al., 2011). In addition, inflammatory cytokines led to up-regulation of the pro-apoptotic BH3-only protein PUMA in primary rat β-cells as well as in human islets through a pathway involving NF-κB signalling, iNOS activation and ER stress (Gurzov et al., 2010). Furthermore, down-regulation of the anti-apoptotic multidomain Bcl-2 family member Mcl-1 turned out to be critically involved in the cytokine-induced apoptosis of the rat insulinoma cell line INS-1E (Allagnat et al., 2011). In summary, exposure to cytokines leads to alterations in expression of several Bcl-2 family members in β-cells in a manner that favours activation of the intrinsic pathway of apoptosis.

3. β-cell stress in type 1 diabetes

3.1 Endoplasmic reticulum stress

It has been suggested that endoplasmic reticulum (ER) stress is involved in β-cell destruction. Pancreatic β-cells are specialised cells that rapidly synthesise and secrete insulin in response to fluctuations in blood glucose levels (Pirot et al., 2007). This imparts a heavy burden on the ER and, consequently, β-cells are particularly susceptible to cellular conditions that impair the ER's ability to correctly fold nascent proteins. Under such conditions, the resultant accumulation of unfolded or damaged proteins within the ER lumen triggers the unfolded protein response (UPR), an adaptive signalling pathway that increases the folding capacity of the ER and restores homeostasis (Szegezdi et al., 2006). Although the initial UPR is a protective response, prolonged ER stress can lead to the initiation of apoptosis. Thus while under physiological conditions the UPR acts as a pro-survival mechanism in β-cells, chronic ER stress can lead to redirection of the UPR towards pro-apoptotic signalling.

Three ER-localized transmembrane proteins sense the accumulation of unfolded proteins in the ER lumen and initiate the UPR, PKR-like ER kinase (PERK), inositol-requiring enzyme 1 α (IRE1α) and activating transcription factor 6 (ATF6). These proteins transduce information from the ER to the nucleus by activating transcription factors that control genes involved in restoring ER function (Szegezdi et al., 2006). The PERK arm of the UPR has been the main focus of studies with regard to β-cell stress in diabetes, therefore this chapter will focus on PERK signalling in more detail. Upon accumulation of unfolded proteins, PERK is activated and induces a translational block by phosphorylating eukaryotic initiation factor 2 α (eIF2α). Phosphorylation of eIF2α by PERK leads to inhibition of cap-dependent protein synthesis. This reduces the protein load of the ER while allowing cap-independent translation to persist and leads to preferential translation of the transcription factor ATF4. One target gene induced by ATF4 (in conjunction with ATF6) is C/EBP homologous protein CHOP, a transcription factor that is known to promote apoptosis (Zinszner et al., 1998).

3.1.1 The role of PERK in β-cell function

The PERK signalling branch of the UPR appears to be essential for the regulation of β-cell function. Stimulation of insulin production in mouse pancreatic islets leads to dephosphorylation of eIF2α (P. Zhang et al., 2002) reversing the translational block caused by PERK signalling and allowing for increased biosynthesis of insulin. Studies with knockout mice showed that PERK is essential for β-cell function and survival (Harding et al., 2001, P. Zhang et al., 2002). Pancreatic β-cells of PERK$^{-/-}$ mice degenerated within the first four weeks after birth, and a diabetic phenotype could be observed (Harding et al.,

2001, P. Zhang et al., 2002). β-cell loss was associated with damaged rough ER and high levels of apoptosis in the pancreas (P. Zhang et al., 2002). However, a subsequent study discovered that the onset of diabetes in PERK-/- mice is due to developmental defects during β-cell proliferation and differentiation leading to a reduction in β-cell mass (W. Zhang et al., 2006). At the molecular level, down-regulation of PERK in rat β-cells was shown to induce deregulation of ER chaperones Grp78 and ERp72 and disruption of ER function leading to reduced insulin production and reduced cell proliferation (Feng et al., 2009).

3.1.2 Involvement of the UPR in cytokine-induced β-cell death

There is some evidence to suggest that cytokines induce β-cell apoptosis by stimulating pro-apoptotic signalling of the UPR. Ca^{2+} levels in the ER are about four times higher than in the cytosol as high Ca^{2+} levels are required for ER function in aiding protein folding and posttranslational processing. Disruption of Ca^{2+} homeostasis causes severe ER stress resulting in accumulation of unfolded proteins in the ER and activation of the UPR. It was shown that cytokine-exposure leads to elevated basal cytosolic Ca^{2+} levels selectively in mouse pancreatic β-cells compared to glucagon-secreting α-cells and this was associated with cytokine-induced apoptosis (L. Wang et al., 1999). In line with these results, it was shown that increased production of NO in rodent β-cells leads to depletion of ER Ca^{2+} levels (Oyadomari et al., 2001). Furthermore, overexpression of the ER-located Ca^{2+}-binding protein, calreticulin increased levels of Ca^{2+} in the ER and made cells more resistant to NO-induced apoptosis (Oyadomari et al., 2001). This suggests that NO-induced apoptosis in rodent β-cells is at least partly caused by ER stress induced by NO-mediated Ca^{2+} depletion.
Some evidence suggests that NO may regulate Ca^{2+} levels in β-cells through down-regulation of the sarcoendoplasmic reticulum Ca^{2+} ATPase 2b (SERCA2b) (Cardozo et al., 2005). SERCA pumps Ca^{2+} from the cytoplasm into the ER thus maintaining ER Ca^{2+} levels. Rodent and human islet cells have been reported to express the isoforms SERCA2b and SERCA3 (Varadi et al., 1996). Treatment of rodent pancreatic β-cells with a combination of IL-1β and IFNγ induced transcriptional down-regulation of SERCA2b and this was partially prevented by inhibition of iNOS. Furthermore, after inhibition of SERCA, the effect of cytokine exposure on ER Ca^{2+} was abolished (Cardozo et al., 2005). This suggests that NO-induced depletion of ER Ca^{2+} is at least in part mediated by SERCA down-regulation. The SERCA isoform SERCA2a has been shown to be specifically inactivated by peroxynitrite ($ONOO^-$)-mediated nitration of a tyrosine residue within the channel-like domain *in vitro* (Viner et al., 1999). Peroxynitrite is produced in cells by a reaction between NO and the free radical superoxide (Pacher et al., 2007). SERCA2a differs from SERCA2b only in regions of the C-terminus (Dode et al., 1998) and it could be hypothesised that cytokine-induced NO production inhibits SERCA2b Ca^{2+}-ATPase activity by peroxynitrite-mediated nitration in the same way. Another possible mechanism by which NO might mediate reduction of ER Ca^{2+} levels is via activation of the ryanodine receptor-2. Ryanodine receptor-2 is a calcium channel located in the ER membrane that releases Ca^{2+} from the ER into the cytosol and has been reported to be expressed in mouse pancreatic β-cells (Islam et al., 1998). NO-induced poly-S-nitrosylation enhances the activity of this calcium channel (Xu et al., 1998) but whether this mechanism is relevant to cytokine-exposed β-cells remains to be determined.
Treatment of rodent β-cells with a combination of IL-1β and IFNγ induces the expression of CHOP in an NO-dependent manner (Fig. 4). This is in line with a number of other reports (Cardozo et al., 2001b, Cardozo et al., 2005). Inhibition of iNOS by N5-(1-iminoethyl)-L-ornithine (L-NIO) or N^G-methyl-L-arginine (LMA) blocked cytokine-induced NO

production and expression of CHOP. In addition to CHOP, the UPR marker proteins Grp78 and phosphorylated eIF2α were also found to be up-regulated after cytokine treatment, without affecting expression of spliced X-box binding protein 1 (sXBP-1) which is induced downstream of IRE1α (Fig. 4). Overexpression of iNOS alone was sufficient for CHOP expression (Fig. 4) and treatment with the NO-donor molecule S-nitroso-N-acetyl-D,L-penicillamine (SNAP) induced expression of Grp78 and CHOP (Oyadomari et al., 2001). This suggests that NO is sufficient to activate the UPR in rodent pancreatic β-cells. Pancreatic islet cells from $CHOP^{-/-}$ mice were shown to be resistant to cytokine- and NO-mediated apoptosis compared to cells from $CHOP^{+/+}$ and $CHOP^{+/-}$ mice (Oyadomari et al., 2001). Together these results suggest that the apoptotic effects of cytokine-induced NO are mediated by activation of CHOP.

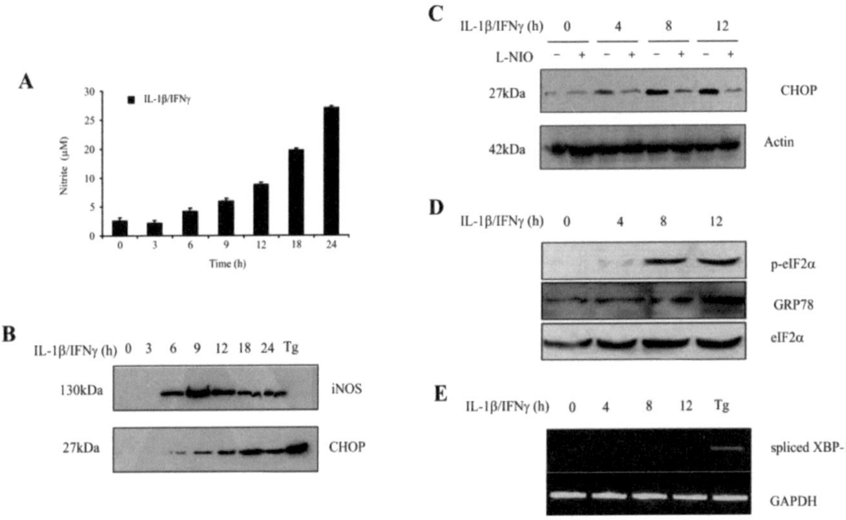

Fig. 4. IL-1β/IFNγ induced the expression of the pro-apoptotic transcription factor CHOP and other UPR markers. (A) A time-course cytokine treatment (IL-1β and IFNγ, 60 U/ml of each) was carried out and samples assayed for NO production. (B) The same samples were then analysed by Western blotting for iNOS and CHOP expression. This data demonstrates an increase in NO production, iNOS expression and CHOP induction occurring at 6 h post cytokine treatment, although CHOP is not strongly expressed until 9 h. (C) Samples were assayed for CHOP expression following cytokine treatment in the presence and absence of the iNOS inhibitor L-NIO. Cytokine-induced CHOP expression was decreased in the presence of L-NIO indicating that this is an NO-dependent process. (D) Alterations in the expression of ER stress-associated proteins after cytokine treatment were analysed by Western blotting. The expression of UPR markers Grp78 and phosphorylated eIF2α (p-eIF2α) were up in response to cytokine treatment. (E) Production of spliced XBP-1 mRNA after cytokine treatment was determined by RT-PCR. Thapsigargin (Tg) treatment was used as a positive control. Cytokine treatment did not show an effect on the level of spliced XBP-1 mRNA. The images presented are representative of three independent experiments.

Conversely, another study suggested that although cytokine signalling induces ER stress as demonstrated by activation of PERK and JNK, induction of CHOP is not required for β-cell death in rodents (Åkerfeldt et al., 2008). In support of these findings, a recent study suggests that CHOP is not required for β-cell death and the development of diabetes in NOD mice (Satoh et al., 2011). However, $CHOP^{-/-}$ NOD mice showed delayed production of insulin autoimmune antibodies (Satoh et al., 2011) suggesting a role for CHOP in the early onset of the autoimmune reaction leading to β-cell destruction. Therefore, cytokine-induced β-cell death may be partly mediated by induction of CHOP.

While a functional UPR (at least the PERK branch) appears to be essential for β-cell function and development, its downstream target CHOP has been associated with cytokine-induced β-cell destruction suggesting that PERK signalling regulates β-cell function and survival under physiological conditions but may switch towards pro-death signalling under conditions of cytokine-induced β-cell stress.

3.2 Oxidative stress

Cytokines induce multiple stress pathways in β-cells. Oxidative stress is induced by increased production of ROS and an imbalanced, low level of antioxidant enzymes (Sies, 1997). IL-1β, TNFα and IFNγ induce the production of ROS and NO by inducing iNOS (Rabinovitch & Suarez-Pinzon, 1998). Free oxygen and nitrogen radicals generated can react to form peroxynitrite, which is a very strong oxidant. Oxygen free radicals, nitrogen free radicals as well as the radical peroxynitrite can react with and damage a range of cellular proteins and in this way block metabolic functions and induce β-cell death (Azevedo-Martins et al., 2003). β-cells have been shown to be especially susceptible to such oxidative stress because they have particularly low levels of antioxidant enzymes (Lenzen et al., 1996, Tiedge et al., 1998).

4. Therapeutic strategies

The number of people affected by T1DM is approximately 20 million worldwide and is rapidly rising (Chabot, 2002). While exogenous administration of insulin is an effective treatment for acute hyperglycaemia in T1DM, it does not prevent secondary complications (White et al., 2008) and can in some cases lead to hypoglycaemia (Kort et al., 2011). Alternative therapeutic strategies include pancreas transplantation and islet transplantation. While whole pancreas transplantation is an invasive surgical method associated with major complications, islet transplantation is less invasive and associated with significantly lower morbidity and mortality. Successful islet transplantation would result in insulin independence, protection from hypoglycaemia, improvement of microvascular complications, improved patient survival and enhanced quality of life (Kort et al., 2011). The method is currently in clinical trials and has been used to treat around 1,000 individuals worldwide (Kort et al., 2011). Islet transplantation has many limitations, including limited availability of suitable islet graft donors, high cost and high rate of partial or total graft failure. Islet graft failure can be caused by allorejection, toxicity of immunosuppressive drugs that are required to reduce immune rejection, glucotoxicity, and recurrence of autoimmunity (Kort et al., 2011).

An approach to reduce β-cell death in islet grafts is the transfer of therapeutically useful genes into islet cells prior to transplantation (McCabe et al., 2006). The development of gene therapy techniques that can protect β-cells from autoimmune destruction may not only improve outcomes after islet transplantation but may also lead to preventive therapies for patients at high risk of developing T1DM (McCabe et al., 2006).

Various candidate transgenes are being examined for their potential in protecting β-cells under various stresses including cytokine-exposure and oxidative stress. The rational choice of therapeutic genes is helped by understanding the mechanism of β-cell destruction which has been the subject of this chapter. Potential targets will be reviewed in this section. Target genes studied to date encode regulators of the cytokine signal transduction pathways, molecules that inhibit β-cell apoptosis, antioxidant enzymes, immunoregulatory proteins and pro-survival cytokines (McCabe et al., 2006).

4.1 Anti-apoptotic gene transfer

Apoptosis plays a major role in β-cell death in T1DM (see section 2.). The transfer of anti-apoptotic genes as a strategy to counteract islet destruction has been explored. Candidate genes include those expressing cytoprotective and anti-apoptotic heat shock proteins (Hsps) and anti-apoptotic Bcl-2 family proteins. Hsp70 is one of the major heat shock proteins in mammals and is thought to be responsible for the relative resistance of human β-cells to cytokine-induced stress and death (Burkart et al., 2000). Hsp70 can protect cells under conditions of stress by directly inhibiting the transduction of the apoptotic signal, by decreasing the amount of oxidative stress and also by reducing ER stress via its chaperone activity. It has been shown that pre-conditioning by heat shock could protect pancreatic islet cells from insults by NO, ROS and the cytotoxic drug streptozocin and this increased resistance correlated with induced expression of Hsp70 (Bellmann et al., 1995). Another Hsp that is potentially capable of protecting β-cells is heme oxygenase (HO-1), also known as Hsp32. HO-1 exerts its cytoprotective effects mainly by reduction of oxidative stress (McCabe et al., 2006) and overexpression of HO-1 could protect cytokine-exposed islet cells from apoptosis (Pileggi et al., 2001, Ye & Laychock, 1998). Bcl-2 family proteins, such as the anti-apoptotic Bcl-2, are major regulators of the apoptotic signalling cascade. It has been suggested that an impaired induction of anti-apoptotic Bcl-2 plays a role in cytokine-induced dysfunction and cell death of human islet cells relative to porcine islets (Piro et al., 2001). Moreover, overexpression of Bcl-2 was shown to protect β-cells from cytokine-induced apoptosis (Y. Liu et al., 1996) and increase the longevity of islet grafts after transplantation (Contreras et al., 2001). Several mechanisms by which Bcl-2 might exert β-cell protection have been suggested (McCabe et al., 2006). These include inhibition of cytochrome c release from mitochondria, inhibition of ER stress-induced apoptosis and blocking of Ca^{2+} release from the ER. It was shown that Bcl-2 overexpression can reduce ER stress-induced apoptosis in islet cells (Contreras et al., 2003). Both of these mechanisms have been associated with cytokine-induced β-cell death. Another candidate transgene may be the gene encoding the cellular FADD-like IL-1β-converting enzyme (FLICE)-like inhibitory protein (cFlip) as its overexpression has been shown to inhibit the activation of caspase-8 in β-cells exposed to TNFα (Cottet et al., 2002).

4.2 Anti-cytokine gene transfer

Inhibition of NF-κB, a main effector of cytokine-signalling, was shown to reduce cytokine-induced apoptosis in rodent β-cells *in vitro* (Baker et al., 2001, Heimberg et al., 2001) and *in vivo* (Eldor et al., 2006) and Fas-induced apoptosis in human islet cells (Giannoukakis et al., 2000). It should be noted that active NF-κB has been shown to be an essential factor in mediating glucose-stimulated insulin secretion (Norlin et al., 2005) and while NF-κB inhibition may protect β-cells from apoptosis it may also interfere with insulin secretion.

JNK is another candidate target for anti-cytokine gene therapy. Inhibition of JNK has been shown to protect pig islet cells from apoptosis and loss of JNK function after isolation and also after transplantation suppresses IL-1β induced apoptosis in insulin-secreting rodent cell lines (Nikulina et al., 2003, Noguchi et al., 2005). Other potential transgenes interfering with cytokine signalling include feedback inhibitors, e.g. SOCS (Yasukawa et al., 2000). It is thought that a compromised ability to up-regulate SOCS in response to cytokine exposure makes β-cells particularly susceptible to cytokine-induced damage (Karlsen et al., 2001, Yasukawa et al., 2000). The overexpression of SOCS-3 in response to IL-1β was shown to be slower in β-cells compared to other cell lines (Karlsen et al., 2001). It was also demonstrated that SOCS-3 overexpression can protect rodent β-cells from cytokine-induced death (Karlsen et al., 2001).

4.3 Anti-oxidant gene transfer

The protective effects of several antioxidant enzymes including catalase, glutathione peroxidase and the superoxide dismutases (SODs) MnSOD and CuZnSOD have been investigated. While results have not been entirely consistent, many studies have demonstrated that activation or overexpression of these enzymes can protect β-cells against oxidative stress or cytokine-induced destruction at least to some extent (Benhamou et al., 1998, Bertera et al., 2003, Hohmeier et al., 1998, Lortz & Tiedge, 2003, Lortz et al., 2000). These studies have shown that antioxidant gene transfer is a promising strategy in prolonging islet graft longevity. However, it has also been observed that transfer of antioxidant genes alone could not protect β-cells long term against toxicity caused by cytokine exposure and oxidative stress.

5. Conclusion

In recent years basic biomedical research has delivered a wealth of knowledge about the pathways by which inflammatory cytokines sensitise β-cells to cell death during the course of T1DM pathogenesis. Although the picture is still incomplete, we have learned about the major stresses to which β-cells are exposed. Some of the molecular players mediating these stresses have been identified. In particular, pro-inflammatory cytokines IL-1β, TNFα and IFNγ have been implicated as main mediators of β-cell stress and death during T1DM. It emerges that these cytokines synergistically activate transcriptional programs that lead to NO signalling, oxidative stress, ER stress, as well as modulation of Bcl-2 family protein expression. How these pathways precisely intersect has not yet been fully clarified. Studies elucidating these mechanisms may provide the knowledge to improve therapy. Islet transplantation, a therapeutic approach that would overcome the need of continuous insulin administration, is still in its infancy. Modern gene transfer techniques offer a huge potential for improvement to islet transplantation as it can help overcoming the cellular and autoimmune-mediated stress transplanted islets are exposed to. The experiments mentioned at the end of this chapter are encouraging that the accumulating knowledge of the molecules and pathways mediating β-cell stress will help to develop gene therapeutic approaches alleviating these stresses, thus improving survival of transplanted islets.

6. Acknowledgement

We are grateful to Dr. Sandra Healy for critical reading of this manuscript and Anna McCormick for providing the microscopy images of mouse pancreatic tissue sections. LV is funded by an Irish Cancer Society Scholarship (CRS10VIN). Our work is in part supported by a grant from Science Foundation Ireland (09/RFP/BIC2371).

7. References

Åkerfeldt, M.C., Howes, J., Chan, J.Y., Stevens, V.A., Boubenna, N., McGuire, H.M., King, C., Biden, T.J. & Laybutt, D.R. (2008). Cytokine-Induced B-Cell Death Is Independent of Endoplasmic Reticulum Stress Signaling. *Diabetes,* Vol. 57, No.11, (Nov), pp.(3034-3044), 1939-327X (Electronic), 0012-1797 (Linking)

Alexander, W.S. (2002). Suppressors of Cytokine Signalling (Socs) in the Immune System. *Nat Rev Immunol,* Vol. 2, No.6, (Jun), pp.(410-416), 1474-1733

Allagnat, F., Cunha, D., Moore, F., Vanderwinden, J.M., Eizirik, D.L. & Cardozo, A.K. (2011). Mcl-1 Downregulation by Pro-Inflammatory Cytokines and Palmitate Is an Early Event Contributing to Beta-Cell Apoptosis. *Cell Death Differ,* Vol. 18, No.2, (Feb), pp.(328-337), 1476-5403 (Electronic), 1350-9047 (Linking)

Azevedo-Martins, A.K., Lortz, S., Lenzen, S., Curi, R., Eizirik, D.L. & Tiedge, M. (2003). Improvement of the Mitochondrial Antioxidant Defense Status Prevents Cytokine-Induced Nuclear Factor-Kb Activation in Insulin-Producing Cells. *Diabetes,* Vol. 52, No.1, (Jan), pp.(93-101), 0012-1797

Baekkeskov, S., Aanstoot, H.-J., Christgai, S., Reetz, A., Solimena, M., Cascalho, M., Folli, F., Richter-Olesen, H. & Camilli, P.-D. (1990). Identification of the 64k Autoantigen in Insulin-Dependent Diabetes as the Gaba-Synthesizing Enzyme Glutamic Acid Decarboxylase. *Nature,* Vol. 347, No.6289, (Sep 13), pp.(151-156), 0028-0836

Baker, M.S., Chen, X., Cao, X.C. & Kaufman, D.B. (2001). Expression of a Dominant Negative Inhibitor of Nf-[Kappa]B Protects Min6 [Beta]-Cells from Cytokine-Induced Apoptosis. *Journal of Surgical Research,* Vol. 97, No.2, (May 15), pp.(117-122), 0022-4804 (Print), 0022-4804 (Linking)

Bellmann, K., Wenz, A., Radons, J., Burkart, V., Kleemann, R. & Kolb, H. (1995). Heat Shock Induces Resistance in Rat Pancreatic Islet Cells against Nitric Oxide, Oxygen Radicals and Streptozotocin Toxicity in Vitro. *The Journal of Clinical Investigation,* Vol. 95, No.6, (Jun), pp.(2840-2845), 0021-9738

Benhamou, P.Y., Moriscot, C., Richard, M.J., Beatrix, O., Badet, L., Pattou, F., Kerr-Conte, J., Chroboczek, J., Lemarchand, P. & Halimi, S. (1998). Adenovirus-Mediated Catalase Gene Transfer Reduces Oxidant Stress in Human, Porcine and Rat Pancreatic Islets. *Diabetologia,* Vol. 41, No.9, (Sep), pp.(1093-1100), 0012-186X

Bertera, S., Crawford, M.L., Alexander, A.M., Papworth, G.D., Watkins, S.C., Robbins, P.D. & Trucco, M. (2003). Gene Transfer of Manganese Superoxide Dismutase Extends Islet Graft Function in a Mouse Model of Autoimmune Diabetes. *Diabetes,* Vol. 52, No.2, (Feb), pp.(387-393), 0012-1797

Bonfoco, E., Krainc, D., Ankarcrona, M., Nicotera, P. & Lipton, S.A. (1995). Apoptosis and Necrosis: Two Distinct Events Induced, Respectively, by Mild and Intense Insults with N-Methyl-D-Aspartate or Nitric Oxide/Superoxide in Cortical Cell Cultures. *Proceedings of the National Academy of Sciences of the United States of America,* Vol. 92, No.16, (Aug 1), pp.(7162-7166), 0027-8424 (Print), 0027-8424 (Linking)

Bruun, C., Heding, P.E., Rønn, S.G., Frobøse, H., Rhodes, C.J., Mandrup-Poulsen, T. & Billestrup, N. (2009). Suppressor of Cytokine Signalling-3 Inhibits Tumor Necrosis Factor-Alpha Induced Apoptosis and Signalling in Beta Cells. *Molecular and Cellular Endocrinology,* Vol. 311, No.1-2, (Nov 13), pp.(32-38), 1872-8057 (Electronic), 0303-7207 (Linking)

Burkart, V., Liu, H., Bellmann, K., Wissing, D., Jäättelä, M., Cavallo, M.G., Pozzilli, P., Briviba, K. & Kolb, H. (2000). Natural Resistance of Human Beta Cells toward Nitric Oxide Is Mediated by Heat Shock Protein 70. *Journal of Biological Chemistry,* Vol. 275, No.26, (Jun 30), pp.(19521-19528), 0021-9258

Burns, K., Clatworthy, J., Martin, L., Martinon, F., Plumpton, C., Maschera, B., Lewis, A., Ray, K., Tschopp, J. & Volpe, F. (2000). Tollip, a New Component of the Il-1ri Pathway, Links Irak to the Il-1 Receptor. *Nat Cell Biol,* Vol. 2, No.6, (Jun), pp.(346-351), 1465-7392

Burns, K., Martinon, F., Esslinger, C., Pahl, H., Schneider, P., Bodmer, J.-L., Di Marco, F., French, L. & Tschopp, J. (1998). Myd88, an Adapter Protein Involved in Interleukin-1 Signaling. *Journal of Biological Chemistry,* Vol. 273, No.20, (May 15), pp.(12203-12209), 0021-9258

Cailleau, C., Diu-Hercend, A., Ruuth, E., Westwood, R. & Carnaud, C. (1997). Treatment with Neutralizing Antibodies Specific for Il-1beta Prevents Cyclophosphamide-Induced Diabetes in Nonobese Diabetic Mice. *Diabetes,* Vol. 46, No.6, (Jun 1), pp.(937-940), 0012-1797

Callewaert, H.I., Gysemans, C.A., Ladrière, L., D'Hertog, W., Hagenbrock, J., Overbergh, L., Eizirik, D.L. & Mathieu, C. (2007). Deletion of Stat-1 Pancreatic Islets Protects against Streptozotocin-Induced Diabetes and Early Graft Failure but Not against Late Rejection. *Diabetes,* Vol. 56, No.8, (Aug), pp.(2169-2173), 1939-327X (Electronic), 0012-1797 (Linking)

Cardozo, A.K., Heimberg, H., Heremans, Y., Leeman, R., Kutlu, B., Kruhøffer, M., Ørntoft, T. & Eizirik, D.L. (2001a). A Comprehensive Analysis of Cytokine-Induced and Nuclear Factor-Kb-Dependent Genes in Primary Rat Pancreatic B-Cells. *Journal of Biological Chemistry,* Vol. 276, No.52, (Dec 28), pp.(48879-48886), 0021-9258

Cardozo, A.K., Kruhoffer, M., Leeman, R., Orntoft, T. & Eizirik, D.L. (2001b). Identification of Novel Cytokine-Induced Genes in Pancreatic Beta-Cells by High-Density Oligonucleotide Arrays. *Diabetes,* Vol. 50, No.5, (May), pp.(909-920), 0012-1797

Cardozo, A.K., Ortis, F., Storling, J., Feng, Y.-M., Rasschaert, J., Tonnesen, M., Van Eylen, F., Mandrup-Poulsen, T., Herchuelz, A. & Eizirik, D.L. (2005). Cytokines Downregulate the Sarcoendoplasmic Reticulum Pump Ca2+ Atpase 2b and Deplete Endoplasmic Reticulum Ca2+, Leading to Induction of Endoplasmic Reticulum Stress in Pancreatic B-Cells. *Diabetes,* Vol. 54, No.2, (Feb 1), pp.(452-461), 0012-1797

Chabot, J.M. (2002). A Report from the World Health Organization. *Rev Prat.,* Vol. 52, No.19, (Dec 1), pp.(2155-2156), 0035-2640

Chong, M.M.W., Chen, Y., Darwiche, R., Dudek, N.L., Irawaty, W., Santamaria, P., Allison, J., Kay, T.W.H. & Thomas, H.E. (2004). Suppressor of Cytokine Signaling-1 Overexpression Protects Pancreatic B Cells from Cd8+ T Cell-Mediated

Autoimmune Destruction. *The Journal of Immunology,* Vol. 172, No.9, (May 1), pp.(5714-5721), 0022-1767

Contreras, J.L., Bilbao, G., Smyth, C.A., Jiang, X.L., Eckhoff, D.E., Jenkins, S.M., Thomas, F.T., Curiel, D.T. & Thomas, J.M. (2001). Cytoprotection of Pancreatic Islets before and Soon after Transplantation by Gene Transfer of the Anti-Apoptotic Bcl-2 Gene 1. *Transplantation,* Vol. 71, No.8, (Apr 27), 0041-1337

Contreras, J.L., Smyth, C.A., Bilbao, G., Eckstein, C., Young, C.J., Thompson, J.A., Curiel, D.T. & Eckhoff, D.E. (2003). Coupling Endoplasmic Reticulum Stress to Cell Death Program in Isolated Human Pancreatic Islets: Effects of Gene Transfer of Bcl-2. *Transplant International,* Vol. 16, No.7, (Jul), pp.(537-542-542-537-542-542), 0934-0874

Cottet, S., Dupraz, P., Hamburger, F., Dolci, W., Jaquet, M. & Thorens, B. (2002). Cflip Protein Prevents Tumor Necrosis Factor-A–Mediated Induction of Caspase-8–Dependent Apoptosis in Insulin-Secreting Btc-Tet Cells. *Diabetes,* Vol. 51, No.6, (Jun), pp.(1805-1814), 0012-1797

Delaney, C.A., Pavlovic, D., Hoorens, A., Pipeleers, D.G. & Eizirik, D.L. (1997). Cytokines Induce Deoxyribonucleic Acid Strand Breaks and Apoptosis in Human Pancreatic Islet Cells. *Endocrinology,* Vol. 138, No.6, (Jun), pp.(2610-2614), 0013-7227

Devin, A., Cook, A., Lin, Y., Rodriguez, Y., Kelliher, M. & Liu, Z.G. (2000). The Distinct Roles of Traf2 and Rip in Ikk Activation by Tnf-R1: Traf2 Recruits Ikk to Tnf-R1 While Rip Mediates Ikk Activation. *Immunity,* Vol. 12, No.4, (Apr), pp.(419-429), 1074-7613

Devin, A., Lin, Y. & Liu, Z.-g. (2003). The Role of the Death-Domain Kinase Rip in Tumour-Necrosis-Factor-Induced Activation of Mitogen-Activated Protein Kinases. *EMBO reports,* Vol. 4, No.6, (Jun), pp.(623-627), 1469-221X

Dinarello, C.A. (1997). Interleukin-1. *Cytokine & Growth Factor Reviews,* Vol. 8, No.4, (Dec), pp.(253-265), 1359-6101

Dode, L., De Greef, C., Mountian, I., Attard, M., Town, M.M., Casteels, R. & Wuytack, F. (1998). Structure of the Human Sarco/Endoplasmic Reticulum Ca2+-Atpase 3 Gene. Promoter Analysis and Alternative Splicing of the Serca3 Pre-Mrna. *J Biol Chem,* Vol. 273, No.22, (May 29), pp.(13982-13994), 0021-9258

Eizirik, D.L. & Darville, M.I. (2001). Beta-Cell Apoptosis and Defense Mechanisms: Lessons from Type 1 Diabetes. *Diabetes,* Vol. 50, No.suppl 1, (Feb), pp.(S64-S64), 0012-1797

Eizirik, D.L. & Mandrup-Poulsen, T. (2001). A Choice of Death - the Signal-Transduction of Immune-Mediated Beta-Cell Apoptosis. *Diabetologia,* Vol. 44, No.12, (Dec), pp.(2115-2133), 0012-186X (Print), 0012-186X (Linking)

Eldor, R., Yeffet, A., Baum, K., Doviner, V., Amar, D., Ben-Neriah, Y., Christofori, G., Peled, A., Carel, J.C., Boitard, C., Klein, T., Serup, P., Eizirik, D.L. & Melloul, D. (2006). Conditional and Specific Nf-Kb Blockade Protects Pancreatic Beta Cells from Diabetogenic Agents. *Proceedings of the National Academy of Sciences of the United States of America,* Vol. 103, No.13, (Mar 28), pp.(5072-5077), 0027-8424

Elias, D., Marcus, H., Reshef, T., Ablamunits, V. & Cohen, I.R. (1995). Induction of Diabetes in Standard Mice by Immunization with the P277 Peptide of a 60-Kda Heat Shock Protein. *European Journal of Immunology,* Vol. 25, No.10, (Oct), pp.(2851-2857), 0014-2980

Emanuelli, B., Glondu, M., Filloux, C., Peraldi, P. & Van Obberghen, E. (2004). The Potential Role of Socs-3 in the Interleukin-1β-Induced Desensitization of Insulin Signaling in Pancreatic Beta-Cells. *Diabetes,* Vol. 53, No.suppl 3, (Dec 1), pp.(S97-S103), 0012-1797

Emanuelli, B., Peraldi, P., Filloux, C., Sawka-Verhelle, D., Hilton, D. & Van Obberghen, E. (2000). Socs-3 Is an Insulin-Induced Negative Regulator of Insulin Signaling. *Journal of Biological Chemistry,* Vol. 275, No.21, (May 26), pp.(15985-15991), 0021-9258

Feng, D., Wei, J., Gupta, S., McGrath, B.C. & Cavener, D.R. (2009). Acute Ablation of Perk Results in Er Dysfunctions Followed by Reduced Insulin Secretion and Cell Proliferation. *BMC Cell Biol,* Vol. 10, (Sep 4), pp.(61), 1471-2121

Flodström-Tullberg, M., Yadav, D., Hägerkvist, R., Tsai, D., Secrest, P., Stotland, A. & Sarvetnick, N. (2003). Target Cell Expression of Suppressor of Cytokine Signaling-1 Prevents Diabetes in the Nod Mouse. *Diabetes,* Vol. 52, No.11, (Nov 1), pp.(2696-2700), 0012-1797

Flodström, M., Welsh, N. & Eizirik, D.L. (1996). Cytokines Activate the Nuclear Factor [Kappa]B (Nf-[Kappa]B) and Induce Nitric Oxide Production in Human Pancreatic Islets. *FEBS Letters,* Vol. 385, No.1-2, (Apr 29), pp.(4-6), 0014-5793

Frigerio, S., Junt, T., Lu, B., Gerard, C., Zumsteg, U., Hollander, G.A. & Piali, L. (2002). [Beta] Cells Are Responsible for Cxcr3-Mediated T-Cell Infiltration in Insulitis. *Nat Med,* Vol. 8, No.12, (Dec), pp.(1414-1420), 1078-8956

Giannoukakis, N., Rudert, W.A., Trucco, M. & Robbins, P.D. (2000). Protection of Human Islets from the Effects of Interleukin-1β by Adenoviral Gene Transfer of an Iκb Repressor. *Journal of Biological Chemistry,* Vol. 275, No.47, (Nov 24), pp.(36509-36513), 0021-9258

Gowda, A., Roda, J., Hussain, S.R., Ramanunni, A., Joshi, T., Schmidt, S., Zhang, X., Lehman, A., Jarjoura, D., Carson, W.E., Kindsvogel, W., Cheney, C., Caligiuri, M.A., Tridandapani, S., Muthusamy, N. & Byrd, J.C. (2008). Il-21 Mediates Apoptosis through up-Regulation of the Bh3 Family Member Bim and Enhances Both Direct and Antibody-Dependent Cellular Cytotoxicity in Primary Chronic Lymphocytic Leukemia Cells in Vitro. *Blood,* Vol. 111, No.9, (May 1), pp.(4723-4730), 1528-0020 (Electronic), 0006-4971 (Linking)

Grunnet, L.G., Aikin, R., Tonnesen, M.F., Paraskevas, S., Blaabjerg, L., Storling, J., Rosenberg, L., Billestrup, N., Maysinger, D. & Mandrup-Poulsen, T. (2009). Proinflammatory Cytokines Activate the Intrinsic Apoptotic Pathway in Beta-Cells. *Diabetes,* Vol. 58, No.8, (Aug), pp.(1807-1815), 1939-327X (Electronic), 0012-1797 (Linking)

Gurzov, E.N., Germano, C.M., Cunha, D.A., Ortis, F., Vanderwinden, J.M., Marchetti, P., Zhang, L. & Eizirik, D.L. (2010). P53 up-Regulated Modulator of Apoptosis (Puma) Activation Contributes to Pancreatic Beta-Cell Apoptosis Induced by Proinflammatory Cytokines and Endoplasmic Reticulum Stress. *J Biol Chem,* Vol. 285, No.26, (Jun 25), pp.(19910-19920), 1083-351X (Electronic), 0021-9258 (Linking)

Gurzov, E.N., Ortis, F., Cunha, D.A., Gosset, G., Li, M., Cardozo, A.K. & Eizirik, D.L. (2009). Signaling by Il-1beta+Ifn-Gamma and Er Stress Converge on Dp5/Hrk Activation:

A Novel Mechanism for Pancreatic Beta-Cell Apoptosis. *Cell Death Differ,* Vol. 16, No.11, (Nov), pp.(1539-1550), 1476-5403 (Electronic), 1350-9047 (Linking)

Gysemans, C., Callewaert, H., Overbergh, L. & Mathieu, C. (2008). Cytokine Signalling in the Β-Cell: A Dual Role for Ifnγ. *Biochemical Society Transactions,* Vol. 36, No.3, (Jun), pp.(328-333), 0300-5127

Gysemans, C.A., Ladrière, L., Callewaert, H., Rasschaert, J., Flamez, D., Levy, D.E., Matthys, P., Eizirik, D.L. & Mathieu, C. (2005). Disruption of the Γ-Interferon Signaling Pathway at the Level of Signal Transducer and Activator of Transcription-1 Prevents Immune Destruction of Β-Cells. *Diabetes,* Vol. 54, No.8, (Aug 1), pp.(2396-2403), 0012-1797

Harding, H.P., Zeng, H., Zhang, Y., Jungries, R., Chung, P., Plesken, H., Sabatini, D.D. & Ron, D. (2001). Diabetes Mellitus and Exocrine Pancreatic Dysfunction in Perk-/- Mice Reveals a Role for Translational Control in Secretory Cell Survival. *Mol Cell,* Vol. 7, No.6, (Jun), pp.(1153-1163), 1097-2765

Heimberg, H., Heremans, Y., Jobin, C., Leemans, R., Cardozo, A.K., Darville, M. & Eizirik, D.L. (2001). Inhibition of Cytokine-Induced Nf-Kapab Activation by Adenovirus-Mediated Expression of a Nf-Kappab Super-Repressor Prevents Beta-Cell Apoptosis. *Diabetes,* Vol. 50, No.10, (Oct), pp.(2219-2224), 0012-1797

Hess, D.T., Matsumoto, A., Kim, S.-O., Marshall, H.E. & Stamler, J.S. (2005). Protein S-Nitrosylation: Purview and Parameters. *Nat Rev Mol Cell Biol,* Vol. 6, No.2, (Feb), pp.(150-166), 1471-0072

Hohmeier, H.E., Thigpen, A., Tran, V.V., Davis, R. & Newgard, C.B. (1998). Stable Expression of Manganese Superoxide Dismutase (Mnsod) in Insulinoma Cells Prevents Il-1beta- Induced Cytotoxicity and Reduces Nitric Oxide Production. *The Journal of Clinical Investigation,* Vol. 101, No.9, (May 1), pp.(1811-1820), 0021-9738

Holohan, C., Szegezdi, E., Ritter, T., O'Brien, T. & Samali, A. (2008). Cytokine-Induced Β-Cell Apoptosis Is No-Dependent, Mitochondria-Mediated and Inhibited by Bcl-Xl. *Journal of Cellular and Molecular Medicine,* Vol. 12, No.2, (Apr), pp.(591-606), 1582-1838

Hoorens, A., Stange, G., Pavlovic, D. & Pipeleers, D. (2001). Distinction between Interleukin-1-Induced Necrosis and Apoptosis of Islet Cells. *Diabetes,* Vol. 50, No.3, (Mar), pp.(551-557), 0012-1797

Hsu, H., Huang, J., Shu, H.-B., Baichwal, V. & Goeddel, D.V. (1996a). Tnf-Dependent Recruitment of the Protein Kinase Rip to the Tnf Receptor-1 Signaling Complex. *Immunity,* Vol. 4, No.4, (Apr), pp.(387-396), 1074-7613

Hsu, H., Shu, H.-B., Pan, M.-G. & Goeddel, D.V. (1996b). Tradd Traf2 and Tradd Fadd Interactions Define Two Distinct Tnf Receptor 1 Signal Transduction Pathways. *Cell,* Vol. 84, No.2, (Jan 26), pp.(299-308), 0092-8674

Hsu, H., Xiong, J. & Goeddel, D.V. (1995). The Tnf Receptor 1-Associated Protein Tradd Signals Cell Death and Nf-ºB Activation. *Cell,* Vol. 81, No.4, (May 19), pp.(495-504), 0092-8674

Igarashi, K., Garotta, G., Ozmen, L., Ziemiecki, A., Wilks, A.F., Harpur, A.G., Larner, A.C. & Finbloom, D.S. (1994). Interferon-Gamma Induces Tyrosine Phosphorylation of Interferon-Gamma Receptor and Regulated Association of Protein Tyrosine

Kinases, Jak1 and Jak2, with Its Receptor. *Journal of Biological Chemistry,* Vol. 269, No.20, (May 20), pp.(14333-14336), 0021-9258

Islam, M.S., Leibiger, I., Leibiger, B., Rossi, D., Sorrentino, V., Ekstrom, T.J., Westerblad, H., Andrade, F.H. & Berggren, P.O. (1998). In Situ Activation of the Type 2 Ryanodine Receptor in Pancreatic Beta Cells Requires Camp-Dependent Phosphorylation. *Proc Natl Acad Sci U S A,* Vol. 95, No.11, (May 26), pp.(6145-6150), 0027-8424

Iwahashi, H., Hanafusa, T., Eguchi, Y., Nakajima, H., Miyagawa, J., Itoh, N., Tomita, K., Namba, M., Kuwajima, M., Noguchi, T., Tsujimoto, Y. & Matsuzawa, Y. (1996). Cytokine-Induced Apoptotic Cell Death in a Mouse Pancreatic Beta-Cell Line: Inhibition by Bcl-2. *Diabetologia,* Vol. 39, No.5, (May), pp.(530-536), 0012-186X

Jun, H.-S. & Yoon, J.-W. (2003). A New Look at Viruses in Type 1 Diabetes. *Diabetes/Metabolism Research and Reviews,* Vol. 19, No.1, (Jan), pp.(8-31), 1520-7560

Kägi, D., Ho, A., Odermatt, B., Zakarian, A., Ohashi, P.S. & Mak, T.W. (1999). Tnf Receptor 1-Dependent ß Cell Toxicity as an Effector Pathway in Autoimmune Diabetes. *The Journal of Immunology,* Vol. 162, No.8, (Apr 15), pp.(4598-4605), 0022-1767

Kägi, D., Odermatt, B., Seiler, P., Zinkernagel, R.M., Mak, T.W. & Hengartner, H. (1997). Reduced Incidence and Delayed Onset of Diabetes in Perforin-Deficient Nonobese Diabetic Mice. *The Journal of Experimental Medicine,* Vol. 186, No.7, (Oct 6), pp.(989-997), 0022-1007

Karlsen, A.E., Rønn, S.G., Lindberg, K., Johannesen, J., Galsgaard, E.D., Pociot, F., Nielsen, J.H., Mandrup-Poulsen, T., Nerup, J. & Billestrup, N. (2001). Suppressor of Cytokine Signaling 3 (Socs-3) Protects Β-Cells against Interleukin-1β- and Interferon-Γ-Mediated Toxicity. *Proceedings of the National Academy of Sciences of the United States of America,* Vol. 98, No.21, (Oct 9), pp.(12191-12196), 0027-8424

Kim, H.-E., Choi, S.-E., Lee, S.-J., Lee, J.-H., Lee, Y.-J., Kang, S.S., Chun, J. & Kang, Y. (2008). Tumour Necrosis Factor-{Alpha}-Induced Glucose-Stimulated Insulin Secretion Inhibition in Ins-1 Cells Is Ascribed to a Reduction of the Glucose-Stimulated Ca2+ Influx. *J Endocrinol,* Vol. 198, No.3, (Sep 1), pp.(549-560), 1479-6805 (Electronic), 0022-0795 (Linking)

Kim, H.S., Han, M.S., Chung, K.W., Kim, S., Kim, E., Kim, M.J., Jang, E., Lee, H.A., Youn, J., Akira, S. & Lee, M.-S. (2007). Toll-Like Receptor 2 Senses [Beta]-Cell Death and Contributes to the Initiation of Autoimmune Diabetes. *Immunity,* Vol. 27, No.2, (Aug), pp.(321-333), 1074-7613

Kim, H.S., Kim, S. & Lee, M.S. (2005). Ifn-Gamma Sensitizes Min6n8 Insulinoma Cells to Tnf-Alpha-Induced Apoptosis by Inhibiting Nf-Kappab-Mediated Xiap Upregulation. *Biochem Biophys Res Commun,* Vol. 336, No.3, (Oct 28), pp.(847-853), 0006-291X

Kim, S., Kim, H.S., Chung, K.W., Oh, S.H., Yun, J.W., Im, S.-H., Lee, M.-K., Kim, K.-W. & Lee, M.-S. (2007). Essential Role for Signal Transducer and Activator of Transcription-1 in Pancreatic Β-Cell Death and Autoimmune Type 1 Diabetes of Nonobese Diabetic Mice. *Diabetes,* Vol. 56, No.10, (Oct), pp.(2561-2568), 1939-327X (Electronic), 0012-1797 (Linking)

Kort, H.d., Koning, E.J.d., Rabelink, T.J., Bruijn, J.A. & Bajema, I.M. (2011). Islet Transplantation in Type 1 Diabetes. *British Medical Journal,* Vol. 342, (Jan 21), pp.(d217-d217), 1468-5833 (Electronic), 0959-535X (Linking)

Kotenko, S.V., Izotova, L.S., Pollack, B.P., Mariano, T.M., Donnelly, R.J., Muthukumaran, G., Cook, J.R., Garotta, G., Silvennoinen, O., Ihle, J.N. & Pestka, S. (1995). Interaction between the Components of the Interferon Receptor Complex. *Journal of Biological Chemistry,* Vol. 270, No.36, (Sep 8), pp.(20915-20921), 0021-9258

Kutlu, B., Cardozo, A.K., Darville, M.I., Kruhøffer, M., Magnusson, N., Ørntoft, T. & Eizirik, D.L. (2003). Discovery of Gene Networks Regulating Cytokine-Induced Dysfunction and Apoptosis in Insulin-Producing Ins-1 Cells. *Diabetes,* Vol. 52, No.11, (Nov 1), pp.(2701-2719), 0012-1797

Kwon, G., Corbett, J., Rodi, C., Sullivan, P. & McDaniel, M. (1995). Interleukin-1 Beta-Induced Nitric Oxide Synthase Expression by Rat Pancreatic Beta-Cells: Evidence for the Involvement of Nuclear Factor Kappa B in the Signaling Mechanism. *Endocrinology,* Vol. 136, No.11, (Nov 1), pp.(4790-4795), 0013-7227

Lenzen, S., Drinkgern, J. & Tiedge, M. (1996). Low Antioxidant Enzyme Gene Expression in Pancreatic Islets Compared with Various Other Mouse Tissues. *Free Radical Biology and Medicine,* Vol. 20, No.3, pp.(463-466), 0891-5849

Lieberman, S.M., Evans, A.M., Han, B., Takaki, T., Vinnitskaya, Y., Caldwell, J.A., Serreze, D.V., Shabanowitz, J., Hunt, D.F., Nathenson, S.G., Santamaria, P. & DiLorenzo, T.P. (2003). Identification of the B Cell Antigen Targeted by a Prevalent Population of Pathogenic Cd8+ T Cells in Autoimmune Diabetes. *Proceedings of the National Academy of Sciences of the United States of America,* Vol. 100, No.14, (Jul 8), pp.(8384-8388), 0027-8424

Liu, D., Pavlovic, D., Chen, M.C., Flodström, M., Sandler, S. & Eizirik, D.L. (2000). Cytokines Induce Apoptosis in Beta-Cells Isolated from Mice Lacking the Inducible Isoform of Nitric Oxide Synthase (Inos-/-). *Diabetes,* Vol. 49, No.7, (Jul), pp.(1116-1122), 0012-1797

Liu, Y., Rabinovitch, A., Suarez-Pinzon, W., Muhkerjee, B., Brownlee, M., Edelstein, D. & Federoff, H.J. (1996). Expression of the Bcl-2 Gene from a Defective Hsv-1 Amplicon Vector Protects Pancreatic B-Cells from Apoptosis. *Human Gene Therapy,* Vol. 7, No.14, (Sep 10), pp.(1719-1726), 1043-0342

Lortz, S. & Tiedge, M. (2003). Sequential Inactivation of Reactive Oxygen Species by Combined Overexpression of Sod Isoforms and Catalase in Insulin-Producing Cells. *Free Radical Biology and Medicine,* Vol. 34, No.6, (May 15), pp.(683-688), 0891-5849

Lortz, S., Tiedge, M., Nachtwey, T., Karlsen, A.E., Nerup, J. & Lenzen, S. (2000). Protection of Insulin-Producing Rinm5f Cells against Cytokine-Mediated Toxicity through Overexpression of Antioxidant Enzymes. *Diabetes,* Vol. 49, No.7, (Jul), pp.(1123-1130), 0012-1797

Mandrup-Poulsen, T. (1996). The Role of Interleukin-1 in the Pathogenesis of Iddm. *Diabetologia,* Vol. 39, No.9, (Sep), pp.(1005-1029), 0012-186X

Mandrup-Poulsen, T., Pickersgill, L. & Donath, M.Y. (2010). Blockade of Interleukin 1 in Type 1 Diabetes Mellitus. *Nat Rev Endocrinol,* Vol. 6, No.3, (Mar), pp.(158-166), 1759-5037 (Electronic), 1759-5029 (Linking)

Mathis, D. & Benoist, C. (2004). Back to Central Tolerance. *Immunity,* Vol. 20, No.5, (May), pp.(509-516), 1074-7613

McCabe, C., Samali, A. & O'Brien, T. (2006). Cytoprotection of Beta Cells: Rational Gene Transfer Strategies. *Diabetes-Metab. Res. Rev.,* Vol. 22, No.3, (May), pp.(241-252), 1520-7552

Mehmeti, I., Lenzen, S. & Lortz, S. (2011). Modulation of Bcl-2-Related Protein Expression in Pancreatic Beta Cells by Pro-Inflammatory Cytokines and Its Dependence on the Antioxidative Defense Status. *Mol Cell Endocrinol,* Vol. 332, No.1-2, (Jan 30), pp.(88-96), 1872-8057 (Electronic), 0303-7207 (Linking)

Moore, F., Naamane, N., Colli, M.L., Bouckenooghe, T., Ortis, F., Gurzov, E.N., Igoillo-Esteve, M., Mathieu, C., Bontempi, G., Thykjaer, T., Ørntoft, T.F. & Eizirik, D.L. (2011). Stat1 Is a Master Regulator of Pancreatic Β-Cell Apoptosis and Islet Inflammation. *Journal of Biological Chemistry,* Vol. 286, No.2, (Jan 14), pp.(929-941), 1083-351X (Electronic), 0021-9258 (Linking)

Muzio, M., Ni, J., Feng, P. & Dixit, V.M. (1997). Irak (Pelle) Family Member Irak-2 and Myd88 as Proximal Mediators of Il-1 Signaling. *Science,* Vol. 278, No.5343, (Nov 28), pp.(1612-1615), 0036-8075

Nakayama, M., Abiru, N., Moriyama, H., Babaya, N., Liu, E., Miao, D., Yu, L., Wegmann, D.R., Hutton, J.C., Elliott, J.F. & Eisenbarth, G.S. (2005). Prime Role for an Insulin Epitope in the Development of Type[Thinsp]1 Diabetes in Nod Mice. *Nature,* Vol. 435, No.7039, (May 12), pp.(220-223), 1476-4687 (Electronic), 0028-0836 (Linking)

Nikulina, M.A., Sandhu, N., Shamim, Z., Andersen, N.A., Oberson, A., Dupraz, P., Thorens, B., Karlsen, A.E., Bonny, C. & Mandrup-Poulsen, T. (2003). The Jnk Binding Domain of Islet-Brain 1 Inhibits Il-1 Induced Jnk Activity and Apoptosis but Not the Transcription of Key Proapoptotic or Protective Genes in Insulin-Secreting Cell Lines. *Cytokine,* Vol. 24, No.1-2, (Oct), pp.(13-24), 1043-4666

Noguchi, H., Nakai, Y., Matsumoto, S., Kawaguchi, M., Ueda, M., Okitsu, T., Iwanaga, Y., Yonekawa, Y., Nagata, H., Minami, K., Masui, Y., Futaki, S. & Tanaka, K. (2005). Cell Permeable Peptide of Jnk Inhibitor Prevents Islet Apoptosis Immediately after Isolation and Improves Islet Graft Function. *American Journal of Transplantation,* Vol. 5, No.8, (Aug), pp.(1848-1855), 1600-6143

Norlin, S., Ahlgren, U. & Edlund, H. (2005). Nuclear Factor-Kb Activity in Β-Cells Is Required for Glucose-Stimulated Insulin Secretion. *Diabetes,* Vol. 54, No.1, (Jan 1), pp.(125-132), 0012-1797

Ortis, F., Cardozo, A.K., Crispim, D., Storling, J., Mandrup-Poulsen, T. & Eizirik, D.L. (2006). Cytokine-Induced Proapoptotic Gene Expression in Insulin-Producing Cells Is Related to Rapid, Sustained, and Nonoscillatory Nuclear Factor-{Kappa}B Activation. *Mol Endocrinol,* Vol. 20, No.8, (Aug 1), pp.(1867-1879), 0888-8809

Ortis, F., Pirot, P., Naamane, N., Kreins, A., Rasschaert, J., Moore, F., Théâtre, E., Verhaeghe, C., Magnusson, N., Chariot, A., Ørntoft, T. & Eizirik, D. (2008). Induction of Nuclear Factor-Kb and Its Downstream Genes by Tnf-Α and Il-1β Has a Pro-

Apoptotic Role in Pancreatic Beta Cells. *Diabetologia,* Vol. 51, No.7, (Jul), pp.(1213-1225), 0012-186X

Oyadomari, S., Takeda, K., Takiguchi, M., Gotoh, T., Matsumoto, M., Wada, I., Akira, S., Araki, E. & Mori, M. (2001). Nitric Oxide-Induced Apoptosis in Pancreatic B Cells Is Mediated by the Endoplasmic Reticulum Stress Pathway. *Proceedings of the National Academy of Sciences of the United States of America,* Vol. 98, No.19, (Sep 11), pp.(10845-10850), 0027-8424

Pacher, P., Beckman, J.S. & Liaudet, L. (2007). Nitric Oxide and Peroxynitrite in Health and Disease. *Physiol Rev,* Vol. 87, No.1, (Jan), pp.(315-424), 0031-9333

Pahl, H.L. (1999). Activators and Target Genes of Rel/Nf-Kappab Transcription Factors. *Oncogene,* Vol. 18, No.49, (Nov 22), pp.(6853-6866), 0950-9232

Paige, J.S., Xu, G., Stancevic, B. & Jaffrey, S.R. (2008). Nitrosothiol Reactivity Profiling Identifies S-Nitrosylated Proteins with Unexpected Stability. *Chemistry & Biology,* Vol. 15, No.12, (Dec 22), pp.(1307-1316), 1074-5521

Pavlovic, D., Andersen, N.A., Mandrup-Poulsen, T. & Eizirik, D.L. (2000). Activation of Extracellular Signal-Regulated Kinase (Erk)1/2 Contributes to Cytokine-Induced Apoptosis in Purified Rat Pancreatic Beta-Cells. *European Cytokine Network,* Vol. 11, No.2, (Jun), pp.(267-274), 1148-5493

Perez-Arana, G., Blandino-Rosano, M., Prada-Oliveira, A., Aguilar-Diosdado, M. & Segundo, C. (2010). Decrease in {Beta}-Cell Proliferation Precedes Apoptosis During Diabetes Development in Bio-Breeding/Worcester Rat: Beneficial Role of Exendin-4. *Endocrinology,* Vol. 151, No.6, (Jun 1), pp.(2538-2546), 1945-7170 (Electronic), 0013-7227 (Linking)

Peter, M.E. & Krammer, P.H. (2003). The Cd95(Apo-1/Fas) Disc and Beyond. *Cell Death Differ,* Vol. 10, No.1, (Jan), pp.(26-35), 1350-9047

Petrovsky, N., Silva, D., Socha, L., Slattery, R. & Charlton, B. (2002). The Role of Fas Ligand in Beta Cell Destruction in Autoimmune Diabetes of Nod Mice. *Annals of the New York Academy of Sciences,* Vol. 958, No.1, (Apr), pp.(204-208), 0077-8923

Pileggi, A., Molano, R.D., Berney, T., Cattan, P., Vizzardelli, C., Oliver, R., Fraker, C., Ricordi, C., Pastori, R.L., Bach, F.H. & Inverardi, L. (2001). Heme Oxygenase-1 Induction in Islet Cells Results in Protection from Apoptosis and Improved in Vivo Function after Transplantation. *Diabetes,* Vol. 50, No.9, (Sept), pp.(1983-1991), 0012-1797

Piro, S., Lupi, R., Dotta, F., Patan, G., Rabuazzo, M.A., Marselli, L., Santangelo, C., Realacci, M., Del Guerra, S., Purrello, F. & Marchetti, P. (2001). Bovine Islets Are Less Susceptible Than Human Islets to Damage by Human Cytokines1. *Transplantation,* Vol. 71, No.1, (Jan 15), 0041-1337

Pirot, P., Ortis, F., Cnop, M., Ma, Y., Hendershot, L.M., Eizirik, D.L. & Cardozo, A.K. (2007). Transcriptional Regulation of the Endoplasmic Reticulum Stress Gene Chop in Pancreatic Insulin-Producing Cells. *Diabetes,* Vol. 56, No.4, (Apr), pp.(1069-1077), 0012-1797

Rabinovitch, A., Suarez-Pinzon, W., Shi, Y., Morgan, A. & Bleackley, R. (1994). DNA Fragmentation Is an Early Event in Cytokine-Induced Islet Beta-Cell Destruction. *Diabetologia,* Vol. 37, No.8, (Aug), pp.(733-738), 0012-186X

Rabinovitch, A., Suarez-Pinzon, W., Strynadka, K., Ju, Q., Edelstein, D., Brownlee, M., Korbutt, G.S. & Rajotte, R.V. (1999). Transfection of Human Pancreatic Islets with an Anti-Apoptotic Gene (Bcl-2) Protects Beta-Cells from Cytokine-Induced Destruction. *Diabetes,* Vol. 48, No.6, (Jun), pp.(1223-1229), 0012-1797

Rabinovitch, A. & Suarez-Pinzon, W.L. (1998). Cytokines and Their Roles in Pancreatic Islet [Beta]-Cell Destruction and Insulin-Dependent Diabetes Mellitus. *Biochemical Pharmacology,* Vol. 55, No.8, (April 15, 1998), pp.(1139-1149), 0006-2952

Reddy, S.A.G., Huang, J.H. & Liao, W.S.-L. (1997). Phosphatidylinositol 3-Kinase in Interleukin 1 Signaling. *Journal of Biological Chemistry,* Vol. 272, No.46, (Nov 14), pp.(29167-29173), 0021-9258

Reddy, S.A.G., Lin, Y.-F., Huang, H.J., Samanta, A.K. & Liao, W.S.L. (2004). The Il-1 Receptor Accessory Protein Is Essential for Pi 3-Kinase Recruitment and Activation. *Biochemical and Biophysical Research Communications,* Vol. 316, No.4, (Apr 16), pp.(1022-1028), 0006-291X

Riedl, S.J. & Salvesen, G.S. (2007). The Apoptosome: Signalling Platform of Cell Death. *Nat Rev Mol Cell Biol,* Vol. 8, No.5, (May), pp.(405-413), 1471-0072

Saldeen, J. (2000). Cytokines Induce Both Necrosis and Apoptosis Via a Common Bcl-2-Inhibitable Pathway in Rat Insulin-Producing Cells. *Endocrinology,* Vol. 141, No.6, (Jun), pp.(2003-2010), 0013-7227

Samali, A., Gorman, A.M. & Cotter, T.G. (1996). Apoptosis -- the Story So Far. *Experientia,* Vol. 52, No.10-11, (Oct 31), pp.(933-941), 0014-4754

Samali, A., Zhivotovsky, B., Jones, D., Nagata, S. & Orrenius, S. (1999). Apoptosis: Cell Death Defined by Caspase Activation. *Cell Death Differ,* Vol. 6, No.6, (Jun), pp.(495-496), 1350-9047

Satoh, T., Abiru, N., Kobayashi, M., Zhou, H., Nakamura, K., Kuriya, G., Nakamura, H., Nagayama, Y., Kawasaki, E., Yamasaki, H., Yu, L., Eisenbarth, G., Araki, E., Mori, M., Oyadomari, S. & Eguchi, K. (2011). Chop Deletion Does Not Impact the Development of Diabetes but Suppresses the Early Production of Insulin Autoantibody in the Nod Mouse. *Apoptosis,* Vol. (Apr), pp.(1-11), 1573-675X (Electronic), 1360-8185 (Linking)

Seewaldt, S., Thomas, H.E., Ejrnaes, M., Christen, U., Wolfe, T., Rodrigo, E., Coon, B., Michelsen, B., Kay, T.W. & von Herrath, M.G. (2000). Virus-Induced Autoimmune Diabetes: Most Beta-Cells Die through Inflammatory Cytokines and Not Perforin from Autoreactive (Anti-Viral) Cytotoxic T-Lymphocytes. *Diabetes,* Vol. 49, No.11, (Nov 1), pp.(1801-1809), 0012-1797

Sies, H. (1997). Oxidative Stress: Oxidants and Antioxidants. *Experimental Physiology,* Vol. 82, No.2, (Mar 1), pp.(291-295), 0958-0670

Stassi, G., De Maria, R., Trucco, G., Rudert, W., Testi, R., Galluzzo, A., Giordano, C. & Trucco, M. (1997). Nitric Oxide Primes Pancreatic Beta Cells for Fas-Mediated Destruction in Insulin-Dependent Diabetes Mellitus. *J Exp Med,* Vol. 186, No.8, (Oct 20), pp.(1193-1200), 0022-1007

Steer, S.A., Scarim, A.L., Chambers, K.T. & Corbett, J.A. (2006). Interleukin-1 Stimulates Beta-Cell Necrosis and Release of the Immunological Adjuvant Hmgb1. *PLoS Med,* Vol. 3, No.2, (Feb), pp.(e17), 1549-1676 (Electronic), 1549-1277 (Linking)

Stephanou, A., Brar, B.K., Knight, R.A. & Latchman, D.S. (2000). Opposing Actions of Stat-1 and Stat-3 on the Bcl-2 and Bcl-X Promoters. *Cell Death Differ,* Vol. 7, No.3, (Mar), pp.(329-330), 1350-9047

Stephanou, A., Brar, B.K., Scarabelli, T.M., Jonassen, A.K., Yellon, D.M., Marber, M.S., Knight, R.A. & Latchman, D.S. (2000). Ischemia-Induced Stat-1 Expression and Activation Play a Critical Role in Cardiomyocyte Apoptosis. *Journal of Biological Chemistry,* Vol. 275, No.14, (Apr 7), pp.(10002-10008), 0021-9258

Storling, J., Binzer, J., Andersson, A.K., Zullig, R.A., Tonnesen, M., Lehmann, R., Spinas, G.A., Sandler, S., Billestrup, N. & Mandrup-Poulsen, T. (2005). Nitric Oxide Contributes to Cytokine-Induced Apoptosis in Pancreatic Beta Cells Via Potentiation of Jnk Activity and Inhibition of Akt. *Diabetologia,* Vol. 48, No.10, (Oct), pp.(2039-2050), 0012-186X

Suk, K., Kim, S., Kim, Y.-H., Kim, K.-A., Chang, I., Yagita, H., Shong, M. & Lee, M.-S. (2001). Ifn-Γ/Tnf-A Synergism as the Final Effector in Autoimmune Diabetes: A Key Role for Stat1/Ifn Regulatory Factor-1 Pathway in Pancreatic B Cell Death. *The Journal of Immunology,* Vol. 166, No.7, (Apr 1), pp.(4481-4489), 0022-1767

Szegezdi, E., Logue, S.E., Gorman, A.M. & Samali, A. (2006). Mediators of Endoplasmic Reticulum Stress-Induced Apoptosis. *EMBO Rep,* Vol. 7, No.9, (Sep), pp.(880-885), 1469-221X (Print), 1469-221X (Linking)

Takeda, K. & Akira, S. (2000). Stat Family of Transcription Factors in Cytokine-Mediated Biological Responses. *Cytokine & Growth Factor Reviews,* Vol. 11, No.3, (Sep 2000), pp.(199-207), 1359-6101

Thiel, D.J., le Du, M.H., Walter, R.L., D'Arcy, A., Chène, C., Fountoulakis, M., Garotta, G., Winkler, F.K. & Ealick, S.E. (2000). Observation of an Unexpected Third Receptor Molecule in the Crystal Structure of Human Interferon-[Gamma] Receptor Complex. *Structure,* Vol. 8, No.9, (Sep 15), pp.(927-936), 0969-2126

Thomas, H.E., Darwiche, R., Corbett, J.A. & Kay, T.W. (2002). Interleukin-1 Plus Gamma-Interferon-Induced Pancreatic Beta-Cell Dysfunction Is Mediated by Beta-Cell Nitric Oxide Production. *Diabetes,* Vol. 51, No.2, (Feb), pp.(311-316), 0012-1797

Tiedge, M., Lortz, S., Munday, R. & Lenzen, S. (1998). Complementary Action of Antioxidant Enzymes in the Protection of Bioengineered Insulin-Producing Rinm5f Cells against the Toxicity of Reactive Oxygen Species. *Diabetes,* Vol. 47, No.10, (Oct), pp.(1578-1585), 0012-1797

Turley, S., Poirot, L., Hattori, M., Benoist, C. & Mathis, D. (2003). Physiological Beta Cell Death Triggers Priming of Self-Reactive T Cells by Dendritic Cells in a Type-1 Diabetes Model. *J Exp Med,* Vol. 198, No.10, (Nov 17), pp.(1527-1537), 0022-1007

Vandenabeele, P., Galluzzi, L., Vanden Berghe, T. & Kroemer, G. (2010). Molecular Mechanisms of Necroptosis: An Ordered Cellular Explosion. *Nat Rev Mol Cell Biol,* Vol. 11, No.10, (Oct), pp.(700-714), 1471-0080 (Electronic), 1471-0072 (Linking)

Varadi, A., Molnar, E., Ostenson, C.G. & Ashcroft, S.J. (1996). Isoforms of Endoplasmic Reticulum Ca(2+)-Atpase Are Differentially Expressed in Normal and Diabetic Islets of Langerhans. *Biochem J,* Vol. 319 (Pt 2), (Oct 15), pp.(521-527), 0264-6021

Viner, R.I., Ferrington, D.A., Williams, T.D., Bigelow, D.J. & Schoneich, C. (1999). Protein Modification During Biological Aging: Selective Tyrosine Nitration of the Serca2a

Isoform of the Sarcoplasmic Reticulum Ca2+-Atpase in Skeletal Muscle. *Biochem J*, Vol. 340 (Pt 3), (Jun 15), pp.(657-669), 0264-6021

Wang, B., Andre, I., Gonzalez, A., Katz, J.D., Aguet, M., Benoist, C. & Mathis, D. (1997). Interferon-Gamma Impacts at Multiple Points During the Progression of Autoimmune Diabetes. *Proc Natl Acad Sci U S A*, Vol. 94, No.25, (Dec 9), pp.(13844-13849), 0027-8424

Wang, L., Bhattacharjee, A., Zuo, Z., Hu, F., Honkanen, R.E., Berggren, P.O. & Li, M. (1999). A Low Voltage-Activated Ca2+ Current Mediates Cytokine-Induced Pancreatic Beta-Cell Death. *Endocrinology*, Vol. 140, No.3, (Mar), pp.(1200-1204), 0013-7227

Wang, P., Qiu, W., Dudgeon, C., Liu, H., Huang, C., Zambetti, G.P., Yu, J. & Zhang, L. (2009). Puma Is Directly Activated by Nf-Kappab and Contributes to Tnf-Alpha-Induced Apoptosis. *Cell Death Differ*, Vol. 16, No.9, (Sep), pp.(1192-1202), 1476-5403 (Electronic), 1350-9047 (Linking)

Welsh, N., Eizirik, D.L. & Sandler, S. (1994). Nitric Oxide and Pancreatic Beta-Cell Destruction in Insulin Dependent Diabetes Mellitus: Don't Take No for an Answer. *Autoimmunity*, Vol. 18, No.4, pp.(285-290), 0891-6934

Wesche, H., Henzel, W.J., Shillinglaw, W., Li, S. & Cao, Z. (1997). Myd88: An Adapter That Recruits Irak to the Il-1 Receptor Complex. *Immunity*, Vol. 7, No.6, (Dec), pp.(837-847), 1074-7613

White, N.H., Sun, W., Cleary, P.A., Danis, R.P., Davis, M.D., Hainsworth, D.P., Hubbard, L.D., Lachin, J.M. & Nathan, D.M. (2008). Prolonged Effect of Intensive Therapy on the Risk of Retinopathy Complications in Patients with Type 1 Diabetes Mellitus: 10 Years after the Diabetes Control and Complications Trial. *Archives of Ophthalmology*, Vol. 126, No.12, (Dec), pp.(1707-1715), 1538-3601 (Electronic), 0003-9950 (Linking)

Xu, L., Eu, J.P., Meissner, G. & Stamler, J.S. (1998). Activation of the Cardiac Calcium Release Channel (Ryanodine Receptor) by Poly-S-Nitrosylation. *Science*, Vol. 279, No.5348, (Jan 9), pp.(234-237), 0036-8075

Yamin, T.-T. & Miller, D.K. (1997). The Interleukin-1 Receptor-Associated Kinase Is Degraded by Proteasomes Following Its Phosphorylation. *Journal of Biological Chemistry*, Vol. 272, No.34, (Aug 22), pp.(21540-21547), 0021-9258

Yasukawa, H., Sasaki, A. & Yoshimura, A. (2000). Negative Regulation of Cytokine Signaling Pathways. *Annu. Rev. Immunol.*, Vol. 18, No.1, (Apr), pp.(143-164), 0732-0582

Ye, J. & Laychock, S.G. (1998). A Protective Role for Heme Oxygenase Expression in Pancreatic Islets Exposed to Interleukin-1{Beta}. *Endocrinology*, Vol. 139, No.10, (Oct), pp.(4155-4163), 0013-7227

Youle, R.J. & Strasser, A. (2008). The Bcl-2 Protein Family: Opposing Activities That Mediate Cell Death. *Nat Rev Mol Cell Biol*, Vol. 9, No.1, (Jan), pp.(47-59), 1471-0080 (Electronic), 1471-0072 (Linking)

Zhang, L., Xing, D. & Chen, M. (2008). Bim(L) Displacing Bcl-X(L) Promotes Bax Translocation During Tnfalpha-Induced Apoptosis. *Apoptosis*, Vol. 13, No.7, (Jul), pp.(950-958), 1573-675X (Electronic), 1360-8185 (Linking)

Zhang, P., McGrath, B., Li, S., Frank, A., Zambito, F., Reinert, J., Gannon, M., Ma, K., McNaughton, K. & Cavener, D.R. (2002). The Perk Eukaryotic Initiation Factor 2

Alpha Kinase Is Required for the Development of the Skeletal System, Postnatal Growth, and the Function and Viability of the Pancreas. *Mol Cell Biol,* Vol. 22, No.11, (Jun), pp.(3864-3874), 0270-7306

Zhang, W., Feng, D., Li, Y., Iida, K., McGrath, B. & Cavener, D.R. (2006). Perk Eif2ak3 Control of Pancreatic Beta Cell Differentiation and Proliferation Is Required for Postnatal Glucose Homeostasis. *Cell Metab,* Vol. 4, No.6, (Dec), pp.(491-497), 1550-4131

Zinszner, H., Kuroda, M., Wang, X., Batchvarova, N., Lightfoot, R.T., Remotti, H., Stevens, J.L. & Ron, D. (1998). Chop Is Implicated in Programmed Cell Death in Response to Impaired Function of the Endoplasmic Reticulum. *Genes Dev,* Vol. 12, No.7, (Apr 1), pp.(982-995), 0890-9369

13

A Novel L-Arginine/L-Glutamine Coupling Hypothesis: Implications for Type 1 Diabetes

Paulo Ivo Homem de Bittencourt Jr.[1,2,3] and Philip Newsholme[4]
[1]*Department of Physiology, Institute of Basic Health Sciences, Federal University of Rio Grande do Sul*
[2]*Federal University of Rio Grande do Sul School of Physical Education, Porto Alegre, RS*
[3]*National Institute of Hormones and Women's Health*
[4]*School of Biomolecular and Biomedical Science and Institute for Sport and Health, UCD Dublin, Belfield, Dublin 4*
[1,2,3]*Brazil*
[4]*Ireland*

1. Introduction

L-Arginine is synthesised *in vivo* from L-glutamine, L-glutamate, or L-proline via the intestinal-renal axis (**Fig. 1A**) in humans and most other mammals (Wu et al., 2009). In humans, plasma L-glutamine is the precursor of 80% of plasma L-citrulline while plasma L-citrulline, in turn, is the precursor of 10% of plasma L-arginine (van de Poll et al., 2007). Although the intestine consumes L-glutamine at a high rates, dependent on L-glutamine supply (and production from the skeletal muscle), approximately 13% of L-glutamine taken up by the intestine is converted to L-citrulline, so that quantitatively, L-glutamine is the major precursor for intestinal release of L-citrulline (van de Poll et al., 2007), which can be further converted to L-arginine. These observations highlight the importance of L-arginine/L-glutamine metabolic coupling, especially as L-arginine is one of the most potent secretagogues of insulin from the pancreatic beta cells (Palmer et al., 1976), whereas L-arginine deficiency is associated with insulinopenia and failure to secrete insulin in response to glucose (Spinas et al., 1999). L-Arginine is essential for metabolism and function of multiple body organs, with decreased plasma and cellular levels of L-arginine reported in type 2 diabetic subjects (Pieper & Dondlinger, 1997).

Since L-arginine is the precursor of nitric oxide (NO)*, which serves as a key cell signalling molecule in pancreatic islet β-cells, restriction in the availability of L-arginine is likely to

---

* **Abbreviations used:** CAT, catalase; GSH, glutathione; GSSG, glutathione disulphide; GSPx, glutathione peroxidase; GSRd, glutathione disulphide reductase; HSP70, 70-kDa member of heat shock protein family; eHSP70, extracellular heat shock protein of 70 kDa; IFN-γ, interferon-γ; IκB, a member of the inhibitors of nuclear factor κB; IKK, inhibitor of κB kinase; IL-1β, interleukin-1β; IL1-ra, IL-1β receptor antagonist; iNOS, inducible nitric oxide synthase; NF-κB, a member of nuclear transcription factor κB; NO, nitric oxide free radical (•N=O); PPAR-γ, peroxisome proliferator activated receptor-γ; RNS, reactive nitrogen species; ROS, reactive oxygen species; SNOG, *S*-nitrosoglutathione; SOD,

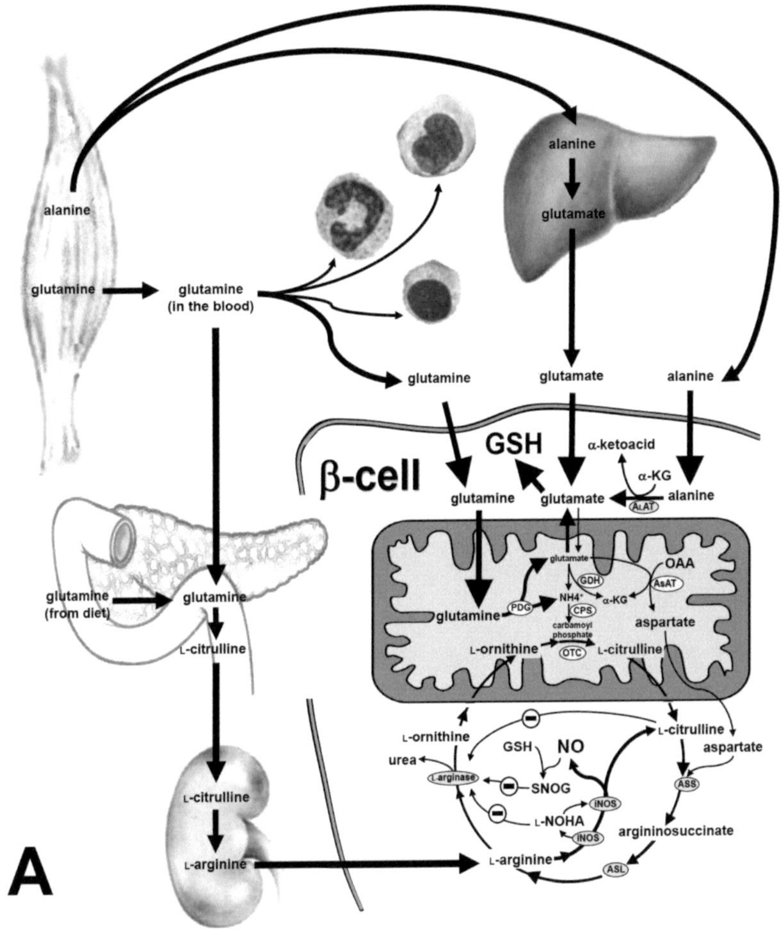

Fig. 1. The l-arginine/l-glutamine coupling hypothesis of insulin-secreting β-cells. (A) Pancreatic islet β-cells utilise l-arginine for the biosynthesis of NO and l-glutamate for GSH generation during secretagogue-stimulated insulin secretion. l-Arginine is provided to the pancreas by the intestinal-renal axis from l-glutamine, while l-glutamate is furnished by the liver mainly from muscle-derived alanine. In the β-cell, NH4+ may contribute to l-arginine biosynthesis, through the concerted action of carbamoyl phosphate synthetase I (CPS), ornithine transcarbamoylase (OTC), argininosuccinate synthetase (ASS) and argininosuccinate lyase (ASL) that eventually produces l-arginine. Skeletal muscle-derived l-glutamine is also substrate for the maintenance of GSH metabolism in β-cells, but rapidly-proliferating cells of the gut as well as immune cells compete with β-cell for the utilisation of l-glutamine. Hence, any minimal reduction in the supply of l-arginine to the pancreas may shift l-glutamate metabolism towards the synthesis of NO instead of GSH, thus leading to oxidative stress, inhibition of insulin secretion and eventually β-cell death. This is the case of undernourishment, cancer states, trauma, sepsis, major burns and low skeletal muscle

---

superoxide dismutase; TBARS, thiobarbituric acid-reactive substances; TNF-α, tumor necrosis factor-α; TNFR, TNF-α receptor; UCP, uncoupling protein-2.

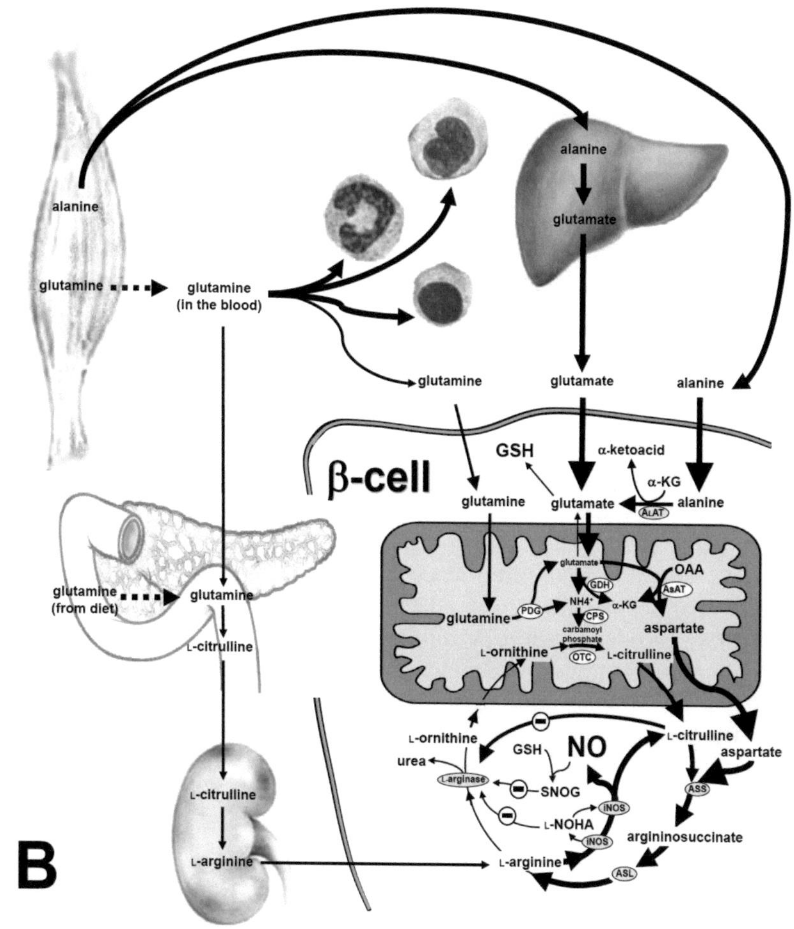

mechanical activity, where blood glutamine stores may be challenged. Metabolic acidosis, by increasing L-glutamine utilisation by the kidney, may also favour glutamine depletion unless enteral supplementation or enhanced physical activity takes place. This is also the case of psychological-stress motivated inflammatory reactions that may underlie by the activation of sympathetic-CRH-histamine system (**Fig. 3**), which ultimately leads to a Th1-centered immune response that augments glutamine utilisation. Therefore, L-glutamine imbalance, by virtue of deficiently supplying L-arginine to the pancreas, deviates β-cell glutamate metabolism from the synthesis of GSH to that of NO, leading to oxidative stress, impairment of insulin release and insulitis. This ongoing inflammation feeds forward NO metabolism, which enhances L-glutamine consumption thus perpetuating this cyclic condition that leads to type 1 diabetes mellitus (T1DM) **(B).** Physical exercise, on the other hand, may improve L-glutamine supply from the skeletal muscle and counteract Th1-mediated inflammation due to the production of type 2 cytokines, such as IL-6. Immunomodulatory action of exercise may also involve heat shock protein production and other anti-inflammatory mediators. Arrow widths indicate the intensity of the metabolic flux through each pathway.

contribute to derangements in the secretion and action of insulin (Newsholme et al., 2009a). Hypertension associated with diabetes is related with a decrease in levels of L-arginine (Spinas, 1999), as are inflammatory conditions characterised by release of L-arginase by activated macrophages (Murphy & Newsholme, 1998). While excessive NO production can trigger oxidative/nitrosative stress and is undoubtedly a key mechanism that results in β-cell death (Newsholme et al., 2009a; Spinas, 1999; Michalska et al., 2010), good evidence now suggests that lesser amounts of cellular NO, produced by the NF-κB-regulated inducible nitric oxide synthase (iNOS, EC 1.14.13.39), encoded by the *NOS-2* gene, serves as an important coupling factor in insulin secreting cells (Newsholme et al., 2009a; Spinas, 1999; Michalska et al., 2010). Recent data from the authors' laboratories has demonstrated that L-arginine is an important stimulator of β-cell glucose consumption and intermediary metabolism (M.S. Krause, N.H. McClenaghan, P.R. Flatt, P.I. Homem de Bittencourt Jr., C. Murphy & P. Newsholme, unpublished results). Such actions lead to increased insulin secretion, enhanced antioxidant and protective responses with greater functional integrity when challenged with pro-inflammatory cytokines. Given that insulin-secreting cells have very low expression levels of antioxidant enzymes, such as catalase (CAT) and glutathione peroxidase (GSPx), β-cells are particularly prone to chemical stress in the diabetogenic or inflammatory environment typical of type 1 and possibly type 2 diabetes (Newsholme et al., 2009a; Spinas, 1999). In fact, the pathogenesis of type 2 diabetes is now recognised to involve both innate and adaptive immunity, since type 2 diabetes is associated with low-grade systemic inflammation, infiltration of adipose tissue and pancreatic islets with $CD8^+$ T lymphocytes that precede invasion by inflammatory macrophages and activation of these cells resulting in pro-inflammatory cytokine secretion (Mandrup-Poulsen, 2010).

In this chapter, we discuss how the continued supply of L-arginine, physiologically provided by the metabolism of L-glutamine via the intestinal-renal axis and from active skeletal muscle (which will be enhanced during exercise) is essential for β-cell functional integrity and indeed for β-cell defence, which will be required to avoid/attenuate islet inflammation associated with the pathogenic mechanisms underlying type 1 and type 2 diabetes (**Fig. 1B**). L-arginine is therefore preserved for essential NO generation and stimulation of glucose metabolism, critical for insulin secretion. Additionally, the role of skeletal muscle (during exercise) on these metabolic processes is discussed.

2. Oxidative metabolism and oxidative stress in β-cells and type 1 diabetes

The intense aerobic metabolism, intrinsic to pancreatic β-cells, exposes these cells to the deleterious effects of high-turnover oxygen-based reactions. In fact, during secretagogue-stimulated insulin secretion, β-cells are associated with accelerated mitochondrial flux of electrons and, consequently, elevated tendency towards reactive oxygen species (ROS) production (Newsholme et al., 2007). However and notably, β-cells present a very low level of expression of antioxidant enzymes such as CAT and GSPx compared with other tissues and this reduced antioxidant activity is associated with significant increases in lipid hydroperoxides, conjugated dienes and protein carbonyls, which are markers for oxidative stress (Santini et al., 1997), so that β-cells are intrinsically prone to oxidative stress.

Moreover, a growing body of evidence indicates that, in the pre-diabetic condition, antioxidant status may be impaired (Rocie et al., 1997). Hence, the low antioxidant defence in certain individuals (even if transiently) may predispose to an enhanced oxidative stress and the eventual β-cell death that categorises the onset of type 1 and type 2 diabetes.

Oxidative stress has long been recognised to play an important role in the development of type 1 diabetes and its subsequent complications (Wierusz-Wysock et al., 1997) which are aggravated due to the low activities of oxygen free radical scavenging enzymes in islet β-cells, especially mitochondrial manganese-type superoxide dismutase (Mn-SOD; Asayama et al., 1986), glutathione peroxidase (GSPx; Malaisse et al., 1982; Mathews & Leiter, 1999) and glutathione disulphide (GSSG) reductase (GSRd; Mathews & Leiter, 1999). Also, the expression of mRNA encoding for several antioxidant enzymes, such as Mn-SOD, cytoplasmic copper-zinc type SOD (Cu/Zn-SOD), GSPx, and catalase (CAT), has been reported to be lower in islets of Langerhans compared with other mouse tissues (Lenzen et al., 1996). Additionally, the administration of antioxidants (nicotinamide, SOD, α-tocopherol, probucol and the 21-aminosteroid lazaroids), as well as oxygen free radical scavengers, have been used in vitro to protect islets from the cytotoxic effects of some pro-inflammatory cytokines (IL-1β, TNFα and INFγ), concurrently providing *in vivo* protection against the development of the autoimmune diabetes process (Nomikos et al., 1986). Conversely, studies on MnSOD and CAT transgenics have shown that protection of islets from oxidative stress does not alter cytokine toxicity (Chen et al., 2005), which indicates that, although related to each other, oxidative stress and cytokine-induced islet toxicity may use specific and diverse pathways to induce β-cell death.

An additional complication to this scenario is the fact that β-cells express mitochondrial uncoupling protein 2 (UCP2) which dissipates the coupling between electron transport from ATP formation favouring O_2^- generation. Since O_2^- anion is a powerful activator of UCP2, a positive feedback mechanism exists in that O2- generation enhances its own formation. This is particularly critical under prolonged hyperglycaemia, where UCP2 activity may be extremely high thus further depressing insulin secretion by β-cells (Newsholme et al., 2007). This situation is probably associated with the development of type 2 diabetes. Furthermore, the high-glucose, high fatty-acid environment created by either insulin-deficiency or insulin-resistance favours the expression of NAD(P)H oxidase with consequently enhanced ROS production and β-cell death (Morgan et al., 2007, Newsholme et al., 2009b).

Type 1 diabetic patients exhibit major defects in antioxidant protection compared with healthy, non-diabetic controls. A significant reduction in total antioxidant status in both plasma and serum samples from these patients is typically observed (Maxwell et al., 1997). Diabetic children show significant reduction in GSH and GSPx in erythrocytes, as well as in plasma α-tocopherol and β-carotene levels (Dominguez et al., 1998). Incubation of rat (Rabinovitch et al., 1992) and human (Rabinovitch et al., 1996) islet cells with a cytotoxic combination of cytokines (IL-1β, TNFα and IFNγ) has been reported as an inducing factor for lipid peroxidation (also known as lipoperoxidation). When individually administered, however, the same cytokines have been shown to inhibit insulin release without any increase in lipid peroxidation or cytodestructive effects in rat islets (Sumoski et al., 1989). Taken together, these findings suggest that cytokine-induced inhibition of insulin release may not be oxygen free radical-mediated, whereas the cytodestructive effects of cytokines on β-cells do appear to involve free radical-mediated events that induce the formation of toxic derivatives within the islets of Langerhans (Suarez-Pinz et al., 1996). This strongly suggests that type 1 cytokines interfere in β-cell metabolism at some point that is intimately related to insulin secretion. But where does reside this extreme sensitivity of β-cells to cytokine signals? The expression of iNOS, necessary for the synthesis of NO during insulin secretion, may provide an explanation.

NO has incontestably been shown to be a physiological regulator of insulin secretion in β-cells, in an elegant experimental protocol designed by Prof. Anne Marie Salapatek's group in Canada and reported in a seminal paper (Smukler et al., 2002). They have also reported that endogenous NO production can be stimulated by glucose, and that this stimulation can be blocked by NOS inhibition, whereas scavenging of NO specifically blocks insulin release stimulated by physiological intracellular concentrations of NO-donors (2 mM), but has no effect on the release stimulated by elevated K^+. It has also been reported that NO donation did not elicit a β-cell intracellular Ca^{2+} ($[Ca^{2+}]_i$) response alone, but was able to potentiate a glucose-induced $[Ca^{2+}]_i$ response. Since NO is a strong heme-reactant, it partially inhibits the mitochondrial respiratory chain by binding to cytochrome *c* and/or cytochrome oxidase. As a consequence, the mitochondrial membrane potential decreases and Ca^{2+} leaves the mitochondria. This is followed by restoration of the mitochondrial membrane potential and Ca^{2+} reuptake by mitochondria (Spinas, 1999). Therefore, overproduction of NO related to inflammatory stimuli may be related to cellular dysfunction but **not** normal levels of NO. As previously argued (Smukler et al., 2002), the precise level of NO is crucial in determining its resultant effect, with low levels being involved in physiological signalling and higher levels becoming cytotoxic (Moncada et al., 1991; Beck et al., 1999). Hence, the supraphysiological elevation of L-arginine, or the application of exogenous NO donors under the condition of already elevated NO, may result in excessive NO production, yielding cytotoxic effects (Smukler et al., 2002).

3. Nuclear factor κB-dependent L-arginine metabolism in β-cells

Pancreatic β-cells have to constantly express NF-κB-regulated iNOS in order to achieve appropriate amounts of NO produced from L-arginine. However, inflammatory cytokines, such as IL-1β and TNF-α, activate NF-κB in rodent and human islet cells (Eizirik & Mandrup-Poulsen, 2001). Contrarily, prevention of NF-κB activation protects pancreatic β-cells against cytokine-induced apoptosis (Giannoukakis et al., 2000; Heimberg et al., 2001). It is impressive that about 70 NF-κB–dependent genes have been currently identified in β-cells, including genes encoding for various inflammatory cytokines and iNOS (Darville & Eizirik, 1998). Remarkably, the expression of *ca.* 50% of the β-cell genes that may be modified after cytokine exposure is secondary to iNOS-mediated NO formation (Kutlu et al., 2003). It is of note that treatment of human, as well as rodent β-cells with purified IL-1β alone is not sufficient to induce apoptosis, but if IL-1β is combined with interferon-γ (IFNγ), β-cells undergo apoptosis after few days in culture (Eizirik & Mandrup-Pouls, 2001). This suggests that an intracellular IFNγ signal must synergise with IL-1β signalling pathways in order to trigger β-cell apoptosis. IFNγ binds to cell surface receptors and activates the Janus tyrosine kinases JAK1 and JAK2. These kinases phosphorylate and activate their downstream transcription factor STAT-1 (for signal transducers and activators of transcription), which dimerises and translocates to the nucleus where binding to γ-activated sites on target genes occurs (Eizirik & Mandrup-Pouls, 2001). STAT-1 mediates the potentiating effect of IFNγ on IL-1β-induced iNOS expression (Darville & Eizirik, 1998). Because excessive activation of JAK/STAT signalling may lead to cell death, STAT transcriptional activity is regulated by multiple negative feedback mechanisms. These include dephosphorylation of JAK and cytokine receptors by cytoplasmic protein-tyrosine phosphatases SHPs (for Src homology 2 domain phosphatases), and inhibition of JAK enzymic activities by the suppressors of cytokine signalling (SOCS) family. Upregulation of either SOCS-1 or SOCS-3 protects β-cells against cytokine-induced cell death in vitro and in vivo (Karlsen et al., 2001; Flodstrom et al., 2003). SOCS-3 also protects insulin-producing cells against IL-1β–mediated apoptosis via NF-κB inhibition (Karlsen et al., 2004). Evidence indicates that the fate of β-cells, after cytokine exposure, depends on the duration and severity of perturbation of key β-cell gene networks.

Besides its activation by cytokines, NF-κB is also a potential target for reactive oxygen/nitrogen species (ROS/RNS). It is noteworthy that NF-κB was the first redox-sensitive eukaryotic transcription factor shown to respond directly to oxidative stress in many types of cells (Dröge, 2002), while its activation leads to the expression of at least a hundred of inducible proteins directly involved in inflammation, such as cyclooxygenase-2 (COX-2), iNOS, TNFα and IL-1β (Moynagh, 2005). Therefore, NF-κB is, at the same time, both a target and an inducer of inflammation and inflammation-induced oxidative stress. In resting (unstimulated) cells, NF-κB dimeric complexes are predominantly found in the cytosol where they are associated with members of the inhibitory IκB family (Moynagh, 2005), so that NF-κB gene products are entirely inducible proteins whose activation is dictated by specific stimuli that activate IκB kinase (IKK) complexes. These stimuli include high intracellular GSSG levels and oxidative stress *per se* (Dröge, 2002). IKKs, in turn, phosphorylate IκB proteins directing them to proteasome-mediated degradation, which sets NF-κB dimers free to bind to DNA in the nucleus.

NF-κB activation is responsible for both initiation and amplification of immune and inflammatory responses in all cells. Actually, NF-κB activation is *sine qua non* for the control of immune and inflammatory responses (Baldwin, 1996; Nakamura et al., 1997; Winyard et al., 1997), and since inflammatory factors, such as pro-inflammatory cytokines, chemokines, adhesion molecules, colony-stimulating factors and inflammatory enzymes, are NF-κB-dependent gene products, dysregulation or aberrant activation of NF-κB could initiate inappropriate autoimmune and inflammatory responses. Conversely, inhibition of NF-κB activation has been argued as a potential therapeutic approach in several immune and inflammatory-related diseases (Chen et al., 1999). This is why cyclopentenone prostaglandins (cp-PGs), which are powerful inhibitors of NF-κB activation (Rossi et al., 2000), are now considered to be the physiological mediators of the "**resolution of inflammation**" (Piva et al., 2005), whereas cp-PG-based pharmacological approaches, *e.g.* LipoCardium technology, which is a liposome contained cp-PG-based formulation specifically directed towards atherosclerotic lesions in arterial walls (Homem de Bittencourt et al., 2007; Gutierrez et al., 2008) have proved to be powerful anti-atherosclerotic strategies (Piva et al., 2005; Ianaro et al., 2003; Homem de Bittencourt Jr., 2007).

Finally, considering that all the known forms of inflammation finish with the formation of naturally-occurring anti-inflammatory agents (e.g. cp-PGs, IL-10), an important question remains as to how does β-cell not resolve inflammation by triggering such responses? A fault in the expression of the anti-inflammatory heat shock proteins may give a clue to this question.

4. Heat shock protein pathways

Heat shock proteins (HSPs) have been found to play a fundamental role in the recovery from multiple stress conditions and to offer protection from subsequent insults (De Maio,

2011). The function of HSPs during stress goes beyond their intracellular localization and chaperone role as they have been detected outside cells activating signaling pathways. Extracellular HSPs are likely to act as indicators of the stress conditions, priming other cells, particularly of the immune system, to avoid the propagation of the insult (see De Maio, 2011 for review). As we shall present below, the delicate balance between the "danger signalling" extracellular HSPs and its intracellular counterparts may dictate pancreatic β-cell response to cytokines and, eventually, the precipitation of diabetes. By regulating L-arginine consumption through iNOS, and, consequently, NO generation, intracellular HSP response (or its deficiency) may unravel unpredicted facets of both type 1 and type 2 diabetes.

Heat shock proteins (HSPs) are a set of highly conserved polypeptides in both eukaryotic and prokaryotic organisms. They are categorised in families according to their molecular sises and include HSP110, HSP100, HSP90, HSP70, HSP60 HSP30 and HSP10 subclasses. By far, the most studied (due to its evident high expression in mammalian cells under stress conditions) and conserved is the 70-kDa family (HSP70), which comprises a number of related proteins whose molecular weights range from 66 to 78 kDa. HSP70 isoforms are encoded by a multigene family consisting presently of, at least, 13 distinct genes in humans so far studied (Kampinga et al., 2009; Henderson, 2010). Human HSP70 is 73% identical to *Drosophila* HSP70 and 47% identical to *E. coli* DnaK (the *E. coli* orthologue of eukaryotic HSP70) while, surprisingly, the nucleotide sequences of the human and *Drosophila* genes are 72% identical and human and *E. coli* genes are 50% identical (Hunt & Morimoto, 1985). HSP70s function as molecular chaperones that facilitate protein transport, prevent protein aggregation during folding, and protect newly synthesised polypeptide chains against misfolding and protein denaturation (Henderson, 2010). While the constitutive form is expressed in a wide variety of cell types at basal levels (being only moderately inducible), the so-called inducible HSP70 forms (which are barely detectable under non-stressful conditions) could be promptly synthesised under a condition of "homeostatic stress", this being any "homeostasis threatening" condition, such as heat, glucose deprivation, lack of growth factors and so forth. Traditionally, research groups indistinctly use HSP70 as a unified term for both inducible (72 kDa, HSP72 encoded by the *HSPA1A* human gene) and constitutive (73 kDa, HSP73 or HSC70, for heat shock cognate protein, encoded by the human *HSPA8* gene whose product differs from *HSPA1A* protein by only 2 amino acids, Kampinga et al., 2009; Tavaria et al., 1996; Arya et al., 2007; Tavaria et al., 1995). However, HSP70 is the preferable form to be used only when one refers to the inducible HSP72 protein encoded by *HSPA1A* gene (Heck et al., 2011).

Many different events can induce HSP expression, among them are environmental, pathological and physiological factors, such as heavy metal exposure, UV radiation, amino acid analogues, bacterial or viral infection, inflammation, cyclo-oxygenase inhibitors (including acetylsalicylic acid), oxidative stress, cytostatic drugs, growth factors, cell differentiation and tissue development, which strongly activate the main eukaryotic heat shock transcription factor, HSF-1, leading to HSP70 expression (Lindquist & Craig, 1988). Physical exercise, even at single low-intensity bouts (Silveira et al., 2007), is able to induce HSP70 expression in different cell types leading to augmented plasma HSP70 concentrations (see Heck et al., 2011 for review). In our hands, rats submitted to swimming sessions of as short as 20 min (2-4% body weight overload, a mild exercise) demonstrate increased HSP72 (mRNA and protein) in circulating monocytes and lymphocytes and in lymph node lymphocytes and peritoneal macrophages, which is paralleled by a rise in plasma HSP70 levels immediately after the exercise (C.M. Schöler, S.P. Scomazzon, P. Renck Nunes, T.G. Heck, P.I. Homem de Bittencourt Jr., unpublished work).

4.1 Intracellular hsp70

Aside the now classical molecular chaperone action, the most remarkable intracellular effect of HSP70s is the inhibition of NF-κB activation, which has profound implications for immunity, inflammation, cell survival and apoptosis. Indeed, HSP70 blocks NF-κB activation at different levels, by inhibiting the phosphorylation of the inhibitor of κB (IκBs), by directly binding to IκB kinase-γ (IKKγ) thus inhibiting tumour necrosis factor-α (TNFα)-induced apoptosis (Ran et al., 2004). In fact, the supposition that HSP70 might act intracellularly as a suppressor of NF-κB pathways has been raised after a number of discoveries in which HSP70 was intentionally induced, such as the suppression of astroglial iNOS expression paralleled by decreased NF-κB activation (Feinstein et al., 1996) and the protection of rat hepatocytes from TNFα-induced apoptosis by treating cells with the NO-donor *S*-Nitroso-*N*-acetylpenicillamine (SNAP), which reacts with intracellular glutathione (GSH) molecules generating *S*-nitrosoglutathione (SNOG) that induces HSP70, and, consequently, HSP70 expression (Kim et al., 1997).

HSP70 confers protection against sepsis-related circulatory mortality via the inhibition of iNOS gene expression in the rostral ventrolateral medulla through the prevention of NF-κB activation, inhibition of IκB kinase activation and consequent inhibition of IκB degradation (Chan et al., 2004). This is corroborated by the finding that HSP72 assembles with hepatocyte NF-κB/IκB complex in the cytosol thus impeding further transcription of NF-κB-depending *TNF-α* and *NOS-2* genes that would worsen sepsis in rats (Chen et al., 2005). This may also be unequivocally demonstrated by treating cells or tissues with HSP70 antisense oligonucleotides that completely reverses the beneficial NF-κB-inhibiting effect of heat shock and inducible HSP70 expression (see, for instance, Kim et al., 1997; Chan et al., 2004). Hence, HSP70 is anti-inflammatory *per se*, when intracellularly located, which also explains why cyclopentenone prostaglandins (cp-PGs) are powerful anti-inflammatory autacoids (Rossi et al., 2000; Homem de Bittencourt & Curi, 2001; Beere, 2004; Gutierrez et al., 2008).

Another striking effect of HSP70 is the inhibition of apoptosis, which occurs via many intracellular downstream pathways (e.g. JNK, NF-κB and Akt) that are both directly and indirectly blocked by HSP70, besides the inhibition of Bcl-2 release from mitochondria (Beere, 2004). Therefore, intracellularly activated HSP70s are cytoprotective and anti-inflammatory by avoiding protein denaturation and excessive NF-κB activation which may be damaging to the cells.

It is strikingly noteworthy that L-glutamine attenuates TNF-α release and enhances HSP72 expression in human peripheral blood mononuclear cells (Wischmeyer et al., 2003). In fact, L-glutamine induces HSP70 expression via *O*-glycosylation and phosphorylation of HSF-1 and Sp1 (Singleton, K.D. & Wischmeyer, P.E., 2008) in a process that is mediated, at least partially, by the increase in the flux through the hexosamine biosynthetic pathway (Hamiel et al., 2009). Also, it has been shown that a single dose of L-glutamine relieve renal ischaemia-reperfusion injury in rats in 24 h by a mechanism associated with enhanced HSP70 expression (Zhang et al., 2009).

4.2 Extracellular hsp70

HSP70s may also be found in the circulation and its presence is associated to oxidative stress. While healthy people usually have low plasma levels of HSP70, the association of increased blood concentrations of such proteins with illness and disease progression has been hypothesised. In this way, oxidative stress, inflammation, cardiovascular disorders and pulmonary fibrosis have been directly correlated with HSP70 concentration in the bloodstream (Ogawa et al., 2008). On the other hand, L-glutamine supplementation, which rises circulating HSP70 levels in critically ill patients, is associated with lower hospital treatment period (Ziegler et al., 2005). Therefore, these studies may suggest that elevation of HSP70 levels could be an important immunoinflammatory response against physiological disorders or disease.

Inasmuch as HSP70s exist in the extracellular space, molecular interactions with cell surface receptors may occur and signalling pathways could be triggered in many cell types, whereas there are a variety of receptors to HSP70 binding, amplifying the possible targets to these extracellular molecules (Calderwood et al., 2007a, 2007b). However, the function of circulating HSP70 is incompletely understood yet. HSP70s are released towards the extracellular space by special mechanisms that include pumping across cell membranes through the highly conserved ABC cassette transport proteins. Recent studies have demonstrated that exosomes provide the major pathway for the vesicular secretory release of HSP70s and that heat stress strikingly enhances the amount of HSP70 secreted per vesicle, but does not influence the efficiency of stress-induced rate of HSP70 release and the number of exosomes neither (Sun et al., 2005; Lancaster & Febbraio, 2005; Multhoff, 2007). A similar profile was observed in our hands (T.G. Heck; P. Renck Nunes; S.P. Scomazzon & P.I. Homem de Bittencourt Jr., manuscript in preparation), in which lymph node lymphocytes from exercised rats submitted to a further (other than the exercise bouts) challenge (heat shock) presented an HSP70 accumulation into the culture medium that is dependent on previous exercise load. Apparently, systemic extracellular HSP70 (eHSP70) could arise from many tissues and different cell types and this may involve distinct mechanisms of release (including necrosis) and a large variety of inducing factors (Mambula et al., 2007). Finally, HSP72 is clearly the major component of the secreted eHSP70 found in the circulation, although recent evidence suggests that other forms may also be released into the blood, as recently pointed out by De Maio (2011). eHSP70 has been shown to bind to type 2 and 4 toll-like receptors (TLR2 and TLR4) on the surface of antigen-presenting cells (APCs) similarly to lipopolysaccharides (LPS), inducing the production of the pro-inflammatory cytokines IL-1β and TNF-α, as well as NO (a product with prominent anti-microbial activity), in an NF-κB-dependent fashion (Ao et al., 2009; Asea, 2003; Asea, 2008).

Taken together, the above findings suggest that the body must attain a precise equilibrium between pro-inflammatory eHSP70 and anti-inflammatory intracellular HSP70 production in order to avoid chronic non-resolved inflammations, such as those observed in sepsis and during the onset of type 1 diabetes. However, why such a balance is not achieved in these illnesses is a matter of intense study.

4.3 Heat shock proteins and exercise

As recently reviewed (Heck et al., 2011), physical exercise and its inherent physiological alterations induce HSP70 expression in many tissues and cell types, not only in the muscle cells. The breakdown of cell homeostasis produced by modifications in temperature, pH, ion concentrations, oxygen partial pressure, glycogen/glucose availability, and ATP depletion are among the factors that activate HSP70 synthesis during exercise (Noble et al., 2008). Rise in core and muscle temperature during exercise seems an obvious way to induce HSP70. However, while skeletal muscle sustains HSP70 expression in the absence of heat stimulus, the heart is not able to do the same, thus suggesting that the mechanisms of HSP70 protein synthesis are specifically driven in each tissue (Harris & Starnes, 2001; Skidmore et al., 2005; Morton et al., 2007; Staib et al., 2007) and that augmented temperature is insufficient to elicit HSP70 synthesis during exercise. Moreover, the susceptibility of tissues to be stressed by the environmental changes elicited by exercise varies enormously and other protective pathways may be activated in the heart, as we have shown for MRP/GS-X pump ATPases whose expression seems to prevent HSP70 expression in the cardiac muscle after exercise bouts (Krause et al., 2007). In spite of free radicals may be produced under normal conditions, a burst in reactive oxygen species does occur during exercise (Fisher-Wellman & Bloomer, 2009). Besides enzymatic and non-enzymatic antioxidant apparatus, studies in both animal models and humans implicate HSP70s as a complementary protection against oxidative damage (Smolka et al., 2000; Silmar et al., 2007; Hamilton et al., 2003), particularly because HSP70s may recover oxidatively denatured proteins. After an acute exercise session, skeletal muscle (Hernando & Manso, 1997), cardiac muscle (Locke et al., 1995) and other tissues, such as the liver (Gonzalez & Manso, 2004; Kregel & Moseley, 1996), have shown a state of oxidative stress, concomitantly to high concentrations of intracellular HSP70 (Salo et al., 1991). Even though oxidative stress is a strong factor to induce HSP70s in response to exercise, free radical production is not the only pathway involved in this process, since sexual hormones and adrenergic stimuli may modulate HSP70 response (Parro & Noble, 1999; Paroo et al., 2002a, 2002b; Paroo et al., 1999) and circulating monocytes from acutely exercised rats do not show appreciable changes in erythrocyte glutathione disulphide (GSSG) to glutathione (GSH) ratio (an index of intracellular redox status) and plasma thiobarbituric acid-reactive substances (TBARS), even in a state of high-profile synthesis of hydrogen peroxide (Silveira et al., 2007).

More recently, however, it has been demonstrated the presence of HSP70s in the circulation in response to exercise (Walsh et al., 2001). Since exercise is able to induce high concentrations of HSP70s in both muscle and plasma, the most obvious hypothesis was, primarily, that skeletal muscle should be the releaser of HSP70 during exercise. However, further studies have revealed that this is not the case, at all. Postural muscles express high levels of HSP70s under basal conditions, which has led to the belief in a preventive role for these proteins against muscle damage through the stabilization of ionic channels (Tupling et al., 2007), as well as myotube development (Kayani et al., 2008). HSP70s were also believed to be an important way to preserve low twitch (oxidative) muscle phenotype after frequent activation, as in physical training (Kelly et al., 1996; Murlasits et al., 2006). Preservation of intracellular muscular function during different exercises, venous-arterial HSP70 differences in different territories (Febbraio et al., 2002a), and the lack of evidence supporting the proposition that the muscle could be the major source of circulatory eHSP70 precluded the 'muscle hypothesis' and suggested that other tissues/cells should be responsible for the increase of eHSP70 in the circulation. Once HSP70 protein release from the muscle to the extracellular fluid could eventually happen by lysis process, and considering that the lysis of muscle fibre occurs only under severe cellular stress condition, the presence of eHSP70 during moderate exercise, as we normally employ, was found to be unfeasible. Though it had been shown that both the intensity and duration of exercise have effects in plasma eHSP70 (Fehrenbach et al., 2005) and muscle (Milne & Noble, 2002) HSP70 immunocontents, this rise in circulating levels of eHSP70 precedes, however, any gene or protein expression of HSP70 in skeletal muscle (Febbraio et al., 2002b), which is another strong argument against the 'muscle hypothesis'. As stated above, other tissues synthesise HSP70s during physiological challenges to the homeostasis, as in an acute physical exercise bout. In this way, after treadmill exercise protocol, the rat liver has been found to enhance the expression of HSP70s (Gonzalez & Manso, 2004). Moreover, and finally, in a human study featuring leg and hepatosplanchnic venous-arterial eHSP70 difference in response to exercise it was unequivocally demonstrated that the contracting muscle does not contribute to eHSP70 circulating levels, while hepatosplanchnic viscera release eHSP70 from undetectable levels at rest to 5.2 pg/min after 120 min of exercise (Febbraio et al., 2002a). Additional studies have shown that oral glucose administration may exclusively reduce HSP70 release from the liver without any effect on muscle glycogen content or intracellular expression of HSP70 (Febbraio et al., 2004). Taken together, these results suggest that other cells may release eHSP70 during exercise, as verified during an experiment that analysed cerebral venous-arterial HSP70 difference (Lancaster et al., 2004). Although the liver seems to participate in this process, the nature of eHSP70-releasing cell(s) during exercise remains to be established.

4.4 HSP70 and glucose/insulin status

Intracellular HSP70 expression produces a clear anti-inflammatory effect by knocking down the expression of pro-inflammatory NF-κB-dependent pathways. However, the activation of HSP70 pathways produces a much more delicate effect. Accordingly, in obese insulin-resistant mice, chronic heat shock treatment has been shown to dramatically reduce insulin resistance by HSP72-specific prevention of c-Jun N-terminal Kinase (JNK) phsophorylation, an effect which is also observed in high-fat fed $HSP72^{+}/^{+}$ transgenic mice (Chung et al., 2008). Also, elevated expression of HSP70 has also been found in circulating mononuclear cells from type 2 diabetic patients (Yabunaka et al., 1995), which, as discussed above, is a immunoinflammatory disease as well. On the other hand, in rat islets, L-glutamine, which is an activator of HSF-1, was shown to attenuate ischaemic injury through the induction of HSP70 (Jang et al., 2008). Moreover, the well known inhibitory effect of IL-1β and TNF-α (alone or combined) on insulin secretion may be completely prevented by a 1-h heat shock (42°C) pre-treatment of both human and rat islets (Scarim et al., 1998). These authors have also shown that the protective effects of heat shock on islet metabolic function are associated with the inhibition of IL-1β- and TNFα-stimulated NF-κB nuclear localization and the consequent iNOS expression. Conversely, NO was found to be one of the triggers of HSP70 expression in human islets (Scarim et al., 1998), which is similar to that previously encountered by Kim et al. (1997), who described a protective effect of NO (via the formation of SNOG that induces HSP70) in rat hepatocytes against TNFα-induced apoptosis. Moreover, J-type cyclopentenone prostaglandins (cp-PGs), which are the most powerful anti-inflammatory substances ever known (see Gutierrez et al., 2008 for review) and natural ligands of peroxisome-proliferator activated receptor-γ (PPAR-γ; Forman et al., 1995; Kliewer et al., 1995), are the strongest inducers of HSP70 expression and consequent NF-κB blockade, a pattern that is shared with synthetic antidiabetic thiazolidinediones (TZDs), such as rosiglitazone, pioglitazone, troglitazone, and ciglitazone (see Zingarelli & Cook, 2005, for review).

The above observations point out again to the importance of poised L-arginine-dependent NO production by β-cells in order to achieve an optimum of HSP70 expression, which may, in turn, allow iNOS expression (needed to NO-assisted insulin secretion) but not at exaggerated ratios that culminate with β-cell death and failure in insulin secretion. In fact, physical exercise, which may also present an anti-inflammatory effect by virtue of its ability to induce the expression of HSP70, is inversely associated with L-arginine utilisation by β-cell iNOS (Atalay et al., 2004). Furthermore, a dramatic scenario does exist in that the susceptibility to oxidative damage to β-cells in type 1 diabetes is associated to the impairment of HSP70-induced cytoprotection, while endurance training may offset some of the adverse effects of diabetes by upregulating tissue HSP70 expression (Atalay et al., 2004). Indeed, in many, if not all, severe inflammatory manifestations of acute nature, such as sepsis or insulitis, the stage of HSP70-based "resolution of inflammation" is simply not seen at all. For instance, in the serum of septic patients with highly oxidative profile (whose prognosis is death), it is observed 30-fold increase in serum HSP70 (eHSP70) compared with control subjects (Gelain et al., 2011), whereas the amount of intracellular HSP70 expressed in the cells of such subjects is, as a rule, lower that that expected. Corroborating this proposition, the expression of HSP70 by pancreatic islets from diabetes-prone BB rats has been found to be lower than that in diabetic-resistant LEW rats of same age and, in the diabetes-prone BB rats, HSP70 expression has shown to be much lower in young as compared to adult animals (Wachlin et al., 2002). Since intracellular HSP70 functions as a potent anti-inflammatory cellular tool due to the impairment over NF-κB downstream pathways, a deficient HSP70 may threaten β-cell survival (see Hooper & Hooper, 2005, for review).

Results from our group have also shown that, besides a reduction in peripheral insulin resistance, heat shock treatment (which also enhances HSP70 export towards the plasma) may impair insulin action under hypoglycaemic conditions in the rat model (M.S. Ludwig.; V.C. Mingueti; P. Renck Nunes; T.G. Heck; R.B. Bazotte & Homem de Bittencourt, P.I. Jr., manuscript in preparation) so that HSP70 balance seems to be crucial for glucose-insulin homeostasis. Now, we are currently evaluating the possibility that exercise may stimulate Th2-based immune response and protect β-cells from pro-inflammatory cytokine pathways through HSP70 induction, which, ultimately, may prevent type 1 diabetes. Since **a)** L-glutamine is a major precursor of L-arginine, which is capital for β-cell survival, **b)** L-arginine-dependent moderate NO synthesis induces HSP70 and **c)** physical exercise is able of directly inducing HSP70 and of enhancing L-glutamine production by the skeletal muscle, both exercise and/or L-glutamine supplementation are argued as preventive agents against the installation of type 1 diabetes by re-establishing the HSP70 equilibrium between the intra and extracellular spaces, as previously hypothesised (Krause & Homem de Bittencourt, 2008).

5. Participation of L-arginine/L-glutamine coupling in diabetes

From the above discussion, it seems clear that the development of diabetes is not simply a question of cytokine imbalance culminating in a redox disruption and consequent oxidative stress that disrupts or kills β-cells. This, in fact, raises another question: is beta cell susceptibility to stress solely a question of compromised antioxidant defence? If this were the case, it would appear preposterous that such a sophisticated cell remains prone to endogenously-generated NO-mediated self-destruction. The intricate metabolism of L-arginine in β-cells may unravel some important points in this regard.

In β-cells, pro-inflammatory cytokines induce the production of NO, synthesised from L-arginine, via a reaction catalysed by iNOS, whose functionality depends on NF-κB-driven gene transcription and *de novo* enzyme synthesis. iNOS also utilises NADPH and O_2 as co-substrates (**Fig. 1A**) and, physiologically, L-arginine is the limiting substrate for NO production. In addition to this, pancreatic β-cells express another L-arginine-metabolising enzyme, *i.e.* L-arginase (L-arginine amidinohydrolase, EC 3.5.3.1), which allows for the completion of urea production through the formation of L-ornithine and urea from L-arginine (Cunningham et al., 1997). Physiologic levels of L-arginase gene expression and activity have been measured in rat β-cells and the insulin-secreting cell line RINm5F (Cunningham et al., 1997; Malaisse et al., 1989; Cardozo et al., 2001; Rieneck et el., 2000). β-Cells express both the cytosolic (L-arginase I) and the mitochondrial (L-arginase II) isoforms of the enzyme. Therefore, under certain circumstances, a true competition may occur in that the activity of iNOS relative to L-arginase dictates either NO or urea production in the pancreas (compare **Fig. 1A and 1B**). Consequently, L-arginase may impair NO production by limiting the availability of L-arginine for iNOS catalysis (Wu & Morris, 1998; Boucher et al., 1999; Mori & Gotoh, 2000). This notion is supported by the finding that inhibition of L-arginase results in enhanced NO synthesis in cytokine-activated cells (Chang et al., 1998; Tenu et al., 1999).

It has been demonstrated that cytokine-elicited co-induction of both NO (iNOS) and urea (argininosuccinate synthetase and argininosuccinate lyase) metabolic pathways occurs in many cell types (Nussler et al., 1994; Hattori et al., 1994; Nagasaki et al., 1996), including β-cells (Flodstrom et al., 1995), *in vitro* as well as *in vivo*. L-Arginase activity may be increased in peritoneal macrophages after exposure to LPS (Currie, 1978), while wound and peritoneal macrophages convert L-arginine to L-citrulline and L-ornithine at comparable rates, indicating that both iNOS and L-arginase pathways are functional (Granger et al., 1990). In clonal β-cells, IL-1β increases L-arginase activity with concomitant increase in NO production (Cunningham et al., 1997), which suggests a kind of coordinated regulation of L-arginase and iNOS in these cells.

There is also evidence for a reciprocal regulation of NOS and L-arginase during immune responses via the antagonistic effects of cytokines released from Th1 and Th2 lymphocytes. While L-arginase activity may be induced by the "anti-inflammatory" Th2 cytokines IL-4, IL-6, IL-10, and IL-13 (Modolell et al., 1995; Waddington et al., 1998; Munder et al., 1999; Wei et al., 2000), the Th1-derived "pro-inflammatory" cytokine IFNγ increases iNOS expression and activity, both alone and in synergy with other pro-inflammatory cytokines, such as IL-1β and TNFα (Gill et al., 1996). Reciprocal effects of Th1- and Th2-derived cytokines on L-arginase and iNOS activities have also been shown by the treatment of murine macrophages with cytokines (Modolell et al., 1995; Corraliza et al., 1995), and by co-culturing murine macrophages with Th1 and Th2 T-cell clones (Munder et al., 1998). In mouse bone marrow-derived macrophages, iNOS and L-arginase activities are regulated reciprocally by Th1 and Th2 cytokines, a strategy that guarantees a precise and efficient production of NO (Modolell et al., 1995).

Because of the above statements, a Th1/Th2 lymphocyte dichotomy has been proposed to play a central role in the pathogenesis of type 1 diabetes (Rabinovitch & Suarez-Pinzon, 1998), whereas evidence suggests that the progression of the disease correlates with a Th1-type immune response (Currie, 1978; Granger et al., 1990; Simmons et al., 1996). Increased generation of NO following cytokine-elicited iNOS induction during insulitis may contribute to β-cell destruction (Modolell et al., 1995; Morris et al., 1998). Therefore, competition between L-arginase and iNOS may be particularly important in protecting β-cells against the establishment of type 1 diabetes.

That macrophages exposed to LPS and IFNγ increase iNOS expression and NO production is well known. A novel clue for the understanding of NO-mediated β-cell damage is that

N^G-hydroxy-L-arginine (L-NOHA), an intermediate in the biosynthesis of NO, is a potent competitive inhibitor of L-arginase I (Boucher et al., 1994; Daghigh et al., 1994). Indeed, substantial amounts of this metabolite are released by LPS-treated rat alveolar macrophages (Hecker et al., 1995), while inhibition of L-arginase by L-NOHA may ensure sufficient availability of L-arginine for high-output production of NO in activated cells. L-Citrulline, the co-product of iNOS catalysis, and *S*-nitrosoglutathione (SNOG), an adduct produced by the reaction of NO with GSH, are also inhibitors of L-arginase in many cell types (Daghigh et al., 1994; Knowles & Moncada, 1994), including β-cells (Cunningham et al., 1997). Hence, intermediates of NO synthesis, as well as NO itself, precisely coordinate a maximum of flux through iNOS in insulin-producing pancreatic cells (**Fig. 1**). Conversely, dexamethasone and dibutyryl cAMP block both iNOS and L-arginase expression, which is paralleled by a strong decrease of NO production (Gotoh & Mori, 1999). Additionally, macrophages treated with LPS and IFNγ undergo NO-dependent apoptosis, which may be prevented by L-arginase DNA plasmid transfection (Gotoh & Mori, 1999). In such cells, L-arginase I and II seem to play a role in determining the route(s) for NO-elicited outcomes.

Competition between L-arginase and iNOS has also been found in activated murine macrophages incubated with another L-arginase inhibitor, nor-L-NOHA (Tenu et al., 1999). Contrarily, L-arginase induction by the type 2 cytokines IL-4 or IL-13 has been shown to inhibit macrophage NO synthesis due to increased L-arginine utilisation by L-arginase (Rutschman et al., 2001). Similar results have been obtained by using different cell types (Gotoh & Mori, 1999; Hecker et al., 1995). In β-cells, both L-arginase I, the major isoform expressed in rodent pancreas, and L-arginase II, the main human isoform, seem to reciprocally regulate iNOS-dependent NO production under physiological L-arginine concentrations (Wu & Morris, 1998; Stickings et al., 2002; Castillo et al., 1993), which suggests that islet L-arginase may be able to compete with iNOS *in vivo*, where L-arginine ranges at non-saturating concentrations for both enzymes. This fact may be of relevance for β-cells during Th1-driven insulitis, since L-arginine concentrations are likely to be reduced at sites of inflammation due to the release of soluble L-arginase from infiltrating macrophages (Albina et al., 1990). Corroborating this proposition is the fact that IL-1β-induction of NO synthesis in RINm5F insulin secreting β-like cells is accompanied by a reduced flux of L-arginine through L-arginase, an effect that appears to be mediated by L-NOHA (Cunningham et al., 1997). Hence, it is likely that, following immune cell-elicited NO production via iNOS, L-NOHA inhibits islet L-arginase activity to some degree *in vivo*, which may be strongly exacerbated by the pro-inflammatory cytokine IL-1β that inhibits L-arginase expression in β-cells (Cardozo et al., 2001; Rieneck et al., 2000). In fact, a remarkable reduction in L-arginase expression has been recently observed during insulitis in the NOD mouse model of type 1 diabetes (Rothe et al., 2002).

In the β-cell, $NH4^+$ may contribute to L-arginine biosynthesis, through the concerted action of carbamoyl phosphate synthetase I, ornithine transcarbamoylase, argininosuccinate synthetase and argininosuccinate lyase that produce L-arginine (**Fig. 1B**). L-Glutamate is also believed to amplify glucose-induced insulin secretion in a K_{ATP} channel-independent way (Brennan et al., 2003). However, L-glutamate is, at the same time, an obligatory substrate for GSH synthesis, which, in turn, enhances the ATP/ADP ratio by optomising mitochondrial function and scavenges ROS/RNS leading to insulin secretion. L-alanine, may replenish the β-cell L-glutamate pool via an L-alanine aminotransferase-catalysed reaction. This explains why L-alanine is cytoprotective to β-cells against cytokine-induced apoptosis (Cunningham et al., 2005), *i.e.*, under cytokine-stimulated NO production,

L-alanine may provide L-glutamate for GSH synthesis thus avoiding oxidative stress and NO-induced apoptosis.

Since, as discussed above, β-cells have poor NADPH-dependent GSSG reductase (GSRd) activity, necessary to regenerate GSH from GSSG in situations of oxidative stress, and NADPH production from the hexose monophosphate shunt is limited because β-cell glycolytic activity is committed to mitochondrial ATP production during glucose-stimulated insulin release, *de novo* GSH biosynthesis from L-glutamate becomes crucial for insulin release and avoidance of β-cell death. Hence, it is easy to envisage that any metabolic disequilibrium in providing L-arginine for NO-assisted insulin secretion, during secretagogue-stimulated insulin release, forces β-cell metabolism to utilise L-glutamine-derived L-glutamate to synthesise GSH, thus ensuring little L-glutamate can undergo oxidative deamination via glutamate dehydrogenase (GDH) in these conditions. The kidney is considered to be the physiological producer of L-arginine since it is the only organ known to take up L-citrulline released from the metabolism of L-glutamine in the gut and release L-arginine into the blood (**Fig. 1 and 2**), although other tissues strongly express argininosuccinate synthetase and lyase but without any net delivery to the circulation (Vermeulen et al., 2007). In fasted humans, the contribution of L-glutamine via L-citrulline to the *de novo* synthesis of L-arginine is about 65% in neonates, where the gut is the major source of systemic L-arginine, even though some residual production in the adult gut could be accounted for by L-arginine release as well (Vermeulen et al., 2007). A minor part of circulating L-arginine may also be provided by the enterocyte metabolism of proline, as stated in the Introduction. Consequently, if, by any chance, the flux through the coupled L-glutamine/L-arginine pathway between intestine and kidney is reduced or lost, then the knock on consequences for NO synthesis are severe (**Fig. 1**). L-Glutamate, however, is a unique source of GSH in β-cells, so that a disruption or hypofunctionality of intestinal-renal L-glutamine/L-arginine axis, would promptly decrease GSH synthesis thus reducing insulin release, leading to oxidative stress and β-cell death. On the other hand, L-glutamine which is a major and immediate L-glutamate precursor, is also a primary nutrient for the maintenance of immune cell function (Curi et al., 1999; Newsholme et al., 2003; Pithon-Curi et al., 2004). Hence, we believe that an immune response triggered by an immune or chemical challenge in a redox-sensitive subject (in which the expression/activity of antioxidant and GSH enzymes is low) might decrease the availability of L-glutamine for GSH generation in β-cells, leading to oxidative stress (**Fig. 1B**). Analogously, it seems likely that other situations, in which the circulating L-glutamine pool is severely endangered (Curi et al., 1999; Newsholme et al., 1987; Lagranha et al., 2008), such as in undernourishment, strenuous-exercise or cancer cachexia-associated muscle loss, chronic inflammatory diseases (including obesity), severe metabolic acidosis, major burns, polytrauma and bacteremia, should result in β-cell dysfunction.

L-Glutamine deficiency can occur during periods of critical illness. In patients with catabolic diseases, plasma and muscle L-glutamine levels are dramatically reduced, which correlates with the poor prognosis and high degree of protein catabolism in those patients. For instance, in patients with major burn injury, plasma L-glutamine concentration is lower than 50% of that in normal controls and it remains low for at least 21 days after the injury (Parry-Billings et al., 1990). Conversely, in LPS-endotoxemic rats, a single dose of L-glutamine, which is known to induce anti-inflammation via HSP70 expression (Wischmeyer et al., 2003; Singleton, K.D. & Wischmeyer, P.E., 2008; Hamiel et al., 2009; Zhang et al., 2009) has been shown to attenuate the release of TNFα and IL-1β and to be associated with a significant decrease in mortality due to the attenuation of pro-inflammatory type 1 cytokines (Wischmeyer et al., 2001), whereas L-arginine-enriched diet limits plasma and muscle L-glutamine depletion in head-injured rats (Moinard et al., 2006). Remarkably, however, **predominately Th1** (but not Th2) cell responses require the presence of optimal concentrations of L-glutamine (Chang et al., 1999). Since β-cell death that accompanies the onset of type 1 diabetes is an essentially Th1-elicited cytotoxic challenge, it is not unreasonable to suppose that the specific recruitment of Th1 cells may greatly enhance L-glutamine and L-arginine utilisation leading to an L-arginine deficit, which causes a reduction of insulin release and redox imbalance.

The positive actions of L-arginine on viability, antioxidant status and insulin secretion are likely to reflect, in large part, the importance of GSH and the glutathione disulphide (GSSG) reductase systems as the main lines of antioxidant defence in β-cells which are characterised by low levels of CAT and GSPx. In order to adequately provide GSH, β-cells may either regenerate GSH from GSSG via a GSSG reductase-catalysed reaction or synthesise it, *de novo*, through the concerted action of γ-glutamylcysteine synthetase (γ-GCS) and GSH synthetase, which are ATP-consuming enzymes (see **Fig. 2** for metabolic schemes). Regeneration of GSH from GSSG, which utilises NADPH as a co-factor but does not require ATP, is metabolically less expensive than the *de novo* synthesis from the constituent amino acids (L-glutamate, L-cysteine and L-glycine). However, unlike the majority of cell types, pentose phosphate shunt activity is relatively low in β-cells (Dröge, 2002), which is exacerbated by the high flux of glucose directed towards ATP production (Spinas, 1999). Therefore, β-cell NADPH must be obtained from the cytosolic malic enzyme (**Fig. 2B**), capable of converting malate to pyruvate with the concomitant production of NADPH from $NADP^+$ (MacDonald, 1995). *De novo* GSH synthesis, on the other hand, is completely dependent on the supply of L-glutamate, not only because this amino acid is a constituent of the GSH molecule, but also because L-glutamate acts as an amino acid donor in the synthesis of serine, which can subsequently, be converted to L-glycine, via a reaction requiring tetrahydrofolate.

We have found that L-arginine significantly increased glucose consumption in β-cells, while decreasing lactate formation, regardless the presence or not of pro-inflammatory cytokines, (unpublished results, also see **Fig. 2B**). This may suggest that L-arginine is able to divert glucose from mitochondrial CO_2 production towards the formation of NADPH via the cytosolic malic enzyme so requiring that glucose-derived malate is transported from the mitochondrial matrix to the cytosol. Indeed, we believe that, in the presence of L-arginine, L-glutamate can be generated from both L-arginine and glucose (via 2-oxoglutarate formation and transamination) and is subsequently utilised for GSH synthesis (please, compare **Fig. 2B and 2C**). L-Arginine addition enhances the conversion of AMPK into its active phosphorylated form, thus favoring fatty acid oxidation and ATP synthesis while glucose metabolism is supporting malate formation and L-glutamate formation for NADPH and GSH generation respectively. This requirement, however, results in a reduction in stimulus-secretion coupling and the associated insulin release.

We have also observed that NOS-2 expression is stimulated by the cytokine cocktail (which enhances iNOS activity) but NO synthesis was not enhanced by changing L-arginine in the culture medium. This suggests that iNOS is saturated with L-arginine which, in turn, results in elevated urea production. This shunt in L-arginine metabolism efficiently preserves β-cell redox status by favoring the production of GSH in conditions which generate excessive levels of NO (**Fig. 2C and 2D**).

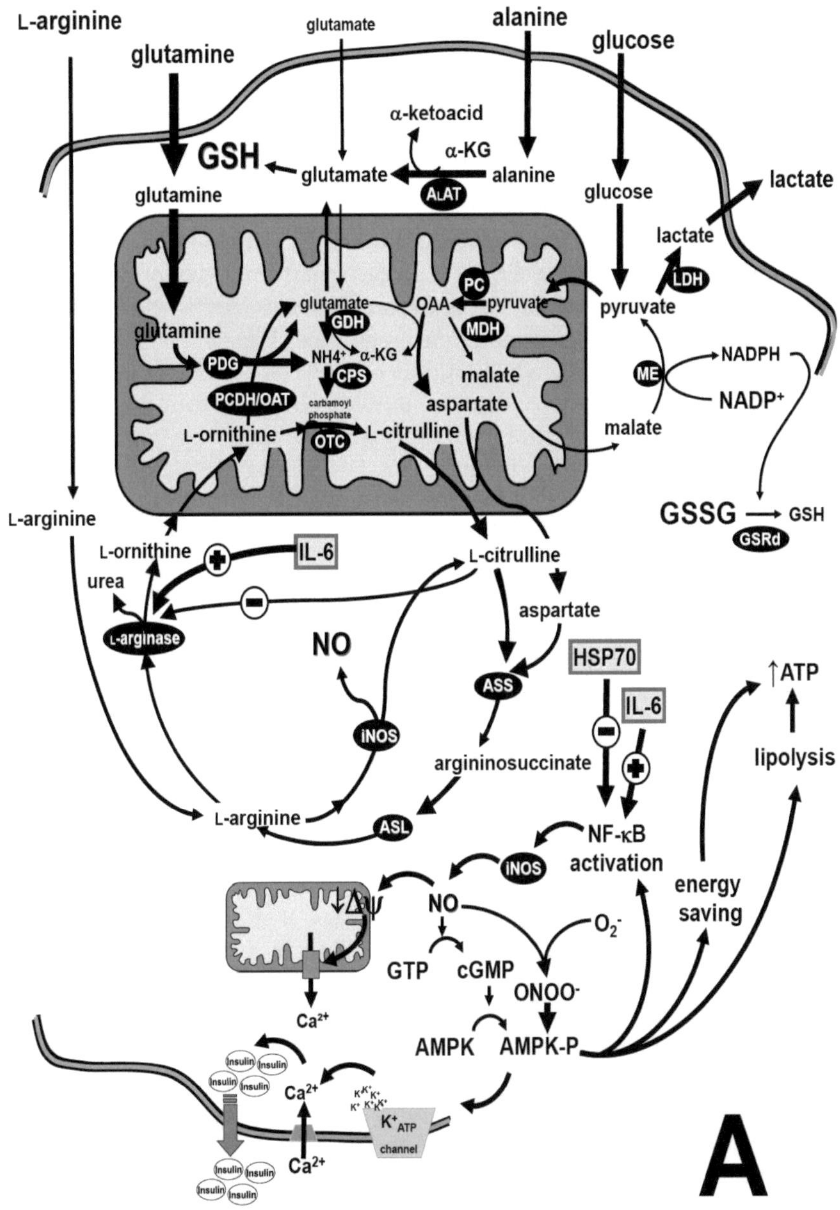
L-arginine
glutamine
glutamate
alanine
glucose
α-ketoacid
α-KG
GSH
glutamate
alanine
ALAT
glutamine
glucose
lactate
lactate
LDH
PC
pyruvate
OAA
pyruvate
glutamate
GDH
MDH
glutamine
PDG
NH4+
α-KG
CPS
malate
ME
NADPH
NADP+
PCDH/OAT
carbamoyl phosphate
aspartate
malate
L-ornithine
OTC
L-citrulline
L-arginine
GSSG
GSH
GSRd
L-ornithine
IL-6
L-citrulline
urea
aspartate
L-arginase
NO
HSP70
ASS
IL-6
↑ATP
iNOS
lipolysis
argininosuccinate
L-arginine
ASL
NF-κB
activation
iNOS
energy
saving
ΔΨ
NO
O2-
GTP
cGMP
ONOO-
Ca2+
AMPK
AMPK-P
Insulin
Ca2+
K+ATP
channel
Ca2+
A

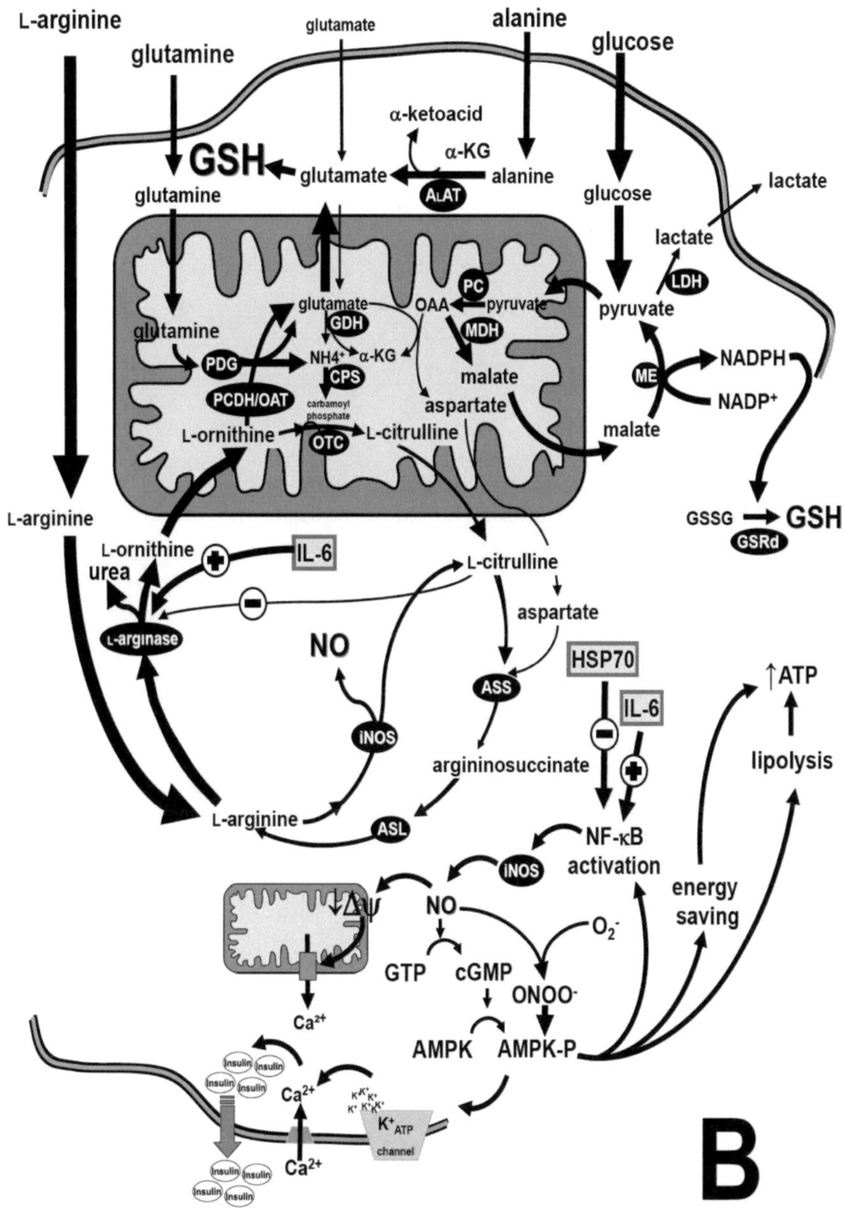
L-arginine
glutamine
glutamate
alanine
glucose
α-ketoacid
α-KG
GSH
glutamate
alanine
ALAT
glutamine
glucose
lactate
lactate
LDH
PC
glutamate
OAA
pyruvate
pyruvate
GDH
MDH
glutamine
PDG
NH4+
α-KG
CPS
malate
ME
NADPH
NADP+
PCDH/OAT
carbamoyl phosphate
aspartate
L-ornithine
OTC
L-citrulline
malate
L-arginine
GSSG
GSH
GSRd
L-ornithine
IL-6
urea
L-citrulline
L-arginase
aspartate
NO
HSP70
ASS
↑ATP
IL-6
iNOS
argininosuccinate
lipolysis
L-arginine
ASL
NF-κB
activation
iNOS
energy
saving
↓Δψ
NO
O2-
GTP
cGMP
ONOO-
Ca2+
AMPK
AMPK-P
insulin
Ca2+
K+ATP
channel
Ca2+
B

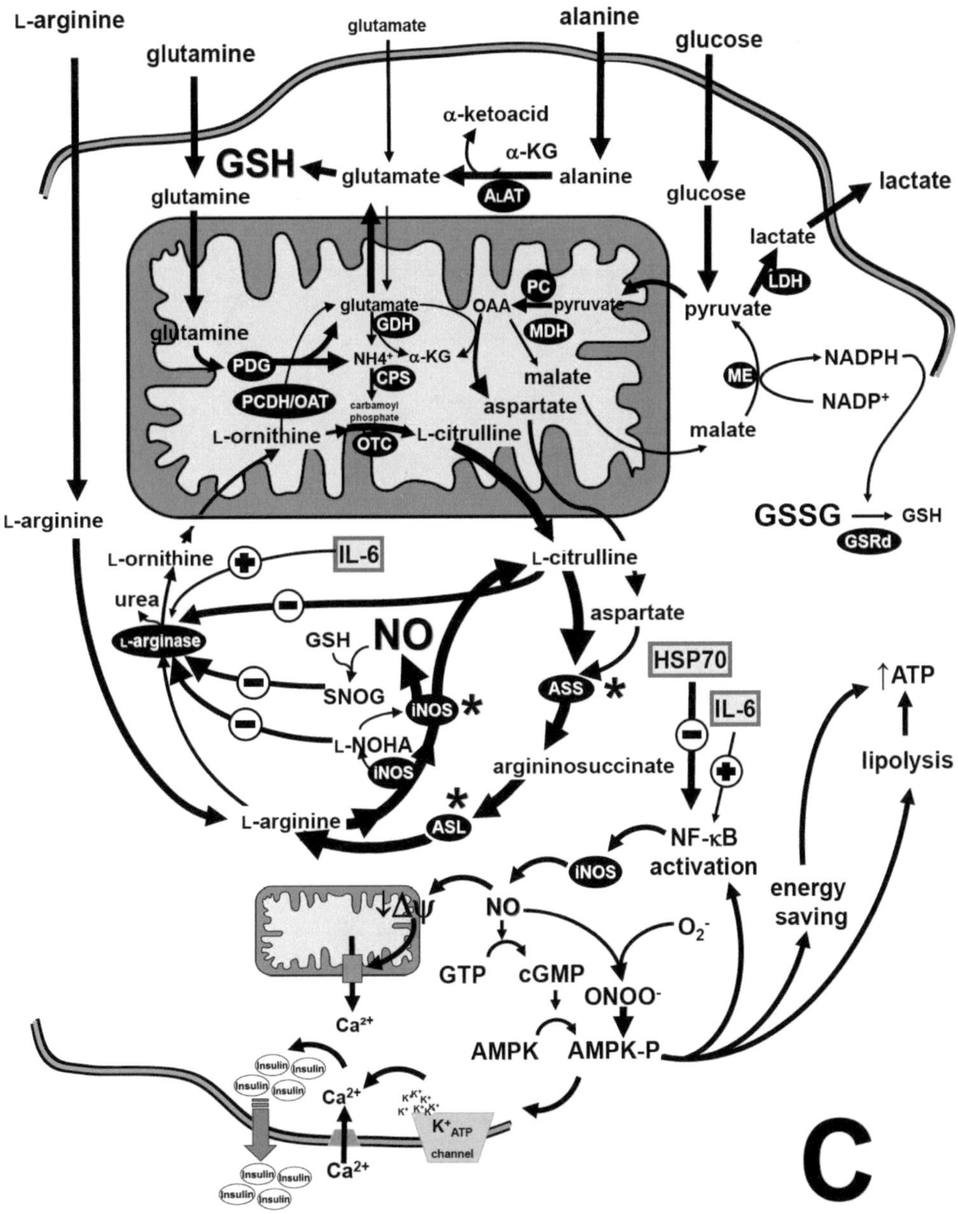
L-arginine
glutamine
glutamate
alanine
glucose
α-ketoacid
α-KG
GSH
glutamate
alanine
ALAT
glutamine
glucose
lactate
lactate
LDH
PC
glutamate
OAA
pyruvate
pyruvate
GDH
MDH
glutamine
NH4+
α-KG
PDG
CPS
malate
NADPH
ME
PCDH/OAT
aspartate
NADP+
carbamoyl phosphate
L-ornithine
OTC
L-citrulline
malate
L-arginine
GSSG
GSH
GSRd
L-ornithine
IL-6
L-citrulline
urea
aspartate
L-arginase
GSH
NO
HSP70
SNOG
ASS
↑ATP
iNOS
IL-6
L-NOHA
argininosuccinate
lipolysis
iNOS
ASL
L-arginine
NF-κB
activation
iNOS
↓Δψ
NO
energy
saving
O2-
GTP
cGMP
ONOO-
Ca2+
AMPK
AMPK-P
Insulin
Ca2+
K+ATP
channel
Ca2+
C

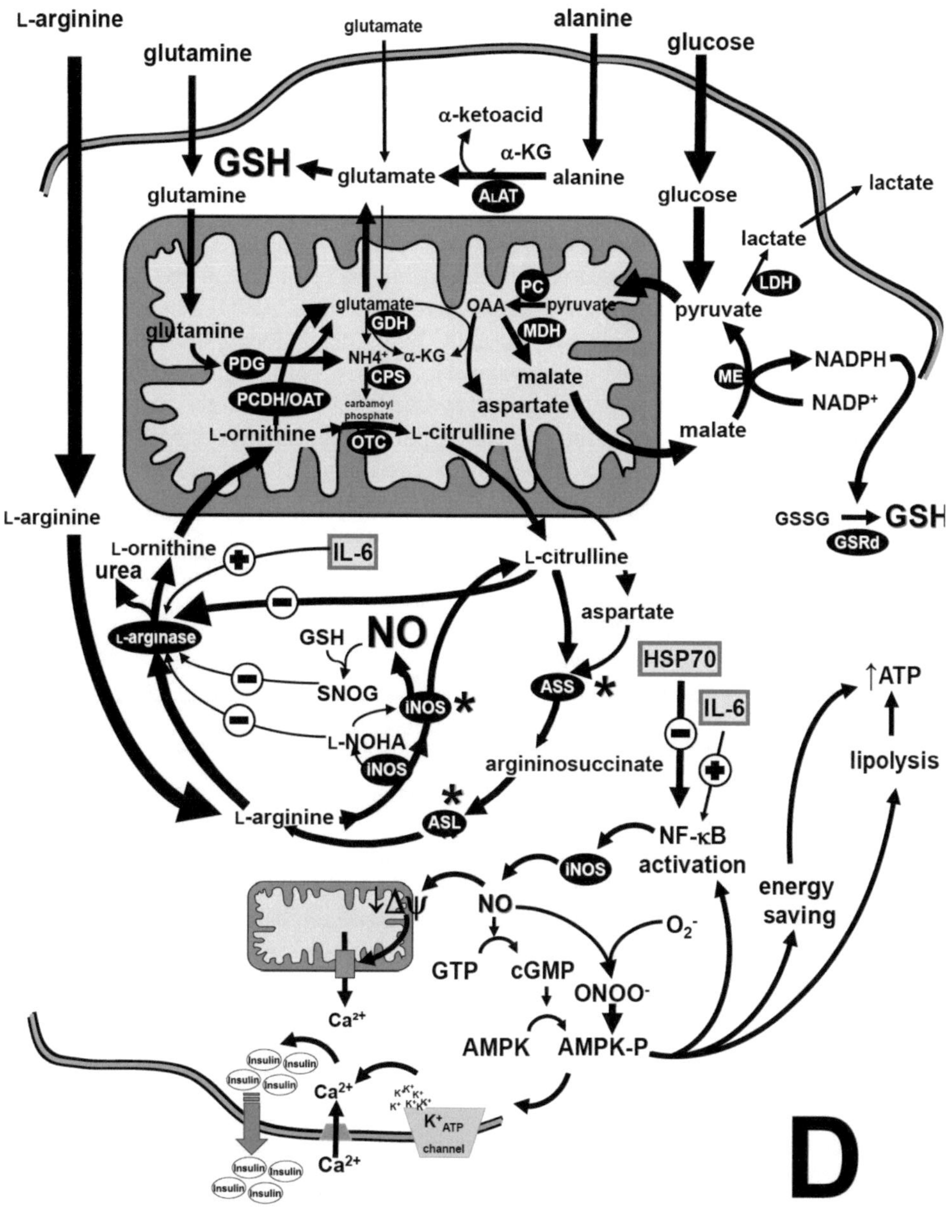

Fig. 2. L-Arginine-glutamate-NO coupling in β-cells. Under physiological secretagogue-mediated insulin release, both NO and GSH are obligatory intermediates. Accordingly, β-cells have an intricate iNOS-cantered machinery to produce NO, which potentiates insulin secretion physiologically. At the same time, insulin-secreting pancreatic cells utilise glutamate-derived GSH in order to maintain redox status needed to allow hormonal secretion and to avoid a possible NO-mediated cytotoxicity. L-Arginine derived from the kidney is the physiological substrate for the NF-κB-dependent iNOS-catalyzed NO production in β-cells. Under insufficient L-arginine supply, however, the high throughput of NO for β-cells may be attained

by the concerted action of phosphate-dependent glutaminase (PDG), glutamate dehydrogenase (GDH), aspartate aminotransferase (not shown), carbamoylphosphate synthetase I (CPS), ornithine transcarbamoylase (OTC), argininosuccinate synthetase (ASS) and argininosuccinate lyase (ASL), which, dramatically enhances the flux of L-glutamate towards NO production. In the presence of an inflammatory NF-κB-centered cytokine insult, multiple negative feedback systems act in β-cells in order to warrant L-arginine entry in iNOS metabolic pathway (lower part of the figure). This is achieved mainly due to the inhibition of L-arginase activity by L-citrulline, N^{G}-hydroxy- L-arginine (L-NOHA, an intermediate in NO synthesis) and *S*-nitrosoglutathione (SNOG), which is formed during NO biosynthesis. On the other hand, β-cells have to synthesize GSH from L-glutamate, L-cysteine and L-glycine, once regeneration of GSH from glutathione disulphide (GSSG) via NADPH-dependent GSSG reductase is relatively low in β-cells because of the high flux of glucose towards ATP production that empty pentose-phosphate shunt impairing NADPH production. In turn, *de novo* GSH synthesis is mainly dependent on liver-emanated supply of glutamate, which is not enough to allow for the enormous flux towards γ-glutamylcysteine synthetase (glutamate-cysteine ligase) and GSH synthetase in the GSH biosynthetic pathway. Therefore, muscle-derived L-alanine and L-glutamine constitute the principal sources of L-glutamate for GSH synthesis. Because of this, any reduction in L-arginine supply to β-cells accounts for a rapid shift in L-glutamate metabolism from GSH synthesis towards NO production. For instance, during Th1-elicited immune responses, the concerted enhancement of NF-κB-mediated (*) expression of ASS, ASL and iNOS dramatically boosts NO production from L-glutamate. If this rise in NO production is not accompanied by an enhanced L-arginine supply to β-cells, NO becomes very cytotoxic. Type 2 cytokines, such as interleukin-6 (IL-6) may alleviate NO toxicity by enhancing L-arginase expression that diverts L-arginine to the formation of L-ornithine and urea. At the same time, intracellular expression of the 70-kDa family of heat shock proteins (HSP70), which blocks a surplus activation of NF-κB-dependent genes, is cytoprotective because it warrants an equilibrium for NO production via NF-κB-dependent iNOS expression thus avoiding NO cytotoxic effects. Results from the present work reveal a novel as yet unpredicted facet of L-arginine metabolism in that an increase in its plasma concentrations (**from A to B**) could drift GSH metabolism from its original main source, via L-glutamine metabolism, towards the production of L-glutamate via the left side of the β-cell urea cycle, by the consecutive action of L-arginase, pyrroline-5-carboxylate dehydrogenase (PCDH), ornithine aminotransferase (OAT), γ-glutamylcysteine synthetase (not shown) and GSH synthetase (not shown). Under inflammatory stimuli (**C and D**), enhancement of L-arginine concentration may alleviate the excessive flux through iNOS by limiting L-arginine availability due to its conversion into GSH. Concomitantly, elevation of L-arginine levels are thought to deviate glucose mitochondrial metabolism towards its cytosolic utilisation as a NADPH precursor via malic enzyme (ME). This favors the regeneration of more GSH molecules from GSSG under oxidative stress conditions. L-Arginine may also stimulate AMPK activation which modulates closure of K_{ATP} channels and insulin secretion. NO is also capable of activating AMPK. However, in a high L-arginine environment, the excessive activation of AMPK may stimulate lipolysis and energy saving at the expense of insulin secretion. Since physical exercise stimulates L-glutamine flux towards L-arginine production, peaks IL-6 secretion by the stretching skeletal muscle and induces HSP70 expression throughout the body tissues, exercise continues to be the cheapest and most efficient way of preventing type-1 diabetes onset. Arrow widths indicate the intensity of the metabolic flux through each pathway.

L-Arginase is normally associated with a K_m value for L-arginine that is much higher than that of iNOS but a greater V_{max} value compared with iNOS (Mori, 2007), so that the V_{max}/K_m ratios of both enzymes are close to each other and thus these enzymes may be expected to compete for L-arginine equally in β-cells. In our hands, iNOS seemed to be saturated in β-cells, regardless of the presence of inflammatory cytokines, so that β-cell urea production is able to furnish L-ornithine and thus L-glutamate for GSH synthesis in appropriate conditions. Moreover, L-arginine may protect β-cells via the induction of haem oxygenase (HO-1) expression (data not shown). HO activity is an important detoxifying enzyme, due to its ability to scavenge haem groups thus providing redox protection (Abraham & Kappas, 2008). However, it is plausible that HO expression in β-cells in response to L-arginine may also play a metabolic role, since one of its direct products, carbon monoxide (CO), has recently been reported to induce insulin secretion and to improve *in vivo* function of β-cells after transplant (Abraham & Kappas, 2008). Moreover, the long-lasting expression of this enzyme has been shown to delay the progression of type 1 diabetes in NOD mice (Li et al., 2007). Hence, L-arginine can be recognised as an antioxidant in its own right, being comparable with known antioxidant stimuli, such as phytochemical supplements (Velmurugan et al., 2009).

Furthermore, and interestingly, chronic hyperlactataemia, in which high plasma levels of lactate block intestinal proline oxidase activity leading to severe hypocitrullinaemia and hypoargininaemia (Dillon et al., 1999), has been described as an independent risk factor for diabetes development, with lactate being an important factor for maintaining insulin resistance (DiGirolamo et al., 1992; Lovejoy et al., 1992). Conversely, L-arginine supplementation to critical care patients did induce L-glutamine rise in the plasma (Loï et al., 2009), which may be related to the fact the L-arginine supplementation spares plasma glutamine pools.

In synthesis, L-arginine derived from the kidney (**Fig. 1**) is the physiological substrate for the NF-κB-dependent iNOS-catalysed NO production in β-cells. Under **insufficient** L-arginine supply, however, the high throughput of NO for β-cells may be attained by the concerted action of phosphate-dependent glutaminase (GDP), glutamate dehydrogenase (GDH), aspartate aminotransferase (AsAT), carbamoylphosphate synthetase (CPS), ornithine transcarbamoylase (OTC), argininosuccinate synthetase (ASS) and argininosuccinate lyase (ASL), which, dramatically enhances the flux of glutamate towards NO production. Multiple negative feedback systems act in β-cells in order to warrant L-arginine entry in iNOS metabolic pathway. This is achieved mainly due to the inhibition of L-arginase activity by L-citrulline, N^G-hydroxy-L-arginine (L-NOHA, an intermediate in NO synthesis) and *S*-nitrosoglutathione (SNOG), which is formed during NO biosynthesis. On the other hand, β-cells have to synthesise GSH from L-glutamate, L-cysteine and L-glycine, because regeneration of GSH from GSSG via NADPH-dependent GSSG reductase is relatively low in β-cells because of the high flux of glucose towards ATP production that empty pentose-phosphate shunt, the major NADPH-producing system. In turn, *de novo* GSH synthesis is mainly dependent on liver-derived supply of glutamate, which is not enough to allow for the enormous flux towards γ-glutamylcysteine synthetase and GSH synthetase in the GSH biosynthetic pathway. Therefore, muscle-derived L-alanine and L-glutamine constitute the principal sources of L-glutamate for GSH synthesis in order to spare β-cell L-arginine stores. In fact, previous reports from our laboratory have highlighted the importance of L-glutamine and L-alanine for GSH generation, insulin secretion and protection against pro-inflammatory cytokines (Brennan et al., 2003; Brennan et a., 2002; Cunninham et al., 2005). Because of this, **any reduction** in L-arginine supply to β-cells accounts for a rapid shift in L-glutamate metabolism from GSH synthesis towards NO production. For instance, during Th1-elicited immune responses (*e.g.* as **in Fig. 2C and 2D**), the concerted enhancement of nuclear factor NF-κB-mediated expression of ASS, ASL and iNOS dramatically boosts NO production from L-glutamate. If this rise in NO production is not accompanied by an enhanced L-arginine supply to β-cells, NO becomes very cytotoxic. Type 2 cytokines (T2-CK) may alleviate NO toxicity by enhancing L-arginase expression that deviates L-arginine to the formation of L-ornithine and urea.

6. Psychological stress and the role peripheral sympathetic nervous system-histamine-CRH axis activation in type 1 diabetes

It has long been recognised that stressful situations are closely related to the onset of type 1 diabetes. In fact, many stressful conditions that are associated with immune system imbalances, including psychological ones, are associated with the incidence of type 1 diabetes (Soltesz, 2003; Dahlquist, 2006). Indeed, it has recently been shown that stressful life events and psychological dysfunctions dramatically augment the likelihood of the incidence of type 1 diabetes in children and adolescents (Sipetic et al., 2007). These include parents' job-related changes or lost job, severe accidents, hospitalization or death of a close friend, quarrels between parents, war, near-drowning in a pool, falling down, being an unhurt participant of an accident, conflicts with parents/teacher/neighbours, to be lost in town, physical attack, failure in competition, penalty, examination, death of pet, presence of lightning strike, loss of housing accommodation and learning problems.

As a general rule, stress is considered as immunosuppressive. Surprisingly, however, a growing body of evidence strongly suggests that acute stress serves as a pro-inflammatory stimulus via the production of corticotropin-releasing hormone (CRH) by peripheral sympathetic nerve terminals (Elenkov et al., 1999). CRH stimulates lymphocyte proliferation (McGillis et al., 1989; Jessop et al., 1997) and secretion of IL-1β and IL-2 by mononuclear cells isolated from the peripheral blood of healthy subjects (Singh & Leu, 1990). Peripheral CRH exerts a pro-inflammatory effect in autoimmune diseases with a selective increase in Th1-type responses, which is mediated by an NF-κB-dependent pathway (Benou et al., 2005). Additionally, it is possible that, upon a stressful situation, peripherally delivered CRH activates mast cells that secrete histamine, which acts via H1 receptors to induce local inflammation (Elenkov et al., 1999). In fact, diabetes is associated with increased basal hypothalamus-pituitary-adrenal (HPA) activity and impaired stress responsiveness (Chan et al., 2005). Therefore, psychological stress may selectively activate Th1 lymphocytes that mediate type-1 cytokine-induced iNOS expression, exacerbated NO production and β-cell cytotoxicity. Enhanced Th1 activity, in turn, increases L-glutamine utilisation with the consequent shift of L-glutamate metabolism from GSH biosynthesis towards NO production, as discussed above (Fig. 2 and 3).

Taken together, these findings suggest that psychological stress may have a dual and cross-potentiating role in determining the onset of type 1 diabetes: an immunoinflammatory (Fig. 3) and a metabolic one (Fig. 2C and 2D). Arguing in proof of such a hypothesis is the observation that orally administered L-arginine supplementation significantly improves patient status in a series of different pathological conditions associated with immune dysfunctions, including in pre-term neonates (Wu et al., 2004), without increasing urea

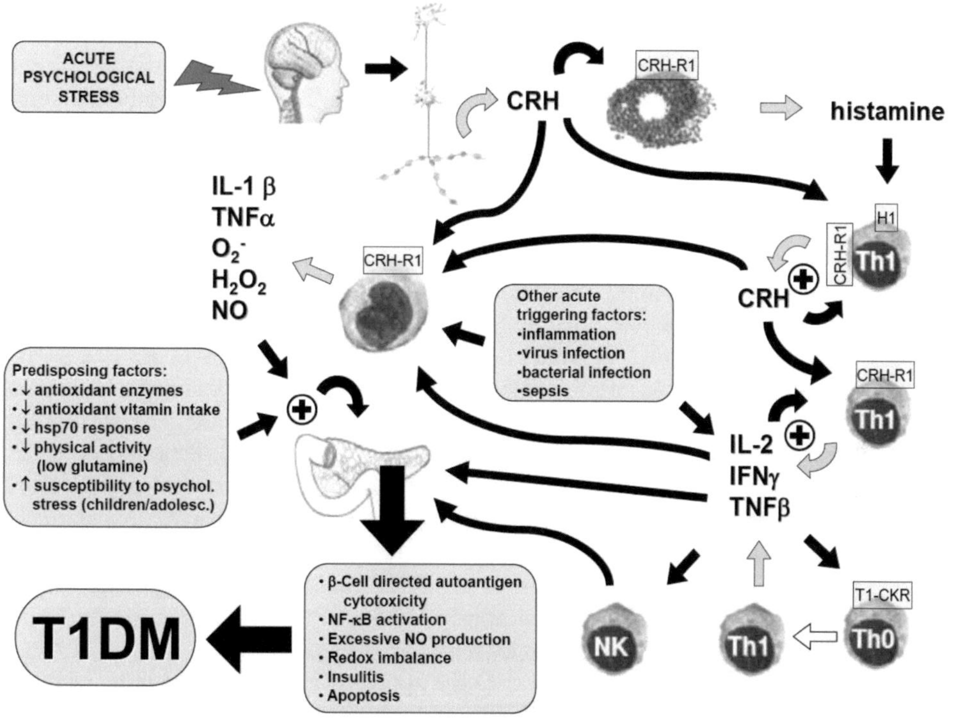

Fig. 3. Psychological stress and autoimmune diabetes. Different stressful situations may lead to the activation of sympathetic-corticotropin-releasing hormone (CRH)-histamine axis that triggers a Th1-specific immunoinflammatory response. Peripheral sympathetic nerve-derived CRH released under acute psychological stressful situations is capable of stimulating mast cells and Th1 lymphocytes, which arm an immunoinflammatory response. Auto-reactive Th1 cell subset and its cytokine products (type 1 cytokines, T1-CK) raised against islet β-cell antigen(s) mediate the activation of macrophages and Th1 lymphocytes, favouring insulitis. Additionally, other predisposing factors may also exacerbate β-cell injury and the onset of type 1 diabetes mellitus (T1DM).

levels (Wilmore, 2004). Curiously, intraperitoneal L-arginine injection, where the physiological coupling of L-glutamine/L-arginine through the intestinal-renal axis is bypassed, does **not** improve diabetes in animal models. On the contrary, it seems to worsen it (Mohan & Das, 1998), while **oral** administration of L-arginine to alloxan-treated rats restores blood glucose and insulin levels (Vasilijevic et al., 2007). Oral L-arginine administration has also been shown to improve, but not completely, peripheral and hepatic insulin sensitivity in type 2 diabetes (Piatti et al., 2001), where oxidative stress (Carvalho-Filho et al., 2005; Oliveira et al., 2003; Hirabara et al., 2006) and NO overproduction (Newsholme et al., 2007; Carvalho-Filho et al., 2005) are also involved. If this is so, nutritional management of L-glutamine and/or L-arginine, **enterally** administered in order to allow for the physiological re-establishment of L-glutamine/L-arginine homeostasis (Vermeulen et al., 2007), may rescue β-cell redox balance in ongoing type 1 diabetes. Additionally, skeletal muscle is a major site for L-glutamine synthesis in the human body and contains over 90% of the whole-body L-glutamine pool. Quantitative studies in humans

(Newsholme et al., 2003) have demonstrated that, in the postabsorptive state, 60% of the amino acids released comprise L-alanine plus L-glutamine (**Fig. 1A**). Therefore, moderate physical exercise, which is known to accelerate the rate of L-glutamine delivery into the circulation, may be of value in protecting L-glutamine/L-arginine metabolic coupling between the gut and β-cells.

7. Influence of regular physical exercise in L-arginine/L-glutamine coupling in β-cells

During physical exercise sessions, pro-inflammatory cytokine production is downregulated and anti-inflammatory cytokines, such as IL-1 receptor antagonist (IL-1ra), IL-10 and IL-6, are upregulated (Drenth et al., 1995; Nieman & Pedersen, 1999; Rohde et al., 1997). In this sense, IL-6 seems to play a capital role during exercise-induced changes in immune function. In fact, the level of circulating IL-6 has been shown to increase dramatically (up to 100-fold) in response to exercise (Pedersen & Hoffman-Goetz, 2000; Febbraio et al., 2002; Pedersen & Steensberg, 2002; Pedersen et al., 2001). Most studies have also reported that exercise, *per se*, does not increase plasma levels of TNFα, although some have shown that strenuous, prolonged exercise, such as marathon running, results in a small increase in the plasma concentration of TNFα (Pedersen et al., 1998; Suzuki et al., 2000). This long-term effect of exercise may be ascribed to the anti-inflammatory response elicited by an acute bout of exercise, which is partly mediated by muscle-derived IL-6.

Physiological concentrations of IL-6 stimulate the appearance, in the circulation, of the anti-inflammatory cytokines IL-1ra and IL-10, and inhibit the production of the pro-inflammatory cytokine TNFα. Hence, exercise-induced IL-6 release downregulates pro-inflammatory cytokine production while increasing anti-inflammatory cytokine production and action, which may induce a very strong anti-inflammatory cytokine response. The main modulator of these responses is likely to be the appearance of IL-6 in the circulation. Since IL-6 strongly downregulates NF-κB activation, we believe that moderate exercise-induced IL-6 production may suppress NF-κB-dependent iNOS while stimulating L-arginase activity/expression with a consequent decrease in NO-dependent β-cell death upon Th1-driven β-cell assault. Therefore, besides any possible beneficial effect that moderate exercise may have on L-glutamine/L-arginine coupling that is responsible for the maintenance of β-cell redox homeostasis and insulin secreting capacity (see above), mild physical exercise may shut off pro-inflammatory cytokine machinery, which gives rise to an additional protection against the development of type 1 diabetes.

Even though the effects of IL-6 on β-cells remains a matter of debate and controversies (Wadt et al., 1998), it has been found that IL-6 hinders the development of type 1 diabetes in different mouse models (Campbell et al., 1994; DiCosmo et al., 1994). Moreover, IL-6 has proven to be effective in protecting insulin-secreting MIN6 cells and freshly isolated pancreatic islets against Th1-derived cytokine (IL-1β, TNFα and IFNγ)-induced apoptosis while improving cellular viability and insulin secretion (Choi et al., 2004). Altogether, the above propositions support an important protective effect of exercise-dependent muscle-derived IL-6 on β-cells against the development of diabetes. Moreover, exercise-induced HSP70 expression in non-muscular cells may have a critical influence in maintaining an anti-inflammatory status, as discussed above. However, exercise-induced HSP70 in pancreatic β-cells has never been addressed. Therefore, we are currently evaluating the effects of acute and chronic (training) exercise sessions (swimming) on HSP70 pathways and L-glutamine/L-arginine coupling enzymes in animal pancreatic islets and isolated β-cells.

8. Conclusion

Continued supply of L-arginine, physiologically provided by the metabolism of L-glutamine via the intestinal-renal axis and from skeletal muscle, which is enhanced during exercise, is essential for β-cell functional integrity and, indeed, for β-cell defence. The dysregulation of immune system function, characteristic of Th1-elicited β-cell toxicity and impaired insulin secretion, which accompany the onset of type 1 diabetes, may be triggered when an individual faces a strong **psychological stress** that determines an enhanced L-glutamine utilisation by Th1 lymphocytes. The oxidative stress that takes place upon reduced intracellular GSH levels allows for the activation of NF-κB, which, in turn, positively feeds back on iNOS expression and activity, thus perpetuating the inflammatory process within β-cells where **excess** NO is harmful. Defective HSP70 induction in response to physiological levels of intraislet NO may also be involved in the pathogenesis of type 1 diabetes. Physical exercise, on the other hand, is capable of inducing a huge production and release of IL-6, which is a key anti-inflammatory mediator that suppresses NF-κB-dependent responses. Moreover, exercise-elicited activation of HSP70 biochemical pathways completely blocks NF-κB activation, impedes apoptosis and is cytoprotective due to HSP70 chaperone activity, which protects against protein denaturation. HSP70 induction is also associated with enhanced Th2 cell activity over Th1. Metabolically, exercise may restore L-glutamine supply thus normalizing pancreatic production of NO from kidney-derived L-arginine, and not from L-glutamate which is necessary for GSH synthesis and antioxidant defence. Thus the enormous changes in human life style, compared with that of our 3-4 million-old ancestors, could be related with our current inability in maintaining healthy β-cells. As previously argued (Krause & Homem de Bittencourt, 2008), we advocate that present-day levels of physical activity and dietary patterns (Simopoulos, 2006; Wisloff et al., 2005) seem to have changed much faster than the time needed to allow evolutionary metabolic changes. In other words, our metabolism evolved to fit a level of physical activity and availability of a variety of food supplies different from those of nowadays (favouring energy conservation and storage). As a corollary, unless humans enhance their pattern of physical activity, diabetes will become more and more of a risk factor in the population. Therefore, the notion that β-cells are solely bystanders of oxidative stress-mediated cell toxicity because their antioxidant defences fail in managing physiological stress is an unfortunate misconception.

Since the L-glutamine/L-arginine duet may influence β-cell function and survival, the knowledge of physiologically adequate levels and fluxes of both amino acids may serve as a predictor of β-cell susceptibility to dysfunction or death in diabetes. Additionally, although the possibility of pharmacologically exploiting Th1/Th2 duality relative to L-arginine metabolism may open new avenues for diabetes therapeutics, physical exercise is still the cheapest and easiest physiological measure to avoid the onset and/or worsening of diabetes. In summary, if the prevention of diabetes is dependent on HSP70 expression and both restoration of adequate L-arginine supply to β-cells and blockage of NF-κB overstimulation, moderate physical exercise is presented as the most convenient solution for these two lacunes.

9. Acknowledgements

We thank UCD School of Biomolecular and Biomedical Science, Science Foundation Ireland and the National Council for Scientific and Technological Development (CNPq), Brazil, for their support of this work.

10. References

Abraham, N.G. & Kappas, A (2008). Pharmacological and clinical aspects of heme oxygenase. *Pharmacological Reviews*, Vol. 60, pp. 79-127

Albina, J.E.; Mills, C.D.; Henry, W.L. & Caldwell, M.D. (1990). Temporal expression of different pathways of L-arginine metabolism in healing wounds. *Journal of Immunology*, Vol. 144, pp. 3877-3880

Ao, L.; Zou, N.; Cleveland, J.C., Jr.; Fullerton, D.A. & Meng, X. (2009). Myocardial TLR4 is a determinant of neutrophil infiltration after global myocardial ischemia: mediating KC and MCP-1 expression induced by extracellular HSC70. *American Journal of Physiology. Heart and Circulatory Physiology*, Vol. 297, N° 1, pp. H21–H28

Arya, R.; Mallik, M. & Lakhotia, S.C. (2007). Heat shock genes—integrating cell survival and death. *Journal of Biosciences*, Vol. 32, N° 3, pp. 595–610

Asayama, K.; Kooy. N;W. & Burr, I.M. (1986). Effect of vitamin E deficiency and selenium deficiency on insulin secretory reserve and free radical scavenging systems in islets: decrease of islet manganosuperoxide dismutase. *Journal Laboratory and Clinical Medicine*, Vol. 107, pp. 459-464

Asea, A. (2003). Chaperokine-induced signal transduction pathways. *Exercise Immunology Review*, Vol. 9, pp. 25–33

Asea, A. (2008). Heat shock proteins and toll-like receptors. *Handbook of Experimental Pharmacology*, Vol. 183, pp. 111–127

Atalay, M.; Oksala, N.K.; Laaksonen, D.E.; Khanna, S.; Nakao, C.; Lappalainen, J.; Roy, S.; Hanninen, O. & Sen, C.K. (2004). Exercise training modulates heat shock protein response in diabetic rats. *Journal of Applied Physiology*, Vol. 97, pp. 605-611

Baldwin, A.S., Jr. (1996). The NF-κB and IκB proteins: new discoveries and insights. *Annual Review of Immunology*, Vol. 14, pp. 649-683

Beck, K.F.; Eberhardt, W.; Frank, S.; Huwiler, A.; Messmer, U.K.; Muhl, H. & Pfeilschifter, J. (1999). Inducible NO synthase: role in cellular signalling. *Journal of Experimental Biology*, Vol. 202, pp. 645-653

Beere, H.M. (2004). "The stress of dying": the role of heat shock proteins in the regulation of apoptosis. *Journal of Cell Science*, Vol. 117, Pt 13, pp. 2641–2651

Benou, C.; Wang, Y.; Imitola, J.; VanVlerken, L.; Chandras, C.; Karalis, K.P. & Khoury, S,J. (2005). Corticotropin-releasing hormone contributes to the peripheral inflammatory response in experimental autoimmune encephalomyelitis. *Journal of Immunology*, Vol. 174, pp. 5407-5413

Boucher, J.L.; Custot, J.; Vadon, S.; Delaforge, M.; Lepoivre, M.; Tenu, J.P.; Yapo, A. & Mansuy, D. (1994). N^{ω}-hydroxyl-L-arginine, an intermediate in the L-arginine to nitric oxide pathway, is a strong inhibitor of liver and macrophage arginase. *Biochemical and Biophysical Research Communications*, Vol. 203, pp. 1614-1621

Boucher, J.L.; Moali, C. & Tenu, J.P. (1999). Nitric oxide biosynthesis, nitric oxide synthase inhibitors and arginase competition for L-arginine utilization. *Cellular and Molecular Life Sciences*, Vol. 55, pp. 1015-1028

Brennan, L.; Corless, M.; Hewage, C.; Malthouse, J.P.; McClenaghan, N.H.; Flatt, P.R. & Newsholme, P. (2003). ^{13}C-NMR analysis reveals a link between L-glutamine metabolism, D-glucose metabolism and gamma-glutamyl cycle activity in a clonal pancreatic β-cell line. *Diabetologia*, Vol. 46, pp. 1512-1521

Brennan, L.; Shine, A.; Hewage, C.; Malthouse, J.P.; Brindle, K.M.; McClenaghan, N.; Flatt, P.R. & Newsholme, P. (2002). A nuclear magnetic resonance-based demonstration of substantial oxidative L-alanine metabolism and L-alanine-enhanced glucose metabolism in a clonal pancreatic beta-cell line: metabolism of L-alanine is important to the regulation of insulin secretion. *Diabetes*, Vol. 51, pp. 1714-1721

Calderwood, S.K.; Mambula, S.S.; Gray, P.J., Jr. & Theriault, J.R. (2007a). Extracellular heat shock proteins in cell signaling. *Federation of European Biochemical Societies Letters*, Vol. 581, N° 19, pp. 3689–3694

Calderwood, S.K.; Theriault, J.; Gray, P.J. & Gong, J. (2007b). Cell surface receptors for molecular chaperones. *Methods*, Vol. 43, N° 3, pp. 199–206

Campbell, I.L.; Hobbs, M.V.; Dockter, J.; Oldstone, M.B. & Allison, J. (1994). Islet inflammation and hyperplasia induced by the pancreatic islet-specific overexpression of interleukin-6 in transgenic mice. *American Journal of Pathology*, Vol. 145, pp. 157-166

Cardozo, A.K.; Kruhoffer, M.; Leeman, R.; Orntoft, T. & Eizirik, D.L. (2001). Identification of novel cytokine-induced genes in pancreatic β-cells by high-density oligonucleotide arrays. *Diabetes*, Vol. 50, pp. 909-920

Carvalho-Filho, M.A.; Ueno, M.; Hirabara, S.M.; Seabra, A.B.; Carvalheira, J.B.; de Oliveira, M.G.; Velloso, L.A.; Curi, R. & Saad, M.J. (2005). *S*-Nitrosation of the insulin receptor, insulin receptor substrate 1, and protein kinase B/Akt: a novel mechanism of insulin resistance. *Diabetes*, Vol. 54, pp. 959-967

Castillo, L.; Chapman, T.E.; Sanchez, M.; Yu, Y.M.; Burke, J.F.; Ajami, A.M.; Vogt, J. & Young, V.R. (1993). Plasma arginine and citrulline kinetics in adults given adequate and arginine-free diets. *Proceedings of the National Academy of Sciences of the U.S.A.*, Vol. 90, pp. 7749-7753

Chan, J.Y.; Ou, C.C.; Wang, L.L. & Chan, S.H. (2004). Heat shock protein 70 confers cardiovascular protection during endotoxemia via inhibition of nuclear factor-κB activation and inducible nitric oxide synthase expression in the rostral ventrolateral medulla. *Circulation*, Vol. 110, N° 23, pp. 3560–3566

Chan, O.; Inouye, K.; Akirav, E.; Park, E.; Riddell, M.C.; Vranic, M. & Matthews, S.G. (2005). Insulin alone increases hypothalamus-pituitary-adrenal activity, and diabetes lowers peak stress responses. *Endocrinology*, Vol. 146, pp. 1382-1390

Chang, C.I.; Liao, J.C. & Kuo, L. (1998). Arginase modulates nitric oxide production in activated macrophages. *American Journal of Physiology. Heart and Circulatory Physiology*, Vol. 274, pp. H342-348

Chang, W.K.; Yang, K.D. & Shaio, M.F. (1999). Effect of glutamine on Th1 and Th2 cytokine responses of human peripheral blood mononuclear cells. *Clinical Immunology*, Vol. 93, pp. 294-301

Chen, F.; Castranova, V.; Shi, X. & Demers, L.M. (1999). New insights into the role of nuclear factor-κB, a ubiquitous transcription factor in the initiation of diseases. *Clinical Chemistry*, Vol. 45, pp. 7-17

Chen, H.; Li, X. & Epstein, P.N. (2005). MnSOD and catalase transgenes demonstrate that protection of islets from oxidative stress does not alter cytokine toxicity. *Diabetes*, Vol. 54, pp. 1437-1446

Chen, H.W.; Kuo, H.T.; Wang, S.J.; Lu, T.S. & Yang, R.C. (2005). In vivo heat shock protein assembles with septic liver NF-κB/I-κB complex regulating NF-κB activity. *Shock*, Vol. 24, N° 3, pp. 232–238

Choi, S.E.; Choi, K.M.; Yoon, I.H.; Shin, J.Y.; Kim, J.S.; Park, W.Y.; Han, D.J.; Kim, S.C.; Ahn, C.; Kim, J.Y.; Hwang, E.S.; Cha, C.Y.; Szot, G.L.; Yoon, K.H. & Park, C.G. (2004). IL-6 protects pancreatic islet β cells from pro-inflammatory cytokines-induced cell death and functional impairment in vitro and in vivo. *Transplantation Immunology*, Vol. 13, pp. 43-53

Chung, J.; Nguyen, A.K.; Henstridge, D.C.; Holmes, A.G.; Chan, M.H.; Mesa, J.L.; Lancaster, G.I.; Southgate, R.J.; Bruce, C.R.; Duffy, S.J.; Horvath, I.; Mestril, R.; Watt, M.J.; Hooper, P.L.; Kingwell, B.A.; Vigh, L.; Hevener, A. & Febbraio, M.A. (2008). HSP72 protects against obesity-induced insulin resistance. *Proceedings of the National Academy of Sciences of the U.S.A.*, Vol. 105, N° 5, pp. 1739-1744.

Corraliza, I.M.; Soler, G.; Eichmann, K. & Modolell, M. (1995). Arginase induction by suppressors of nitric oxide synthesis (IL-4, IL-10 and PGE_2) in murine bone-marrow-derived macrophages. *Biochemical and Biophysical Research Communications*, Vol. 206, pp. 667-673

Cunningham, G.A.; McClenaghan, N.H.; Flatt, P.R. & Newsholme, P. (2005). L-Alanine induces changes in metabolic and signal transduction gene expression in a clonal rat pancreatic β-cell line and protects from pro-inflammatory cytokine-induced apoptosis. *Clinical Science (London)*, Vol. 109, pp. 447-455

Cunningham, J.M.; Mabley, J.G. & Green, I.C. (1997). Interleukin 1β-mediated inhibition of arginase in RINm5F cells. *Cytokine*, Vol. 9, pp. 570-576

Curi, R.; Newsholme, P.; Pithon-Curi, T.C.; Pires-de-Melo, M.; Garcia, C.; Homem-de-Bittencourt, P.I., Jr.; Guimarães, A.R. (1999). Metabolic fate of glutamine in lymphocytes, macrophages and neutrophils. *Brazilian Journal of Medical and Biological Research*, Vol. 32, pp. 15-21

Currie, G.A. (1978). Activated macrophages kill tumour cells by releasing arginase. *Nature*, Vol. 273, pp. 758-759

Daghigh, F.; Fukuto, J.M. & Ash, D.E. (1994). Inhibition of rat liver arginase by an intermediate in NO biosynthesis, N^G-hydroxy-L-arginine: implications for the regulation of nitric oxide biosynthesis by arginase. *Biochemical and Biophysical Research Communications*, Vol. 202, pp. 174-180

Dahlquist, G. (2006). Can we slow the rising incidence of childhood-onset autoimmune diabetes? The overload hypothesis. *Diabetologia*, Vol. 49, pp. 20-24

Darville, M.I. & Eizirik, D.L. (1998). Regulation by cytokines of the inducible nitric oxide synthase promoter in insulin-producing cells. *Diabetologia*, Vol. 41, pp. 1101-1108

De Maio A. (2011). Extracellular heat shock proteins, cellular export vesicles, and the Stress Observation System: A form of communication during injury, infection, and cell damage : It is never known how far a controversial finding will go! Dedicated to Ferruccio Ritossa. *Cell Stress and Chaperones*, Vol. 16, N° 3, pp. 235-249

DiCosmo, B.F.; Picarella, D. & Flavell, R.A. (1994). Local production of human IL-6 promotes insulitis but retards the onset of insulin-dependent diabetes mellitus in non-obese diabetic mice. *International Immunology*, Vol. 6, pp. 1829-1837

DiGirolamo, M.; Newby,F.D. & Lovejoy, J. (1992). Lactate production in adipose tissue: a regulated function with extra-adipose implications. *Federation of American Societies for Experimental Biology Journal*, Vol. 6, N° 7, pp. 2405-2412

Dillon, E.L.; Knabe, D.A. & Wu, G. (1999). Lactate inhibits citrulline and arginine synthesis from proline in pig enterocytes. *American Journal of Physiology. Gastrointestinal and Liver Physiology*, Vol. 276, N°5 Pt 1, pp. G1079-G1086

Domínguez, C.; Ruiz, E.; Gussinye, M. & Carrascosa A. (1998). Oxidative stress at onset and in early stages of type I diabetes in children and adolescents. *Diabetes Care*, Vol. 21, pp. 1736-1742

Drenth, J.P.; Van Uum, S.H.; Van Deuren, M.; Pesman, G.J.; Van der Ven-Jongekrijg, J. & Van der Meer, J.W. (1995). Endurance run increases circulating IL-6 and IL-1ra but downregulates ex vivo TNF-α and IL-1β production. *Journal of Applied Physiology*, Vol. 79, pp. 1497-1503

Dröge, W. (2002). Free radicals in the physiological control of cell function. *Physiological Reviews*, Vol. 82, pp. 47-95

Eizirik, D.L. & Mandrup-Poulsen, T. (2001). A choice of death - the signal-transduction of immune-mediated β-cell apoptosis. *Diabetologia*, Vol. 44, pp. 2115-2133

Elenkov, I.J. & Chrousos, G.P. (1999). Stress hormones, Th1/Th2 patterns, pro/anti-inflammatory cytokines and susceptibility to disease. *Trends in Endocrinology and Metabolism*, Vol. 10, N° 9, pp. 359-368

Elenkov, I.J.; Webster, E.L.; Torpy, D.J. & Chrousos, G.P. (1999). Stress, corticotropin-releasing hormone, glucocorticoids, and the immune/inflammatory response: acute and chronic effects. *Annals of the New York Academy of Sciences*, Vol. 876, pp. 1-11 (see discussion in pp. 11-13)

Febbraio, M.A.; Mesa, J.L.; Chung, J.; Steensberg, A.; Keller, C.; Nielsen, H.B.; Krustrup, P.; Ott, P.; Secher, N.H. & Pedersen, B.K. (2004). Glucose ingestion attenuates the exercise-induced increase in circulating heat shock protein 72 and heat shock protein 60 in humans. *Cell Stress and Chaperones*, Vol. 9, N° 4, pp. 390–396

Febbraio, M.A.; Ott, P.; Nielsen, H.B.; Steensberg, A.; Keller, C.; Krustrup, P.; Secher, N.H. & Pedersen, B.K. (2002a). Exercise induces hepatosplanchnic release of heat shock protein 72 in humans. *Journal of Physiology*, Vol. 544, Pt 3, pp. 957–962

Febbraio, M.A.; Steensberg, A.; Walsh, R.; Koukoulas, I; Van Hall, G.; Saltin, B. & Pedersen, B.K. (2002b). Reduced glycogen availability is associated with an elevation in HSP72 in contracting human skeletal muscle. *Journal of Physiology*, Vol. 538, Pt 3, pp. 911–917

Fehrenbach, E.; Niess, A.M.; Voelker, K.; Northoff, H. & Mooren, F.C. (2005). Exercise intensity and duration affect blood soluble HSP72. *International Journal of Sports Medicine*, Vol. 26, N° 7, pp. 552–557

Feinstein, D.L; Galea, E.; Aquino, D.A.; Li, G.C.; Xu, H. & Reis DJ. (1996). Heat shock protein 70 suppresses astroglial-inducible nitric-oxide synthase expression by decreasing NF-κB activation. *Journal of Biological Chemistry*, Vol. 271, N° 30, pp. 17724–17732

Fisher-Wellman, K. & Bloomer, R.J. (2009). Acute exercise and oxidative stress: a 30 year history. Dynamic Medicine, Vol. 8, pp. 1

Flodstrom, M.; Niemann, A.; Bedoya, F.J.; Morris, S.M. & Eizirik, D.L. (1995). Expression of the citrulline-nitric oxide cycle in rodent and human pancreatic β-cells: induction of argininosuccinate synthetase by cytokines. *Endocrinology*, Vol. 136, pp. 3200-3206

Flodstrom, M.; Tsai, D.; Fine, C.; Maday, A. & Sarvetnick, N. (2003). Diabetogenic potential of human pathogens uncovered in experimentally permissive β-cells. *Diabetes*, Vol. 52, pp. 2025-2034

Forman, B.M.; Tontonoz, P.; Chen, J.; Brun, R.P.; Spiegelman, B.M. & Evans RM. (1995). 15-deoxy-$\Delta^{12,14}$-prostaglandin J_2 is a ligand for the adipocyte determination factor PPARγ. *Cell*, Vol. 83, pp. 803-812

Gelain, D.P.; de Bittencourt Pasquali, M.A.; Comim, C.; Grunwald, M.S.; Ritter, C.; Tomasi, C.D.; Alves, S.C.; Quevedo, J.; Dal-Pizzol, F.; Fonseca Moreira, J.C. (2011). Serum HSP70 Levels, Oxidant Status and Mortality in Sepsis. *Shock*, Feb 15 [Epub ahead of print], DOI: 10.1097/SHK.0b013e31820fe704

Giannoukakis, N.; Rudert, W.A.; Trucco, M. & Robbins, P.D. (2000). Protection of human islets from the effects of interleukin-1β by adenoviral gene transfer of an IκB repressor. *Journal of Biological Chemistry*, Vol. 275, pp. 36509-36513

Gill, D.J.; Low, B.C. & Grigor, M.R. (1996). Interleukin-1β and tumor necrosis factor-α stimulate the cat-2 gene of the L-arginine transporter in cultured vascular smooth muscle cells. *Journal of Biological Chemistry*, Vol. 271, pp. 11280-11283

Gonzalez, B. & Manso, R. (2004). Induction, modification and accumulation of HSP70s in the rat liver after acute exercise: early and late responses. *Journal of Physiology*, Vol. 556, N° Pt 2, pp. 369–385

Gotoh, T. & Mori, M. (1999). Arginase II downregulates nitric oxide (NO) production and prevents NO-mediated apoptosis in murine macrophage-derived RAW 264.7 cells. *Journal of Cell Biology*, Vol. 144, pp. 427-434

Granger, D.L.; Hibbs, J.B.; Perfect, J.R. & Durack, D.T. (1990). Metabolic fate of L-arginine in relation to microbiostatic capability of murine macrophages. *Journal of Clinical Investigation*, Vol. 85, pp. 264-273

Gutierrez, L.L.P.; Maslinkiewicz, A.; Curi, R. & Homem de Bittencourt, P.I., Jr. (2008). Atherosclerosis: a redox-sensitive lipid imbalance suppressible by cyclopentenone prostaglandins. *Biochemical Pharmacology*, Vol. 75, N° 12, pp. 2245-2262

Hamiel, C.R.; Pinto, S.; Hau, A. & Wischmeyer, P.E. (2009). Glutamine enhances heat shock protein 70 expression via increased hexosamine biosynthetic pathway activity. *American Journal of Physiology. Cell Physiology*, Vol. 297, N° 6, pp. C1509-C1519

Hamilton, K.L.; Staib, J.L.; Phillips, T.; Hess, A.; Lennon, S.L. & Powers, S.K. (2003). Exercise, antioxidants, and HS P72: protection against myocardial ischemia/reperfusion. *Free Radical Biology and Medicine*, Vol. 34, N° 7, pp. 800–809

Harris, M.B. & Starnes, J.W. (2001). Effects of body temperature during exercise training on myocardial adaptations. *American Journal of Physiology. Heart and Circulatory Physiology*, Vol. 280, N° 5, pp. H2271–H2280

Hattori, Y.; Campbell, E.B. & Gross, S.S. (1994). Argininosuccinate synthetase mRNA and activity are induced by immunostimulants in vascular smooth muscle. Role in the regeneration or arginine for nitric oxide synthesis. *Journal of Biological Chemistry*, Vol. 269, pp. 9405-9408

Heck, T.G.; Schöler, C.M. & Homem de Bittencourt, P.I., Jr. (2011). HSP70 expression: does it a novel fatigue signalling factor from immune system to the brain? *Cell Biochemistry and Function*, Vol. 29, N° 3, pp. 215-26

Hecker, M.; Nematollahi, H.; Hey, C.; Busse, R. & Racke, K. (1995). Inhibition of arginase by N^G-hydroxy-L-arginine in alveolar macrophages: implications for the utilization of L-arginine for nitric oxide synthesis. *Federation of European Biochemical Societies Letters*. Vol. 359, pp. 251-254

Hecker, M.; Schott, C.; Bucher, B.; Busse, R. & Stoclet, J.C. (1995). Increase in serum N^G-hydroxy-L-arginine in rats treated with bacterial lipopolysaccharide. *European Journal of Pharmacology*, Vol. 275, pp. R1-R3.

Heimberg, H.; Heremans, Y.; Jobin, C.; Leemans, R.; Cardozo, A.K; Darville, M. & Eizirik, D.L. (2001). Inhibition of cytokine-induced NF-κB activation by adenovirus-mediated expression of a NF-κB super-repressor prevents β-cell apoptosis. *Diabetes*, Vol. 50, pp. 2219-2224

Henderson, B. (2010). Integrating the cell stress response: a new view of molecular chaperones as immunological and physiological homeostatic regulators. *Cell Biochemistry and Function*, Vol. 28, N° 1, 1–14

Hernando, R. & Manso, R. (1997). Muscle fibre stress in response to exercise: synthesis, accumulation and isoform transitions of 70-kDa heat-shock proteins. *European Journal of Biochemistry*, Vol. 243, N° 1–2, pp. 460–467

Hirabara, S.M.; Silveira, L.R.; Alberici, L.C.; Leandro, C.V.; Lambertucci, R.H.; Polimeno, G.C.; Cury Boaventura, M.F.; Procopio, J.; Vercesi, A.E. & Curi, R. (2006). Acute effect of fatty acids on metabolism and mitochondrial coupling in skeletal muscle. *Biochimica et Biophysica Acta*, Vol. 1757, pp. 57-66

Homem de Bittencourt, P.I., Jr. & Curi, R. (2001). Antiproliferative prostaglandins and the MRP/GS-X pump role in cancer immunosuppression and insight into new strategies in cancer gene therapy. *Biochemical Pharmacology*, Vol. 62, N° 7, pp. 811-819.

Homem de Bittencourt, P.I., Jr.; Lagranha, D.J.; Maslinkiewicz, A.; Senna, S.M.; Tavares, A.M.; Baldissera, L.P.; Janner, D.R.; Peralta, J.S.; Bock, P.M.; Gutierrez, L.L.; Scola, G.; Heck, T.G.; Krause, M.S.; Cruz, L.A.; Abdalla, D.S.; Lagranha, C.J.; Lima, T. & Curi, R. (2007). LipoCardium: endothelium-directed cyclopentenone prostaglandin-based liposome formulation that completely reverses atherosclerotic lesions. *Atherosclerosis*, Vol. 193, pp. 245-258

Hooper, P.L. & Hooper, J.J. (2005). Loss of defense against stress: diabetes and heat shock proteins. *Diabetes Technology and Therapeutics*, Vol. 7, N° 1, pp. 204-208

Hunt, C. & Morimoto, R.I. (1985). Conserved features of eukaryotic hsp70 genes revealed by comparison with the nucleotide sequence of human hsp70. *Proceedings of the National Academy of Sciences of the U.S.A.*, Vol. 82, N° 19, pp. 6455-6459

Ianaro, A.; Ialenti, A.; Maffia, P.; Di Meglio, P.; Di Rosa, M. & Santoro, M.G. (2003). Anti-inflammatory activity of 15-deoxy-$\Delta^{12,14}$-PGJ_2 and 2-cyclopenten-1-one: role of the heat shock response. *Molecular Pharmacology*, Vol. 64, pp. 85-93

Jang, H.J.; Kwak, J.H.; Cho, E.Y; We, Y.; Lee, Y.H.; Kim, S.C. & Han, D.J. (2008). Glutamine induces heat-shock protein-70 and glutathione expression and attenuates ischemic damage in rat islets. *Transplantation Proceedings*, Vol. 40, N°8, pp. 2581-2584

Jessop, D.S.; Douthwaite, J.A.; Conde, G.L.; Lightman, S.L.; Dayan, C.M. & Harbuz, M.S. (1997). Effects of Acute Stress or Centrally Injected Interleukin-1β on Neuropeptide Expression in the Immune System. *Stress*, Vol. 2, pp. 133-144

Kampinga, H.H.; Hageman, J.; Vos, M.J.; Kubota, H.; Tanguay,R.M.; Bruford, E.A.; Cheetham, M.E.; Chen, B. & Hightower, L.E. (2009). Guidelines for the nomenclature of the human heat shock proteins. *Cell Stress and Chaperones*, Vol. 14, N° 1, pp. 105-111.

Karlsen, A.E.; Heding, P.E.; Frobose, H.; Ronn, S.G.; Kruhoffer, M.; Orntoft, T.F.; Darville, M.; Eizirik, D.L.; Pociot, F.; Nerup, J.; Mandrup-Poulsen, T. & Billestrup, N. (2004). Suppressor of cytokine signalling (SOCS)-3 protects β cells against IL-1β-mediated toxicity through inhibition of multiple nuclear factor-κB-regulated pro-apoptotic pathways. *Diabetologia*, Vol. 47, pp. 1998-2011

Karlsen, A.E.; Ronn, S.G.; Lindberg, K.; Johannesen, J.; Galsgaard, E.D.; Pociot, F.; Nielsen, J.H.; Mandrup-Poulsen, T.; Nerup, J. & Billestrup, N. (2001). Suppressor of cytokine signaling 3 (SOCS-3) protects β-cells against interleukin-1β- and interferon-γ-mediated toxicity. *Proceedings of the National Academy of Sciences of the U.S.A.* Vol. 98, pp. 12191-12196

Kayani, A.C.; Close, G.L.; Broome, C.S.; Jackson, M.J. & McArdle, A. (2008). Enhanced recovery from contraction-induced damage in skeletal muscles of old mice following treatment with the heat shock protein inducer 17-(allylamino)-17-demethoxygeldanamycin. *Rejuvenation Research*, Vol. 11, N° 6, pp. 1021–1030

Kelly, D.A.; Tiidus, P.M.; Houston, M.E. & Noble, E.G. (1996). Effect of vitamin E deprivation and exercise training on induction of HSP70. *Journal of Applied Physiology*, Vol. 81, N° 6, pp. 2379–2385

Kim, Y.M.; de Vera, M.E.; Watkins, S.C. & Billiar, T.R. (1997). Nitric oxide protects cultured rat hepatocytes from tumor necrosis factor-α-induced apoptosis by inducing heat shock protein 70 expression. *Journal of Biological Chemistry*, Vol. 272, N° 2, pp. 1402–1411

Kliewer, S.A.; Lenhard, J.M.; Willson, T.M.; Patel, I.; Morris, D.C. & Lehmann JM (1995). A prostaglandin J_2 metabolite binds peroxisome proliferator-activated receptor γ and promotes adipocyte differentiation. *Cell*, Vol. 83, pp. 813–819

Knowles, R.G. & Moncada, S. (1994). Nitric oxide synthases in mammals. *Biochemical Journal*, Vol. 298, Pt 2, pp. 249-258

Krause, M.S. & Homem de Bittencourt, P.I., Jr. (2008). Type 1 diabetes: can exercise impair the autoimmune event? The L-arginine/glutamine coupling hypothesis. *Cell Biochemistry and Function*, Vol. 26, N° 4, pp. 406-433

Krause, M.S.; Oliveira Junior, L.P.; Silveira, E.M.; Vianna, D.R.; Rossato, J.S.; Almeida, B.S.; Rodrigues, M.F.; Fernandes, A.J.M.; Costa, J.A.B.; Curi, R. & Homem de Bittencourt, P.I., Jr. (2007). MRP1/GS-X pump ATPase expression: is this the explanation for the cytoprotection of the heart against oxidative stress-induced redox imbalance in comparison to skeletal muscle cells? *Cell Biochemistry and Function*, Vol. 25, N° 1, pp. 23–32

Kregel, K.C. & Moseley, P.L. (1996). Differential effects of exercise and heat stress on liver HSP70 accumulation with aging. *Journal of Applied Physiology*, Vol. 80, N° 2, pp. 547–551

Kutlu, B.; Cardozo, A.K.; Darville, M.I.; Kruhoffer, M.; Magnusson, N.; Orntoft, T. & Eizirik, D.L. (2003). Discovery of gene networks regulating cytokine-induced dysfunction and apoptosis in insulin-producing INS-1 cells. *Diabetes*, Vol. 52, pp. 2701-2719

Lagranha, C.J.; Levada-Pires, A.C.; Sellitti, D.F.; Procópio, J.; Curi, R. & Pithon-Curi, T.C. (2008). The effect of glutamine supplementation and physical exercise on neutrophil function. *Amino Acids*, Vol 34, N°3, pp. 337-346

Lancaster, G.I. & Febbraio, M.A. (2005). Exosome-dependent trafficking of HSP70: a novel secretory pathway for cellular stress proteins. *Journal of Biological Chemistry*, Vol. 280, N° 24, pp. 23349–23355

Lancaster, G.I.; Moller, K.; Nielsen, B.; Secher, N.H.; Febbraio, M.A. & Nybo, L. (2004). Exercise induces the release of heat shock protein 72 from the human brain in vivo. Cell Stress and Chaperones, Vol. 9, N° 3, pp. 276–280

Lenzen, S.; Drinkgern, J. & Tiedge, M. (1996). Low antioxidant enzyme gene expression in pancreatic islets compared with various other mouse tissues. *Free Radical Biology and Medicine*, Vol. 20, pp. 463-466

Li, M.; Peterson. S.; Husney, D.; Inaba, M.; Guo, K.; Kappas, A.; Ikehara, S. & Abraham, N.G. (2007). Long-lasting expression of HO-1 delays progression of type I diabetes in NOD mice. *Cell Cycle*, Vol. 6, pp. 567-571

Ligthart-Melis, G.C.; van de Poll, M.C.; Boelens, P.G.; Dejong, C.H.; Deutz, N.E. & van Leeuwen, P.A. (2008). Glutamine is an important precursor for de novo synthesis of arginine in humans. *American Journal of Clinical Nutrition*, Vol. 87, N° 5, pp. 1282-1289

Lindquist, S. & Craig, E.A. (2004). The heat-shock proteins. *Annual Review of Genetics*, Vol. 22, pp. 631–677

Locke, M.; Noble, E.G.; Tanguay, R.M.; Field, M.R.; Ianuzzo, S.E. & Ianuzzo, C.D. (1995). Activation of heat-shock transcription factor in rat heart after heat shock and exercise. *American Journal of Physiology. Cell Physiology*, Vol. 268, N° 6 Pt 1, pp. C1387–C1394

Loï, C.; Zazzo, J.F.; Delpierre, E.; Niddam, C.; Neveux, N.; Curis, E.; Arnaud-Battandier, F. & Cynober, L. (2009). Increasing plasma glutamine in postoperative patients fed an arginine-rich immune-enhancing diet - a pharmacokinetic randomized controlled study. *Critical Care Medicine*, Vol. 37, N° 2, pp. 501-509.

Lovejoy, J.; Newby, F.D.; Gebhart, S.S. & DiGirolamo, M. (1992). Insulin resistance in obesity is associated with elevated basal lactate levels and diminished lactate appearance following intravenous glucose and insulin. *Metabolism*, Vol. 41, N°1, pp. 22-27

MacDonald, M.J. (1995). Feasibility of a mitochondrial pyruvate malate shuttle in pancreatic islets. Further implication of cytosolic NADPH in insulin secretion. *Journal of Biological Chemistry*, Vol. 270, pp. 20051-20058

Malaisse, W.J.; Blachier, F.; Mourtada, A.; Camara, J.; Albor, A.; Valverde, I. & Sener, A. (1989). Stimulus-secretion coupling of arginine-induced insulin release. Metabolism of L-arginine and L-ornithine in pancreatic islets. *Biochimica et Biophysica Acta*, Vol. 1013, pp. 133-143

Malaisse, W.J.; Malaisse-Lagae, F.; Sener, A. & Pipeleers, D.G. (1982). Determinants of the selective toxicity of alloxan to the pancreatic B cell. *Proceedings of the National Academy of Sciences of the U.S.A.*, Vol. 79, pp. 927-930

Mambula, S.S.; Stevenson, M.A.; Ogawa, K. & Calderwood, S.K. (2007). Mechanisms for Hsp70 secretion: crossing membranes without a leader. *Methods*, Vol. 43, N° 3, pp. 168–175

Mandrup-Poulsen, T. (2010). IAPP boosts islet macrophage IL-1 in type 2 diabetes. *Nature Immunology*, Vol. 11, N°10, pp. 881-883

Mandrup-Poulsen, T.; Helqvist, S.; Wogensen, L.D.; Mølvig, J.; Pociot, F.; Johannesen, J. & Nerup, J. (1990). Cytokine and free radicals as effector molecules in the destruction of pancreatic β cells. *Current Topics in Microbiology and Immunology*, Vol. 164, pp. 169-193

Mathews, C.E. & Leiter, E.H. (1999). Constitutive differences in antioxidant defense status distinguish alloxan-resistant and alloxan-susceptible mice. *Free Radical Biology and Medicine*, Vol. 27, pp. 449-455

Matthews, G.D.; Gould, R.M. & Vardimon, L. (2005). A single glutamine synthetase gene produces tissue-specific subcellular localization by alternative splicing. *Federation of European Biochemical Societies Letters*. Vol. 579, pp. 5527-5534

Maxwell, S.R.; Thomason, H.; Sandler, D.; Leguen, C.; Baxter, M.A.; Thorpe, G.H. & Jones, A.F. (1997). Antioxidant status in patients with uncomplicated insulin-dependent and non-insulin-dependent diabetes mellitus. *European Journal of Clinical Investigation*, Vol. 27, N°6, pp. 484-490

McGillis, J.P.; Park, A.; Rubin-Fletter, P.; Turck, C.; Dallman, M.F. & Payan, D.G. (1989). Stimulation of rat B-lymphocyte proliferation by corticotropin-releasing factor. *Journal of Neuroscience Research*, Vol. 23, pp. 346-352

Michalska, M.; Wolf, G.; Walther, R. & Newsholme, P. (2010). Effects of pharmacologic inhibition of NADPH oxidase and iNOS on pro-inflammatory cytokine, palmitic acid or H_2O_2-induced mouse islet or clonal pancreatic beta cell dysfunction. *Bioscience Reports*, Vol. 30, pp. 445-453

Milne, K.J. & Noble, E.G. (2002). Exercise-induced elevation of HSP70 is intensity dependent. *Journal of Applied Physiology*, Vol. 93, N° 2, pp. 561–568

Modolell, M.; Corraliza, I.M.; Link, F.; Soler, G. & Eichmann, K. (1995). Reciprocal regulation of the nitric oxide synthase/arginase balance in mouse bone marrow-derived macrophages by TH1 and TH2 cytokines. *European Journal of Immunology*, Vol. 25, pp. 1101-1104

Mohan, I.K. & Das, U.N. (1998). Effect of L-arginine-nitric oxide system on chemical-induced diabetes mellitus. *Free Radical Biology and Medicine*, Vol. 25, pp. 757-765

Moinard, C.; Belabed, L.; Gupta, S.; Besson, V.; Marchand-Verrecchia, C.; Chaumeil, J.C.; Cynober, L. & Charrueau, C. (2006). Arginine-enriched diet limits plasma and muscle glutamine depletion in head-injured rats. *Nutrition*, Vol. 22, pp. 1039-1044

Moncada, S.; Palmer, R.M. & Higgs, E.A. (1991). Nitric oxide: physiology, pathophysiology, and pharmacology. *Pharmacological Reviews*, Vol. 43, pp. 109-142

Morgan, D.; Oliveira-Emilio, H.R.; Keane, D.; Hirata, A.E.; Santos da Rocha, M.; Bordin, S.; Curi, R.; Newsholme, P. & Carpinelli, A.R. (2007). Glucose, palmitate and pro-inflammatory cytokines modulate production and activity of a phagocyte-like NADPH oxidase in rat pancreatic islets and a clonal β cell line. *Diabetologia*, Vol. 50, pp. 359-369

Mori, M. & Gotoh, T. (2000). Regulation of nitric oxide production by arginine metabolic enzymes. *Biochemical and Biophysical Research Communications*, Vol. 275, pp. 715-719

Mori, M. (2007). Regulation of nitric oxide synthesis and apoptosis by arginase and arginine recycling. *Journal of Nutrition*, Vol. 137, pp. 1616S-1620S

Morris, S.M.; Kepka-Lenhart, D. & Chen, L.C. (1998). Differential regulation of arginases and inducible nitric oxide synthase in murine macrophage cells. *American Journal of Physiology. Endocrinology and Metabolism*, Vol. 275, pp. E740-E747

Morton, J.P.; Maclaren, D.P.; Cable, N.T.; Campbell, I.T.; Evans, L.; Bongers, T.; Griffiths, R.D.; Kayani, A.C.; McArdle, A. & Drust, B. (2007). Elevated core and muscle temperature to levels comparable to exercise do not increase heat shock protein content of skeletal muscle of physically active men. *Acta Physiologica* (Oxford), Vol. 190, N° 4, pp. 319–327

Moynagh, P.N. (2005). The NF-κB pathway. *Journal of Cell Science*, Vol. 118, pp. 4589-4592

Multhoff, G. (2007). Heat shock protein 70 (Hsp70): membrane location, export and immunological relevance. *Methods*, Vol. 43, N° 3, pp. 229–237

Munder, M.; Eichmann, K. & Modolell, M. (1998). Alternative metabolic states in murine macrophages reflected by the nitric oxide synthase/arginase balance: competitive regulation by $CD4^+$ T cells correlates with Th1/Th2 phenotype. *Journal of Immunology*, Vol. 160, pp. 5347-5354

Munder, M.; Eichmann, K.; Moran, J.M.; Centeno, F.; Soler, G. & Modolell, M. (1999). Th1/Th2-regulated expression of arginase isoforms in murine macrophages and dendritic cells. *Journal of Immunology*, Vol. 163, pp. 3771-3777

Murlasits, Z.; Cutlip, R.G.; Geronilla, K.B.; Rao, K.M.; Wonderlin, W.F. & Always, S.E. (2006). Resistance training increases heat shock protein levels in skeletal muscle of young and old rats. *Experimental Gerontology*, Vol. 41, N° 4, pp. 398–406

Murphy, C. & Newsholme, P. (1998). Importance of glutamine metabolism in murine macrophages and human monocytes to L-arginine biosynthesis and rates of nitrite or urea production. *Clinical Science* (London), Vol. 95, pp. 397-407

Murphy, C. & Newsholme, P. (1998). Importance of glutamine metabolism in murine macrophages and human monocytes to L-arginine biosynthesis and rates of nitrite or urea production. *Clinical Science (London)*, Vol. 95, pp. 397-407

Nagasaki, A.; Gotoh, T.; Takeya, M.; Yu, Y.; Takiguchi, M.; Matsuzaki, H.; Takatsuki, K. & Mori, M. (1996). Coinduction of nitric oxide synthase, argininosuccinate synthetase, and argininosuccinate lyase in lipopolysaccharide-treated rats. RNA blot, immunoblot, and immunohistochemical analyses. *Journal of Biological Chemistry*, Vol. 271, pp. 2658-2662

Nakamura, H.; Nakamura, K. & Yodoi, J. (1997). Redox regulation of cellular activation. *Annual Review of Immunology*, Vol. 15, pp. 351-369

Newsholme P.; Homem de Bittencourt, P.I., Jr.; O' Hagan, C.; DeVito, G.; Murphy, C. & Krause, M.S. (2009a). Exercise and possible molecular mechanisms of protection from vascular disease and diabetes: the central role of ROS and nitric oxide. *Clinical Science* (London), Vol. 118, pp. 341–349

Newsholme P., Morgan D., Rebelato, E., Oliveira-Emilio H.C., Procopio J., Curi R. and Carpinelli A. (2009b) Insights into the critical role of NADPH oxidase(s) in the normal and dysregulated pancreatic beta cell. *Diabetologia*, Vol.52, pp. 2489-2498

Newsholme, P.; Gordon, S. & Newsholme, E.A. (1987). Rates of utilization and fates of glucose, glutamine, pyruvate, fatty acids and ketone bodies by mouse macrophages. *Biochemical Journal*, Vol. 242, pp. 631-636

Newsholme, P.; Haber, E.; Hirabara, S.; Rebelato, E.; Propcopio, J.; Morgan, D.; Oliveira-Emilio, H.; Carpinelli, A & Curi, R. (2007). Diabetes associated cell stress and dysfunction - Role of mitochondrial and non-mitochondrial ROS production and activity. *Journal of Physiology*, Vol. 583, pp. 9-24

Newsholme, P.; Lima, M.M.; Procopio, J.; Pithon-Curi, T.C.; Doi, S.Q.; Bazotte, R.B. & Curi, R. (2003). Glutamine and glutamate as vital metabolites. *Brazilian Journal of Medical and Biological Research*, Vol. 36, pp. 153-163

Newsholme, P.; Procópio, J.; Lima, M.M.; Pithon-Curi, T.C. & Curi R. (2003). Glutamine and glutamate - their central role in cell metabolism and function. *Cell Biochemisry and Function*, Vol. 21, pp. 1-9

Nieman, D.C. & Pedersen, B.K. (1999). Exercise and immune function. Recent developments. *Sports Medicine*, Vol. 27, pp. 73-80

Noble, E.G.; Milne, K.J. & Melling, C.W. (2008). Heat shock proteins and exercise: a primer. *Applied Physiology, Nutrition and Metabolism*, Vol. 33, N° 5, pp. 1050–1065

Nomikos, I.N.; Prowse, S.J.; Carotenuto, P. & Lafferty, K.J. (1986). Combined treatment with nicotinamide and desferrioxamine prevents islet allograft destruction in NOD mice. *Diabetes*, Vol. 35, pp. 1302-1304

Nussler, A.K.; Billiar, T.R.; Liu, Z.Z. & Morris, S.M., Jr. (1994). Coinduction of nitric oxide synthase and argininosuccinate synthetase in a murine macrophage cell line. Implications for regulation of nitric oxide production. *Journal of Biological Chemistry*, Vol. 269, pp. 1257-1261

Ogawa, F.; Shimizu, K.; Hara, T. ; Muroi, E.; Hasegawa, M.; Takehara, K. & Sato, S. (2008). Serum levels of heat shock protein 70, a biomarker of cellular stress, are elevated in patients with systemic sclerosis: association with fibrosis and vascular damage. *Clinical and Experimental Rheumatology*, Vol. 26, N° 4, pp. 659–662

Oliveira, H.R.; Verlengia, R.; Carvalho, C.R.; Britto, L.R.; Curi, R. & Carpinelli, A.R. (2003). Pancreatic β-cells express phagocyte-like NAD(P)H oxidase. *Diabetes*, Vol. 52, pp. 1457-1463

Palmer, J.P.; Benson, J.W.; Walter, R.M. & Ensinck, J.W. (1976). Arginine-stimulated acute phase of insulin and glucagon secretion in diabetic subjects. *Journal of Clinical Investigation*, Vol. 58, pp. 565-570

Paroo, Z. & Noble, E.G. (1999). Isoproterenol potentiates exercise-induction of Hsp70 in cardiac and skeletal muscle. *Cell Stress and Chaperones*, Vol. 4, N° 3, pp. 199–204

Paroo, Z.; Dipchand, E.S. & Noble, E.G. (2002b). Estrogen attenuates postexercise HSP70 expression in skeletal muscle. *American Journal of Physiology. Cell Physiology*, Vol. 282, N° 2, pp. C245–C251

Paroo, Z.; Haist, J.V.; Karmazyn, M. & Noble, E.G. (2002a). Exercise improves postischemic cardiac function in males but not females: consequences of a novel sex-specific heat shock protein 70 response. *Circulation Research*, Vol. 90, N° 8, pp. 911–917

Paroo, Z.; Tiidus, P.M. & Noble, E.G. (1999). Estrogen attenuates HSP 72 expression in acutely exercised male rodents. *European Journal of Applied Physiology and Occupational Physiology*, Vol. 80, N° 3, pp. 180–184

Parry-Billings, M.; Leighton, B.; Dimitriadis, G.D.; Bond, J. & Newsholme, E.A. (1990). Effects of physiological and pathological levels of glucocorticoids on skeletal muscle glutamine metabolism in the rat. *Biochemical Pharmacology*, Vol. 40, pp. 1145-1148

Pedersen, B.K. & Hoffman-Goetz, L. (2000). Exercise and the immune system: regulation, integration, and adaptation. *Physiological Reviews*, Vol. 80, pp. 1055-1081

Pedersen, B.K. & Steensberg, A. (2002). Exercise and hypoxia: effects on leukocytes and interleukin-6-shared mechanisms? *Medicine Science in Sports and Exercise*, Vol. 34, pp. 2004-2013

Pedersen, B.K.; Ostrowski. K.; Rohde, T. & Bruunsgaard, H. (1998). The cytokine response to strenuous exercise. Canadian Journal of Physiology and Pharmacology, Vol. 76, N° 5, pp. 505-511

Pedersen, B.K.; Steensberg, A. & Schjerling, P. (2001). Muscle-derived interleukin-6: possible biological effects. *Journal of Physiology*, Vol. 536, pp. 329-337

Piatti, P.M.; Monti, L.D.; Valsecchi, G.; Magni, F.; Setola, E.; Marchesi, F.; Galli-Kienle, M.; Pozza, G. & Alberti, K.G. (2001). Long-term oral L-arginine administration improves peripheral and hepatic insulin sensitivity in type 2 diabetic patients. *Diabetes Care*, Vol. 24, pp. 875-880

Pieper, G.M. & Dondlinger, L.A. (1997). Plasma and vascular tissue arginine are decreased in diabetes: acute arginine supplementation restores endothelium-dependent relaxation by augmenting cGMP production. *Journal of Pharmacology and Experimental Therapeutics*, Vol. 283, pp. 684-691

Pithon-Curi, T.C.; De Melo, M.P. & Curi, R. (2004). Glucose and glutamine utilization by rat lymphocytes, monocytes and neutrophils in culture: a comparative study. *Cell Biochemistry and Function*, Vol. 22, pp. 321-326

Piva, R.; Gianferretti, P.; Ciucci, A.; Taulli, R.; Belardo, G. & Santoro, M.G. (2005). 15-Deoxy-$\Delta^{12,14}$-prostaglandin J_2 induces apoptosis in human malignant B cells: an effect associated with inhibition of NF-κB activity and down-regulation of antiapoptotic proteins. *Blood*, Vol. 105, pp. 1750-1758

Rabinovitch, A. & Suarez-Pinzon, W.L. (1998). Cytokines and their roles in pancreatic islet β-cell destruction and insulin-dependent diabetes mellitus. *Biochemical Pharmacology*, Vol. 55, pp. 1139-1149

Rabinovitch, A.; Suarez, W.L.; Thomas, P.D.; Strynadka, K. & Simpson, I. (1992). Cytotoxic effects of cytokines on rat islets: evidence for involvement of free radicals and lipid peroxidation. *Diabetologia*, Vol. 35, pp. 409-413

Rabinovitch, A.; Suarez-Pinzon, W.L; Strynadka, K.; Lakey, J.R. & Rajotte, R.V. (1996). Human pancreatic islet β-cell destruction by cytokines involves oxygen free radicals and aldehyde production. *Journal of Clinical Endocrinology and Metabolism*, Vol. 81, pp. 3197-3202

Ran, R.; Lu, A.; Zhang, L.; Tang, Y.; Zhu, H.; Xu, H.; Feng, Y.; Han, C.; Zhou, G.; Rigby, A.C. & Sharp, F.R. (2004). Hsp70 promotes TNF-mediated apoptosis by binding IKK gamma and impairing NF-kappa B survival signaling. *Genes and Development*, Vol. 18, N° 12, pp. 1466–1481

Rieneck, K.; Bovin, L.F.; Josefsen, K.; Buschard, K.; Svenson, M. & Bendtzen, K. (2000). Massive parallel gene expression profiling of RINm5F pancreatic islet β-cells stimulated with interleukin-1β. *Acta Pathological, Microbiologica, et Immunologica Scandinavica*, Vol. 108, pp. 855-872

Rocič, B.; Vucič, M.; Knezevič-Cuča, J.; Radica, A.; Pavlič-Renar, I.; Profozič, V. & Metelko, Z. (1997). Total plasma antioxidants in first-degree relatives of patients with insulin-dependent diabetes. *Experimental and Clinical Endocrinology and Diabetes*, Vol. 105, N° 4, pp. 213-217

Rohde, T.; MacLean, D.A.; Richter, E.A.; Kiens, B. & Pedersen, B.K. (1997). Prolonged submaximal eccentric exercise is associated with increased levels of plasma IL-6. *American Journal of Physiology. Endocrinology and Metabolism*, Vol. 273, pp. E85–E91

Rossi, A.; Kapahi, P.; Natoli, G.; Takahashi, T.; Chen, Y.; Karin, M. & Santoro, M.G. (2000). Anti-inflammatory cyclopentenone prostaglandins are direct inhibitors of IκB kinase. *Nature*, Vol. 403, N° 6765, pp. 103–108

Rothe, H.; Hausmann, A. & Kolb, H. (2002). Immunoregulation during disease progression in prediabetic NOD mice: inverse expression of arginase and prostaglandin H synthase 2 *vs.* interleukin-15. *Hormone and Metabolic Research*, Vol. 34, pp. 7-12

Rutschman, R.; Lang, R.; Hesse, M.; Ihle, J.N.; Wynn, T.A. & Murray, P.J. (2001). Cutting edge: Stat6-dependent substrate depletion regulates nitric oxide production. *Journal of Immunology*, Vol. 166, pp. 2173-2177

Salo, D.C.; Donovan, C.M. & Davies, K.J. (1991). HSP70 and other possible heat shock or oxidative stress proteins are induced in skeletal muscle, heart, and liver during exercise. *Free Radical Biology and Medicine*, Vol. 11, N° 3, pp. 239–246

Santini, S.A.; Marra, G.; Giardina, B.; Cotroneo, P.; Mordente, A.; Martorana, G.E.; Manto, A. & Ghirlanda, G. (1997). Defective plasma antioxidant defenses and enhanced susceptibility to lipid peroxidation in uncomplicated IDDM. *Diabetes*, Vol. 46, pp. 1853-1858

Scarim, A.L.; Heitmeier, M.R. & Corbett, J.A. (1998). Heat shock inhibits cytokine-induced nitric oxide synthase expression by rat and human islets. *Endocrinology*, Vol. 139, N° 12, pp. 5050-5057

Silveira, E.M.; Rodrigues, M.F.; Krause, M.S.; Vianna, D.R.; Almeida, B.S.; Rossato, J.S.; Oliveira Junior, L.P.; Curi, R. & Homem de Bittencourt, P.I., Jr. (2007) Acute exercise stimulates macrophage function: possible role of NF-κB pathways. *Cell Biochemistry and Function*, Vol. 25, N° 1, pp. 63–73

Simar, D.; Malatesta, D.; Badiou, S.; Dupuy, A.M. & Caillaud, C. (2007). Physical activity modulates heat shock protein-72 expression and limits oxidative damage accumulation in a healthy elderly population aged 60-90 years. *Journals of Gerontology. Series A, Biological Sciences and Medical Sciences*, Vol. 62, N° 12, pp. 1413–1419

Simmons, W.W.; Closs, E.I.; Cunningham, J.M.; Smith, T.W. & Kelly, R.A. (1996). Cytokines and insulin induce cationic amino acid transporter (CAT) expression in cardiac myocytes. Regulation of L-arginine transport and no production by CAT-1, CAT-2A, and CAT-2B. *Journal of Biological Chemistry*, Vol. 271, pp. 11694-11702

Simopoulos, A.P. (2006). Evolutionary aspects of diet, the ω-6/ω-3 ratio and genetic variation: nutritional implications for chronic diseases. *Biomedicine and Pharmacotherapy*, Vol. 60, pp. 502-507

Singh, V.K. & Leu, S.J. (1990). Enhancing effect of corticotropin-releasing neurohormone on the production of interleukin-1 and interleukin-2. *Neuroscience Letters*, Vol. 120, pp. 151-154

Singleton, K.D. & Wischmeyer, P.E. (2008). Glutamine induces heat shock protein expression via O-glycosylation and phosphorylation of HSF-1 and Sp1. Journal of Parenteral and Enteral Nutrition, Vol. 32, N° 4, pp. 371-376

Sipetic, S.; Vlajinac, H.; Marinkovi, J.; Kocev, N.; Milan, B.; Ratkov, I. & Sajic, S. (2007). Stressful life events and psychological dysfunctions before the onset of type 1 diabetes mellitus. *Journal of Pediatric Endocrinology and Metabolism*, Vol. 20, pp. 527-534

Skidmore, R.; Gutierrez, J.A.; Guerriero, V., Jr. & Kregel, K.C. (1995). HSP70 induction during exercise and heat stress in rats: role of internal temperature. *American Journal of Physiology. Regulatory, Integrative and Comparative Physiology*, Vol. 268, N° 1 Pt 2, pp. R92–R97

Smolka, M.B.; Zoppi, C.C.; Alves, A.A.; Silveira, L.R.; Marangoni, S.; Pereira-Da-Silva, L.;Novello, J.C. & Macedo, D.V. (2000). HSP72 as a complementary protection against oxidative stress induced by exercise in the soleus muscle of rats. *American Journal of Physiology. Regulatory, Integrative and Comparative Physiology*, Vol. 279, N° 5, pp. R1539–R1545

Smukler, S.R.; Tang, L.; Wheeler, M.B. & Salapatek, A.M. (2002). Exogenous nitric oxide and endogenous glucose-stimulated β-cell nitric oxide augment insulin release. *Diabetes*, Vol. 51, pp. 3450-3460

Soltesz, G. (2003). Diabetes in the young: a paediatric and epidemiological perspective. *Diabetologia*, Vol. 46, pp. 447-454

Spinas, G.A. (1999). The Dual Role of Nitric Oxide in Islet β-Cells. *News in Physiological Sciences*, Vol. 14, pp. 49-54

Staib, J.L.; Quindry, J.C.; French, J.P.; Criswell, D.S. & Powers, S.K. (2007). Increased temperature, not cardiac load, activates heat shock transcription factor 1 and heat shock protein 72 expression in the heart. *American Journal of Physiology. Regulatory, Integrative and Comparative Physiology*, Vol. 292, N° 1, pp. R432–R439

Stickings, P.; Mistry, S.K.; Boucher, J.L.; Morris, S.M. & Cunningham, J.M. (2002). Arginase expression and modulation of IL-1β-induced nitric oxide generation in rat and human islets of Langerhans. *Nitric Oxide*, Vol. 7, pp. 289-296

Suarez-Pinzon, W.L.; Strynadka, K. & Rabinovitch, A. (1996). Destruction of rat pancreatic islet β-cells by cytokines involves the production of cytotoxic aldehydes. *Endocrinology*, Vol. 137, pp. 5290-5296

Sumoski, W.; Baquerizo, H. & Rabinovitch, A. (1989). Oxygen free radical scavengers protect rat islet cells from damage by cytokines. *Diabetologia*, Vol. 32, pp. 792-796

Sun, Y. & MacRae, T.H. (2005). The small heat shock proteins and their role in human disease. *Federation of European Biochemical Societies Letters*, Vol. 272, N° 11, pp. 2613–2627.

Suzuki, K.; Yamada, M.; Kurakake, S.; Okamura, N.; Yamaya, K.; Liu, Q.; Kudoh, S.; Kowatari, K.; Nakaji, S. & Sugawara, K. (2000). Circulating cytokines and hormones with immunosuppressive but neutrophil-priming potentials rise after endurance exercise in humans. *European Journal of Applied Physiology*, Vol. 81, pp. 281-287

Tavaria, M.; Gabriele, T.; Anderson, R.L.; Mirault, M.E.; Baker, E.; Sutherland, G. & Kola, I. (1995). Localization of the gene encoding the human heat shock cognate protein, HSP73, to chromosome 11. *Genomics*, Vol. 29, N° 1, pp. 266–268

Tavaria, M.; Gabriele, T.; Kola. I & Anderson, R.L. (1996). A hitchhiker's guide to the human Hsp70 family. *Cell Stress and Chaperones*, Vol. 1, N° 1, pp. 23–28

Tenu, J.P.; Lepoivre, M.; Moali, C.; Brollo, M.; Mansuy, D. & Boucher, J.L. (1999). Effects of the new arginase inhibitor N^{ω}-hydroxy-nor-L-arginine on NO synthase activity in murine macrophages. *Nitric Oxide*, Vol. 3, pp. 427-438

Tupling, A.R.; Bombardier, E.; Stewart, R.D.; Vigna, C. & Aqui, A.E. (2007). Muscle fiber type-specific response of Hsp70 expression in human quadriceps following acute isometric exercise. *Journal of Applied Physiology*, Vol. 103, N° 6, pp. 2105–2111

Vabulas, R.M.; Ahmad-Nejad, P.; Ghose, S.; Kirschning, C.J.; Issels, R.D & Wagner. H. (2002). HSP70 as endogenous stimulus of the Toll/interleukin-1 receptor signal pathway. *Journal of Biological Chemistry*, Vol. 277, N° 17, pp. 15107–15112

Van de Poll, M.C.; Ligthart-Melis, G.C.; Boelens, P.G.; Deutz, N.E.; van Leeuwen, P.A. & Dejong, C.H. (2007). Intestinal and hepatic metabolism of glutamine and citrulline in humans. *Journal of Physiology*, Vol. 581(Pt 2), pp. 819-827

Vasilijevič, A.; Buzadzič, B.; Korač, A.; Petrovič, V.; Jankovič, A.; Micunovič, K. & Korač, B. (2007). The effects of cold acclimation and nitric oxide on antioxidative enzymes in rat pancreas. *Comparative Biochemistry and Physiology. C: Toxicology and Pharmacology*, Vol. 145, pp. 641-647

Velmurugan, K.; Alam, J.; McCord, J.M. & Pugazhenthi, S. (2009). Synergistic induction of heme oxygenase-1 by the components of the antioxidant supplement Protandim. *Free Radical Biology and Medicine*, Vol. 46, pp. 430-440

Vermeulen, M.A.; van de Poll, M.C.; Ligthart-Melis, G.C.; Dejong, C.H.; van den Tol, M.P.; Boelens, P.G. & van Leeuwen, P.A. (2007). Specific amino acids in the critically ill patient--exogenous glutamine/arginine: a common denominator? *Critical Care Medicine,* Vol. 35, pp. S568-S576

Wachlin, G.; Heine, L.; Klöting, I.; Dunger, A.; Hahn, H.J. & Schmidt, S. (2002). Stress response of pancreatic islets from diabetes prone BB rats of different age. *Autoimmunity,* Vol. 35, N° 6, pp. 389-395

Waddington, S.N.; Mosley, K.; Cook, H.T.; Tam, F.W. & Cattell, V. (1998). Arginase AI is upregulated in acute immune complex-induced inflammation. *Biochemical and Biophyssical Research Communications,* Vol. 247, pp. 84-87

Wadt, K.A.; Larsen, C.M.; Andersen, H.U.; Nielsen, K.; Karlsen, A.E. & Mandrup-Poulsen, T. (1998). Ciliary neurotrophic factor potentiates the β-cell inhibitory effect of IL-1β in rat pancreatic islets associated with increased nitric oxide synthesis and increased expression of inducible nitric oxide synthase. *Diabetes,* Vol. 47, pp. 1602-1608

Walsh, R.C.; Koukoulas, I.; Garnham, A.; Moseley, P.L.; Hargreaves, M. & Febbraio, M.A. (2001). Exercise increases serum Hsp72 in humans. *Cell Stress and Chaperones,* Vol. 6, pp. 386–393

Wei, L.H.; Jacobs, A.T.; Morris, S.M., Jr. & Ignarro, L.J. (2000). IL-4 and IL-13 upregulate arginase I expression by cAMP and JAK/STAT6 pathways in vascular smooth muscle cells. *American Journal of Physiology. Cell Physiology.* Vol. 279, pp. C248-C256

Wierusz-Wysocka, B.; Wysocki, H.; Byks, H.; Zozulińska, D.; Wykretowicz, A. & Kaźmierczak, M. (1997). Metabolic control quality and free radical activity in diabetic patients. *Diabetes Research and Clinical Practice,* Vol. 27, pp. 193-197

Wilmore, D. (2004). Enteral and parenteral arginine supplementation to improve medical outcomes in hospitalized patients. *Journal of Nutrition,* Vol. 134, pp. 2863S-2867S (see discussion in 2895S)

Winyard, P.G. & Blake, D.R. (1997). Antioxidants, redox-regulated transcription factors, and inflammation. *Advances in Pharmacology,* Vol. 38, pp. 403-421

Wischmeyer, P.E.; Kahana, M.; Wolfson, R.; Ren, H.; Musch, M.M. & Chang, E.B. (2001). Glutamine reduces cytokine release, organ damage, and mortality in a rat model of endotoxemia. *Shock,* Vol. 16, pp. 398-402

Wischmeyer, P.E.; Riehm, J.; Singleton, K.D.; Ren, H.; Musch, M.W.; Kahana, M. & Chang, E.B. (2003). Glutamine attenuates tumor necrosis factor-alpha release and enhances heat shock protein 72 in human peripheral blood mononuclear cells. *Nutrition,* Vol. 19, N° 1, pp. 1-6

Wisloff, U.; Najjar, S.M.; Ellingsen, O.; Haram, P.M.; Swoap, S.; Al-Share, Q.; Fernstrom, M.; Rezaei, K.; Lee, S.J.; Koch, L.G. & Britton, S.L. (2005). Cardiovascular risk factors emerge after artificial selection for low aerobic capacity. *Science,* Vol. 307, pp. 418-420

Wu, G. & Morris, S.M. (1998). Arginine metabolism: nitric oxide and beyond. *Biochemical Journal,* Vol. 336, Pt 1, pp. 1-17

Wu, G.; Bazer, F.W.; Davis, T.A.; Kim, S.W.; Li, P.; Marc Rhoads, J.; Carey Satterfield, M.; Smith, S.B.; Spencer, T.E. & Yin, Y. (2009). Arginine metabolism and nutrition in growth, health and disease. *Amino Acids,* vol 37, pp. 153-168

Wu, G.; Knabe, D.A. & Kim, S.W. (2004). Arginine nutrition in neonatal pigs. *Journal of Nutrition,* Vol. 134, pp. 2783S-2790S (see discussion in 2796S-2797S)

Yabunaka, N.; Ohtsuka, Y.; Watanabe, I.; Noro, H.; Fujisawa, H. & Agishi, Y. (1995). Elevated levels of heat-shock protein 70 (HSP70) in the mononuclear cells of patients with non-insulin-dependent diabetes mellitus. *Diabetes Research and Clinical Practice*, Vol. 30, N° 2, pp. 143-147

Zhang, Y.; Zou, Z.; Li, Y.K.; Yuan, H.B. & Shi, X.Y. (2009). Glutamine-induced heat shock protein protects against renal ischaemia-reperfusion injury in rats. *Nephrology* (Carlton), Vol. 14, N° 6, pp. 573-580

Ziegler, T.R.; Ogden, L.G.; Singleton, K.D.; Luo, M.; Fernandez-Estivariz, C.; Griffith, D.P.; Galloway, J.R. & Wischmeyer, P.E. (2005). Parenteral glutamine increases serum heat shock protein 70 in critically ill patients. *Intensive Care Medicine*, Vol. 31, N° 8, pp. 1079-1086

Zingarelli, B.& Cook, J.A. (2005). Peroxisome proliferator-activated receptor-gamma is a new therapeutic target in sepsis and inflammation. *Shock*, Vol. 23, N° 5, pp. 393-399

Part 4

Identification and Monitoring of Diabetes Mellitus

Diabetes Type 1 and 2: What is Behind a Classification?

Adriana Mimbacas[1] and Gerardo Javiel[2,3]
[1]*Instituto de Investigaciones Biológicas Clemente Estable, Department of Genetics, Human Genetic Group*
[2]*ASSE-Ministry of Health, Hospital Pasteur*
[3]*IAMPP-Centro de Asistencia del Sindicato Médico del Uruguay,(CASMU), Diabetologic Service*
Uruguay

1. Introduction

At present, we wonder if the current classification of diabetes agrees with the new advances At the molecular genetic level. Every day we can see an exponential increase of type 1 and 2 diabetes anywhere in the world. On the other hand, although several clinical and biochemical characteristics have been described in order to differentiate between both types of diabetes, this does not seem satisfactory for all cases when facing the patient. These characteristics are: (a) The presence of a strong familiar history of diabetes, obesity, *acanthosis nigricans*, and lack of ketoacidosis and auto-antibodies against antigens of pancreatic b-cells islets supports the diagnosis of type 2 diabetes; (b) In contrast, patients with type 1 diabetes are usually thin and with ketoacidosis; almost 90% of them have auto-antibodies at the onset of the disease.

Nevertheless, in the last decades numerous reports described adults and adolescents (usually from minority groups) presenting ketoacidosis with lack of antibodies and characteristics of type 2 diabetes such as obesity, *acanthosis nigricans* and/or one significant familiar history of diabetes (Pinhas-Hamiel et al., 1997; Pinhas-Hamiel & Zeitler, 1999;).

Until very recently, most children and adolescents diagnosed with the disease were diagnosed as type 1 diabetes; however, there have recently been numerous reports describing an increase in the number of cases of type 2 diabetes in youngsters (Dabelea et al., 1998; Hathout et al., 2001; Neufeld et al., 1998; Pinhas Hamiel et al., 1996; Scott et al., 1997). Epidemiological data suggests that type 1 and 2 diabetes can coexist in the same family (Kolb & Mandrup-Poulsen, 2005; Libman & Becker, 2003).

The potential importance of formulating a specific diagnosis has been emphasized, as this could determine the type of treatment, associated complications, and outcomes (Fagot et al., 2001; Pinhas-Hamiel & Zeitler, 1999). The current criteria for defining diabetes (Asociación Latinoamericana de Diabetes [ALAD], 2010; American Diabetes Association [ADA], 2010) do not always explain neither the evolution of the disease in different patients or the different responses of individuals to treatments. These facts are suggesting the importance

of considering the genetic background of individuals for their categorization and subsequent treatment. A highly controversial topic has recently aroused worldwide: is there a new type of diabetes with mixed characteristics of both types? Different authors have identified this variety as "Double Diabetes" or "Hybrid Diabetes" (Libman & Becker, 2003; Mimbacas et al., 2011; Pozzilli & Buzzetti; 2007; Pozzilli & Guglielmi., 2007); but, are we really facing a new type of diabetes unknown before?, or is it a phenomenon not demonstrated until present due to the use of former inappropriate methodologies or instrumentations? If it is a new expression, why does it appear now? Is there an evolutionary process involved? How?
We will try to discuss these subjects in this chapter.

2. Brief history of diabetes mellitus and the evolution of the classification

In order to understand our point of view we must begin with a brief description of diabetes history and classification. The term diabetes (Greek: διαβητη) was coined by Aretaues of Cappadocia. It is derived from the Greek word διβαινειν, diabaínein that literally means "passing through" or "siphon", a reference to one of diabetes' major symptoms—excessive urine production. In 1675, Thomas Willis added the word mellitus, from the Latin meaning "honey", as a reference to the sweet taste of the urine. Matthew Dobson (1776) confirmed that the sweet taste was due to an excess of a kind of sugar in the urine and blood of people with diabetes. The ancient Indians tested for diabetes by observing whether ants were attracted to a person's urine, and called the ailment "sweet urine disease". The Korean, Chinese, and Japanese words for diabetes are based on the same ideographs (糖尿病), which mean "sugar urine disease".
As stated above, although diabetes has been recognized since antiquity, and treatments of different efficiencies have been known in several regions since the Middle Ages and for much longer in legends, the pathogenesis of diabetes has only been understood experimentally since about 1900 (Patlak, 2002a; 2002b). The endocrine role of the pancreas in metabolism, and indeed the existence of insulin, was not further clarified until 1922, when Banting and Best demonstrated that they could reverse induced diabetes in dogs by giving them a pancreatic islets of Langerhans extract of healthy dogs (Banting et al., 1922). However the precise molecular mechanism of the disease is just beginning to be unraveled. Fortunately, the increasing inventory of human genetic variation is easing our understanding of why susceptibility to the common disease varies between individuals and populations (Rotimi & Jorde, 2010), as we shall see.
In terms of classification, the first distinction between different presentations of the disease, as it is currently known, was clearly established by Sir H P Himsworth, and published in January 1936 (Himsworth, 1936). From its very beginning, the different classifications have undergone changes in the attempt to obtain a better adjustment of the organization of diabetes' nosology (Alberti & Zimmet, 1998): (1) Age, which was the main criterion of the first classification, was quickly abandoned because the different forms can appear at any age, although one is more frequently observed in childhood and youth and the other one in adults (at present, type 1 and 2 respectively); (2) Insulin dependence was the new clinical criterion taken into consideration, because it was easy to use in clinical practice and allowed to consider sub-groups with different pathogenic mechanisms; for several years insulin dependence was an indicator of the auto-immune process.

Currently, the classification of Diabetes mellitus (ADA, 2010; ALAD, 2010) contemplates four well-known major groups: (a) Type 1 Diabetes (T1DM), (b) Type 2 (T2DM), (c) Other specific types of diabetes, and (d) Gestational diabetes.

However, on the basis of clinical observations, genetics and molecular research studies carried out in some mixed populations such as those in Latin America (as we shall see below) would point out that this classification is not always adequate; phenotype does not always reflect genotype (Mimbacas et al., 2009).

3. Miscegenated population

In order to support our hypothesis that phenotype is not always a proper indicator of genotype, mainly in miscegenated populations (particularly in multifactorial diseases such as diabetes), we will focus our analysis on the research carried out in our population. We believe that the current classification does not always allow an accurate diagnosis, and therefore the treatment plan is not always the correct one.

Previous research has shown that the Uruguayan population has a particular genetic behavior; in addition to its small size (three millions inhabitants), it presents such a high level of miscegenation that there are individuals that cannot currently identify their ancestors' origin. It has a tri-hybrid origin (Caucasoid, African and Amerindian) but, unlike other Latin-American countries, we do not isolate Amerindian groups (Cardoso et al., 2004; Gascue et al., 2005; Mimbacas et al., 2003, 2004, 2007, 2009; Sans et al., 2011). Thus, this would permit us to think a priori that ethnological factors would (at least in part) cancel each other, therefore eliminating their possible blurring effect on the analysis. When we consider these factors, we can look at our population as an interesting source of information for the study of different issues on diabetes.

Several years ago, we focused our investigation on HLA genes associated with type 1 diabetes; our studies (Mimbacas et al., 2003, 2004) were done both by case-control and parent-cases design. We found a very high frequency of specific alleles (DQB1*0201, DQB1*0302, DR3, DR4) in our population; although the associated alleles were the same as those of the Caucasian population, their frequencies were different; additionally, we also found that almost all of the patients had associated DR3 and DR4 alleles. Continuing with our investigations, we observed that different polymorphisms of other analyzed genes also showed variations when compared with Caucasian populations or with populations from other origin (Fernández et al., 2009; Mimbacas et al., 2007; Soto et al., 2004; Zorrilla et al., 2006).

Conversely, there have been numerous reports describing an increasing number of type 2 diabetes cases in youngsters (Dabelea et al., 1998; Neufeld et al., 1998; Pinhas-Hamiel et al., 1996; Scott et al., 1997). Recently, Lidman and Becker (2003) described the coexistence of types 1 and 2 diabetes in a non-Caucasian individual; afterwards, Pozzili and Buzzetti (2007) described more cases and defined the possibility of a new type of diabetes, proposing more characterization studies in different ethnic groups. In a recent paper (Mimbacas et al., 2011) we described a case report that, according to our criteria, showed this type of presentation of the disease.

In what it has to do with this possibility of a new expression of diabetes, it is important to determine the influence of the genetic and auto-immune factors underlying the consequent destruction of the beta islets, which would pass unnoticed in a classic phenotype.

In the light of an emerging expression of diabetes, and in an attempt to link genetics to the clinic, we continued with our research. On the basis of previous findings and in the clinical evolution of patients, we began to see that in many cases it was very difficult to classify patients into one of the 2 main groups of the current diabetes classification (type 1 or type 2). Another associated observation was that, despite following the international protocols, patients did not always show a good response to treatment.
Therefore, we were interested in testing the hypothesis that genotype does not necessarily result in the disease phenotype. For this purpose, we proposed to determine whether a genetic profile is useful for providing the clinician and the patient with more accurate information, not only for knowing the specific type of diabetes, but also to understand the hyperglycemia pathogenesis and thus treat it more effectively.
For five years we examined a dynamic cohort of clinical histories of diabetes' patients, with a follow up of 86.6% (Mimbacas et al., 2009). At first, patients were classified into two groups: type 1 diabetes and type 2 diabetes according to the American Diabetes Association criteria (ADA, 2004). We analyzed HLADQB1*/DR in all samples and studied the presence of autoantibodies glutamic acid decarboxylase (GADA) and islet cell (ICA). We found surprising results, specifically in patients diagnosed as type 2 diabetes. When we applied the classification grouping the patients as type 1 and type 2 to our data, we found that the phenotype was not correlated with the expected data in all cases. In order to improve our knowledge of the pathogenesis of hyperglycemia and thus implement a more accurate treatment for the patients, we reclassified our sample according to the presence or absence of the genetic and immunological markers (Figure 1).

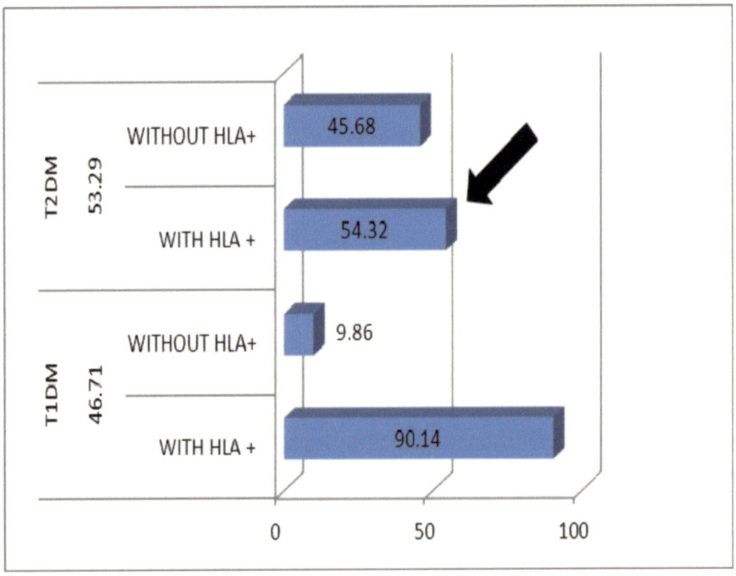

Fig. 1. A high percent of type 2 diabetes have HLA susceptibility gene for type 1 diabetes.

The data obtained shows statistical significant differences, implying that the clinical classification is probably not discriminatory enough for an accurate classification of different types of diabetes (Mimbacas et al., 2009). The methodology implemented in this investigation permitted us to establish that the phenotypic classification did reflect neither the genetic profile nor the immunological disease. The genetic data can help us to provide an accurate definition of the disease, and would therefore give the physician a better possibility of providing an adequate treatment.

Today, a proper differentiation between the different types of diabetes is becoming an increasingly challenging task. The effect of genetic variables on diabetes has been studied for several decades, but there are only a few consistent risk factors identified up to date.

Most of the large scale studies on candidate genes for diabetes published so far have not performed a combined analysis of both types of diabetes; moreover, there are a high number of published papers dealing with this subject but whose populations are not admixed like the Uruguayan one. Thus, we consider that the Uruguayan population is an interesting one to accomplish epidemiological studies, and that it will therefore contribute to the discussion.

Unfortunately, currently there are a very few researchers using new advanced methodology, such as genome wide association, in non-Caucasian population; nearly 90% of genome scan studies have been carried out in populations of European ancestry (Rotimi & Jorde, 2010).

4. Overweight and obesity mask a genetic profile associated to type 1 diabetes

As stated above, once diabetes diagnosed, proper classification is the first difficulty of this disease in clinical practice, as future treatment will depend on this. This is partly due to a lack of correlation between phenotype and genotype, and to the possible existence of a new form of diabetes, or a different expression, called "hybrid or double". This may pass inadvertently if the corresponding genetic and immunological analyses are not carried out.

Overweight or obesity is one phenotypic trait that is part of the definition of type 2 diabetes. In our study (Mimbacas et al., 2009) we observed that many patients clinically diagnosed as type 2 with positive HLA show overweight or obesity; we therefore suggested looking for a genetic explanation for this apparent contradiction. Overweight or obesity is indicative of insulin-resistance. The primary disorder type 2 diabetes is considered as an insulin-resistant one with an increase in insulin secretion and a decrease in beta cell secretion after several years (Ruiz, 2011).

On the other hand, the importance of a study on insulin resistance lies in the fact that the underlying process would be a cardiovascular risk factor per se (Howard et al., 1996; Yip et al., 1998).

Despite evidence of a genetic influence, bibliography suggests that the genetic contribution to insulin resistance is the result of several gene variants that are relatively common in the population, each one with only a moderate influence, but with much more stronger effects when they interact. The heterogeneous and polygenic nature of insulin resistance has made the identification of these gene variants a challenging task. However, once these insulin-resistance susceptibility gene variants are identified, they will have far-reaching implications for our comprehension of the molecular and pathophysiologic basis of insulin resistance, type 2 diabetes and related clustered traits, and thus for the treatment and prevention of these endemic disorders (Mercado et al., 2002).

From the molecular point of view, Insulin-Resistance is caused by different metabolic pathways with gene-gene and gene-environment interactions. In order to begin our study, we selected some of the genes found within these pathways; the first selected gene was the Peroxisome Proliferator-Activated Receptor (PPARγ2) gene, which is in turn one of the strongest candidate genes contributing to the susceptibility of type 2 diabetes, especially the

Pro12Ala polymorphism (de Dios & Frechtel, 2011). The PPARγ gene is a key regulator of lipid metabolism and energy balance, and it is implicated in the development of insulin resistance and obesity. It is a member of the nuclear hormone receptor family involved in adipocyte differentiation and gene expression regulation, and it is a transcriptional factor involved in adipogenesis and regulation of adipocyte gene expression. PPARγ plays a role in insulin signaling, insulin resistance and the development of type 2 diabetes mellitus (Chawla et al., 1994; Auwerx, 1999; Zhang et al., 2007)

A splice variant of this gene contains a common amino acid polymorphism, Pro12Ala (carrier frequencies 8–20%, depending on the population) that, depending on the cell lines, reduces the ligand-induced activity of the PPARγ protein by 30–50% (Altshuler et al., 2000; Deeb et al., 1998; Hansen et al., 2006). This missense mutation (involving a C to G substitution at nucleotide 34) results in the exchange of a proline for an alanine in position 12 of the PPARγ2 protein (Yen et al., 1997). This polymorphism has been associated with a reduced risk of development of a type 2 diabetes mellitus (Altshuler et al., 2000; Stumvoll et al., 2001). Many studies have suggested that the mechanism of reduction of the risk of type 2 diabetes mellitus by this polymorphism involves enabling greater insulin sensitivity. The Pro12Ala polymorphism produces a PPARγ2 protein with lower transcriptional activity (Deeb et al., 1998; Kang et al., 2005). The Diabetes Prevention Program (DPP) found that the Ala12 allele influences central obesity and that it is associated with the differences seen in the different treatment groups regarding polyunsaturated fatty acid intake (DPP, 2008).

In recent years, research has identified PPARs as pivotal actors in the transcriptional control of the Uncoupling Protein genes (UCP) (Villarroya et al., 2007). Thus we selected this one as a possible second gene responsible for IR. UCP-2 are mitochondrial transporters present in the inner membrane of the mitochondria of several cells (Das & Elbein, 2006; Villaroya et al., 2007). Their main function is the uncoupling of oxidative phosphorylation in the respiratory chain, preventing the formation of ATP from the energy released by substrate oxidation, and promoting its dissipation as heat.

The UCP would be in charge of the so-called adaptive thermogenesis, i.e. the generation or dissipation of heat to certain stimuli, such as overeating, cold and exercise, thus regulating temperature and body weight. Other functions have been described, in the case of UCP-2, that takes part in the regulation of insulin secretion (inhibiting its secretion by lowering the ATP synthesis through uncoupling), in immunity, and decreased oxidative stress. Their presence in different tissues, together with their energy dissipating role, could be crucial in explaining not only the genesis of obesity, but certain co morbidities (diabetes mellitus type 2) and their treatment.

A common polymorphism (-866G/A) has been associated with obesity, insulin secretion, and type 2 diabetes (Bell et al., 2005; Freeman and Cox, 2006). In what it has to do with the genetic-environmental interaction, several evidences indicate a fatty acid-dependent activation of UCP-2. Direct analysis of regulation of the promoter of the UCP-2 gene in muscle cells indicated that PPARγ and their ligands induce promoter activity (Aubert et al., 1997), while PPAR activators induce UCP-2 mRNA expression in brown adipocytes. Adipose tissue contains large amounts of endogenous triglycerides, which are capable of causing the local generation of free fatty acids after lipolysis. PPAR receptors can provide a mechanism for responsiveness of UCP-2 expression to intracellularly-derived fatty acid.

Thus cross-talk between adrenergic regulation of adipose tissue lipolysis and PPAR induction mechanisms of UCP-2 gene expression may occur, especially in response to noradrenergic stimulus in brown adipocytes (Carmona et al., 1998; Villaroya et al., 2007).

With regard to diabetes, the overexpression of PPARγ causes up regulation of UCP-2 expression and suppresses glucose-stimulated insulin secretion (Ito et al., 2004).

However, there are situations where patients can, due to these genes, present the wild type variant and yet remain with their obesity and IR unchanged. Because of this, we selected another gene that may cause IR on the other metabolic pathway: IRS-1.

IRS-1: Genetic variance in the insulin receptor substrate-1 is thought to play a key role in the insulin resistance that characterizes type 2 diabetes. Transfection studies have demonstrated that the most common IRS-1 variant, Arg972, which involves a Gly 224 Arg substitution at codon 972, impairs insulin signaling via the phosphatidylinositol-3 (PI3)-kinase pathway, and in some (but not all) studies this variant has been found with an increased frequency among type 2 diabetic patients (Almind et al., 1993, 1996; Imai et al., 1994; Sesti et al., 2001; Sigal et al., 1996; Zhang et al., 1996). Interestingly, carriers of the Arg972 substitution have been found to have lower fasting insulin and C-peptide levels than noncarriers (Clausen et al., 1995; Stumvoll et al., 2001), suggesting that this IRS-1 variant might also play a role in the secretory capacity of the beta-cells. Indeed, impaired insulin secretion has also been observed in rat insulinoma (RIN) cells overexpressing the Arg972 IRS-1 polymorphism (Porzio et al., 1999), in human islets naturally carrying the variant (Marchetti et al., 2002), and even in normal glucose-tolerant subjects with the Arg972 variant. These observations raise the intriguing hypothesis that genetic defects in the IRS-1/PI3 kinase pathway might also be involved in the inadequate insulin secretion that characterizes type 2 diabetes. More recent studies suggest that the Arg972 IRS-1 variant also plays a role in beta cell survival.

The human Arg972 islets contain a significantly higher number of apoptotic cells than their wild-type counterparts, and they are also resistant to the antiapoptotic effects of insulin (Federici et al., 2003). It has been speculated that apoptosis plays a crucial role in the autoimmune destruction of beta cells characterizing type 1 diabetes (Mathis et al., 2001). An increase in apoptosis might have pathological consequences in diabetes prone individuals, who have an auto-reactive T-cell repertoire that may be activated by the exposed beta-cell antigens. The Arg972 variant of the IRS-1 seems to play a complex role in the pathogenesis of diabetes, affecting both peripheral insulin sensitivity and the functional capacities of the pancreatic beta-cells themselves. In the light of our findings, it is possible to speculate that the same mechanisms —in the presence of a genetically determined predisposition— might also result in, or contribute to, different clinical manifestations of diabetes.

Once we have identified the genes to be analyzed, we decided to test our hypothesis: there are patients with a complex clinical autoimmune disease masked by insulin-resistance which in turn is genetically determined.

The results of our research, although not published yet, were presented in recent meetings in our country and international events as the "1st Latin American Congress: Controversies to Consensus in Diabetes, Obesity and Hypertension [CODHy]" and the "XIV Latin-American Congress of Asociación Latinoamericana de Diabetes [ALAD]" (Fabregat et al., 2010; Farias et al., 2010; Fernández et al., 2010; Mimbacas et al., 2010; Reyes et al., 2010; Souto et al., 2010).

Indeed, all patients tested (presence of HLA and positive susceptibility to type 1 diabetes antibody) with a body mass index >25kg/m^2 and clinical diagnosis of type 2 diabetes were overweight or obese with mutations in one or more of the analyzed genes. Our results indicated that insulin resistance in patients with complex diagnosis may be explained by the occurrence of a mutation in one or more of the analyzed single nucleotide polymorphisms (SNPs).

5. Importance of genetics for the clinician

In the last 15 to 20 years, clinicians have been concerned with grasping the increasing complexity of this disease, with a gradual worldwide increase of its prevalence that has turned it into a pandemic disease. The latest evidence shows that, despite correcting their lifestyle, we cannot always achieve good metabolic control in patients in complex clinical situations.

There is a population, which is probably formed by most of our patients, with clinical features where their phenotype is a good reflection of their genotype; but we are finding with increasingly frequency clinical cases that are difficulty to classify with the current criteria.

In these cases, a high percentage of patients had severe difficulties with their metabolic control. It is precisely here where we need to carry out a proper genetic diagnosis, and eventually an immunologic one, to allow us a broader view of their pathology. Several clinical observations and systematic studies have shown that classical type 1 diabetes, whether in children, late onset in adults, or individuals over 65, can coexist in the same individual with "classic" type 2 diabetes where insulin secretion deficiency and insulin resistance are detected simultaneously (Serrano Rios, 2009). This group of patients is usually referred to a diabetes specialist because the primary care physician cannot decide about or control them. Once reached this stage and after correcting the variables that affect proper metabolic control, such as nutritional plan and regular physical activity, we can see that many of these patients keep having a poor metabolic control. These patients are usually overweight and / or obese with a very erratic response to anti-diabetic drugs alone or in combination, both between them and with insulin.

Complying with the algorithms, we almost always end up giving insulin to our patients, but in many cases this is probably done too late. This was analyzed by many authors that described as final: "therapeutic inertia". They are usually described as patients with a poor adherence to the treatment plan. Also, on average they start insulin treatment before the classical diabetes type 2 patients.

Thus, we are planning to deepen into genetic typing, in order to see if it may help us to understand the etiopathogenesis of these patients, and why they do not have the expected response to the drug treatment.

As stated above, these patients surprisingly had a genotype that does not agree with their phenotype. This was what allowed us as clinicians to begin to understand these facts and to find an explanation (albeit partial) of the poor outcome of each patient.

What are the issues that the clinician should consider for further study of certain patients?

a. Obese patients showing good response to insulin during intercurrence: many of these patients had an intercurrent disease, and with the temporary insulin treatment they achieved a good control (especially in early stages of diagnosis) that may be explained by an improvement in glucotoxicity and / or moderate insulinopenia. In these patients the insulin will be removed based on these myths: (1) Insulin is "ineffective"; (2) Insulin injection increases cardiovascular diseases and hyperinsulinemia; and (3) Insulin causes weight gain. The reluctance we see in these patients insulin is based on misguided or questionable in view of the genetic results we are finding and the matching clinical trials.
b. Poor response to insulin sensitizers: in particular thiazolidinedione but also biguanides.
c. Poor response to secretagogues: it is usually attributed to glucotoxicity, but how much influence does drug response have?

d. Obese patients without dyslipidemia or other elements of metabolic syndrome.
e. Overweight or obese type 2 diabetes patients with hypoglycemia episodes, especially at night.
f. Type 2 Diabetic patients with microangiopathic complications preceding or concomitant to the macrovascular complications.

Already, Nolan and Murphy (2001) posed an approach to the phenotypic and metabolic characterization of insulin-resistant patients, impaired glucose tolerance, or type 2 diabetes, and the use of glutamic acid decarboxylase antibodies (GADA), genetic markers, and models to estimate the insulin-resistance should be considered. These authors discuss the utility of using genetic markers based on population studies for type 2 diabetes mellitus. In what it has to do with the poor response to treatment, we must remember that both therapeutic inefficiency and drug toxicity, which have been seen in some individuals, have been frequently observed. Due to the presence of some drug metabolizing enzymes, drugs can participate as inhibitors or inducers of these enzymes, thereby their variation in activity between individuals. This variability in enzyme activity may reflect the existence of mutations in their genes.

6. Conclusion: What is happening?

The above mentioned points will lead us to review the different mechanisms that may have taken place in the evolutionary processes leading to the current status of this disease. We will consider some possible situations.

a. Researchers are considering the way natural selection is currently operating in humans. The concept of "the survival of the strongest individual" perhaps is no longer valid in the 21st century. Quintana Murci et al. (2007), at the Pasteur Institute (Paris), have looked for answers regarding the mechanisms of human evolution by comparing whole genomes of different populations. They analyzed more than 2.8 million genetic markers in different populations from different ethnic groups collected in the HAPMAP project. They found that 582 genes were subject to "strong selective pressures" during the last 60,000 to 10,000 years. Some of these genes are strongly associated to external features (e.g.: hair, skin color); others are to the response to pathogenic agents or drugs; and others to diseases with different incidences between populations, like diabetes, obesity, or hypertension. Barreiro pointed out that "it is the first time that it can be demonstrated, concerning the whole genome that natural selection participates in the differentiation of the populations" This work is not only useful to satisfy our curiosity, but also to aid in the identification of genes implied in different diseases (Barreiro et al., 2005; 2008).

Well defined since the XV century, clinical knowledge on diabetes gradually increased, and in the end two major distinct types of this pathology were described (1 and 2). In order to understand the current increase of chronic diseases, it is necessary to consider the important relationship between human feeding and human evolution. The regular offer of food that seemed to help human evolution so greatly in the past is also generating a great amount of diseases and their corresponding incapacities (like hemiplegics, aphasia, amputations, etc.). This fact is a true evolutionary paradox (Insua & Fuks, 2003).

Initially, we must consider the importance of the neutralization of positive selective pressure introduced by the availability of nutrients as consequence of human civilization. A good example of the relationship between nutritional factors, diabetes, and population genetics is Szathmary's hypothesis (Marrodán, 2000) for explaining the high incidence of diabetes in several Amerindian populations (USA and Canada), either in reservations or in those adapted to western life.

Diabetes is a genetic-based disease whose manifestation is partly favored by excessive carbohydrate consumption. Possibly, several individuals with a specific genotype would produce insulin faster when faced with higher glucose levels than others; and they would also store this glucose as glycogen or fat more efficiently. This genotype would have been positively selected in a nutritional environment where periods of abundant or shortage of foods oscillate in a critical form. But this capacity for a faster answer to carbohydrate stimulus has a biological cost when food intake is constant. Under this situation, genes increasing insulin production are no longer beneficial to the individual because their carriers become obese, exhausting the physiological capacity of the pancreas, and leading to the subsequent development of diabetes (Marrodán, 2000; Harris, 2002). Variations in diabetes or obesity genes imply that adaptation to fasting was also an important selective agent. Quintana-Murci et al. (2007) pointed out that insulin-regulating genes have been positively selected. Thus, for instance, the ENPP1 gene has a mutation protecting against obesity and type II diabetes. This variant is present in 90% of non-African individuals and it is almost absent in African ones.

The susceptible genotype may have been selected in these populations because unusually frequent fasting periods may have taken place during the initial colonization of 'new worlds'. The abovementioned non-insulin dependent diabetes mellitus has shown a strong genetic component that may include a 'thrifty' genotype(s) (Neel 1962; Zimmet et al., 1990).

The 'thrifty' genotype(s) may have once allowed founding populations to survive both 'feast' and 'famine' conditions for several generations. Individuals carrying these genes would have had an increased efficiency for energy extraction (nutrition) from environmental scarce resources. During times of abundance those individuals with this predisposition would store more energy than those lacking it. When the progress of human civilization assured continuous fat-rich and fiber-poor diets, and a sedentary lifestyle, the 'thrifty' genotype(s) became disadvantageous, leading to obesity, increased insulin resistance, beta cell misbalance, and finally diabetes (Wendorf, 1991; 1992).

What was a selective advantage in past environments is currently, for most people in industrialized countries, an undesired condition. The result is obesity, diabetes, and the metabolic syndrome. For many years, diabetes was considered as a lethal or near-fatal disease by death simply by complications or by difficulties in the reproductive stages, both for men and women. More recently —the use of insulin is a landmark in this subject— reproductive problems and some of their related complications have been solved.

In conclusion, evolutionary or Darwinian medicine considers that many contemporary diseases are associated to incompatibility between current human lifestyles and environments, and those under which human biology was shaped. As the observed difference between the incremental rates of both civilization and evolution is so great, most human evolutionary changes took place when our ancestors were gatherer-hunters. Thus, many characteristics and conducts that had adaptive value in the past may currently have non-adaptive value. Medicine has always tried to improve and look for the patient's cure. It really improved people's health, but in this process populational issues that are beyond the epidemiologic point of view were overlooked. This medical conduct may be explained by the lack of information, or misinterpretation, of the importance of the genetic components of the disease. But this disregarding could be considered also as having iatrogenic elements: we improve the current patient's quality of life, but on the other hand we hamper that of future persons. This process implies the emergence of currently unknown entities. New discoveries have allowed life extension for affected people, with the subsequent appearance of new pathological complications that were not seen before simply because affected individuals passed away before their onset.

b. Are we witnessing a new type of diabetes, called "double o hybrid" by some authors? We believe that the phenomenon we are watching is simply another expression of the multifactorial nature of this disease. When we analyze populations with an ethnic mixture or of different ethnic origins, we begin to get a glimpse of the products of genetic admixture. This leads us to find a higher proportion of problematic patients that are difficult to classify because, when examining their phenotype, they are affected by certain genes that are masked by others. Hence, we can see families where, according to traditional classification, both entities (type 1 and type 2) coexist. This fusion would be associated with a new and intermediate phenotype (Tuomi, 2005). There are a few studies identifying patients where both type of diabetes overlap (Libman &. Becker, 2003; Pozzilli & Guglielmi, 2009); moreover, Pozzilli and Gugliemi (2007) place this entity in the middle of the double "rainbow" (made up of type 1 and type 2 diabetes).

The "accelerator hypothesis" is a theory that shares this vision. It is a singular, unifying concept, which states that type 1 and type 2 diabetes are the same insulin-resistance disorder set against different genetic backgrounds. This hypothesis does not deny the role of autoimmunity, only its primacy in the process. It distinguishes type 1 and 2 diabetes only by tempo, the faster tempo reflecting the (inevitably) earlier presentation in the more susceptible genotype (Wilkin, 2009).

Recognition that susceptibility arises through the combination of multiple genetic pathways influencing hazardous factors in a nonlinear manner suggests that a 'decanalization' process contributes to the epidemic nature of common genetic diseases. The evolution of the human genome, combined with a marked environmental and cultural perturbation in the past two generations, might lead to the uncovering of cryptic genetic variations that are a major source of disease susceptibility (Gibson, 2009).

This would be also favored by others processes such as an increase of life expectancy and fertility of affected individuals, the globalization phenomena, and increased admixture of different ethnic groups when compared with the past. The last phenomenon is clearly seen in Latin America and mainly in the Uruguayan population as it was stated above.

Regardless of all the arguments presented in this chapter, we think that it is extremely important to introduce the genetic risk profile into the present diabetes classification criteria. This will clearly improve our capability of distinguishing between different types of diabetes or specific presentations.

The effects of genetic traits in diabetes had been studied for decades, but few consistent risk factors have been well established. Currently, most of large scale studies on candidate genes do not combine the analysis of both types of diabetes. Establishing the association between genotype and phenotype would allow a deeper insight into the pathogenesis of the disease. Screening of associated anomalies and the possibility of anticipating future outcomes would be consequently improved.

While for many countries, especially in Latin-America, individual genetic diagnosis can be very expensive to implement, we must realize that we are facing a multifactorial disease.

Thus, although classifications may be useful, they only have relative value. We must keep an open mind to the fact that there are patients that do not fall in any of them, and we must remember that genetics is at the base of diabetes, as there are multiple genes that interact both with the environment and between them. These interactions can result in a somewhat "liar" phenotype. In the preceding sections we saw how mutations in a few genes associated to insulin resistance may mask the presence and/or action of genes causing autoimmune disorders. Moreover, if we take into account the modifications observed with genome scanning, where there are millions of Single Nucleotide Polymorphisms, it is virtually impossible to make a phenotype-based classification.

Although we are aware that understanding the pathogenesis of hyperglycemia or the basis for an effective treatment may be deemed as more important than knowing the type of diabetes we are dealing with, we are currently persuaded that the distinguishing between different types or presentation forms of diabetes based on genetic information is an important task that has turned into our great challenge.

7. Acknowledgment

This chapter could not have been written without the valuable collaboration of graduate and postgraduate students that are part of our research group (in alphabetic list): Br. Matías Fabregat, B.S. Joaquina Farías, MSc. Mariana Fernández, B.S. Ana Laura Reyes, Br. Jorge Souto, MSc. Pilar Zorrilla.

8. References

ADA (2004). American Diabetes Association. Diagnosis and Classification of Diabetes Mellitus, American Diabetes Association. *Diabetes Care* Vol. 27 (s1), (January, 2004), pp.55-60, ISSN 0149-5992

ADA (2010). American Diabetes Association (2010). Diagnosis and Classification of Diabetes Mellitus. *Diabetes Care*, Vol.33, (January, 2010), pp.S62-S69; doi:10.2337/dc10-S062, ISSN 0149-5992.

ALAD (2010). Asociación Latinoamericana de Diabetes. Guías ALAD de diagnóstico control y tratamiento de la Diabetes Mellitus Tipo 2. pp 1-78 http://www.revistaalad.com.ar/guias/GuiasALAD_DMTipo2_v3.pdf.

Alberti, K.G. & Zimmet, P.Z. (1998). For the WHO Consultation: Definition, diagnosis and classification of diabetes mellitus and its complications. I. Diagnosis and classification of diabetes mellitus: provisional report of a WHO Consultation. *Diabetes Medicine*, Vol.15, N°7, (July 1998), pp.539 -553, ISSN 1464-5491.

Almind, K.; Bjorbaek, C.; Vestergaard, H.; Hansen, T.; Echwald, S. & Pedersen, O. (1993) Amino-acid polymorphisms of insulin-receptor substrate-1 in non-insulin-dependent diabetes-mellitus. *Lancet*, Vol.342, N° 8875, (October 1993), pp.828-832, ISSN 1474-4422.

Almind, K.; Inoue, G.; Pedersen, O. & Kahn, C.R. (1996) A common amino acid polymorphism in insulin-receptor substrate-1 causes impaired insulin signalling evidence from transfection studies. *Journal Clinical Investigation*, Vol.97, N°11, (Jun 1996), pp.2569-2575, ISSN 1365-2362

Altshuler, D.; Hirschhorn, J.N.; Klannemark, M.; lindgren C.M.; Vohl, M.C.; Nemesh, J.; Lane, C.R.; Schaffner, S.F.; Bolk, S.; Brewer, C.; Tuomi, T.; Gaudet, D.; Hudson, T.J.;

Daly, M.; Groop, L. & Lander, L.S. (2000). The common PPARgamma Pro12Ala polymorphism is associated with decreased risk of type 2 diabetes. *Nature Genetics* Vol.26, N°.1, (September 2000), pp.76-80. ISSN 1061-4036.

Aubert, J.; Champigny, O.; Saint-Marc P.; Negrel, R.; Collins, S.; Ricquier, D. & Ailhaud, G. (1997). Up-regulation of UCP-2 gene expression by PPAR agonists in preadispose and adipose cell. *Biochemical Biophysical Research Communications*, Vol.238, N°2, (September 1997), pp.606-611, ISSN. 1090-2104.

Auwerx, J. (1999). PPARgamma, the ultimate thrfty gene. *Diabetologia*, Vol. 42, N°.9, (September 1999), pp.1033-1049, ISSN 0012-186X

Banting, F.G.; Best, C.H.; Collip, J.B.; Campbell, W.R. & Fletcher, A.A. (1922). Pancreatic extract in the treatment of diabetes mellitus. *Canadian Medical Association Journal*, Vol. 12, N°3, (March 1922), pp.141–146, ISSN. 0008-4409

Barreiro, L.B.; Patin, E.; Neyrolles, O.; Cann, H.M.; Gicquel, B. & Quintana-Murci, L. (2005). The heritage of pathogen pressures and ancient demography in the human innate immunity *CD209/CD209L* region. *American Journal of Human Genetic*, Vol.77, N°5, (August 2005), pp. 869-886, ISSN 1537-6605.

Barreiro, L.B.; Laval, G.; Quach, H.; Patin, E. & Quintana Murci, L. (2008). Natural selection has driven population differentiation in modern humans *Nature genetics*, Vol.40, N°.3, (February 2008), pp.340-345, ISSN 1061-4036.

Bell, Ch.G.; Walley, A.J. & Froguel Ph. (2005). The genetics of human obesity. *Nature Reviews Genetics*, Vol. 6, N°.3, (March 2005), pp.221-234, doi:10.1038/nrg1556, ISSN 1061-4036

Cardoso, H.; Crispino, B.; Mimbacas, A. & Cardoso, E. (2004). A low prevalence of cystic fibrosis in Uruguayans of mainly European descent. *Genetics Molecular Research* Vol.3, N°.2, (March 2004) pp.258-263 ISSN 1676-5680.

Carmona, M.C.; Valmaseda, A.; Iglesias, R.; Mampel, T.; Viñas, O.; Giralt, M. & Villaroya, F. (1998). 9-cis retinoic acid induces the expression of uncoupling protein-2 gene in brown adipocytes. *Federation of European Biochemical Societies*, Vol.441, N°.3, (December 1998), pp.447-450, ISSN 1873-3468.

Chawla, A.; Schwarz, E.J.; Dimaculangan, D.D. & Lazar, M.A. (1994) Peroxisome proliferator-activated receptor (PPAR) gamma: adipose-predominant expression and induction early in adipocyte differentiation. *Endocrinology*, Vol. 135, N°2, (August 1994), pp.798-800, ISSN. 0013-7227.

Clausen, J.; Hansen, T.; Bjoerbaek, C.; Echwald, S.; Urhammer, S.; Rasmussen, S.; Andersen, C.; Hansen, L.; Almind, K.; Winther, K.; Haraldsdottir, J.; Borch-Johnsen, K. & Pedersen, O. (1995). Insulin resistance: Interactions between obesity and a common variant of the insulin receptor substrate-1. *Lancet*, Vol.346, N°8972, (August 1995), pp.397–402, ISSN 0140-6736.

Dabelea, D.; Hanson, R.; Bennett, P.H.; Roumain, J.; Knowler, W.C. & Pettitt, D.J. (1998). Increasing prevalence of type 2 diabetes in American Indian children. *Diabetologia*, Vol.41, N°8, (August 1998), pp. 904–910, ISSN 0012-186X.

Das, S.K. & Elbein, S.C. (2006). The Genetic Basis of Type 2 Diabetes. *Cellscience*, Vol.2, No.4, (August 1994), pp.100–131, ISSN 1742-8130.

De Dios A. & Frechtel G. Ruiz M. (2011). Genética molecular de la diabetes y sus complicaciones. In: *Diabetes mellitus*, M. Ruiz & M.L. Ruiz Morosini, pp.27-31, Acadia, ISBN 978-987-570-153-3, Buenos Aires, Argentina.

Deeb, S.S.; Fajas, L.; Nemoto, M.; Pihlajamäki, J.; Mykkänen, L.; Kuusisto, J.; Laakso, M.; Fujimoto, W & Auwerx, J. (1998). A Pro12Ala substitution in PPARgamma2 associated with decreased receptor activity, lower body mass index and improved insulin sensitivity. *Nature Genetics*, Vol.20, No.3, (November 1998), pp. 284-287, ISSN 1061-4036.

Dobson, M. Nature of the urine in diabetes. Medical Observations and Inquiries, 1776, Vol.5. pp.298–310 In: Goldfine ID & Youngre JF. (1998). Contributions of the American Journal of Physiology to the discovery of insulin. *Endocrinology Metabolism* Vol.37, (February 1998), E207–E209, 1998, ISSN 94143-161

DPP (Clinical Trils.gov ID n°: NCT00004992). NIH Publication No. 06–5099 http://ndep.nih.gov/media/DPP_FactSheet.pdf, July 2008, http://diabetes.niddk.nih.gov/dm/pubs/preventionprogram/

Fabregat, M.; Javiel, G.; Vitarella, G. & Mimbacas, A. (2010). Estudio de frecuencias génicas del SNP -23Hph1 como segundo loci de susceptibilidad en la población con diabetes en el Uruguay. XIV Congreso de la Asociación Latinoamericana de Diabetes (ALAD), Santiago de Chile, Chile, 7-11 Noviembre http://www.congresoaladchile2010.com/pdfs/trabajos_modalidad_oral.pdf .

Farias, J.; Fabregat, M.; Reyes, A.L.; Souto, J.; Fernandez, M.; Javiel, G.; Vitarella, G. & Mimbacas, A. (2010). El perfil genético como herramienta en la identificación de pacientes con Doble Diabetes. V Congreso Uruguayo de Endocrinología y Metabolismo (SUEM) Montevideo 2-4 de Setiembre, Montevideo, Uruguay http://www.congresoaladchile2010.com/pdfs/trabajos_modalidad_poster.pdf

Federici, M.; Pertrone, A.; Porzio, O.; Bizzarri, C.; Lauro, D.; Alfonso, R.; Patera, I.; Cappa, M.; Nistico, L.; Baroni, M.; Sesti, G.; Di Mario, U.; Lauro, R. & Buzzetti, R. (2003) The Gly9723Arg IRS-1 Variant Is Associated with Type 1 Diabetes in Continental Italy. *Diabetes*,Vol.52, N°3, (March 2003), pp.887–890, ISSN. 0012-1797

Fernández, M.; Acosta, M.; Airaudo, C.; Fernández, J.; Ferrero, R.; Javiel, G.; Pena, A.; Simonelli, B.; Soto, E.; Vitarella, G. & Mimbacas. A. (2009). Estudio comparativo de prevalencia del gen de la ECA en muestras de diabéticos y población general. Revista Médica del Uruguay, Vol.25, N°2 (June 2009), pp. 110-115, ISSN 1688-0390.

Fernández, M.; Javiel, G.; Vitarella, G. & Mimbacas, A. (2010) Estudio preliminar de test genético moleculares sencillos que permitan determinar si el paciente tendrá una buena respuesta al tratamiento inicial con metformina. XIV Congreso de la Asociación Latinoamericana de Diabetes (ALAD), Santiago de Chile, Chile, 7-11 Noviembre http://www.congresoaladchile2010.com/pdfs/trabajos_modalidad_poster.pdf.

Freeman, H. & Cox, R.D. (2006). Type-2 diabetes: a cocktail of genetic discovery. *Human Molecular Genetics*, Vol. 15, N°2, (July 2006), pp. R202–R209, ISSN 1460-2083.

Gascue, C.; Mimbacas, A.; Sans, M.; Gallino, J.P.; Bertoni, B.; Hidalgo, P. & Cardoso, H. (2005). Frequencies of the four major Amerindian mtDNA haplogroups in the population of Montevideo, Uruguay. *Human Biology*, Vol.77, N°.6, (December 2005), pp. 873-878, ISSN 0018-7143, Copyright 48201-1309

Gibson, G. (2009). Decanalization and the origin of complex disease. *Nature Review Genetic*, Vol.10, N°2, (February 2009), pp.134-140, ISSN 1471-0056.

Hansen, L.; Ekstrøm C.T.; Tabanera y Palacios, R.; Anant, M.; Wassermann, K. & Reinhardt, R.R. (2006). The Pro12Ala variant of the PPARG gene is a risk factor for Peroxisome Proliferator-Activated Receptor Agonist-Induced edema in type 2 diabetic patients. *The Journal of Clinical Endocrinology & Metabolism*, Vol.91, N°.9, (September 2996), pp.3446–3450, ISNN 1945-7197

Harris, M. (2002). *Buenos para comer. Enigmas de la Alimentación*, Alianza Editorial S.A., pp.1-336, ISBN: 84-206-3977-X

Hathout, E.H.; Thomas, W.; El-Shahawy, M.; Nahab, F. & Mace, J.W. (2001). Diabetic autoimmune markers in children and adolescents with type 2 diabetes. *Pediatrics*, Vol. 107, N°.6, (June 2001), pp. 1-4, ISSN 1098-4275

Himsworth, A. (1936) Diabetes mellitus: its differentiation into insulin-sensitive and insulin-insensitive types. *Lancet* Vol.227, N°5864, (January 1936), pp.127-130, ISSN 1474-4465

Howard, G.; O'Leary, D.; Zaccaro, D.; Haffner, S.; Rewers, M.; Hamman, R.; Selby J.V.; Saad, M.F.; Savage, P. & Bergman,R. (1996). Insulin sensitivity and atherosclerosis. *Circulation*, Vol.93, N°10, (May 1996), pp.1809-1817, ISSN 1524-4539

Imait, Y.; Fusco, A.; Suzuki, Y.; Lesniak, M.A.; D'Alfonso, R.; Sesti, G.; Bertoli, A.; Lauro, R.; Accili, D. & Taylor; S.I. (1994). Variant sequences of Insulin Receptor Substrate-1 in patients with noninsulin-dependent Diabetes Mellitus. *Journal of Clinical Endocrinology and Metabolism*, Vol.79, N°.6, (December 1994), pp.1655-1658, ISSN 1945-7197

Insúa, M.F. & Fuks, K. (2011). Evolución humana y dieta Introducción: Paradoja evolutiva Nutriinfo.com.ar http://nutrinfo.com/pagina/info/evolucio.html (14/2/2011).

Ito, E.; Ozawa, S.; Takahashi, K.; Tanaka, T.; Katsuta, H.; Yamaguchi, S.; Maruyama, M.; Takizawa, M.; Katahira, H.; Yoshimoto, K.; Nagamatsu, S. & Ishida, H. (2004). PPAR-gamma overexpression selectively suppresses insulin secretory capacity in isolated pancreatic islet through induction of UCP-2 protein. Biochemical and *Biophysical Research Communications* Vol.324, N°22, (November 2004), pp.810-814. ISSN 1090-2104

Kang, E.S.; Park, S. Y.; kim, H.J.; Ahn, C.W.; Cha, B.S.; Lim, S.K.; Nam. C.M. & Lee, H.C. (2005). Effects of Pro12Ala polymorphism of peroxisome proliferator-activated receptor γ 2 gene on rosiglitazone response in type 2 diabetes. *Clinical Pharmacology and Therapeutics*, Vol.78, N°2, (August 2005), pp.202-208, ISSN 1532-6535

Kolb, T. & Mandrup-Poulsen, T. (2005)An immune origen of type 2 diabetes? Diabetologia, Vol.48, (March 2005), pp.1038–1050. DOI 10.1007/s00125-005-1764-9n

Libman, I.M. & Becker, D.J. (2003). Coexistence of type 1 and type 2 diabetes mellitus: double diabetes? *Pediatric Diabetes*, Vol.4, (March 2003), pp. 110-113. ISSN 1399-543X

Marchetti, P.; Lupi, R.; Federici, M.; Marselli, L.; Masini, M.; Boggi, U.; Del Guerra, S.; Patanè, G.; Piro, S.; Anello, M., Bergamini, E.; Purrello, F.; Lauro, R. & Mosca, F. (2002) Insulin secretory function is impaired in isolated human islets carrying the Gly9723Arg IRS-1 polymorphism. *Diabetes*, Vol.51, N°5, (May 2002), pp.1419–1424, ISSN 1939-327X

Marrodán, M.D. (2000). La alimentación en el contexto de la evolución biocultural de los grupos humanos. *Zairak*, Vol.20, pp.109-121 ISSN 1137-439X.

Mercado, M.M.; McLenithan, J.C.; Silver, K.D. & Shuldiner, A.R. (2002). Genetics of Insulin Resistance. *Current Diabetes Reports*, Vol.2, N°1, (February 2002), pp.83–95, ISSN 1539-0829

Mimbacas, A.; Pérez-Bravo, F.; Hidalgo, P.C.; Javiel, G.; Pisciottano, C.; Grignola, R.; Jorge, A.M., Gallino, J.; Gasagoite, J. & Cardoso, H. (2003). Association between type 1 diabetes and DQB1* alleles in a case-control study conducted in Montevideo, Uruguay. *Genetics and Molecular Research*, Vol.2, N°1, (September 2002), pp. 29-35, ISSN 1676-5680.

Mimbacas, A.; Pérez-Bravo, F.; Santos, J.L.; Pisciottano, C.; Grignola, R.; Javiel, G.; Jorge, A.M. & Cardoso, H. (2004). The association between HLA-DQ genetic polymorphism and type 1 diabetes in a case-parent study conducted in an admixed population. *European Journal of Epidemiology*, Vol.19, N°10, (March 2004), pp. 931-934, ISSN 0393-2990

Mimbacas, A.; Trujillo, J.; Gascue, C.; Javiel, G. & Cardoso, H. (2007). Prevalence of vitamin D receptor gene polymorphism in a Uruguayan population and its relation to type 1 diabetes mellitus. *Genetics and Molecular Research*, Vol. 6, N°3, (July 2007), pp. 534-542, ISSN 1676-5680.

Mimbacas, A.; García, L.; Zorrilla, P.; Acosta, M.; Airaudo, C.; Ferrero, R.; Pena, A.; Simonelli, B.; Soto, E.; Vitarella, G.; Fernández, J. & Javiel, G. (2009). Genotype and phenotype correlations in diabetic patients in Uruguay. *Genetics and Molecular Research*, Vol.8, N°4, (September 2009), pp. 1352-1358, ISSN 1676-5680.

Mimbacas, A.; Fernández M.; Souto, J.; Farias, J.; Reyes, A.; García, L.; Acosta, M.; Airaudo, C.; Ferrero, R.; Simonelli, B.; Soto, E.; Vitarella, G.; Fernández, J. & Javiel, G. (2010). Genotype and phenotype correlations in diabetic patients in Uruguay. The 1st Latin American Congress: Controversies to Consensus in Diabetes, Obesity and Hypertension (CODHy). Hilton Hotel, Buenos Aires, Argentina, March 11-14.

Mimbacas, A.; Vitarella G.; Souto, J.; Reyes, AL.; Farías, J.; Fernández, M.; Fabregatm M. & Javiel G. (2011). The phenotype mask the genotype: a posible new diabetes expression. Journal of Pediatric Genetic. In press.

Neel, J.V. (1962). Diabetes mellitus: a "thrifty" genotype rendered detrimental by 'progress'? *American Journal of Human Genetics*, Vol.14, N° 4, (December 1962), pp.353-362. ISSN 1537-6605.

Neufeld, N.; Raffael, L.; Landon, C.; Chen, Y. & Valdheim, C. (1998). Early presentation of type 2 diabetes in Mexican-American youth. *Diabetes Care* Vol.21, N°1, (January 1998), pp. 80-86, ISSN 1935-5548

Nolan J.J. & Murphy E. (2001). ¿Existe la intolerancia oral a la glucosa y, en tal caso, qué hay que hacer?. In: *Diabetes Aspectos difíciles y controvertidos*. G. V. Gill, J.C. Pickup & G. Williams, pp.25-39, Ars Médica, Barcelona, ISBN 0-632-05324-0, España.

Patlak, M. (2002). Combating diabetes. *Federation of American Societies for Experimental Biology Journal (FASEB)*, Vol. 16, N°.14,(December 2002), pp.1853, ISSN 1530-6860.

Patlak, M. (2002). New weapons to combat an ancient disease: treating diabetes. Breakthroughs in Bioscience, *Federation of American Societies for Experimental Biology Journal (FASEB)*, (December 2002), pp. 1-13, ISSN 1530-6860

Pinhas-Hamiel, O.; Dolan, L.M.; Daniels, S.R.; Standiford, D.; Khoury, R. & Zitler, P. (1996) Increased incidence of non-insulin dependent diabetes mellitus among adolescents. *The Journal of Pediatric*, Vol.128, N°5, (May 1996), pp. 608-615, ISSN 1097-6833.

Pinhas-Hamiel, O. & Zeitler, P. (1999). The importance of a name. *The New England Journal of Medicine*, Vol.340, (May 1999), pp. 1418-1421, ISSN 0028-4793

Pinhas-Hamiel, O.; Dolan, L.M. & Zeitler, P. (1997). Diabetic ketoacidosis among obese African-American adolescents with NIDDM. *Diabetes Care*, Vol.20, N°4, (April 1997), pp. 484-486, ISSN 0149-5992

Porzio, O.; Federici, M.; Hribal, M.L.; Lauro, D.; Accili, D.; Lauro, R.; Borboni, P. & Sesti, G. (1999). The Gly972Arg amino acid polymorphism in IRS-1 impairs insulin secretion in pancreatic β cells. The *Journal Clinical Investigation*, Vol.104, N°3, (August 1999), pp.357-364, ISSN 1558-8238 (

Pozzilli, P. & Buzzetti, R. (2007). A new expression of diabetes: double diabetes *Trends in Endocrinology and Metabolism*, Vol.18, N°.2, (January 2007), pp.52-57, ISSN 1879-3061

Pozzilli, P.; Guglielmi, C.; Pronina, E.; Petraikina, E. (2007). Double or hybrid diabetes associated with an increase in type 1 and type 2 diabetes in children and youths. *Pediatric Diabetes*, Vol.8, N°.S9, (December 2007), pp.88–95. ISSN 1399-5448

Pozzilli, P. & Guglielmi C. (2009). Double Diabetes: A Mixture of Type 1 andType 2 Diabetes in Youth. Endocr Dev. Basel, Karger, 2009, vol 14, pp 151–166 In *Endocrine Involvement in Developmental Syndromes*, Cappa M, Maghnie M, Loche S, Bottazzo GF ISBN: 978-3-8055-9042-6 retrieved from http://content.karger.com/

Quintana-Murci, L.; Alcaïs, A.; Abel, L. & Casanova, J.L. (2007). Immunology in natura: clinical, epidemiological and evolutionary genetics of infectious diseases. *Nature Immunology*, Vol.8, N°11, (November 2007), pp.1165-1171, ISSN 1529-2908

Reyes, A.L.; Farias, J.; Fernández, M.; Souto, J.; Fabregat, M.; Javiel, G.; Vitarella, G. & Mimbacas, A. (2010). La genética como potente herramienta para el diagnóstico y clasificación de pacientes diabéticos de clínica compleja. XIV Congreso de la Asociación Latinoamericana de Diabetes (ALAD), Santiago de Chile, Chile, 7-11 Noviembre
http://www.congresoaladchile2010.com/pdfs/trabajos_modalidad_poster.pdf

Rotimi, C.N. & Jorde, L.B. (2010). Ancestry and disease in the age of genome medicine. New England Journal of Medicine, Vol.363, N°16, (October 2010), pp.1551-1558, ISSN 0028-4793.

Ruiz M. (2011). Etiopatogenia de la diabetes tipo 2. In: Diabetes mellitus, M. Ruiz & M.L. Ruiz Morosini, 27-31, Acadia, ISBN 978-987-570-153-3, Buenos Aires, Argentina

Sans, M.; Figueiro, G.; Ackermann, E.; Barreto, I.; Egaña, A.; Bertoni, B.; PoittevinGilmet, E.; Maytia, D. & Hidalgo, P.C. (2011). Mitochondrial DNA in Basque-descendants from the city of Trinidad, Uruguay: Uruguayan- or Basque-like population?. Human Biology, Vol.83, No1, (in press)

Scott, C.; Smith, J.; Cradock, M. & Pihoker, C. (1997). Characteristics of youth-onset non-insulin dependent diabetes mellitus and insulin-dependent diabetes mellitus at diagnosis. Pediatrics, Vol.100, N°1, (July 1997), pp.84-91, ISSN 0031-4005

Serrano Ríos M. (2009). Etiopatogenia de la diabetes mellitus tipo 1. In: La diabetes mellitus en la práctica clínica, F.J. Tëbar Massó & F. Escobar Jiménez, pp.31-45, Editorial Panamericana, ISBN978-84-7903-450-4, Madrid.

Sesti, G.; Federici, M.; Hribal, M.L.; Lauro, D.; Sbraccia, P. & Lauro, R. (2001). Defects of the insulin receptor substrate (IRS) system in human metabolic disorders. The Federation of American Societies for Experimental Biology Vol.15, N°12, (October 2001), pp.2099-2111, ISSN 1530-6860

Sigal, R.J.; Doria, A.;Warram J.H. & Krolewski, A.S. (1996) Codon 972 polymorphism in the insulin receptor substrate-1 gene, obesity, and risk of noninsulin-dependent diabetes mellitus. Journal Clinical Endocrinoly and Metabolism, Vol.81, N°.4, (April, 1996), pp. 1657-1659, ISSN 1945-7197

Soto, E.; Mimbacas, A.; Gascue, C.; Javiel, G.; Ferrero, R.; Vitarella, G. & Cardoso, H. (2004). Asociación entre hiperhomocisteinemia, cardiopatía isquémica y diabetes tipo 2. Revista Uruguaya de Cardiología, Vol.19, pp.101-106, ISSN 0797-0048

Souto,J.; Javiel, G.; Fernández, J. & Mimbacas A. (2010). Contribución de la Genética en la toma de decisiones terapéuticas, a propósito de 2 casos clínicos. XIV Congreso de la Asociación Latinoamericana de Diabetes (ALAD), Santiago de Chile, Chile, 7-11

Noviembre http://www.congresoaladchile2010.com/pdfs/trabajos_modalidad_poster.pdf

Stumvoll, M.; Wahl, H.G.; Löblein, K.; Becker, R.; Machicao, F.; Jacob, S. & Häring H. (2001) Pro12Ala Polymorphism in the Peroxisome Proliferator-Activated Receptor-g2 gene is associated with increased antilipolytic insulin sensitivity. Diabetes Vol.50, N°4, (April 2001), pp.876–881, ISSN 0012-1797

Tuomi, T. (2005). Type 1 and Type 2 Diabetes What do they have in common? Diabetes, Vol. 54, NoS2, (December 2005), pp.S40-S45, ISSN 0012-1797

Villaroya, F.; Iglesisas, R. & Giralt, M. (2007), PPARs in the control of Uncoupling Gene expression. Hindawi Publishing Corporation Peroxsimone proliferator-activated receptors research, Vol. 2007, (October 2006), pp74364-74376, ISSN 1637-4765.

Wendorf, M. & Goldfine, I.D. (1991). Archaeology of NIDDM: excavation of the "thrifty" genotype. Diabetes, Vol.40, N°2, (February 1991), pp.161-165, ISSN 0012-1797

Wendorf, M. (1992). Archaeology and the "Thrifty" Non Insulin Dependent Diabetes Mellitus (NIDDM) Genotype. Advances in peritoneal dialysis. Vol.992, N°8, pp.201-2077, ISSN. 1197-8554

Wilkin, T.J. (2009). The accelerator hypothesis: a review of the evidence for insulin resistance as the basis for type I as well as type II diabetes. International Journal of Obesity, Vol.33, N°7, (July 2009), pp.716-726, ISSN 1476-5497

Yen, C.J.; Beamer, B.A.; Negri, C.; Silver, K.; Brown, K.A.; Yarnall, D.P.; Burns D.K., Roth, J. & Shuldiner, A.R. (1997). Molecular scanning of the human peroxisome proliferator activated receptor gamma (hPPAR gamma) gene in diabetic Caucasians: identification of a Pro12Ala PPAR gamma 2 missense mutation. Biochemical Biophysical Research Community. Vol.18, N°2, (December 1997), pp.270-274, ISSN 1090-2104

Yip, J.; Facchini, F.S. & Reaven, G.M. (1998). Resistance to insulin-mediated glucose disposal as a predictor of cardiovascular disease. Journal Clinical Endocrinology Metabolism, Vol.83, N°.8, (August 1998), pp.2773-2776, ISSN 1945-7197

Zhang, Y.; Wat, N.; Stratton, I.M.; Warren-Perry, M.G.; Orho, M.; Groop, L. & Turner, R.C. (1996). UKPDS 19: heterogeneity in NIDDM: separate contributions of IRS-1 and beta 3-adrenergic-receptor mutations to insulin resistance and obesity respectively with no evidence for glycogen synthase gene mutations. UK Prospective Diabetes Study. Diabetologia, Vol.39, N°12, (December 1996), pp.1505-1511, ISSN 0012-180X

Zhang, F.; Lavan, B.E. & Gregoire, F.M. (2007). Selective Modulators of PPAR-γ Activity: Molecular Aspects Related to Obesity and Side-Effects. Peroxsimone proliferator-activated receptors research, (2007), pp.1-7, doi:10.1155, ISSN 1687-4765

Zimmet, P.; Dowse, G. & Finch, C. (1990). The Epidemiology and natural history of NIDDM -lessons from the South Pacific. Diabetes Metabolism Reviews, Vol.6, N°2, (March 1990), pp.91-124, ISSN 0742-4221

Zorrilla, P.; Mimbacas, A.; Gascue, C.; Javiel, G. & Cardoso, H. (2006). Prevalencia del polimorfismo I/D del gen de la enzima convertidora de angiotensina (ECA) en la población de Montevideo. Revista Médica del Uruguay, Vol.12, N°.1, (Octubre 2005), pp.17-21 ISSN 1688-0390.

15

The Enlarging List of Phenotypic Characteristics That Might Allow the Clinical Identification of Families at Risk for Type 1 Diabetes

Elena Matteucci and Ottavio Giampietro
Department of Internal Medicine, University of Pisa
Italy

1. Introduction

Type 1 diabetes is a chronic metabolic disease whose aetiology and pathogenesis remain not completely understood. Current criteria for the diagnosis of diabetes are: 1) haemoglobin A1c ≥ 6.5% (assayed using a method that is certified by the National Glycohemoglobin Standardization Program, NGSP, and standardised or traceable to the Diabetes Control and Complications Trial, DCCT, reference assay), 2) fasting plasma glucose (FPG) ≥ 126 mg/dl, 3) 2-hour plasma glucose ≥ 200 mg/dl during an oral glucose tolerance test (OGTT, 75 g), 4) a random plasma glucose ≥ 200 mg/dl (American Diabetes Association, 2011). The classification of diabetes includes: type 1 diabetes, type 2 diabetes, other specific types of diabetes due to other causes, and gestational diabetes mellitus. Type 2 diabetes, which is usually associated with obesity and older age, results from insulin resistance and progressive failure of pancreatic beta-cell function. Type 1 diabetes, which has usually an abrupt onset in younger people, is an organ-specific autoimmune disease characterised by absolute insulin deficiency resulting from beta-cell destruction. However, autoimmunity may not be the primary cause: environmental triggers are believed to precipitate type 1 diabetes in genetically susceptible individuals (van Belle et al., 2011). The overall incidence of type 1 diabetes is increasing; the majority of the increase is observed in the youngest age group, which also appeared to be the heaviest (Evertsen et al., 2009). Indeed, the accelerator hypothesis (Wilkin, 2009) suggests that type 1 and type 2 diabetes are the same disorder of insulin resistance set against different genetic backgrounds. Three processes could variably accelerate the loss of beta cells through apoptosis: constitution, insulin resistance, and autoimmunity. None of these accelerators leads to diabetes without excess weight, which causes an increase in insulin resistance and, thus, the weakening of glucose control. In turn, the glucotoxicity accelerates beta-cell apoptosis directly and by inducing beta-cell immunogens and autoimmunity in genetically predisposed subjects. Insulitis is commonly observed in recent-onset type 1 diabetes, but it does not uniformly affect all insulin-containing islets (differences in islet function?). It has been suggested that under increased insulin demand (puberty, adolescence, high sugar intake, etc.) a population of islets may be more prone to dysfunction or death, thereby attracting antigen presenting cells and promoting insulitis in susceptible individuals (Rowe et al., 2011). In a genome-wide association study, 41 distinct genomic locations provided evidence for association with type 1 diabetes in the meta-analysis (Barrett et al., 2009). The Type 1 Diabetes Genetics Consortium (T1DGC) has recruited families with at least two siblings who have type 1 diabetes in order to identify genes that determine an individual's risk of type 1 diabetes. T1DBase is the web-based resource focused on the genetics and genomics of type 1 diabetes susceptibility (https://www.t1dgc.org) that provides the updated table of human loci associated with type 1 diabetes (Table 1).

Chromosome	**Gene of interest**	**Abbreviation**
1p13.2	Protein tyrosine phosphatase, non-receptor type 22	PTPN22
1q31.2	Regulator of G-protein signalling 1	RGS1
2q12	Interleukin 18 receptor accessory protein	IL18RAP
2q24.2	Interferon induced with helicase C domain 1	IFIH1
2q33.2	Cytotoxic T-lymphocyte-associated protein 4	CTLA4
3p21.31	Chemokine (C-C motif) receptor 5	CCR5
4q27	Interleukin 2	IL2
5p13		
6p21.31 6p21.33	Major histocompatibility complexes	HLA-B, -A, -DRB1, -DQB1, -DPB1
6q15	similar to BTB and CNC homology 1, basic leucine zipper transcription factor 2	BACH2
6q23.3	similar to Tumor necrosis factor, α-induced protein 3	TNFAIP3
6q25.3	T-cell activation Rho GTPase-activating protein	TAGAP
10p15.1	Interleukin 2 receptor, α	IL2RA
10p15.1	Protein kinase C, θ	PRKCQ
11p15.5	Insulin II	INS
12q13.2		
12q13.3	Kinesin family member 5A	KIF5A
12q24.12		
15q25.1		
16p13.3		
18p11.21	Protein tyrosine phosphatase, non-receptor type 2	PTPN2
18q22.2	CD226 antigen	CD226
21q22.3		
22q13.1		

(from: http://t1dbase.org/page/PosterView/display/poster_id/386)

Table 1. Human loci associated with type 1 diabetes.

With regards to the causative environmental triggers that have been implicated in the pathogenesis of type 1 diabetes, they have been recently reviewed (van Belle et al., 2011; Vehik & Dabelea, 2011) and include particularly viral infections, gut microbic flora and other bacteria, early life feeding patterns, wheat proteins, and vitamin D.

2. Identifying individuals at risk for type 1 diabetes

In Europe, the number of adults with diabetes was expected to reach 55.2 million (8.5% of the adult population) in 2010; about 112,000 children and adolescents were estimated to have type 1 diabetes mellitus (http://www.diabetesatlas.org/content/europe).

Most diabetic cases are complex diseases resulting from interactions between genetic and environmental determinants in genetically predisposed individuals. Empirical evidence suggests a architecture of many genetic loci with many variants of small effect (Wray & Goddard, 2010). Genome-wide association studies have suggested that the majority of susceptible loci have small contributions to phenotypic variation and therefore there should be a large number of susceptibility loci involved in the genetic basis of complex diseases (consistent with the polygenic model). Moreover, the differentiation of sporadic and familial cases has implied that most complex diseases are genetically heterogeneous. Family history has a high positive predictive value, but a low negative predictive value. Yang et al. (2010) have shown that 1) the proportion of sporadic cases depends on disease prevalence and heritability of the underlying liability scale, and 2) a large proportion of sporadic cases is expected under the polygenic model due to the low prevalence rates of common complex genetic diseases. Thus, the causal mechanisms cannot be inferred from the observed proportion of sporadic cases alone. The prediction of disease risk to relatives from many risk loci or markers requires a model that combines the effects of these loci. The constrained multiplicative, Odds and Probit models fitted data on risk to relatives, but it is difficult to distinguish between them until genetic variants that explain the majority of the known genetic variance are identified (Wray & Goddard, 2010). Hence, genetic risk modelling to derive prediction of individual risk and risk to relatives are still difficult to reconcile.

In most individuals with autoimmune type 1 diabetes, beta cell destruction is a chronically progressive and very slow process that starts long before overt disease. During this "silent" phase, autoantibodies are produced and self-reactive activated lymphocytes infiltrate the islets of Langerhans (Rowe et al., 2011). Autoantibodies that target self-antigens in the insulin-secreting beta cells of the pancreas include: islet cell autoantibodies (ICA), insulinoma-associated antigen-2 antibodies (IA-2A), antibodies against the related antigen IA-2 beta (IA-2β), insulin autoantibodies (IAA), autoantibodies to the 65kDa isoform of glutamic acid decarboxylase 65 (GADA), and the recently identified autoantibodies to the zinc transporter 8 (ZnT8A) (Table 2).

Islet autoantibodies are potent tools for the prediction of type 1 diabetes and are the basis for recruitment in prevention trials and immunointervention trials. In the general childhood population in Finland, one-time screening for GADA and IA-2A was capable of identifying about 60% of those individuals who will develop type 1 diabetes over the subsequent 27 years; both positive and negative seroconversions occurred over time reflecting a dynamic process of beta cell autoimmunity, but positivity for at least two diabetes-associated autoantibodies represented in most cases a point of no return (Knip et al., 2010). So far, however, the place of autoantibody-based risk assessment in routine clinical practice is limited because no proven therapeutic interventions is available for people at high risk of progression to type 1 diabetes. Until therapies modulating the disease process become available, the benefit to individual patients is questionable - awareness of risk is rather useless or even stressful - and diabetes antibody testing does not yet have a role in clinical care (Bingley, 2010). It is considered likely that islet-related autoantibodies are not directly pathogenetic, whereas autoreactive CD4 and CD8 T cells mediate beta cell damage.

Therefore, standardised autoantibody screenings should be combined with the detection of autoreactive T cells. Unfortunately, none of the currently available T cell assays satisfies all the features of a good assay: small blood sample required, simplicity, specificity, low intra- and inter-assay variability (Fierabracci, 2011). Notwithstanding recent developments based on immunosorbent spot and immunoblotting techniques, the International Workshops of the Immunology Diabetes Society concluded that T cell results are still inconclusive and novel approaches are currently being investigated.
In conclusion, it may be that in the future combination screening predicts type 1 diabetes clinical onset, but actually genetic risk, serum autoantibody profiling and T cell assays are uneconomical when applied in the general population.

Autoantibodies against	**Abbreviation**	**Method**
38-kDa glycated islet cell membrane-associated protein	GLIMA	Immunoprecipitation
51-kDa aromatic-L-amino-acid decarboxylase	AADC	Immunoprecipitation
52-kDa rat insulinoma	52-kDa RIN	Immunoblot
Aminoacyl-tRNA synthetase	ARS	ELISA*
Carbonic anydrase II	CA II	ELISA*
Carboxypeptidase H	CPHA	Radiobinding assay
Chymotrypsinogen-related 30-kDa pancreatic		Immunoblot analysis
DNA topoisomerase II	TopIIA	ELISA* and Western blot
Ganglioside GM2-1	GM2-1	Indirect immunoperoxidase technique
Gangliosides GM1, 2, 3, etc.		*ELISA
Glucose type-2 transporter	GLUT2	Western blot
Glutamic acid decarboxylase	GADA	Radiobinding assay, ELISA*
Heat shock proteins	HSP	*ELISA
Insulin	IAA	Radiobinding assay
Insulinoma-associated antigen-2	IA-2A	Radiobinding assay, ELISA*
Insulinoma-associated antigen 2β	IA-2β	Radiobinding assay
Islet cell	ICA	Indirect immunofluorescence
Islet cell surface	ICSA	Radiobinding assay
Proinsulin	PIAA	Radiobinding assay
Zinc transporter 8	ZnT8	Radiobinding assay

* Enzyme linked immunosorbent assay

Table 2. List of islet autoantibodies detected in type 1 diabetes (modified from Winter & Schatz, 2011).

3. Phenotyping type 1 diabetes families

Translational research aims to integrate basic life science (genomics, transcriptomics, proteomics, and metabolomics) with insights gained from clinical experience to comprehensively study complex biological system and complex human diseases. Translation requires, among others, methods that relate molecular and cellular phenotypes to clinical characteristics (Bebek et al., 2011). Indeed, the correlation between quantitative phenotypes and traits allows for a more efficient use of the genetic information; hence the importance of accurate family phenotyping studies. Unaffected family members can contribute as much to the analysis as individuals with the disease diagnosis. For example, the finding of cognitive deficits in individuals with schizophrenia and in the clinically unaffected relatives of these individuals suggested that these deficits are part of the innate underlying distinct differences that make some individuals vulnerable to schizophrenia. Examining these complementary biological phenotypes in genetic studies has been found to provide valuable information about the pathway that connects genotype to clinical disease (Almasy et al., 2008). Similarly, large-scale genetic fine mapping and genotype-phenotype associations implicated polymorphisms in the IL2RA region in type 1 diabetes: IL2RA type 1 diabetes susceptibility genotypes were associated with lower circulating levels of the biomarker, soluble IL-2RA (Lowe et al., 2007). However, despite the theoretical advantages of quantitative trait analysis and testing of multiple plausible domains, some matters have emerged since quantitative traits may not be the most relevant phenotypes to investigate in search for the genetic etiology of disease. Identifying the "best" phenotype for genetic studies needs to survey family members and examine coexisting features and familial segregation patterns. A focus on careful assessment of the most genetically relevant phenotypes has been recommended (Brzustowicz & Bassett, 2008).

Over the years, our research efforts have sought primarily to gain a comprehensive understanding of the common phenotypic elements that characterise families with a sporadic case of type 1 diabetes. Here we provide a research-based overview of these familial peculiarities that include multifaceted, easily detectable, clinical perturbations: physical (BMI), cardiovascular (blood pressure response to exercise and circadian blood pressure pattern), biochemical (fasting plasma glucose, HbA1c, lipids, homeostasis model assessment of insulin sensitivity, plasma markers of oxidative damage), cellular (cellular markers of oxidative damage, transplasma membrane electron transport systems, mitochondrial membrane potential), and immunological (lymphocyte subsets).

4. Body weight in type 1 diabetes families

According to epidemiological findings and the accelerator hypothesis, the prevalence of overweight in preadolescent children is increasing, it tracks into adulthood and may increase diabetes and cardiovascular disease risk in adulthood. The risk of childhood obesity seems to increase with exposure to diabetes or cigarette smoke in utero, high birth weight, rapid weight gain in infancy, and shorter breastfeeding duration. The Diabetes Autoimmunity Study in the Young (DAISY) examined longitudinally 1,718 children from birth that were at increased risk for type 1 diabetes (Lamb et al., 2010). Gender, diabetes exposure in utero, size for gestational age, weight gain in the first year of life, and total breastfeeding duration (inverse) showed significant association with higher childhood BMI. Mediation analysis suggested that 1) the protective effect of breastfeeding duration on childhood BMI was largely mediated by slower infant weight gain, and 2) the increased risk of higher childhood BMI associated with exposure to diabetes in utero was partially explained by greater birth size. Maternal obesity before pregnancy and weight gain during pregnancy significantly predicted increased risk of persistent multiple positivity for islet autoantibodies in offspring with high genetic susceptibility for type 1 diabetes (Rasmussen et al., 2009). A systematic review and meta-analysis (12 studies) indicated that high birth weight and increased weight gain during the first year of life were associated with an increased risk of type 1 diabetes in later life (Harder et al., 2009).

Metabolic demand and insulin resistance have been suggested to be involved in the development of type 1 diabetes (Evertsen et al., 2009; Wilkin, 2009), but the evidence is not consistent across the studies. In 1650 prospectively followed children of mothers or fathers with type 1 diabetes (BABYDIAB cohort), islet autoantibodies-positive children were not insulin resistant (based on homeostasis model assessment of insulin resistance, HOMA-IR) and did not have increased BMI around and early after seroconversion (Winkler at al., 2009). In this study, of 777 children with HOMA-IR measurements, 84 developed islet antibodies during the study: analysis of HOMA-IR by age showed no significant difference between islet autoantibody-positive and islet autoantibody-negative children, with a tendency towards a lower HOMA-IR in the antibody-positive children compared with the antibody-negative children.

In a primary school health program in Pisa we screened 869 primary school children (448 M, 421 F, mean age 118±5 months): height, weight, four skinfolds, and four circumferences were measured; a family-reported questionnaire was used to determine family composition, history, and lifestyle (Giampietro et al., 2002). The percentages of children who could be considered overweight (BMI ≥ 95th percentile of age- and sex-specific National Health and Nutrition Examination Survey I, NHANES I, reference data) were boys, 10.0%, and girls, 9.3%. It emerged that offspring BMI was correlated with birth weight, parental BMI and scholarship level, children blood pressure, and hours per day spent in television viewing. Family history for diabetes was associated with higher BMI, skinfold thickness at the subscapular area (SSF), waist circumference, and upper thigh. Family history for hypertension was associated with higher SSF/skinfold thickness at the triceps area (TCF) ratio. We concluded that anthropometric and anamnestic data on child and family yield more accurate estimates of risk profile: fat distribution seems relevant for metabolic and cardiovascular disorders.

Since our initial investigations on type 1 diabetes families, we found that first degree relatives' BMI tended to be higher when compared with healthy control subjects who had no first-degree relative with type 1 diabetes, although the difference did not always reach statistical significance (Matteucci & Giampietro, 2000a; Matteucci et al. 2004a, 2004b; Matteucci et al. 2006). In recent years, on the contrary, the difference in BMI between unaffected siblings of type 1 diabetic probands and healthy control subjects has reached the statistical significance (Figure 1, Matteucci et al., 2010).

This finding probably reflects the trend toward increasing body weight and obesity in the general population, declining physical activity and unhealthy dietary habits that we have documented (Matteucci et al., 2004b, 2007, 2008). However, the emerging difference in BMI between unaffected relatives and control subjects suggests that additional factors are operative in type 1 diabetes families, which remain unknown. The single nucleotide polymorphism rs9939609 in the fat mass and obesity associated gene (FTO) region on chromosome 16q12, which increases the risk of childhood obesity and type 2 diabetes, did not alter susceptibility to type 1 diabetes (Field et al., 2007). Although increased early growth was associated with disease risk in various European populations, any role of infant feeding in this association remained unclear (EURODIAB Substudy 2 Study Group, 2002). Scientific evidences suggested associations of allelic variations in the Vitamin D receptor gene and phenotypes related to body weight, glucose homeostasis, diabetes and its vascular complications (Reis et al., 2005). Whatever the case, our data in adult members of type 1 diabetes families highlight that the 'familial' predisposition to overweight remains throughout life.

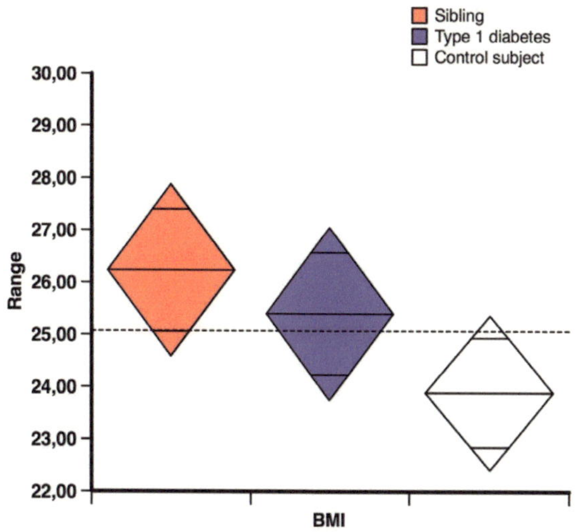

Fig. 1. Body mass index (BMI) in control subjects, type 1 diabetic patients and their siblings (Matteucci et al., 2010).

5. Familial cardiovascular abnormalities

Diabetes and hypertension are strongly associated although the role of glycaemia in promoting hypertension is a matter of debate (Invitti, 2003). HbA1c variability predicts not only incident microalbuminuria and progression of established renal disease but also cardiovascular disease events in patients with type 1 diabetes (Wadén et al., 2009). Moreover, HbA1c concentration predicts cardiovascular disease and all-cause mortality in adults without diabetes (Khaw et al., 2004). In healthy non-diabetic and non-hypertensive men, fasting plasma glucose is independently associated with blood pressure at rest and during exercise and development of elevated blood pressure after 7-years follow-up (Biornholt et al., 2003). Usually, in type 1 diabetes families, parental hypertension has been associated with diabetic nephropathy in adult and young offspring (Viberti et al., 1987; Marcovecchio et al., 2010), but the familial/hereditary factors that have an impact on diabetic nephropathy have not been so far identified. In a large homogeneous population from the Finnish Diabetic Nephropathy study, a cluster of parental hypertension, cardiovascular disease, cardiovascular mortality, and type 1 diabetes was associated with diabetic nephropathy in offspring with type 1 diabetes. It seemed that the more the traits clustered in family, the higher the risk for diabetes nephropathy (Thorn et al., 2007).

In this regard it is noteworthy that enhanced sodium/lithium countertransport and sodium/hydrogen exchange had been suggested to predict diabetic nephropathy (Walker et al., 1990; Ng et al, 1990). However, we found evidence contradicting this favourite hypothesis. Indeed, our data demonstrated convincingly that sodium/hydrogen exchange activity was significantly higher in type 1 diabetes with no difference among the two groups of diabetic patients with and without nephropathy. Moreover, enhanced sodium/hydrogen exchange activity was also a common feature of nondiabetic first-degree relatives of type 1 diabetic patients with no difference among the corresponding groups of relatives. The association between antiport activities of diabetic probands and their relatives suggested that the altered activity of the transporter was primarily determined by familial factors whose nature remained to be clarified (Matteucci & Giampietro, 2000b).

Generally, the observation of raised arterial blood pressure in relatives of type 1 diabetes patients was based on history, a single measurement of arterial blood pressure, or a 24-h ambulatory record; we were first to evaluate the response to ergometer exercise (Matteucci et al., 2006). Blood pressure response to exercise had been evaluated as a predictor of future hypertension and cardiovascular disease (Sharabi et al., 2001). Moreover, the heritability for resting blood pressure and blood pressure response to exercise was under investigation (An et al., 2000). We identified an abnormal blood pressure response to exercise testing not only in type 1 diabetic probands but also in asymptomatic normotensive non-diabetic relatives of type 1 diabetics, in which it was associated with indices of metabolic syndrome and oxidative damage. Furthermore, in healthy normotensive non-diabetic control subjects without family history of type 1 diabetes, strong associations were found 1) between resting systolic blood pressure and fasting plasma glucose as well as fasting plasma insulin levels, and 2) between systolic blood pressure response to exercise and HbA1c levels (Matteucci et al., 2006).

In a recent study, we performed 24-hour ambulatory blood pressure monitoring in type 1 diabetes families with the primary aim of investigating the circadian variability of blood pressure and the ambulatory arterial stiffness index in healthy siblings of type 1 diabetes patients vs healthy control subjects who had no first-degree relative with type 1 diabetes (Matteucci et al., 2010). Secondary aims of the study were to explore the influence of both cardiovascular autonomic function and erythrocyte electron transfer activity as oxidative marker on the ambulatory blood pressure profile. Indeed, human erythrocytes possess a transplasma ferricyanide reductase activity (measured as the erythrocyte velocity of ferricyanide reduction) that transfers reducing equivalents from intracellular reductants to extracellular oxidants (Matteucci & Giampietro, 2000c) and belongs to the ubiquitous transplasma membrane electron transport systems. Transplasma membrane electron transport activities have been related to the regulation of vital cellular processes and to the pathogenesis of various human disorders (Lane & Lawen, 2009) and exist also in endothelial cells where they have been suggested to regulate redox status and possibly atherogenesis through regulation of haeme oxygenase-1 expression (Lee et al., 2009).

We found that systolic blood pressure midline-estimating statistic of rhythm and pulse pressure were higher in type 1 diabetes patients and correlated positively with diabetes duration and the rate of oxidant-induced erythrocyte electron transfer to extracellular ferricyanide. Autonomic dysfunction was associated with diastolic blood pressure ecphasia and increased ambulatory arterial stiffness index. Siblings had higher BMI (Figure 1), lower insulin sensitivity (Figure 2), larger systolic blood pressure amplitude (Figure 3), and higher ambulatory arterial stiffness index than controls. Daytime systolic blood pressure was positively, independently associated with BMI and erythrocyte electron transfer to extracellular ferricyanide. Among non-diabetic people, there was a significant correlation between ambulatory arterial stiffness index and fasting plasma glucose. We concluded that siblings of type 1 diabetes patients exhibited a cluster of sub-clinical metabolic abnormalities associated with consensual perturbations in blood pressure variability. Moreover, our findings supported, in a clinical setting, the proposed role of transplasma membrane electron transport systems in vascular pathobiology.

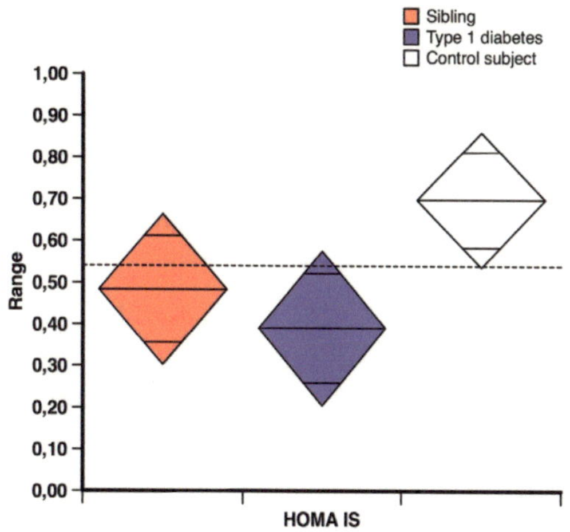

Fig. 2. Homeostasis model assessment of insulin sensitivity (HOMA-IS) in the same study groups (Matteucci et al., 2010).

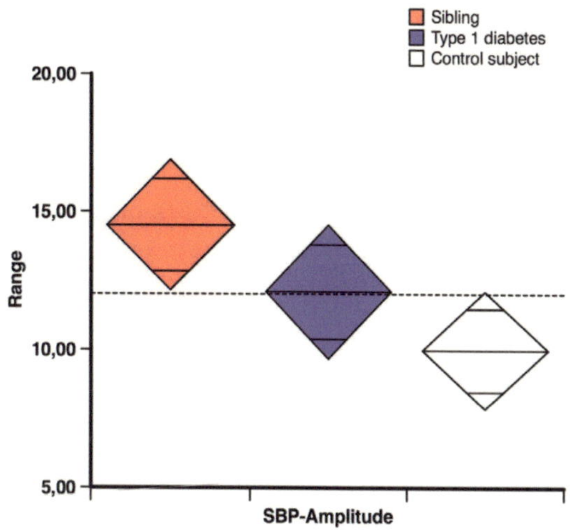

Fig. 3. Systolic blood pressure amplitude (SBP-Amplitude) in the same study groups (Matteucci et al., 2010).

6. Biochemical phenotype and redox balance in type 1 diabetes relatives

Our studies over the years have linked family history of type 1 diabetes (first-degree kinship) with multiple biochemical abnormalities. Since 2000 we documented metabolic perturbations in nondiabetic relatives: parents differed from age-matched control subjects in the higher plasma concentrations of glucose and Lipoprotein (a); their fibrinogen was borderline but did not reach any statistical significance; in turn, siblings of type 1 diabetes patients differed from age-matched control subjects in the higher levels of Lipoprotein (a) (Matteucci et al., 2000a). In the same study, we investigated the redox status and antioxidant defences in these families.

The premises were the following:

- enhanced levels of free radicals found in diabetes mellitus and impaired glucose tolerance has long been assumed to be related to chronically elevated glucose levels (Baynes and Thorpe, 1999; Vijayalingam et al., 1996),
- oxidative stress was suggested to play a primary role in the pathogenesis of diabetes and its complications but Authors still discussed whether oxidation preceded the appearance of complications or it merely reflected their presence (Baynes and Thorpe, 1999).

We suggested an alternative hypothesis, i.e. that oxidative stress preceded diabetes mellitus. In the case, indirect evidence for increased oxidative stress could be also detectable in non-diabetic relatives of type 1 diabetic patients. In order to provide evidence of a familial imbalance between radical production and antioxidant defences, we investigated indices of glucose and lipid metabolism, markers of plasma and cell lipid peroxidation, a novel marker of oxidant-induced protein damage, and the effects of oxygen radicals on erythrocytes of patients with type 1 diabetes and their relatives. We measured blood creatinine, glucose, HbA1c, cholesterol, triglycerides, Lipoprotein (a), fibrinogen, malondialdehyde, and advanced oxidation protein products. Erythrocyte response to oxidative stress (3-h-incubation at 37°C with or without a radical generating system) was evaluated by measuring erythrocyte glutathione, erythrocyte malodialdehyde, and haemolysis. Plasma and erythrocyte malodialdehyde were found to be significantly elevated in diabetics and relatives than in controls. Basal erythrocyte glutathione was lower in diabetics and incubations of cells caused in diabetics a decrease in erythrocyte glutathione of lesser degree than in control subjects, while a significant increase in haemolysis. Among relatives, haemolysis was increased both at baseline and after incubation. Plasma malodialdehyde was associated with blood glucose, creatinine, and fibrinogen; basal erythrocyte malodialdehyde with plasma Lipoprotein (a), fibrinogen, and plasma malodialdehyde. Basal erythrocyte glutathione content correlated with serum glucose and erythrocyte malodialdehyde production.

In that occasion, we were pioneers of the research on redox balance in type 1 diabetes families. We presented first evidence that markers of lipoprotein metabolism (Lipoprotein (a)), oxidative stress (plasma and erythrocyte malodialdehyde), and cellular fragility (haemolysis) are abnormal in non diabetic relatives of type 1 diabetics supporting the view that familial elements even precede diabetes. It seemed reasonable that the same biologic markers considered major predictors of cardiovascular disease could also trace familial susceptibility to type 1 diabetes, just as they have been associated with the development of type 2 diabetes (Matteucci et al., 2000a).

Based on the finding of elevated circulating markers of lipid peroxidation and increased cellular fragility, we decided to complete and integrate our investigation with further biochemical measurements of possible first-chain initiating or stimulating factors in order to evaluate, in the same families, the contribution of extracellular antioxidants to the increased oxidative stress. We also aimed to understand the eventual relationship between oxidative stress and the abnormal sodium/hydrogen exchange activity previously observed

(Matteucci et al., 2001). We were unable to find out any abnormalities in circulating metal ions (such as iron, transferrin, ferritin, copper, and ceruloplasmin) or extracellular antioxidant defences (such as serum uric acid, albumin, bilirubin,) that could favour oxidative stress in non-diabetic relatives of type 1 patients. On the contrary, we confirmed our previous finding of a generalised increase in sodium/hydrogen exchange activity. The rate of amiloride-sensitive hydrogen efflux from erythrocytes was significantly associated with both erythrocyte glutathione content and some markers of radical-induced damage such as plasma advanced oxidation protein products and malondialdehyde, erythrocyte osmotic fragility, and erythrocyte malondialdehyde accumulation under oxidative stress. Hence, this additional study provided the first *in vivo* demonstration of a significant association between oxidative stress and sodium/hydrogen exchange upregulation. The familiarly overactive sodium/hydrogen exchange itself could be viewed as further evidence pointing to the presence in these families of a redox disequilibrium where oxidation seems to be prevailing.

Taken into account that:

- mitochondria are the cellular site of oxidation-reduction reactions and energy transfer processes; mitochondrial dysfunction is believed to play a role in the development of diabetes and its complications because of the active generation of free radicals (Maiese et al., 2007),
- a reactive oxygen species-mediated long-term 'memory' of hyperglycaemic stress has been reported in the mitochondria of endothelial cells (Ihnat et al., 2007), but impairment of mitochondrial function has been also observed in subjects with family history of type 2 diabetes before the onset of impaired glucose tolerance (Petersen et al., 2004),

in the last step of our research we measured the mitochondrial membrane potential in peripheral blood granulocytes from type 1 diabetic patients and their unaffected siblings using the mitochondrial indicator 5,5′,6,6′-tetra chloro-1,1′,3,3′-tetraethylbenzimidazolyl-carbocyanine iodide (JC-1) in conjunction with flow cytometry (Matteucci et al., 2011). This was the first study to examine mitochondrial membrane potential of circulating leukocytes in type 1 diabetes families and to document consistent evidence for mitochondrial hyperpolarisation that was highest in type 1 diabetic patients and intermediate in their siblings. Fasting plasma glucose was the only correlate of leukocyte mitochondrial membrane potential. Confirming previous observations in type 1 diabetes families, siblings had fasting plasma glucose slightly higher than control subjects yet lower HbA1c levels. The combination of higher mean fasting plasma glucose, lower homeostasis model assessment of insulin sensitivity (HOMA-IS) and lower HbA1c levels suggested that siblings had both impaired basal glucose clearance rate and enhanced insulin-stimulated muscle glucose disposal.

We hypothesised that in type 1 diabetes families, radical-induced mitochondrial membrane potential oscillations may be synchronized toward polarized states. The positive association between mitochondrial membrane potential oscillations and fasting plasma glucose within the range from normal to dysglycemic conditions suggested that hyperglycaemic challenge implied increased glucose metabolisation, enhanced oxidant formation and hyperpolarisation of the mitochondrial membrane.

It is noteworthy that succination of proteins, which is an irreversible chemical modification of cysteine by the Krebs cycle intermediate fumarate, is increased by hyperpolarisation of the inner mitochondrial membrane and develops in concert with mitochondrial and oxidative stress in diabetes (Frizzell et al., 2011).

7. Immunological functions in type 1 diabetes families

Although type 1 diabetes is a T-cell–mediated autoimmune disease, until a few years ago relatively few studies have attempted to associate T-cell autoreactivity with disease progression, in comparison with efforts directed on monitoring autoantibodies, and those that have been performed were largely limited to CD4 T-cells (Roep, 2008). Currently, islet epitope-specific CD8 T cells are believed to have a pivotal role in the destruction process. Unfortunately, monitoring multiple epitope-specific CD8 T cell populations poses many technical problems. Recently, monitoring of CD8 T cells reactive to beta-cell-derived antigens has been performed using the combinatorial quantum dot technique, which has been validated using peripheral blood cells from recent-onset type 1 diabetic patients, their siblings, and control subjects (Velthuis et al., 2010). Moreover, during the progression of autoimmune diabetes, memory autoreactive regulatory CD8 T cells can be expanded that could effectively suppress the expansion of dominant and subdominant effectors (Khadra et al., 2010). Increasing evidence shows the significance of CD4 and CD8 regulatory T cells, expressing the marker CD25 or IL-2 receptor, in autoimmune disease models. On the contrary, very few study have dealt with the role of CD23 or low affinity IgE receptor. In 2004, given that abnormalities in redox balance clustered in type 1 diabetes families and the intracellular redox status seemed to modulate immune function, we aimed to investigate the relationship between oxidative stress and immunologic features. We measured oxidative markers, serum pro-inflammatory cytokines, soluble cytokine receptors, and subsets of peripheral blood lymphocytes (by varying combinations of CD4, CD8, CD23, and CD25) from type 1 patients, low-risk (i.e. without underlying islet autoimmunity) non-diabetic first-degree relatives of diabetic patients, and healthy subjects (Matteucci et al., 2004a). In these families, protein and lipid oxidation was confirmed from reduced sulfhydryl groups, increased advanced oxidation protein products, increased plasma and erythrocyte malondialdehyde. Relatives had decreased counts of monocytes, of cells coexpressing CD23 and CD25, and of $CD25^+$ cells in peripheral blood. Patients with type 1 diabetes had similar defects and, in addition, showed decreased counts of peripheral $CD4^+CD8^+$ lymphocytes and increased serum levels of soluble receptors for IL-6 and IL-2. This was the first demonstration of leukocyte abnormalities in low-risk T1DM relatives, also presenting signs of oxidative stress. Moreover, our study reported first evidence that the oxidative stress observed in type 1 diabetes families was correlated to immunological hallmarks suggestive of different immunoregulatory mechanisms. A crucial question remained open: did the alteration in immune functions follow the altered intracellular redox status or vice versa?

More recently, we have characterised CD26 expression of T cell subsets in patients with type 1 diabetes because 1) high expression of CD26 among $CD8^+$ T cells has been suggested to be a marker of effective long-term memory T cell formation typical of acute resolved viral infections (Ibegbu et al., 2009), and 2) an increased risk of persistent viral infections, such as hepatitis C (HCV), was reported among diabetic patients (Lonardo et al., 2009).

No significant difference was seen in percentages or absolute numbers of $CD4^+CD26^+$, $CD4^+CD26^-$, $CD8^+CD26^+$, and $CD8^+CD26^-$ between type 1 diabetes and control people.

However, the fluorescence intensity of CD26 expression on $CD8^+$ lymphocytes revealed a significant decrease in type 1 diabetic patients compared with control subjects. Mean fluorescence of $CD8^+CD26^+$ cells was inversely correlated with the absolute number of $CD4^+CD26^-$ cells (Matteucci et al., 2010). We interpreted the finding (low expression of CD26 among $CD8^+$ T cells in type 1 diabetes) as indicating a defect in successfully developed long-term memory $CD8^+$ T cells or in $CD8^+$ T cells activation, even though the negative association with the number of $CD4^+CD26^-$ T cell does not support a recent activation of peripheral T cells. We intend to continue research in this field in consideration of the immunomodulating role of the multifunctional CD26 (Ohnuma et al., 2011).

8. Concluding remarks

Today, there is a great need to integrate molecular biology with whole organ physiology. Findings from molecular and cellular studies must be brought back to intact organ systems without loosing the physiological context (Königshoff et al., 2011). This is especially true in the field of metabolic diseases where the study of individual proteins and signalling pathways in detail may not be easily translated to the intact organism. Taken into account the enlarging list of phenotypic characteristics that might allow the early clinical identification of families possibly at risk for sporadic cases of type 1 diabetes, many questions await an answer. We suggest the two main (in our opinion) issues.

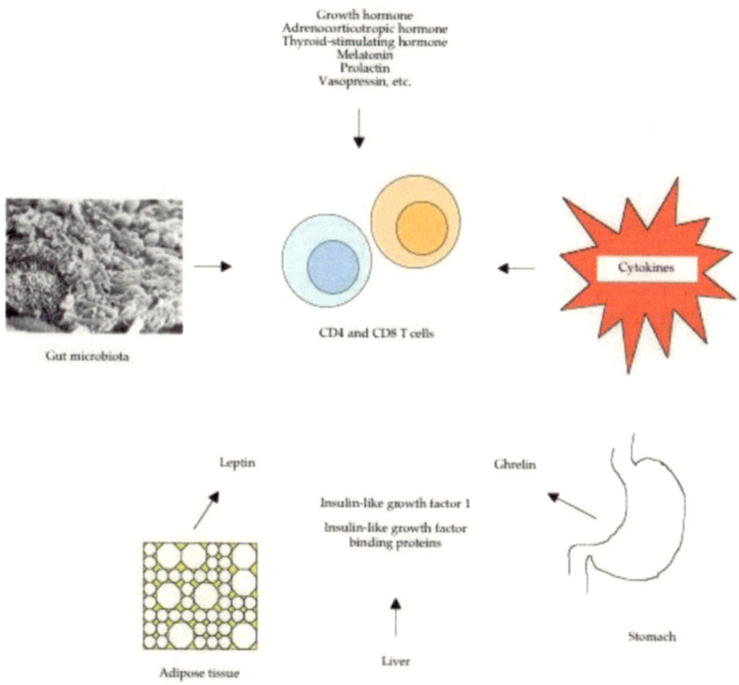

Fig. 4. Some of the potential mechanisms linking metabolic syndrome and T cell maintenance.

First question: may insulin-resistance be the common denominator of the observed familial peculiarities? And therefore, second question: could an early correction of one/some of these common clinical abnormalities modify the natural history of the disease and thence its epidemiology? The data above summarised suggest to consider also alternative ways beyond the traditional immuno-based interventions so far extensively investigated in the field of type 1 diabetes. There is increasing attention to the role of metabolic syndrome and immune responses as well as to the relation between the immune and neuroendocrine systems (Figure 4). The adipocyte-derived proinflammatory hormone leptin can affect the survival and proliferation of autoreactive CD4 T cells (Matarese et al., 2008; Galgani et al., 2010). Immune and neuroendocrine systems have bidirectional communications (Kelley et al., 2007; Berczi et al., 2009). Growth hormone and ghrelin are expressed in immune cells, which in turn bear receptors for these hormones (Hattori, 2009). Leptin, ghrelin, insulin-like growth factor 1, insulin-like growth factor binding protein 3, and cytokines regulate both thymopoiesis and maintenance of T cells. Therefore, elucidation of metabolic syndrome, T cell metabolism, hormones, and microbiota may lead to new insights into the maintenance of proper immune responses (Hsu & Mountz, 2010).

At the present state of knowledge and given the current diabetes epidemic, it would seem reasonable that proper, more realistic, public health interventions (by general and family practitioners) are designed that address general issues such as feeding, lifestyle, overweight, 'borderline' blood pressure, impaired fasting glucose, etc. These health interventions, beyond the conventional boundaries that have for so long limited the visual field, might have a favourable cost-benefit ratio.

9. References

Almasy, L., Gur, R.C., Haack, K., Cole, S.A., Calkins, M.E., Peralta, J.M., Hare, E., Prasad, K., Pogue-Geile, M.F., Nimgaonkar, V., Gur, RE. (2008). A genome screen for quantitative trait loci influencing schizophrenia and neurocognitive phenotypes. *The American Journal of Psychiatry*, Vol. 165, N. 9: 1185–1192.

American Diabetes Association. (2011). Standards of medical care in diabetes-2011. *Diabetes Care*, Vol. 34, N. Supplement 1: S11-S61.

An, P., Rice, T., Pérusse, L., Borecki, I.B., Gagnon, J., Leon, A.S., et al. (2000). Complex segregation analysis of blood pressure and heart rate measured before and after a 20-week endurance exercise training program: the HERITAGE Family Study. *American Journal of Hypertension,* Vol. 13, N. 5 Pt1: 488-497.

Barrett, J.C., Clayton, D.G., Concannon, P., Akolkar, B., Cooper, J.D., Erlich, H.A., Julier, C., Morahan, G., Nerup, J., Nierras, C., Plagnol, V., Pociot, F., Schuilenburg, H., Smyth, D.J., Stevens, H., Todd, J.A., Walker, N.M., Rich, S.S.; Type 1 Diabetes Genetics Consortium. (2009). Genome-wide association study and meta-analysis find that over 40 loci affect risk of type 1 diabetes. *Nature Genetics*, Vol. 4, N. 6: 703-707.

Baynes, J.W., Thorpe, S.R. (1999). Role of oxidative stress in diabetic complications. A new perspective on an old paradigm. *Diabetes*, Vol. 48, N. 1: 1-9.

Bebek, G., Koyutürk, M., Chance, M.R., Price, N.D. (2011). Integrative -omics for translational sciente. In: *Biocomputing 2011. Proceedings of Pacific Symposium*, date of access 2011-03-17, available from: <http://eproceedings.worldscinet.com/9789814335058/9789814335058_0001.html>. Berczi, I., Quintanar-Stephano, A., Kovacs, K. (2009). Neuroimmune regulation in immunocompetence, acute illness, and healing. *Annals of the New York Academy of Sciences*, Vol. 1153: 220-239.

Bingley, P. J. (2010). Clinical application of diabetes antibody testing. *The Journal of Clinical Endocrinology and Metabolism*, Vol. 95, N. 1: 25-33.

Biornholt, J., Erikssen, G., Kjeldsen, S.E., Bodegård, J., Thaulow, E., Erikssen, J. (2003) Fasting blood glucose is independently associated with resting and exercise blood pressure and development of elevated blood pressure. *Journal of Hypertension*, Vol. 21, N. 7: 1383-1389.

Brzustowicz, L.M., Bassett, A.S. (2008). Phenotype matters: the case for careful characterization of relevant traits. *The American Journal of Psychiatry*, Vol. 165, N. 9: 1196–1198.

EURODIAB Substudy 2 Study Group. (2002). Rapid early growth is associated with increased risk of childhood type 1 diabetes in various European populations. *Diabetes Care*, Vol. 25, N. 10: 1755-1760.

Evertsen, J., Alemzadeh, R., Wang, X. (2009). Increasing incidence of pediatric type 1 diabetes mellitus in Southeastern Wisconsin: relationship with body weight at diagnosis. *PLoS ONE*, Vol. 4, N. 9: e6873.

Field, S.F., Howson, J.M., Walker, N.M., Dunger, D.B., Todd, J.A. (2007). Analysis of the obesity gene FTO in 14,803 type 1 diabetes cases and controls. *Diabetologia*, Vol. 50, N. 10: 2218-2220.

Fierabracci, A. (2011). The potential of multimer technologies in type 1 diabetes prediction strategies. *Diabetes/Metabolism Research and Reviews*, Vol. 27, N. 3: 216-229.

Frizzell, N., Lima, M., Baynes, J.W. (2011). *Free Radical Research*, Vol. 45, N. 1: 101-109.

Galgani, M., Procaccini, C., De Rosa V., Carbone, F., Chieffi, P., La Cava, A., Matarese, G. (2010). Leptin modulates the survival of autoreactive CD4+ T cells through the nutrient/energy-sensing mammalian target of rapamycin signaling pathway. *Journal of Immunology*, Vol. 185, N. 12: 7474-7479.

Giampietro, O., Virgone, E., Carneglia, L., Griesi, E., Calvi, D., Matteucci, E. (2002). Anthropometric indices of school children and familiar risk factors. *Preventive Medicine*, Vol. 32, N. 5: 492-498.

Harder, T., Roepke, K., Diller, N., Stechling, Y., Dudenhausen, J.W., Plagemann, A. (2009). Birth weight, early weight gain, and subsequent risk of type 1 diabetes: systematic review and meta-analysis. *American Journal of Epidemiology*, Vol. 169, N. 12: 1428-1436.

Hattori, N. (2009). Expression, regulation and biological actions of growth hormone (GH) and ghrelin in the immune system. *Growth hormone and IGF Research*, Vol. 19, N. 3: 187-197.

Hsu, H.C., Mountz, J.D. (2010). Metabolic syndrome, hormones, and maintenance of T cells during aging. *Current Opinion in Immunology*, Vol. 22, N. 4: 541-548.

Ibegbu, C.C., Xu, Y.X., Fillos, D., Radziewicz, H., Grakoui, A., Kourtis, A.P. (2009). Differential expression of CD26 on virus-specific CD8(+) T cells during active, latent and resolved infection. *Immunology*, Vol. 126, N. 3:346-353.

Ihnat, M.A., Thorpe, J.E., Kamat, C.D., Szabó, C., Green, D.E., Warnke, L.A., et al. (2007). Reactive oxygen species mediate a cellular 'memory' of high glucose stress signalling. *Diabetologia*, Vol. 50, N. 7: 1523-1531.

Invitti, C. (2003). Can glycaemia affect blood pressure? *Journal of Hypertension*, Vol. 21, N. 7: 1265-1267.

Kelley, K.W., Weigent, D.A., Kooijman, R. (2007). Protein hormones and immunity. *Brain, Behavior, and Immunity*, Vol. 21, N. 4: 384-392.

Khadra, A., Tsai, S., Santamaria, P., Edelstein-Keshet, L. (2010). On how monospecific memory-like autoregulatory CD8+ T cells can blunt diabetogenic autoimmunity: a computational approach. *Journal of Immunology*, Vol. 185, N. 10: 5962-5972.

Khaw, K.-T., Wareham, N., Bingham, S., Luben, R., Welch, A., Day, N. (2004). Association of hemoglobin A1c with cardiovascular disease and mortality in adults: the European Prospective Investigation into cancer in Norfolk. *Annals of Internal Medicine*, Vol. 141, N. 6: 413-420.

Knip, M., Korhonen, S., Kulmala, P., Veijola, R., Reunanen, A., Raitakari, O.T., Viikari, J., Akerblom, H.K. (2010). Prediction of type 1 diabetes in the general population. *Diabetes Care*, Vol. 33, N. 6: 1206-1212.

Königshoff, M., Uhl, F., Gosens, R. (2011). From molecule to man: integrating molecular biology with whole organ physiology in studying respiratory disease. *Pulmonary Pharmacology & Therapeutics*, doi:10.1016/j.pupt.2011.02.002.

Lamb, M.M., Dabelea, D., Yin, X., Ogden, L.G., Klingensmith, G.J., Rewers, M., Norris, J.M. (2010). Early-life predictors of higher body mass index in healthy children. *Annals of Nutrition & Metabolism*, Vol. 56, N. 1: 16-22.

Lane, D.J., Lawen, A. (2009). Ascorbate and plasma membrane electron transport-Enzymes vs efflux. *Free Radical Biology & Medicine,* Vol. 47, N. 5:485-495.

Lee, S., Li, R., Kim, B., Palvolgyi, R., Ho, T., Yang, Q.Z., Xu, J., Szeto, W.L., Honda, H., Berliner, J.A. (2009). Ox-PAPC activation of plasma membrane electron transport (PMET) system increases expression of heme oxygenase 1 (HO-1) in human aortic endothelial cell (HAEC). *Journal of Lipid Research,* Vol. 50, N. 2:265-274.

Lonardo, A., Adinolfi, L.E., Petta, S., Craxì, A., Loria, P. (2009). Hepatitis C and diabetes: the inevitable coincidence? *Expert Review of Anti-Infective Therapy*, Vol. 7, N. 3:293-308.

Lowe, C.E., Cooper, J.D., Brusko, T., Walker, N.M., Smyth, D.J., Bailey, R., Bourget, K., Plagnol, V., Field, S., Atkinson, M., Clayton, D.G., Wicker, L.S., Todd, J.A. (2007). Large-scale genetic fine mapping and genotype-phenotype associations implicate polymorphism in the IL2RA region in type 1 diabetes. *Nature Genetics*, Vol. 39, N. 9: 1074-1082.

Maiese, K., Morhan, S.D., Chong, Z.Z. (2007). Oxidative stress biology and cell injury during type 1 and type 2 diabetes mellitus. *Current Neurovascular Research*, Vol. 4, N. 1: 63-71.

Marcovecchio, M.L., Tossavainen, P.H., Acerini, C.L., Barrett, T.G., Edge, J., Neil, A., Shield, J., Widmer, B., Dalton, R.N., Dunger, D.B. (2010). Maternal but not paternal association of ambulatory blood pressure with albumin excretion in young offspring with type 1 diabetes. *Diabetes Care*, Vol. 33, N. 2: 366-371.

Matarese, G., Procaccini, C., De Rosa V. (2008). The intricate interface between immune and metabolic regulation: a role for leptin in the pathogenesis of multiple sclerosis? *Journal of Leukocyte Biology*, Vol. 84, N. 4: 893-899.

Matteucci, E., Consani, C., Masoni, M.C., Giampietro, O. (2010). Circadian blood pressure variability in type 1 diabetic subjects and their nondiabetic siblings - influence of erythrocyte electron transfer. *Cardiovascular Diabetology*, 9: 61 (http://www.cardiab.com/content/9/1/61).

Matteucci, E., Ghimenti, M., Consani, C., Di Beo, S., Giampietro, O. (2010). About CD26 CD8 lymphocytes in type 1 diabetes. *Scandinavian Journal of Immunology*, Vol. 71, N. 2: 123-124.

Matteucci, E., Ghimenti, M., Consani, C., Masoni, M.C., Giampietro, O. (2011). Exploring mitochondrial membrane potential in type 1 diabetes families. *Cell Biochemistry and Biophysics*, Vol. 59, N. 2: 121-126.

Matteucci, E., Giampietro, O. (2000a). Oxidative stress in families of type 1 diabetic patients. *Diabetes Care*, Vol. 23, N. 8, 1182-1186.

Matteucci, E., Giampietro, O. (2000b). Erythrocyte sodium/hydrogen exchange activity and albuminuria in families of type 1 diabetic patients. *Diabetes Care*, Vol. 23, N. 3, 418-420.

Matteucci, E., Giampietro, O. (2000c). Transmembrane electron transfer in diabetic nephropathy. *Diabetes Care*, Vol. 23, N. 7, 994-999.

Matteucci, E., Giampietro, O. (2001). Oxidative stress in families of type 1 diabetic patients: further evidence. *Diabetes Care*, Vol. 24, N. 1, 167-168.

Matteucci, E., Giampietro, O. (2007). Central Italy: unexpected macro- and micro-nutrient deficiencies in regular diet of residents from Pisa province. The potential role of medical education in young people; In: *Malnutrition in the 21th century*, Editor Vesler L.W., pp. 127-145, Nova Science Publishers, Hauppauge NY, U.S.A.

Matteucci, E., Giampietro, O. (2008). Central Italy: physical activity of female residents from Pisa province, In: *Progress in exercise and women's health research*, Editor Coulter J. P., pp. 241-253, Nova Science Publishers, Hauppauge NY, U.S.A.

Matteucci, E., Malvaldi, G., Fagnani, F., Evangelista, I., Giampietro, O. (2004a). Redox status and immune function in type I diabetes families. *Clinical and Experimental Immunology*, Vol. 136, N. 3: 549-554.

Matteucci, E., Passerai, S., Mariotti, M., Fagnani, F., Evangelista, I., Rossi, L., Giampietro, O. (2004b). Dietary habits and nutritional biomarkers in Italian type 1 diabetes families: evidence of unhealthy diet and combined-vitamin-deficient intakes. *European Journal of Clinical Nutrition*, Vol. 59, N. 1: 114-122.

Matteucci, E., Rosada, J., Pinelli, M., Giusti, C., Giampietro, O. (2006). Systolic blood pressure response to exercise in type 1 diabetes families compared with healthy control individuals. *Journal of Hypertension*, Vol. 24, N. 9: 1745-1751.

Ng, L.L., Simmons, D., Frighi, V., Garrido, M.C., Bomford, J., Hockaday, T.D. (1990). Leukocyte Na+/H+ antiport activity in type 1 (insulin-dependent) diabetic patients with nephropathy. *Diabetologia*, Vol. 33, N. 6: 371-377.

Ohnuma, K., Hosono, O., Dang, N.H., Morimoto, C. (2011). Dipeptidyl peptidase in autoimmune pathophysiology. *Advances in Clinical Chemistry*, Vol. 53: 51-84.

Petersen, K.F., Dufour, S., Befroy, D., Garcia, R., Shulman, G.I. (2004). Impaired mitochondrial activity in the insulin-resistant offspring of patients with type 2 diabetes. *The New England Journal of Medicine*, Vol. 350, N. 7: 664-671.

Rasmussen, T., Stene, L.C., Samuelsen, S.O., Cinek, O., Wetlesen, T., Torjesen, P.A., Rønningen, K.S. (2009). Maternal BMI before pregnancy, maternal weight gain during pregnancy, and risk of persistent positivity for multiple diabetes-associated autoantibodies in children with the high-risk HLA genotype: the MIDIA study. *Diabetes Care*, Vol. 32, N. 10: 1904-1906.

Reis, A.F., Hauache, O. M., Velho, G. (2005). Vitamin D endocrine system and the genetic susceptibility to diabetes, obesity and vascular disease. A review of evidence. *Diabetes & Metabolism*, Vol. 31, N. 4: 318-325.

Roep, B.O. (2008). Islet autoreactive CD8 T-cells in type 1 diabetes: licensed to kill? *Diabetes*, Vol. 57, N. 5: 1156.

Rowe, P.A., Campbell-Thompson, M.L., Schatz, D.A., Atkinson, M.A. (2011) The pancreas in human type 1 diabetes. *Seminars in Immunopathology*, Vol. 33, N. 1: 29-43.

Sharabi, Y., Ben-Cnaan, R., Hanin, A., Martonovitch, G., Grossman, E. (2001). The significance of hypertensive response to exercise as a predictor of hypertension and cardiovascular disease. *Journal of Human Hypertension*, Vol. 15, N. 5: 353-356.

Thorn, L.M., Forsblom, C., Fagerudd, J., Pettersson-Fernholm, K., Kilpikari, R., Groop, P.H.; FinnDiane Study Group. (2007). Clustering of risk factors in parents of patients with type 1 diabetes and nephropathy. *Diabetes Care*, Vol. 30, N. 5 :1162-1167.

van Belle, T.L., Coppieters, K.T., von Herrath, M.G. (2011). Type 1 diabetes: etiology, immunology, and therapeutic strategies. *Physiological Reviews*, Vol. 91, N. 1: 79-118.

Vehik, K., Dabelea, D. (2011). The changing epidemiology of type 1 diabetes: why is it going through the roof? *Diabetes/Metabolism Research and Reviews*, Vol. 27, N. 1: 3-13.

Velthuis, J.H., Unger, W.W., Abreu, J.R., Duinkerken, G., Franken, K., Peakman, M., Bakker, A.H., Reker-Hadrup, S., Keymeulen, B., Drijfhout, J.W., Schumacher, T.N., Roep, B.O. (2010). Simultaneous detection of circulating autoreactive CD8+ T-cells specific for different islet cell-associated epitopes using combinatorial MHC multimers. *Diabetes*, Vol. 59, N. 7: 1721-1730.

Viberti, G.C., Keen, H., Wiseman, M.J. (1987). Raised arterial pressure in parents of proteinuric insulin dependent diabetics. *British Medical Journal*, Vol. 295, N. 6597: 515–51.

Vijayalingam, S., Parthiban, A., Shanmugasundaram, K.R., Mohan, V. (1996). Abnormal antioxidant status in impaired glucose tolerance and non-insulin-dependent diabetes mellitus. *Diabetic Medicine*, Vol. 13, N. 8: 715-719.

Wadén, J., Forsblom, C., Thorn, L.M., Gordin, D., Saraheimo, M., Groop, P.H.; Finnish Diabetic Nephropathy Study Group. (2009). A1C variability predicts incident cardiovascular events, microalbuminuria, and overt diabetic nephropathy in patients with type 1 diabetes. *Diabetes*, Vol. 58, N. 11: 2649-2655.

Walker, J.D., Tariq, T., Viberti, G. (1990). Sodium-lithium countertransport activity in red cells of patients with insulin-dependent diabetes and nephropathy and their parents. *British Medical Journal*, Vol. 301, N. 6753: 635-638.

Wilkin, T.J. (2009) The accelerator hypothesis: a review of the evidence for insulin resistance as the basis for type I as well as type II diabetes. *International Journal of Obesity*, Vol. 34, N:1: 210-211.

Winkler, C., Marienfeld, S., Zwilling, M., Bonifacio, E., Ziegler, A.G. (2009). Is islet autoimmunity related to insulin sensitivity or body weight in children of parents with type 1 diabetes? *Diabetologia*, Vol. 51, N. 10: 2072-2078.

Wray, N.M., Goddard, M.E. (2010). Multi-locus models of genetic risk of disease. *Genome Medicine*, Vol. 2 (N. 2): 10.

Yang, J., Visscher, P.M., Wray, N.M. (2010). Sporadic cases are the norm for complex disease. *European Journal of Human Genetics*, Vol. 18, N. 9: 1039-1044.

16

Altering Trends in the Epidemiology of Type 1 Diabetes Mellitus in Children and Adolescents

Elisavet Efstathiou and Nicos Skordis
Paediatric Endocrine Unit, Department of Paediatrics,
Makarios Hospital, Nicosia
Cyprus

1. Introduction

Diabetes mellitus is a group of metabolic diseases characterised by chronic hyperglycemia resulting from defects in insulin secretion and/or insulin action, or both [1]. The history of diabetes dates back to 1550 BC as the polyuric states were described in an Egyptian papyrus, where treatment was given with a four day decoction of bones, wheat, grain, grit and earth. The term diabetes was coined by Aretaeus of Cappadocia in the 2nd century AD for conditions causing increased urine output. The sweet taste of diabetic urine was noted in the 5th century AD by Indian physicians and in 1776, Matthew Dobson confirmed that diabetic serum and urine contained sugar. The revolution in the history of Diabetes was the discovery of insulin by Banting, Best and colleagues in 1922 (http://wwunix.oit.umass.edu/~abhu000/diabetes/index.html).

Type 1 diabetes mellitus (T1DM) is one of the most common endocrine metabolic disorders in children and adolescence worldwide with serious acute and chronic complications. It has been proven that T1DM represents the ending result of an autoimmune destruction of the pancreatic islet beta cells in genetically susceptible individuals exposed to certain but still unclear environmental factors. The precise cause of T1DM is not known. However, multiple genetic and environmental risk factors seem to play an important role in the genesis of the disease. The genetic background is complex and difficult to be explained by the involvement of HLA gene region alone. On the other hand viral and nutritional factors changing continuously from country to country, may contribute to the etiology of T1DM. There is no doubt that monitoring temporal trends and incidence of T1DM contribute to the international effort to determine the exact pathogenesis of the disease and it is of critical public health importance. All these temporal trends in the incidence of T1DM have provided significant clues for understanding the disease, most likely reflecting environmental changes more than genetic changes and detecting the factors that implicated in this increase.

In this chapter we review the changing trends in the epidemiology of T1DM and we present data on the rising incidence of T1DM in Greek Cypriot population.

2. Incidence-changing trends

The prevalence of T1DM greatly varies between different countries, within countries, and between different ethnic populations. The global variation of the incidence of T1DM is evaluated by grouping the populations with very low (<1/100.000 per yr), low (1-4/100.000 per yr), intermediate (5-9.99/100.000 per yr), high (10-19.99/100.000 per yr) and very high (>20/100.000 per yr) incidence [2]. The different annual incidence rates of T1DM comparing different countries of the world (0.1 to 57.6 per 100000) are displayed in figure 1 [1]. The highest incidence is observed in the Scandinavian countries, where Finland has the highest one reported while there is a gradual decrease in countries located closer to equator [3]. However in some areas such as Puerto Rico, Kuwait and Sardinia there is an unexplained highly increased incidence [4]. The lowest incidence in the world is observed in China, where an enormous geographic variation in the development risk is observed [5]. A long time ago, during the 5th century BC, Hippocrates described diabetes as a 'rare condition' while later on Arataeus the Cappadocian described it as 'not being frequent among men' (http://wwunix.oit.umass.edu/~abhu000/diabetes/index.html). Nowadays the incidence of T1DM increases dramatically throughout the world and it is estimated that it may reach the status of an epidemic in the 21st century [6].

A number of 37 studies from 27 countries confirmed the increased incidence for the period 1960-96 in T1DM with an upward tendency in another 12 countries. The global average annual increase was 3.0% per year with a more pronounced relative increase in the populations with lower incidence [7]. If these trends continue, the number of new cases T1DM in children younger than five years of age may double in some regions between 2005 and 2020 and prevalent cases in children under 15 years will rise by 70 % [8].

The need for rigorous epidemiological studies to monitor the trends of T1DM in children less than 15 year of age led to the creation of the World Health Organization (WHO) - sponsored Diabetes Mondiale (DIAMOND) [2] Project and the EURODIAB study [9].

The data from the WHO project for the incidence of T1DM worldwide DIAMOND showed a large geographic variability. This study group was based on 43,013 cases of T1DM from a study population of 84 million children aged 14 year old or less during the period 1990-1999 in 114 populations from 57 countries. During this time the average annual increase in incidence was 2.8% (95% CI 2.4%-3.2%) with a slightly higher rate during 1995 to 1999, 3.4% (95% CI 2.7%-4.3%) than during 1990 to 1994, 2.4% (95% CI 1.3%-3.4%). An increase in the incidence of T1DM was observed in the populations studied (4.0% in Asia, 3.2% in Europe, and 5.3% in North America) with the exception of Central America and the West Indies, where T1D is less prevalent, and where the trend was a decrease of 3.6% [10].

It is of interest that several reports have shown an increase in the incidence of T1DM worldwide. This tendency implicates an increasing influence of environmental trigger factors against a background of genetic susceptibility. The geographic and ethnic variations mirror the prevalence of susceptibility genes or that of contributing environmental factors, or both. Nevertheless this increasing incidence rate in such a short period cannot be solely attributed to genetic shifts.

The EURODIAB ACE study group examined the trends in the incidence of T1DM from 1989 to 1994. The study was based on 16,362 cases of T1D in 44 European centres and Israel covering a population of 28 million children [9]. There were enormous variations in the annual incidence rate with 3.2/100,000 person-years in the Former Yugoslav Republic of Macedonia to 40.2/100,000 person-years in two regions of Finland. During this time the annual increase in the incidence rate of T1D was 3.4% (95% CI 2.5%-4.4%) although the rate of increase was noted to be higher in some central European countries. The rates of increase were found to be the highest in the youngest age group: ages 0 to 4 years (6.3%, 95% CI 1.5%-8.5%), 5 to 9 years (3.1%, 95% CI 1.5%-4.8%), and 10 to 14 years (2.4%, 95% CI 1.0%-3.8%).

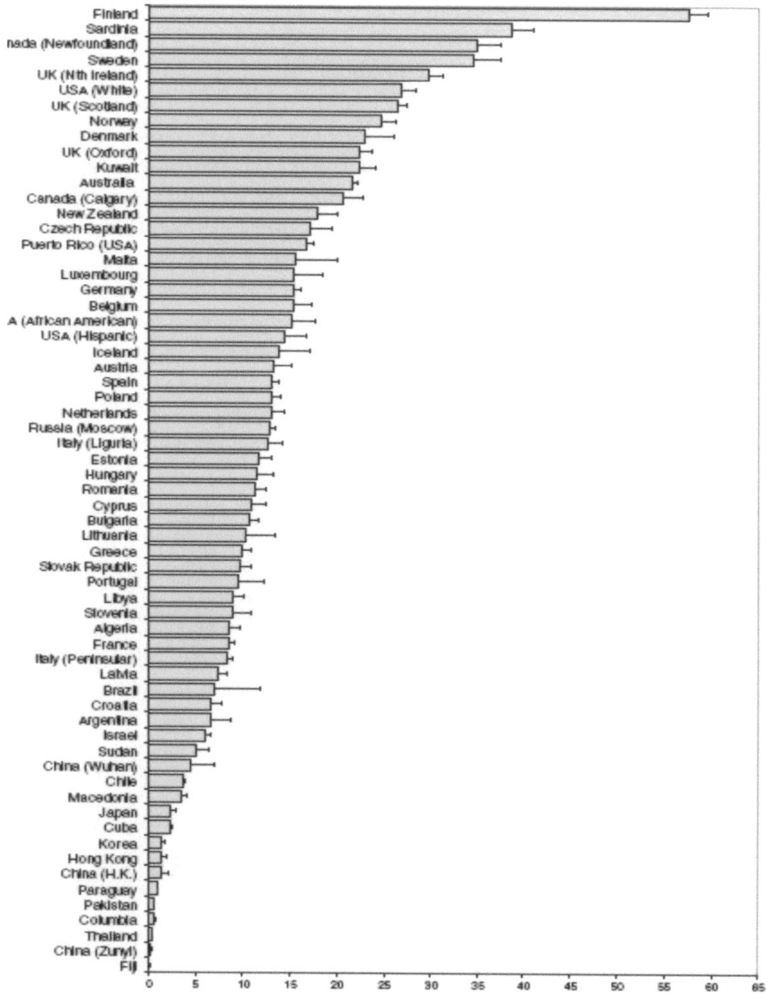

Fig. 1. Mean Annual Incidence rates for T1DM comparing different countries in the world as seen in reference 1.

Furthermore one of the most notable and recent, in the United States, includes a population-based study of incidence rates of T1DM from 10 study locations by The SEARCH for Diabetes in Youth Study. The Search Group found an overall incidence of T1DM in children 0–19 of 24.3 per 100,000 person years with the highest rates observed among the 5–9 and 10–14 age groups with rates of 22.9 and 33.9 per 100,000 respectively [11].

A recent study from Saudi Arabia over an 18 year period, has shown an average incidence of 27.52/100000/year increasing from 18.05/100000/year in the first 9 years of the study period to 36.99/100000/year in the next 9 years [12]. Significant increase in incidence of T1DM was also observed in Lower Silesia during the period 2000-2005 with an increase from 10.43/100000 in 2000 to 13.49/100000 in 2005 [13].

Additionally in Scotland two studies by Patterson and co-workers [14-15] have shown an increasing incidence from 13, 8/100000/year between 1968 and 1976 and up to

21,0/100000/year from 1977 to 1983 for children aged less than 19 year old. Another study for the same population found that the incidence of T1DM had increased from 22,7/100000 in 1984 to 26,0/100000 in 1993 and this increase of about 2% a year, though small, is statistically significant and the effect over 10 years is a large increase [16]. An important increase in incidence of T1DM was also observed in Saxony between the five year periods 1999-2003 and 2004-2008 with estimated rates 15.7/100000 and 19.2/100000 respectively [17].

In our study we have ascertained the mean annual incidence on T1DM in the Greek Cypriot population during the period 1990 - 1999 in children younger than 15 years of age. During this period the incidence of T1DM was 10.76 /100000[18]. In order to identify an increase in the incidence of T1DM in our country, as occurred in the majority of the populations worldwide, we had performed an analysis of the newly diagnosed cases until the end of the year 2004. There was a statistically significant increase in the incidence during the period 2000-2004 with an estimated mean overall incidence 11.9/100000[19]. We had subsequently extended this work by adding the new cases of the five year period 2005 – 2009 in order to document this rising trend by comparing the incidence between the two decades (1990-1999 vs 2000-2009). We have observed a rising trend of the mean incidence from 10.76/100.000 at the first decade (1990-1999) of the study up to 14.4/100.000 at the second decade (2000-2009). According to Wilcoxon two-sample test this increasing trend of incidence during the 20 years analysed is statistically significant (p-value=0.0091). The mean incidence rate for each 5 year- period in accordance with the population data (population below the age of 15yr) is presented in figure 2. The overall mean incidence of T1DM, in the Greek Cypriot population was 12.46/100000 during the twenty-year period 1990-2009. This raised incidence classifies Cyprus among the countries with high incidence of T1DM.

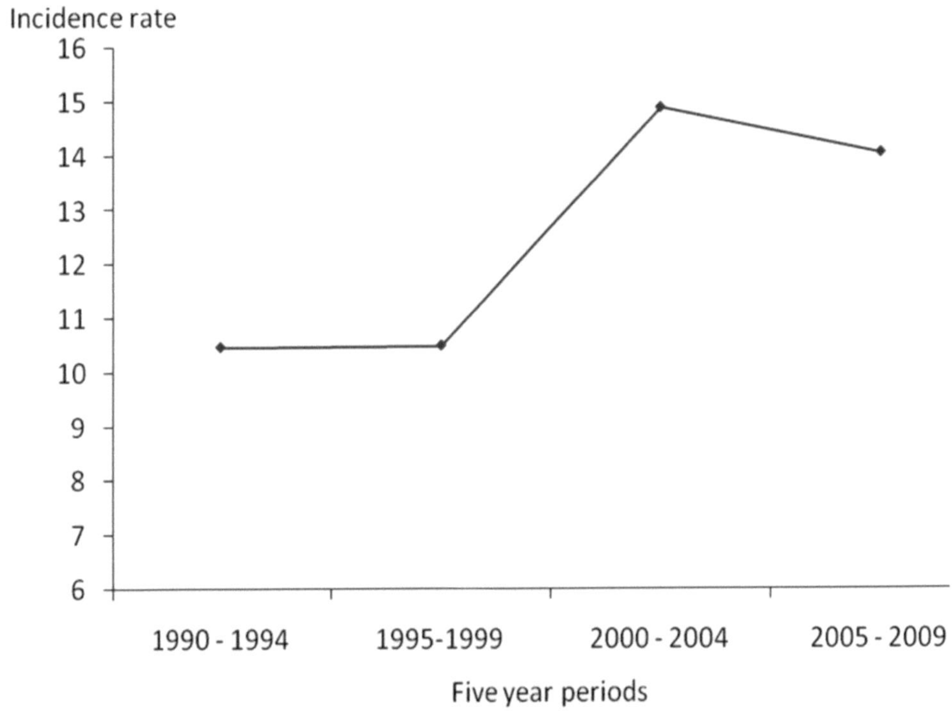

Fig. 2. Different annual incidence rates during five year periods.

Additionally this rising incidence was more pronounced among children who manifested the disease before the age of 5yr. Table 1 shows the percentage of newly diagnosed T1DM cases expressed as age group in accordance with the international standards.

Period at Diagnosis	Age Group (years)					
	0-4		5-9		10-14	
	n	%	n	%	n	%
1990-1999	31	19.0 (13.0-25.0)	66	40.5 (33.0-48.0)**	66	40.5 (33.0-48.0)**
2000-2009	55	26.4 (20.4-32.4)	77	37.0 (30.4-43.6)*	76	36.5 (30.0-43.0)*
1990-2009	*86*	*23.2 (18.9-27.5)*	*143*	*38.5 (33.5-43.5)***	*142*	*38.3 (33.4-43.2)***

Table 1. Age of diagnosis in total and in the three age groups. Binomial test performed to compare proportions compared to "0-4 year" age group: * $p<0.01$, ** $p<0.001$

3. Age of onset

T1DM formerly called as juvenile diabetes it is one of the most common chronic disease of youth as 80% of individuals with T1DM are younger than 20 year of age [20-21]. The age of manifestation of childhood onset T1DM has a bimodal allotment with one peak at 4 to 6 years of age and a second in early puberty (10 to 14 years of age) [22-23]. Recent studies report a higher rate of increase among children younger than 5 years than in children between 5 and 15 years of age [24-25]. This may be related to an earlier onset of clinical manifestation or to a true increase in the causative factors of the disease.

Although the clinical appearance occurs at all ages [21] one fourth of individuals with T1DM are diagnosed as adults [26]. Up to 10% of adults primarily supposed to have type 2 diabetes are found to have antibodies associated with T1D [27] and beta cell destruction in adults seems to take place at a much slower rate than in young T1D cases, often delaying the need for insulin therapy after diagnosis.

4. Gender differences

Although most autoimmune diseases are more common in females, there appears to be no gender difference in the overall incidence of childhood T1DM [11].

However, a gender influence on the age of onset has been reported, in select populations. Some data reported from Europe suggest a female predominance in lower risk populations, and slight male excess in the high risk groups [3]. Furthermore many reports showed that older male adults of European origin (≥15 to 40 years of age) are more likely to develop T1DM than females of similar age and geographic location with an approximate 3:2 male to female ratio [28-30]. The same 3:2 male to female ratio also was reported in children younger than 6 years of age in an observational study from Boston [31]. Based on our data it seems that more males develop T1DM at younger age, whereas female predominate during the peripubertal period as shown in figure 3.

5. Seasonal variation at onset and birth

The first report of seasonal variation in the manifestation of T1DM was presented by Franklin Adams in 1926[32] although a consistent picture on the real seasonality of the disease has not been established. The increased incidence of T1DM diagnosis during

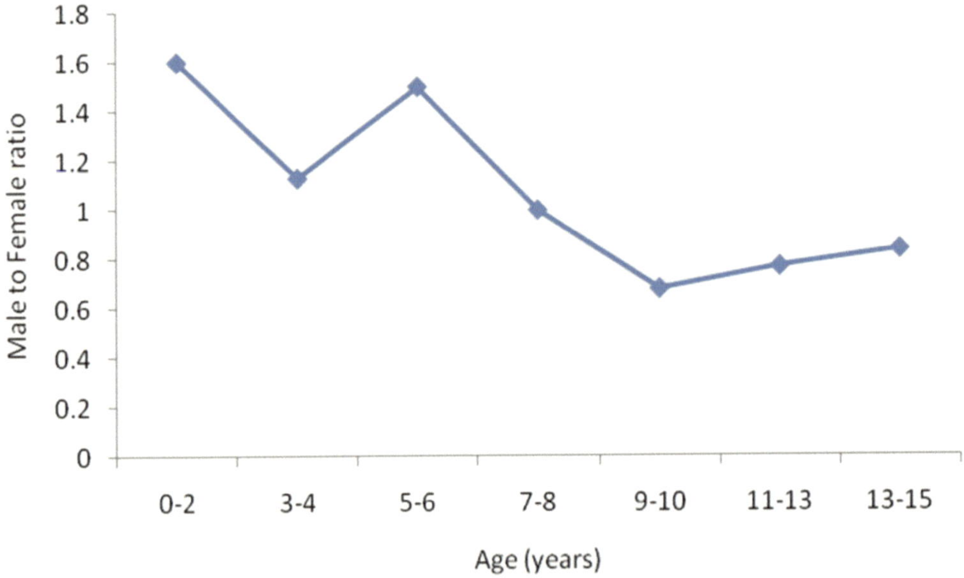

Fig. 3. Ratio of males and females in relation to year of diagnosis (at 2-yr intervals).

Autumn and Winter months could support the hypothesis that infections may act as participating factors in the clinical onset of the disease, possibly accelerating an autoimmune process that may have been initiated months or years before [33]. Based on the average temperature record in our island, the newly diagnosed cased were grouped according to the month of diagnosis as follow: November, December, January, and February were defined as cold months, October, March, April and May as neutral months and, June, July , August and September, as warm months. More children were significantly diagnosed with T1DM during the cold months compared to those who manifested the disease during the warm months (p<0.001), whereas no difference was observed in the incidence between neutral and cold months ((p>0.05) throughout the study period (1990-2009) as depicted in Table 2. A recent study on seasonal variation in DM in 53 countries has suggested that seasonality in the diagnosis of T1DM occurs and that the pattern of seasonality appears to be related to the geographical position, at least as far as the northern/southern hemisphere dichotomy is concerned [34].

Period at Diagnosis	Month at Diagnosis					
	Cold Months		Neutral Months		Warm Months	
	n	%	n	%	n	%
1990-1999	64	38.6 (31.2-46.0)	61	36.7 (29.4-44.0)*	41	24.7 (18.1-31.3)****
2000-2009	82	39.4 (32.8-46.0)	67	32.2 (25.9-38.5)**	59	28.4 (22.3-34.5)***
1990-2009	*146*	*39.0 (34.1-43.9)*	*128*	*34.2 (29.4-39.0)**	*100*	*26.7 (22.2-31.2)*****

Table 2. Percentage of children diagnosed with T1DM at cold months, neutral months and warm months. Binomial test performed to compare proportions compared to "Cold Months" group: * NS (p>0.05), ** p<0.05, *** p<0.01, ****p<0.001

A seasonal variation of birth has been also observed in children who developed T1DM later in life in many countries, which suggests that environmental factors during pregnancy, in the neonatal period or very early in life play a role in its development. Several studies from Europe [35-37] and Israel [38] showed higher rates of T1DM among youth born in spring and lower rates among youth born in winter. Although McKinney maintained that there is no relationship between T1DM diagnosis and date of birth[39]. It has been suggested that seasonability pattern may be explained by reduced vitamin D production [40] during the critical intrauterine and neonatal periods of life.

6. Genotype

The genetics of T1DM cannot be classified according to a specific model of inheritance. Susceptibility to autoimmune T1DM is determined by multiple genes with HLA genes having the strongest known association. HLA antigens are present on the surface of the leucocytes and participate in some immune reactions. The genes coding for these antigens are located on chromosome 6. The class II sub region of HLA consists of the DR, DQ, and DP loci. These class II molecules are involved to the immune destruction of the pancreatic beta cells because they participate in the presentation of the antigen to the helper T cell, which initiates the immune reaction.

Inheritance of HLA-DR3 and HLA-DR4 appears to confer a 2 to 3 fold increased risk for the development of T1DM. When both HLA-DR3 and HLA-DR4 are inherited the relative risk for the development of T1DM is increased by 7-10 folds. It is estimated that 48 percent of the familial aggregation can now be ascribed to known loci, and the Major Histocompatibility Complex (MHC) contributes 41 percent [41]. As an example, siblings with the highest risk HLA DR and DQ alleles, who inherit both HLA regions identical by descent to their diabetic sibling, may have a risk of developing anti-islet autoimmunity as high as 80 percent and a similar long-term risk of diabetes[42]. Moreover HLA DR2 and HLA DR5 are both protective in most studies. Furthermore, stronger associations of DM1 have been reported with other MHC loci: HLA-DQA1 and DQB1 antigens[43].

In our effort to detect the genetic susceptibility of Greek Cypriot population to DM1, we studied 101 DM1 patients with age of onset less than 15 years through HLA serological typing for the DR and DQ1 alleles and compared them to 209 healthy controls. Our findings support the strong association of HLA-DR4 and DR3 with DM1. The most frequent allelic combination was that of HLA-DR3/DR4 (27%) followed by that of DR2/DR4 (21.6%). The percentage of HLA antigens in patients with DM1 and controls are shown in figure 4. The protective role of HLA-DR5 was shown, whereas the presence of HLA-DR2 is neutral, in contrast with most findings among Caucasian population where DR2 is protective. In addition, high resolution testing of the DR4 and DR3 alleles revealed the predominant presence of the DRB1*0403 (0% vs 36%), similar frequency of the DRB1*0402 in both groups (19% vs 14%) and that the DRB1*301 was the only DR3 allele detected. The DQB1 alleles present in our T1DM patients as shown in figure 5 were nearly exclusively DQB1*0201 and DQB1*0302 [44]. The relative risk of developing T1DM in children carrying the DQB1*0201 and the DQB1*0302 alleles is 5.05 and 2.56 respectively whereas the protective role of DQB1*0301 is documented.

Furthermore, although most T1D cases occur in individuals without a family history of the disease, T1D is strongly influenced by genetic factors. The lifelong risk of T1DM is markedly

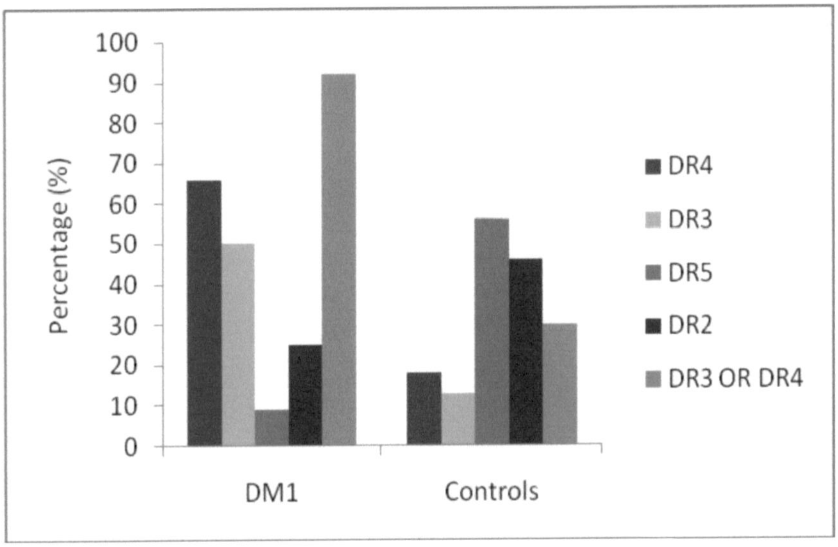

Fig. 4. HLA antigens in DM1 patients and controls.

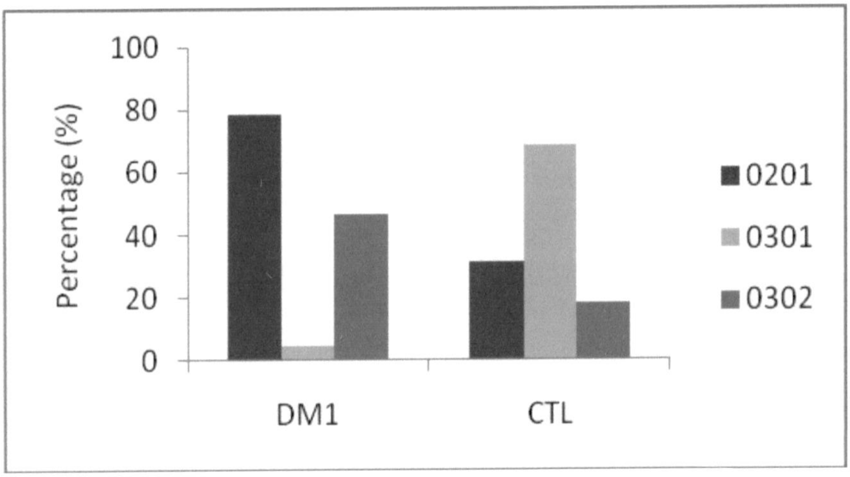

Fig. 5. HLA DQ B1 alleles in DM1 patients and controls.

increased in close relatives of a patient with T1DM, averaging about 6 percent in offspring, 5 percent in siblings and 50 percent in identical twins (versus 0.4 percent in subjects with no family history) [45-46]. T1DM is 2-3 times more common in the offspring of diabetic men (3.6-8.5%) compared with diabetic woman (1.3-3.6%) [1]. A monozygotic twin of a patient with type 1 diabetes has a higher risk of diabetes than a dizygotic twin, and the risk in a dizygotic twin sibling is similar to that in non-twin siblings [46].

Additionally age at onset is inversely related to the proportion of HLA haplotypes, and young children with T1DM show the greatest HLA-associated genetic risk. Siblings of children with onset of T1D before the age of 5 years have a 3- to 5-fold greater cumulative risk of diabetes by age 20 years compared with siblings of children diagnosed between 5 and 15 years of age [47]. Several reports suggest a higher proportion of lower risk haplotypes

and in association with the decreased age at onset of T1DM are consisted with a major environmental effect on the development of the disease [48-51].
T1DM is associated with other autoimmune diseases such as thyroiditis, celiac disease, autoimmune gastritis and Addison disease [52]. The coexistence of these autoimmune diseases is associated to genes within the MHC complex [52].

7. Other risk factors

The variations in the incidence of T1DM in different countries its rising in rich and developed countries have raised questions about changes in environmental risk factors that may either initiate or accelerate the autoimmune process leading to pancreatic β-pancreatic cell destruction.
Reports have linked several environmental factors to an increased risk of T1DM; however, none of these have associations have verified and many have been contradicted by other studies. They include: viral infections in infancy and early childhood, maternal viral infection during pregnancy [53], early exposure to cow's milk and other nutritional factors [54], chemical contamination of food and water [55], high birth weight and an increase in body mass index [56].
Viruses that have been associated with T1DM as environmental triggers include enteroviruses, mumps, rubella, cytomegalovirus, rotavirus and Epstein-Barr virus. The one proven environmental virus trigger T1DM is congenital rubella [57]. Many epidemiological studies have been supported the involvement of enteroviruses, especially the Coxsackie B viruses in the aetiology which appears to trigger β cell autoimmunity [58-59]. Furthermore it has been hypothesized that excessive weight gain and increase in insulin resistance in early childhood is trigger event which initiates the autoimmunity leading to β cell destruction and this Accelerator Hypothesis has been supported by several epidemiological studies [56, 60-61].
A number of dietary factors may influence the development of T1DM in infants at high risk for T1DM. Early introduction to the infant diet of cattle proteins, lack or short lasting breast feeding might be reasons for development of immunological reaction leading to the destruction of pancreatic beta cells [62]. In two large prospective cohort studies of newborns at high risk for T1DM diabetes (either a first degree relative [63-64] or a high risk HLA genotype) [63], first exposure to cereal before age three months [63-64] or after seven months [63] was associated with an increased risk of developing autoantibodies (IA) compared to infants whose first exposure was between ages four to six months. The increased risk was associated with gluten-containing cereals in one study [64], but with either gluten or rice-containing cereals in the other [63].
On the other hand Vitamin D and omega-3 fatty acids may have a protective role. A case control study in seven European countries suggested that supplementation with vitamin D in early infancy can protect against development of T1DM [65]. A similar protective effect was found in a birth-cohort study of over 10,000 children [66]. Moreover preliminary studies in animals sustain a protective role of omega-3 fatty acids in the inflammatory reaction associated with autoimmune islet cell damage [67-68].
In conclusion there is no doubt that the incidence of T1DM is increasing dramatically. Data from large epidemiological studies worldwide indicate that the incidence of T1DM has been increasing by 2% to 5% worldwide [69] and this is of concern because of its health and resource implications. This rising incidence of T1DM in young children has been confirmed

to a genetically susceptible subgroup of the population (48). The heightened proportion of lower risk hapltotypes and decreased median age at onset of T1DM within the subgroup are consistent with a major environmental effect on Diabetes development (50).

8. Epilogue

It is a an actuality that significant advances have been made in the clinical care of T1DM, which ultimately improved the clinical outcomes. However much more need to be done to find a cure for T1DM. In the absence of an ideal therapy Diabetes will always be a hurdle in the quality of life of these children. Moreover the increasing incidence is of concern because of its health and resource implications. There is a great research potential and more studies are required to identify the environmental factors that trigger the autoimmune destruction of the pancreatic beta cell particularly in some populations and individuals, who are not genetically predisposed to develop T1DM. These environmental triggers if ever identified could potentially be targeted for new preventive strategies and optimal intervention.

9. References

[1] Craig, M.E., A. Hattersley, and K.C. Donaghue, *Definition, epidemiology and classification of diabetes in children and adolescents.* Pediatr Diabetes, 2009. 10 Suppl 12: p. 3-12.

[2] Karvonen, M., et al., *Incidence of childhood type 1 diabetes worldwide. Diabetes Mondiale (DiaMond) Project Group.* Diabetes Care, 2000. 23(10): p. 1516-26.

[3] Green, A., E.A. Gale, and C.C. Patterson, *Incidence of childhood-onset insulin-dependent diabetes mellitus: the EURODIAB ACE Study.* Lancet, 1992. 339(8798): p. 905-9.

[4] Eisenbarth, G.S., *Immunology of type 1 diabetes.* 2nd ed. 2004: Plenum Publishers.

[5] Yang, Z., et al., *Childhood diabetes in China. Enormous variation by place and ethnic group.* Diabetes Care, 1998. 21(4): p. 525-9.

[6] Silink, M., *Childhood diabetes: a global perspective.* Horm Res, 2002. 57 Suppl 1: p. 1-5.

[7] Onkamo, P., et al., *Worldwide increase in incidence of Type I diabetes--the analysis of the data on published incidence trends.* Diabetologia, 1999. 42(12): p. 1395-403.

[8] Patterson, C.C., et al., *Incidence trends for childhood type 1 diabetes in Europe during 1989-2003 and predicted new cases 2005-20: a multicentre prospective registration study.* Lancet, 2009. 373(9680): p. 2027-33.

[9] *Variation and trends in incidence of childhood diabetes in Europe. EURODIAB ACE Study Group.* Lancet, 2000. 355(9207): p. 873-6.

[10] *Incidence and trends of childhood Type 1 diabetes worldwide 1990-1999.* Diabet Med, 2006. 23(8): p. 857-66.

[11] Dabelea, D., et al., *Incidence of diabetes in youth in the United States.* JAMA, 2007. 297(24): p. 2716-24.

[12] Al-Mendalawi, M.D., et al., *Incidence trends of childhood type 1 diabetes in eastern Saudi Arabia.* Saudi Med J, 2010. 31(9): p. 1074-5; author reply 1074-5.

[13] Zubkiewicz-Kucharska, A. and A. Noczynska, *[Epidemiology of type 1 diabetes in Lower Silesia in the years 2000-2005].* Pediatr Endocrinol Diabetes Metab, 2010. 16(1): p. 45-9.

[14] Patterson, C.C., et al., *Increasing prevalence of diabetes mellitus in children.* Br Med J (Clin Res Ed), 1983. 287(6386): p. 213-4.

[15] Patterson, C.C., et al., *Geographical variation in the incidence of diabetes mellitus in Scottish children during the period 1977-1983.* Diabet Med, 1988. 5(2): p. 160-5.

[16] Rangasami, J.J., et al., *Rising incidence of type 1 diabetes in Scottish children, 1984-93. The Scottish Study Group for the Care of Young Diabetics.* Arch Dis Child, 1997. 77(3): p. 210-3.

[17] Galler, A., et al., *Incidence of childhood diabetes in children aged less than 15 years and its clinical and metabolic characteristics at the time of diagnosis: data from the Childhood Diabetes Registry of Saxony, Germany.* Horm Res Paediatr, 2010. 74(4): p. 285-91.

[18] Skordis, N., et al., *The incidence of type 1 diabetes mellitus in Greek-Cypriot children and adolescents in 1990-2000.* Pediatr Diabetes, 2002. 3(4): p. 200-4.

[19] Toumba, M., et al., *Rising incidence of type 1 diabetes mellitus in children and adolescents in Cyprus in 2000-2004.* Pediatr Diabetes, 2007. 8(6): p. 374-6.

[20] Liese, A.D., et al., *The burden of diabetes mellitus among US youth: prevalence estimates from the SEARCH for Diabetes in Youth Study.* Pediatrics, 2006. 118(4): p. 1510-8.

[21] Thunander, M., et al., *Incidence of type 1 and type 2 diabetes in adults and children in Kronoberg, Sweden.* Diabetes Res Clin Pract, 2008. 82(2): p. 247-55.

[22] Felner, E.I., et al., *Genetic interaction among three genomic regions creates distinct contributions to early- and late-onset type 1 diabetes mellitus.* Pediatr Diabetes, 2005. 6(4): p. 213-20.

[23] Elamin, A., et al., *Epidemiology of childhood type I diabetes in Sudan, 1987-1990.* Diabetes Care, 1992. 15(11): p. 1556-9.

[24] Karvonen, M., J. Pitkaniemi, and J. Tuomilehto, *The onset age of type 1 diabetes in Finnish children has become younger. The Finnish Childhood Diabetes Registry Group.* Diabetes Care, 1999. 22(7): p. 1066-70.

[25] Schoenle, E.J., et al., *Epidemiology of type I diabetes mellitus in Switzerland: steep rise in incidence in under 5 year old children in the past decade.* Diabetologia, 2001. 44(3): p. 286-9.

[26] Haller, M.J., M.A. Atkinson, and D. Schatz, *Type 1 diabetes mellitus: etiology, presentation, and management.* Pediatr Clin North Am, 2005. 52(6): p. 1553-78.

[27] Turner, R., et al., *UKPDS 25: autoantibodies to islet-cell cytoplasm and glutamic acid decarboxylase for prediction of insulin requirement in type 2 diabetes. UK Prospective Diabetes Study Group.* Lancet, 1997. 350(9087): p. 1288-93.

[28] Gale, E.A. and K.M. Gillespie, *Diabetes and gender.* Diabetologia, 2001. 44(1): p. 3-15.

[29] Weets, I., et al., *The incidence of type 1 diabetes in the age group 0-39 years has not increased in Antwerp (Belgium) between 1989 and 2000: evidence for earlier disease manifestation.* Diabetes Care, 2002. 25(5): p. 840-6.

[30] Pundziute-Lycka, A., et al., *The incidence of Type I diabetes has not increased but shifted to a younger age at diagnosis in the 0-34 years group in Sweden 1983-1998.* Diabetologia, 2002. 45(6): p. 783-91.

[31] Quinn, M., et al., *Characteristics at diagnosis of type 1 diabetes in children younger than 6 years.* J Pediatr, 2006. 148(3): p. 366-71.

[32] Adams, F., *The seasonal variation in the onset of acute diabetes. The age and sex factors in 1000 diabetic patients.* Arch Intern Med, 1926. 37: p.:861-864.

[33] Jun, H.S. and J.W. Yoon, *A new look at viruses in type 1 diabetes.* Diabetes Metab Res Rev, 2003. 19(1): p. 8-31.

[34] Moltchanova, E.V., et al., *Seasonal variation of diagnosis of Type 1 diabetes mellitus in children worldwide.* Diabet Med, 2009. 26(7): p. 673-8.

[35] Vaiserman, A.M., et al., *Seasonality of birth in children and young adults (0-29 years) with type 1 diabetes in Ukraine.* Diabetologia, 2007. 50(1): p. 32-5.

[36] Jongbloet, P.H., et al., *Seasonality of birth in patients with childhood diabetes in The Netherlands.* Diabetes Care, 1998. 21(1): p. 190-1.

[37] Samuelsson, U., C. Johansson, and J. Ludvigsson, *Month of birth and risk of developing insulin dependent diabetes in south east Sweden.* Arch Dis Child, 1999. 81(2): p. 143-6.

[38] Laron, Z., et al., *Month of birth and subsequent development of type I diabetes (IDDM).* J Pediatr Endocrinol Metab, 1999. 12(3): p. 397-402.

[39] McKinney, P.A., *Seasonality of birth in patients with childhood Type I diabetes in 19 European regions.* Diabetologia, 2001. 44 Suppl 3: p. B67-74.

[40] Mohr, S.B., et al., *The association between ultraviolet B irradiance, vitamin D status and incidence rates of type 1 diabetes in 51 regions worldwide.* Diabetologia, 2008. 51(8): p. 1391-8.

[41] Todd, J.A., et al., *Robust associations of four new chromosome regions from genome-wide analyses of type 1 diabetes.* Nat Genet, 2007. 39(7): p. 857-64.

[42] Aly, T.A., et al., *Extreme genetic risk for type 1A diabetes.* Proc Natl Acad Sci U S A, 2006. 103(38): p. 14074-9.

[43] Thorsby, E. and K.S. Ronningen, *Particular HLA-DQ molecules play a dominant role in determining susceptibility or resistance to type 1 (insulin-dependent) diabetes mellitus.* Diabetologia, 1993. 36(5): p. 371-7.

[44] Stylianou, C.H., Apsiotou, N., Stavrou, S., Demetriades, M., Kyriakou, A., Costeas, P., Skordis, N., *Detection of HLA-DR and DQB1 alleles, which predispose to diabetes mellitus type 1 in the Greek Cypriot population.* Hormone Research, 2003. 60((Suppl I)): p. 136.

[45] Atkinson, M.A. and N.K. Maclaren, *The pathogenesis of insulin-dependent diabetes mellitus.* N Engl J Med, 1994. 331(21): p. 1428-36.

[46] Redondo, M.J., et al., *Genetic determination of islet cell autoimmunity in monozygotic twin, dizygotic twin, and non-twin siblings of patients with type 1 diabetes: prospective twin study.* BMJ, 1999. 318(7185): p. 698-702.

[47] Gillespie, K.M., E.A. Gale, and P.J. Bingley, *High familial risk and genetic susceptibility in early onset childhood diabetes.* Diabetes, 2002. 51(1): p. 210-4.

[48] Gillespie, K.M., et al., *The rising incidence of childhood type 1 diabetes and reduced contribution of high-risk HLA haplotypes.* Lancet, 2004. 364(9446): p. 1699-700.

[49] Hermann, R., et al., *Temporal changes in the frequencies of HLA genotypes in patients with Type 1 diabetes--indication of an increased environmental pressure?* Diabetologia, 2003. 46(3): p. 420-5.

[50] Gale, E.A., *The rise of childhood type 1 diabetes in the 20th century.* Diabetes, 2002. 51(12): p. 3353-61.

[51] Vehik, K., et al., *Trends in high-risk HLA susceptibility genes among Colorado youth with type 1 diabetes.* Diabetes Care, 2008. 31(7): p. 1392-6.

[52] Tsirogianni, A., E. Pipi, and K. Soufleros, *Specificity of islet cell autoantibodies and coexistence with other organ specific autoantibodies in type 1 diabetes mellitus.* Autoimmun Rev, 2009. 8(8): p. 687-91.

[53] Dahlquist, G.G., et al., *Maternal enteroviral infection during pregnancy as a risk factor for childhood IDDM. A population-based case-control study.* Diabetes, 1995. 44(4): p. 408-13.

[54] Akerblom, H.K., et al., *Dietary manipulation of beta cell autoimmunity in infants at increased risk of type 1 diabetes: a pilot study.* Diabetologia, 2005. 48(5): p. 829-37.

[55] Longnecker, M.P. and J.L. Daniels, *Environmental contaminants as etiologic factors for diabetes.* Environ Health Perspect, 2001. 109 Suppl 6: p. 871-6.

[56] Hypponen, E., et al., *Obesity, increased linear growth, and risk of type 1 diabetes in children.* Diabetes Care, 2000. 23(12): p. 1755-60.

[57] McIntosh, E.D. and M.A. Menser, *A fifty-year follow-up of congenital rubella.* Lancet, 1992. 340(8816): p. 414-5.

[58] Rewers, M. and P. Zimmet, *The rising tide of childhood type 1 diabetes--what is the elusive environmental trigger?* Lancet, 2004. 364(9446): p. 1645-7.

[59] Salminen, K., et al., *Enterovirus infections are associated with the induction of beta-cell autoimmunity in a prospective birth cohort study.* J Med Virol, 2003. 69(1): p. 91-8.

[60] Betts, P., et al., *Increasing body weight predicts the earlier onset of insulin-dependant diabetes in childhood: testing the 'accelerator hypothesis' (2).* Diabet Med, 2005. 22(2): p. 144-51.

[61] Evertsen, J., R. Alemzadeh, and X. Wang, *Increasing incidence of pediatric type 1 diabetes mellitus in Southeastern Wisconsin: relationship with body weight at diagnosis.* PLoS One, 2009. 4(9): p. e6873.

[62] Virtanen, S.M. and M. Knip, *Nutritional risk predictors of beta cell autoimmunity and type 1 diabetes at a young age.* Am J Clin Nutr, 2003. 78(6): p. 1053-67.

[63] Norris, J.M., et al., *Timing of initial cereal exposure in infancy and risk of islet autoimmunity.* JAMA, 2003. 290(13): p. 1713-20.

[64] Ziegler, A.G., et al., *Early infant feeding and risk of developing type 1 diabetes-associated autoantibodies.* JAMA, 2003. 290(13): p. 1721-8.

[65] *Vitamin D supplement in early childhood and risk for Type I (insulin-dependent) diabetes mellitus. The EURODIAB Substudy 2 Study Group.* Diabetologia, 1999. 42(1): p. 51-4.

[66] Hypponen, E., et al., *Intake of vitamin D and risk of type 1 diabetes: a birth-cohort study.* Lancet, 2001. 358(9292): p. 1500-3.

[67] Kleemann, R., et al., *Impact of dietary fat on Th1/Th2 cytokine gene expression in the pancreas and gut of diabetes-prone BB rats.* J Autoimmun, 1998. 11(1): p. 97-103.

[68] Krishna Mohan, I. and U.N. Das, *Prevention of chemically induced diabetes mellitus in experimental animals by polyunsaturated fatty acids.* Nutrition, 2001. 17(2): p. 126-51.

[69] Maahs, D.M., et al., *Epidemiology of type 1 diabetes.* Endocrinol Metab Clin North Am, 2010. 39(3): p. 481-97.

17

Genetic Testing of Newborns for Type 1 Diabetes Susceptibility – The MIDIA Study

Kjersti S. Rønningen
Department of Pediatric Research
Oslo University Hospital, Rikshospitalet, Oslo
Norway

1. Introduction

Type 1 Diabetes (T1D) is one of the most common chronic diseases with childhood onset, and the disease has increased two to threefold over the past half century by yet unknown means. Recently it was showed that if the present trend continues, the prevalence of cases younger than 5 years of age will rise by 70% within year 2020 (Patterson et al., 2009).

1.1 Background and status of knowledge

Type 1 Diabetes (T1D) is a T-cell mediated autoimmune disease that develops in genetically susceptible individuals whose immune system destroys the majority of insulin-secreting β-cells in pancreatic islets (Eizirik et al., 2009). The incidence of T1D has increased more than two- to threefold over the past half century, the most striking example being Finland where it has risen from 12 to 63/100,000 (Knip & Siljander, 2008; Patterson et al., 2009). This increase in incidence has not been paralleled by an increase in the frequency of major risk genes, including HLA class II, insulin, PTPN22, CTLA-4 and IL2RA (Barrett et al., 2009). Indeed, the prevalence of the classical HLA class II genes, which account for approximately 40% of genetic risk, appears to be decreasing (Gillespie et al., 2004; Fourlanos et al., 2008). There are now more than 40 risk loci associated with T1D with the majority of non-HLA genes displaying odds ratio <1.2. (Barrett et al., 2009). Moreover, most individuals who possess T1D risk genes do not develop the disease. Importantly, the concordance rate among monozygotic twins ranges from as low as 25 to 65% (Redendo et al., 1999, 2008; Hyttinen et al., 2003) and is approximately 6% in siblings. A common explanation has been that changes in environment must contribute to the increase in the disease. In particular, environmental exposures to dietary antigens and microbes have been implicated (Knip et al., 2005; Lefebvre et al., 2006). However, no single pathogenic environmental agent has been identified that explain all cases. In all likelihood, T1D develops by various combinations of pathways in response to commonly encountered environmental exposures.

1.2 Nutritional related factors and type 1 diabetes risk

The Norwegian Institute of Public Health is currently running two large prospective cohort studies; "Environmental Triggers of Type 1 Diabetes" (MIDIA) (www.fhi.no/midia) and "The Norwegian Mother and Child Cohort Study" (MoBa) (www.fhi.no/morogbarn). In MIDIA we will be able to study the impact of the dietary intake in children as well as mothers during the breast-feeding period and in MoBa we will be able to study the dietary intake of the mother during pregnancy for development of T1D in the child. These two studies will be linked to allow several approaches to be tested in the role of early diet and development of T1D. In the MIDIA study newborns have been identified by testing for the high-risk genotype (DRB1*03-DQA1*05-DQB1*02/ DRB1*04:01-DQA1*03-DQB1*03:02) in the HLA-system (Cinek et al., 2000). The MIDIA study is unique compared to the few other ongoing worldwide cohorts because of pregnancy data from the Norwegian Mother and Child Cohort Study (MoBa). Information from questionnaires, public records as well as blood samples from mothers (twice during pregnancy) and children (cord blood) have been collected from 107,000 pregnancies (Magnus et al., 2006; Rønningen et al., 2006). 50% of the children participating in MIDIA have a mother who also participates in MoBa, and consent has been given for linking information from the two studies and using biological specimens (Stene et al., 2007).

1.2.1 Foetal exposure and early life exposure to nutritional factors

Many nutritional factors may operate in uteri (measured as the mother's exposure during pregnancy), and also during postnatal life, and the status of the child is often influenced both by the maternal intake during pregnancy and postnatal exposures. Because the most relevant timing of exposure and possible induction times are unknown for T1D, an approach addressing both intrauterine and postnatal exposure to hypothetical risk factors or protective factors is most sensible.

1.2.2 Breast-feeding and cow's milk

Several epidemiological studies indicate that the risk of T1D is lower in children that have been breast-fed compared to children given breast-milk substitute produced from cow's milk (Norris & Scott., 1996), and recent data also indicate that for avoiding early autoimmunity the duration of breastfeeding is of importance (Rosenbauer et al., 2008). But most case-control studies suffer from potential recall bias, and prospective studies up to now have been few and very small. Case-control studies have also found associations between cow's milk antibodies and T1D see e.g. (Sarugeri et al., 1999; Monetini et al., 2002), but some form of reverse causality cannot be excluded as alternative explanations for the association described in these studies. Although an early study indicated a role of so-called molecular mimicry between a protein in cow's milk and a β-cell antigen (Karjalainen et al., 1992), it was subsequently refuted (Rønningen et al., 1998). Multiple other biologically plausible mechanisms have also been proposed for the possible relation between short duration of breast-feeding or early introduction of cow's milk.

1.2.3 Introduction of solid food

Studies indicate that the time point for introduction of solid food, especially with regard to cereal products, may have an influence on the development of autoimmunity (Norris et al., 2003; Ziegler et al., 2003). Early exposure to cereals is against generally accepted recommendations on infant nutrition in all developed countries and occurs infrequently. For example, Scandinavian babies are rarely exposed to cereals before the age of 4 months. A prospective analysis of data from the Finnish Diabetes Prediction and Prevention (DIPP) study showed no relation between early or late introduction of cereals and emergence of advanced β-cell autoimmunity. Another study from Finland suggests that an early introduction of fruit, berries and roots associated independently with β-cell autoimmunity

(Virtanen et al., 2006). While a recent study found that higher maternal intake of potatoes in the last trimester of pregnancy was associated with delayed onset of autoimmunity in the offspring (Lamb et al., 2008). Inconsistencies between the studies indicate that additional studies are required, including resolving the question of what aspects of cereals or other solid food items which are involved.

1.2.4 Cod liver oil, vitamin D and omega-3 fatty acids

A Norwegian study found intake of cod liver oil by the mothers during pregnancy or possibly by the child during the first year of life to be associated with lower risk of T1D in the child (Stene et al., 2000), but a subsequent larger study indicated that the child's intake was most important (Stene & Joner, 2003). Other vitamin D supplements were not associated in the Norwegian studies, pointing towards a possible effect of long-chain omega-3 fatty acids. Such fatty acids (e.g. EPA, DHA) have anti-inflammatory effects and potentially preventive effects for T1D (Chase et al., 1979). Results from a case-control study indicated, however, that vitamin D supplementation in early childhood could protect against T1D , and this has also been supported both from an European collaborative study (EURODIAB, 1999) as well as in a prospective study of children born in 1965 in Finland (Hyppönen et al., 2001). The longitudinal, observational study, the Diabetes Study in the Young (DAISY), conducted in Denver, Colorado, between January 1994 and November 2006, suggested that higher consumption of total omega-3 fatty acids, which was reported by a food frequency questionnaire, was associated with a lower risk of autoimmunity in children at increased genetic risk for type 1 diabetes. This association was further sustained by the observation of a higher proportion of omega-3 fatty acids found in the erythrocyte membranes in a subset of the children. Given that fish are a source of both omega-3 fatty acids and vitamin D, vitamin D was initially included in the analysis, but no association was found (Norris et al., 2007). Neither was it support for an effect of marine omega-3 fatty acids analysed separately. Pilot data from the MIDIA study do, however, indicate a protective effect against progression from autoimmunity to development of T1D (unpublished data). Although epidemiological studies can suggest possible associations, randomized clinical trials are necessary to prove a cause and effect. The pilot trial Nutritional Intervention to Prevent (NIP) T1D among babies with high genetic risk was therefore recently initiated (Chase et al., 2009).

1.2.5 Vitamin E

Hypothesising that antioxidants may protect against destruction of β-cells, Finnish researchers measured serum α-tocopherol concentration in frozen sera from 19 cases who developed T1D and in about 60 individually matched controls from a prospective cohort of individuals aged above 20 years (Knekt et al., 1999). Higher α-tocopherol was associated with a significantly lower risk of T1D. Another study from Finland, attempted to replicate this finding in siblings of persons with T1D, and found partial support, although the results were not significant (Uusitalo et al., 2005). Recently both concentration of α- and γ-tocopherol were studied in the Type 1 Diabetes Prediction and Prevention project (DIPP). Although it seemed unlikely that high concentration of α- or γ-tocopherol protect against advanced β–cell autoimmunity in young children, there was a suggestive protective effect of high levels of γ-tocopherol at the age of 1 year on development of autoimmunity, which needs to be replicated (Uusitalo et al., 2008).

1.2.6 Sugar

A Norwegian study shows that children receive from 9% to 24% of their energy from added sugar in the diet, where a major part comes from soft drinks (Øverby et al., 2004). Despite the fact that the increase in intake of simple sugar (in the form of sweets and drinks) in ecological studies correlate with increasing incidence of T1D, only a couple of studies have attempted to investigate this at the individual level. In one study an association between sugar intake and T1D incidence was not found (Dahlquist et al., 1990), but in two more recent studies a correlation was found (Pundziute-Lycka et al., 2004; Benson et al., 2008). Both studies used a case-control design which is likely to suffer from recall bias. Prospective studies with proper registration of dietary habits are therefore needed. The role of diet at different ages in a child's life may also be important.

1.2.7 Overweight

A few studies have observed an association between high birth weight and increased risk of T1D (Stene et al., 2001), although the relation is not very strong, but overweight and obesity are increasing. Gestational diabetes in the mother is a risk factor for a high birth weight and gestational diabetes has increased the last decades. Today a considerable proportion of pregnant women have gestational diabetes. Gestational diabetes may be a consequence of increased body weight in connection with the increased insulin resistance following pregnancies in general. Data from the MIDIA study indicate that both the mothers Body Mass Index (BMI) before getting pregnant as well as high weight gain during pregnancy increase the risk for autoimmunity at an early age for the offspring (Rasmussen et al., 2009). Obesity during childhood is emerging as a possible risk factor for T1D (EURODIAB, 2002; Pundziute-Lycka et al., 2004), but further studies are needed, including to find what particular aspects of body size/obesity (such as inflammatory cytokines or other markers) are most relevant in this relation. Since all the potential relations described above have very important public health implications, the different factors need to be investigated in larger well-designed prospective studies.

1.3 The hygiene hypothesis

The hygiene hypothesis states that the lack of exposure to parasites, symbiotic organisms and infectious agents in early childhood increases the susceptibility to allergic and autoimmune diseases (Zazdanbakhsh et al., 2001). Since humans have evolved coexisting in a shared environment with microbial agents throughout much of our evolutionary history, these agents might be necessary for the development of a balanced and regulated immune system (Stoll, 1947). The decline in non-specific infectious and microbial exposure in many populations is thus proposed to be the cause of the concomitant increase in atopic disorder over the past few decades (Bachlin & Degremont, 1997), and this hypothesis has been extended to autoimmune diseases such as T1D (Kyronseppa, 1993).

1.3.1 The hygiene hypothesis and epidemiology

The hygiene hypothesis is supported by epidemiological studies that show higher prevalence of autoimmune diseases in North America and Europe compared to South America and Africa, higher incidence associated with increased material wealth and higher risk for autoimmune diseases for third world immigrants to the industrialized countries (Herrström et al., 2001). There are also many studies showing that some infections and microbial agents reduce the incidence of autoimmune diabetes in experimental animals

(Blaser, 1998; Malaty, 1994). There are fewer studies in man suggesting protective effect of childhood infections against T1D (Sepp et al., 1997; Samulsson & Ludvigsson, 2003; Horman et al., 2004).

1.3.2 Intestinal parasites

Since immunomodulatory effects of parasites have been reported (Samulsson & Ludvigsson, 2003), and there is evidence that infections protect against the development of allergic disorders, parasites become obvious and major candidates for the hygiene hypothesis. In 1947 it was reported that 40-60% of European children were positive for helminths (Horman et al., 2004), while in recent years only 5-23% are found positive (Strachan, 1989; Jones et al., 2000; Yazdanbakhsh et al., 2002; Cooke, 2009; Bach, 2002; Honeyman, 2005; van der Werf et al., 2007; Gibbon et al., 1997; Parslow et al., 2001; Pundziute-Lycka et al., 2003; Round & Mazmanian, 2009). The most prevalent of the helminths is Enterobius Vermicularis (pinworm) which is usually asymptomatic and each bout is self-limiting since the worms cannot reproduce within the gut. Most common of the water borne parasites are Cryptosporium and Giardia. While the genus Giardia comprises six species, more than 20 variants of Cryptosporium are known (Nygard et al., 2003).

1.3.3 Bacterial colonization and virus infection in the intestines

Another interesting possibility is that the age at infection makes a difference in the pathology. In a similar fashion, it has been shown that colonization of the gut and intestines in early infancy by bacteria plays a role in the development of the adaptive immune system and structural development of the gut (Strachan, 1989). It is well known that due to improved hygiene some viral infections that would normally occur in early life are encountered for the first time at a later stage. For example, mononucleosis is associated with late infection of Epstein-Barr virus (EBV) (Pohl, 2009). Mononucleosis is rare in third world countries. Similarly, hepatitis A and B are less likely to cause disease if exposed to at an early age, and chickenpox (caused by varicella-zoster virus) is more severe in adults. Apparently, late infections typically give rise to a more severe pathology and concomitant increased activation of the immune system. The increased activation of the immune system may dispose for the establishment of an autoimmune condition. This hypothesis would explain the apparent conflict in data indicating that viral infections may confer protection and susceptibility. The MIDIA study offers a unique possibility to test this hypothesis.

1.4 Viral infections as triggers of type 1 diabetes

Viral infections have long been considered as triggers of T1D, and there are several lines of evidence implying virus infections in utero or early life in the aetiology of T1D . The high frequency of T1D in children with congenital rubella syndrome was the first indication of a viral involvement, and hinted towards the importance of the intra-uterine environment (Menser et al., 1978). Intra-uterine rubella infection is now rare in Scandinavia due to vaccination, but the incidence of T1D is high and continues to rise. Mumps and measles were also suspected of playing a role in T1D (Vuorinen et al., 1992), and a plateau in T1D incidence in Finland was also noted after measles, mumps and rubella vaccine was introduced (Hyöty et al., 1993). Measles vaccination was also suggested to be protective in a Swedish study (Dahlquist et al., 1991). Another interesting observation is that acute viral infections can be associated with disease onset (Elfaitouri et al., 2007; Frisk et al., 1992; Osame et al., 2007). There is also a seasonal correlation between periods of viral infections and onset of T1D (Jun & Yoon, 2003; Richer & Horwitz, 2003). Several viruses have been implicated as having an association with T1D, amongst them members of the picornaviridae and other viruses.

1.4.1 Mechanisms proposed for viral triggering of autoimmunity

There is unfortunately limited data on viral infections in young children (and infection load in early life), but there are several proposed mechanisms for how viruses might be associated with T1D. Viruses can activate polyclonal cells and trigger production of autoantibodies (Hiemstra et al., 2001), viruses can directly infect and lyse cells, viral antigens might mimic self-antigens, inflammatory responses stemming from viral infections might trigger autoimmunity (Horwitz et al., 1998), or as predicted in the hygiene hypothesis, viruses might be needed for proper maturation and regulation of the immune response.

1.4.2 Picornavirus

Picornaviruses are small RNA viruses that replicate mainly in the gut, and are spread by the fecal-oral route. The family has several well-known human and animal pathogens, but also many viruses without any known pathology. Human picornaviruses are known to be mostly asymptomatic and are common in infancy, with a prevalence of 10-12% in stool samples for human enterovirus (Cinek et al., 2006), human parechovirus (Tapia et al., 2008) and cardiovirus (Blinkova et al., 2009). The picornaviridae family currently consists of 8 current genera and 4 proposed genera.

The enterovirus genus consists of ten species, with six of them having human hosts (human enteroviruses A-D, rhinovirus A-B). Human enteroviruses are the most promising candidates, with two case-control studies that have shown an association between maternal enterovirus infection during pregnancy or enterovirus infection in children and risk of T1D (Dahlquist et al., 1995; Viskari et al., 2005). There are also studies that showed no association (Richer & Horwitz, 2009). In particular, Coxsackievirus (a member of human enterovirus B) is suspected of having a role in the development of autoimmunity (reviewed in Graves et al., 2003). In addition, enteroviruses have been shown to be more present in the sera (Elfving et al., 2008; Oikarinen et al., 2008), small intestine (Richardson et al., 2009) and pancreatic islets (Harvala & Simmonds, 2009) of recently diagnosed T1D patients (Clements et al., 1995; Andreoletti et al., 1997). A recent study by our group suggest that there is less enterovirus infections among children with high genetic risk for T1D compared with control children, although the difference is not statistically significant due to the low number of children presently tested (Tapia et al., 2011). Moreover, there appear to be a higher prevalence of enterovirus infections during early life in children who do not develop autoimmunity later, suggesting that enteroviral infections confer a protective effect against the development of autoimmunity (Wolthers et al., 2008). The parechovirus genus consists of two species, the murine virus Ljungan virus (LV) and human parechovirus (HPeV). Human parechovirus 1 and 2 have been known since the 1960s, and were originally classified with the enteroviruses as echovirus 22 and 23. Several new parechoviruses have recently been reported, with HPeV3-8 being described from 2004 to 2009 and HPeV9-14 recently announced. They are common in children, uncommon in adults and are present worldwide. Our previous data show that human parechoviruses are present in approximately 12% of stool samples from infants without causing symptoms (Tapia et al., 2008). There are, however, studies linking them to several serious conditions. Our most recent case-control study shows no difference in positivity for human parechovirus infections in stool samples (Tapia et al., 2010). Ljungan virus has earlier been shown to cause diabetes-like condition in rodents (Niklasson et al., 2006), but was not identified in samples from children in our studies (Tapia et al., 2008, Tapia et al., 2010). HPeV1 has been reported to show no association with T1D (Tauriainen et al., 2007), but there is no data on the other types of HPeVs. However, sequencing should be done to see if there is any difference in strains, and to test for all the new human Parechoviruses. Human parechoviruses seem to be asymptomatic, common viruses in childhood, and data on their epidemiology (and of other common asymptomatic viruses) will be used to test the hygiene hypothesis.

1.4.3 Cardiovirus

The genus Cardiovirus consists of 2 species, encephalomyocarditis virus and theliovirus (Liang et al., 2008). Until recently only rodent cardioviruses have been known. Encephalomyocarditis virus has been shown to induce diabetes in mice, and thelioviruses have been associated with myocarditis, and MS like symptoms in mice (Chiu et al., 2008). Recently, human thelioviruses, termed Saffold virus 1-8, have been discovered (Drexler et al., 2008). There is little known about them, but a serological study shows that SAFV3 are ubiquitous and cause infection early in life (Zoll et al., 2009), but are apparently asymptomatic. Being a recently discovered virus, only a few studies have detected it with molecular methods (Abed & Boivin, 2008; Jones et al., 2007; Day, 2009; Coulson et al., 2002), so making assumptions about its epidemiology may be premature. Being in the picornaviridae family, and being closely related to rodent pathogens suggest they might be unknown human pathogens, and they should be studied both to get a clear picture of infections in early childhood and if there is any association with T1D in humans. The MIDIA study offers an excellent opportunity to study these viruses.

1.4.4 Reovirus

The family reovirus consists of six genera. Two of these genera, rotavirus and reovirus, have been shown to infect β-cells, and are of interest to the project. They are double-stranded RNA viruses, also known to be common and ubiquitous (Honeyman et al., 1998). Rotaviruses are the single most important cause of severe diarrheal illness in infancy in both the developed and undeveloped world. They are spread through the fecal-oral route. Studies in mice have shown infection of β-cells (Comins et al., 2008) indicating molecular mimicry (Toniolo et al., 1980). These viruses are being studied by a post doc. in the MIDIA project, and we will pool our data to study the infections in childhood.

The name reovirus is a derivation of respiratory enteric orphan viruses, acknowledging that they can infect the respiratory and gastrointestinal system, but are not associated with any known disease (Wetzel et al., 2006). They are generally regarded as benign, but have also been associated with symptoms. In mice, they have been shown to infect β-cells, but have also been shown to delay overt diabetes in mice. Screening longitudinally collected stool samples for these viruses will show whether they are associated with any disease in human infants, and also be used to test the hygiene hypothesis.

1.4.5 Other viruses

Our results show that infections in early life are much more prevalent and asymptomatic than previously known, but also highlight the need for more studies on viral infections in children. There are several viruses that are considered common in childhood that should be studied to test the hygiene hypothesis, and viruses that have been implicated with T1D, or human strains of animal viruses associated with T1D, should be studied. In addition, newly discovered viruses will also be evaluated as candidates for testing. However, these viruses will have a lower priority than the candidates listed above.

1.5 Psychosocial effects of risk information

We are all born with variants in our genes which make us susceptible to diseases. With the developments in biotechnology and increasing knowledge about the relation between genes and diseases, we are faced with both new opportunities and new dilemmas. The use of tests that provide knowledge about risks and possibilities for illness in the future raises many fundamental questions of ethical, legal and psychosocial character.

1.5.1 Cohort studies giving risk information

In the MIDIA study parents were informed about that their child had the high-risk genotype for T1D (babies carrying HLA-DRB1*03-DQA1*05-DQB1*02/ DRB1*04:01-DQA1*03-DQB1*0302) or not. 2.1% of Norwegian newborns carry the high-risk genotype, and this group represents approximately 34% of future cases of T1D. Children with the high-risk genotype have 7% risk for getting T1D before 15 years of age and a lifetime risk at 20% (Rønningen et al., 1991; Undlien et al., 1997; Joner & Søvik, 1982, 1989; Mølbak et al., 1994). Several other studies have used predictive genetic testing of newborns as a strategy to solve research questions about environmental factors contributing to T1D, including BABYDIAB in Germany (Ziegler et al.; 2011, Schatz et al.; 2000), DIPP in Finland (Kimpimaki et al.; 2001), PANDA in Florida (Carmichael et al., 2003, Krischer, 2007), DiPiS in Sweden (Lernmark et al., 2004), DAISY in Colorado (Rewers et al., 1996), and the multinational TEDDY study in the USA and Europe (Kiviniemi et al.; 2007, TEDDY study group; 2008). The main advantage for study participants identified as having increased risk for T1D is the possibility of early detection of the destruction of the insulin producing cells by autoantibodies, resulting in a milder disease onset having parents who are prepared in advance for the possibility of T1D onset, and therefore will handle the new life situation with a child with T1D better than other parents. In addition children with known increased genetic risk for T1D who also have developed autoantibodies will be the first to participate in intervention studies when possible preventive get available. However, there may be disadvantages of living with the knowledge of an increased susceptibility to a disease with no prevention. Thus, even though predictive testing is highly acknowledged as a valuable research method per se, the predictive testing has given rise to concerned debate.

1.5.2 Particular aspects for the Norwegian MIDIA and MoBa studies

With the widespread and increasing use of genetic tests, assessing the adverse effects of information about susceptibility genes for disease on the tested subject is important. The MIDIA study aimed to estimate the effect on maternal mental health from receiving genetic risk information about their newborns. Outcome measurements were maternal self-reported scores of anxiety and depression symptoms, satisfactory with life, self-esteem, and serious worry about their child. A number of previous studies (Hood et al., 2005; Johnson et al., 2004; Kerrush et al., 2007) have examined maternal reactions after being informed about their children having elevated genetic risk for T1D. None of these studies have shown a significant effect on symptoms of anxiety or other mental health disorders as result of the testing, though a few mothers did seem to react strongly. Previous studies were conducted in a setting in which the mothers were asked questions about it in connection with the genetic testing project. The MIDIA study was designed differently. When completing the questionnaire the mothers were not aware that their answers were going to be used for any particular comparisons, though they were rightfully informed that the personal data would be used for multiple research purposes. Thus, our results were not affected by reporting bias associated with maternal attitudes towards genetic risk information or other factors motivating to under- or over-report poor mental health. Since 50% of mothers who got their child tested for genetic high-risk for T1D also participated in the Norwegian Mother and Child Cohort (MoBa) study, all data used came from MoBa. In MoBa data was available both from the 30th week of pregnancy and when the child was 6 months of age. These data therefore permit to answer the main question to what extent receiving information about a young child having high risk for T1D changes maternal well being and health.

2. Material and methods

2.1 Research design and subjects

The MIDIA study is a longitudinal cohort study with inclusion of children with the high-risk HLA genotype (DRB1*04:01-DQA1*03-DQB1*03:02/DRB1*03-DQA1*05-DQB1*02), with follow-up from three months of age up to 15 years of age. Recruitment to MIDIA started in small scale in the summer of 2001, covered the whole country of Norway from March 2006 (60,000 births per year) and was stopped in December 2007 since it was suddenly found to be against the Norwegian Biotechnology Law. Both approvals from the Regional Medical Committee and the Norwegian Data Inspectorate had been given before recruitment to MIDIA started. In December 2007 close to 48,000 children were recruited to MIDIA. Of those 1,047 were identified with the high-risk genotype. Approval from the government was given for further follow-up of those already identified with the high-risk genotype. At the end of March 2011, 19 of these children had got Type 1 Diabetes, 33 were confirmed positive for two or three autoantibodies and 24 for one. A total of 4,829 blood samples, 18,275 stool samples and 4,412 questionnaires are presently available for analysis in the cohort.
A questionnaire summarizing weekly diaries was filled out at 3, 6, 9 and 12 months of age. Blood samples were taken at the same intervals. After this period, a questionnaire and a blood sample are asked for annually (Stene et al., 2007). For more information on MIDIA, see www.fhi.no/midia. In The Norwegian Mother and Child Cohort Study (MoBa), questionnaires have been asked for at 17th, 22nd and 30th week of pregnancy, and when the child is 6 and 18 months old as well as then the child get 3, 5, 7 years of age (Magnus et al., 2006) . Blood samples were asked for at 17th week of pregnancy and at the time of delivery from the mother and cord blood was taken from the baby (Rønningen et al., 2006). For more information on MoBa, see www.fhi.no/morogbarn.

2.2 Outcome measurements

The incoming blood samples in the MIDIA study are immediately tested at the Hormone Laboratory, Aker Hospital, for diabetes associated autoantibodies as marker of β-cell autoimmunity, autoantibodies against insulin, anti-glutamic acid decarboxylase (GAD), and against the protein tyrosine kinase related protein IA-2 (Petersen et al., 1994; Bingley et al., 2001). High titres of one autoantibody or titres above the cut-off for two or three autoantibodies on at least two consecutive time periods (3-6 months apart) is defined as islet autoimmunity for the purpose of data analysis, and will be used as the first outcome (optimal cut-off values for the autoantibodies has been defined after participation by the Hormone laboratory in international autoantibody standardisation workshops; DASPs). Clinical diagnosis of T1D will also be used as outcome, and analysis will be performed when a sufficient number of children have developed either autoimmunity or T1D.

2.3 Measurement of nutrition-related factors ("exposures")

2.3.1 Questionnaires

A questionnaire summarising weekly diaries were filled out when the children were 3, 6, 9 and 12 months old, and annually thereafter. The questionnaires include for examples detailed information about dietary habits of the mother and the child (detailed information about diet for the mother as long as she breast-fed and intake of specific food items, etc.). Since few studies have been conducted on children's diet in Norway, new dietary questions had to be developed for both the MIDIA and the MoBa study. Validation of various aspects of dietary habits of pregnant women has recently been undertaken within the MoBa study. Blood samples and questionnaires from MIDIA can be used to assess validity of relevant information in childhood (Brantsæter et al., 2007a, 2007b, 2008, 2009; Willett, 1998; Serdula et al., 2001).

2.3.2 Biomarkers: Fatty acids, vitamin D and E

The distribution of fatty acids in the plasma phospholipid fraction as well as Vit D and Vit E will be analyzed in plasma samples from the same aliquots at a commercial laboratory in Oslo (AS Vitas; http://www.vitas.no/) using solid phase extraction and gas chromatography.

2.4 Measurement of exposure to virus (viral infections)

2.4.1 Real-time PCR

The real-time PCR have been run on ABI7300 real times machines according to earlier publications (Cinek et al., 2006). Primers were first designed for main type of virus and thereafter for subtypes (serotypes) and optimalisation was performed for each of the reactions.

2.4.2 Sequencing

Sequencing for enterovirus, picornavirus and E.coli as well as other bacterial species will be done as earlier published (Tapia et al., 2011; Witsø et al., 2006, 2007; Muinck et al., 2011). Deep sequencing will be performed on at 454 machines at the Centre for Ethological and Evolutional Sciences (CEES), Institute of Biology, University of Oslo according to the manufacture instructions.

2.4.3 Questionnaires

Data from questionnaires will be used to test association between viral RNA/DNA in stool and symptoms reported by the parents (coughing, diarrhea, vomiting), and will be used to search for risk factors of viral infection, such as breastfeeding, number of siblings and socioeconomic status.

2.5 Identification of eggs from enterobius vermicularis

Parents of children participating in MIDIA have been asked to collect tape samples touching the anal region on three following mornings. They have then sent the samples in specially designed containers for tape sampling to the central laboratory in Oslo. Here all the tape samples have been examined by two scientists at different times. A child has been regarded as positive if down to one egg have been identified on one of the tapes.

3. Results

3.1 Psychosocial effects of risk information

3.1.1 Effects of genetic risk information on mental health variables among MIDIA mothers

In the study of mothers who had participated in both MIDIA and MoBa (N=166 for those having a child with high genetic risk for T1D and N=7,224 for those who had been told that their child did not have the high-risk genotype) there were no sosiodemographic characteristics differences between those who had got the risk-information and those who had let their child be genotyped in MIDIA, but had been told that their child did not carry the high-risk genotype. Information on genetic risk in newborns was found to have no significant impact on maternal symptoms of anxiety and depression, self-esteem, satisfaction with life, or serious worry about their child. Mental health before birth was strongly associated with mental health after birth, see Table 1. Maternal symptoms of anxiety and depression were assed using a short version of SCL-25, including 4 question for anxiety and 4 for depression (Aas et al., 2010). The five-item Satisfaction With Life (SWLS) was developed to measure the cognitive component of subjective well-being. The short-form of the Rosenberg Self-Esteem Scale (RSES) used in the MoBa study includes four items. Maternal worry about their child was one of the items in an 11-item checklist of life events experienced during the last year, given in the 6 month questionnaire. The question was phased "Have you been serious worried that there is something wrong with your child?" Responses were coded as "yes" or "no". A dichotous variable was constructed to indicate the presence of maternal T1D. The variable was based on health questions from both The Medical Birth Registry of Norway (MBRN) and the MoBa questionnaires. The results from the linear regression analyses of the association between genetic risk information and change in maternal mental health are shown as unstandardized (B) and standard (β) coefficients in Table 1. The upper part of the table shows the results from the regression analysis with symptoms of anxiety and depression (SCL) as the dependent variable. The estimated regression coefficient (B=-0.001, p=0.95) for child's genetic risk indicate no effect of genetic information on changes in maternal mental health from baseline to post-disclosure. The maternal T1D status had neither any effect (B=0.040, p=0.409). However, as expected, the baseline anxiety/depression score was strongly associated with post-disclosure scores (B=0.536, p<0.001).

3.1.2 How often do parents think on that they have a child with high genetic risk for T1D

Although 5% of mothers and 2% of fathers did think of their child's high genetic risk for T1D when they filled out the 3 month questionnaire, usually just 2 week after they had got the information, very few parents continued to think often about their child's high genetic risk for T1D. To answer the questionnaire with the same questions each time needs that you sometimes think about having a high-risk child for T1D, see Figure 1 and 2.

Effects of maternal diabetes and genetic risk information on mental health variables	B (95% CI)	*β*	*p*	Adjusted R^2
Symptoms of anxiety and depression				
Child's genetic risk	-0.001 (-0.047 - 0.044)	-0.001	0.953	
Maternal type 1 diabetes	0.040 (-0.055 - 0.135)	0.008	0.409	
Baseline anxiety/depression	0.536 (0.517 - 0.555)	0.544	< 0.001	
				0.296
Self esteem				
Child's genetic risk	0.037 (-0.022 - 0.097)	0.011	0.218	
Maternal type 1 diabetes	-0.040 (-0.164 - 0.083)	-0.006	0.521	
Baseline self esteem	0.682 (0.664 - 0.700)	0.651	< 0.001	
				0.423
Satisfaction with life scale				
Child's genetic risk	-0.080 (-0.198 - 0.039)	-0.013	0.187	
Maternal type 1 diabetes	0.016 (-0.231 - 0.263)	0.001	0.902	
Baseline SWLS	0.609 (0.590 - 0.628)	0.587	< 0.001	
				0.345

Table 1.

3.2 Nutrition-related factors

Cohort design was used for assessing whether BMI before pregnancy and weight gain during pregnancy predicted the risk of islet autoimmunity in 885 children who were followed with serial blood samples and questionnaires. 36 of the children developed autoimmunity, of whom 10 developed Type 1 Diabetes. Both maternal BMI before pregnancy and weight gain < or = 15 kg predicted increased risk for islet autoimmunity, significant hazard ratio at 2.5 for both situations (Rasmussen et al., 2009).

3.3 Virus in stool samples

Among 911 children, were stool samples were available, 27 had developed autoimmunity in two or more consecutive samples (case children) in December 2008. In the pilot study based on these cases two control children per case were matched by follow-up time, day of birth, and county of residence. The frequency of human enterovirus RNA in stool samples from cases before seroconversion (43 of 339, 12.7%) did not differ from the frequency in control subjects (94 of 692, 13.2%) (Tapia et al., 2011a). There was neither any difference in the prevalence of human parechovirus when cases and controls were compared: 13.0% and 11.1%, respectively (Tapia et al., 2011b). None of the 3,803 samples analysed were positive for rodent parechovirus-Ljungan virus (Tapia et al., 2008, Tapia et al., 2010). Indicating that Ljungan virus is rare among Norwegian children, and in contract to what have been reported earlier does not seem to be involved in T1D susceptibility.

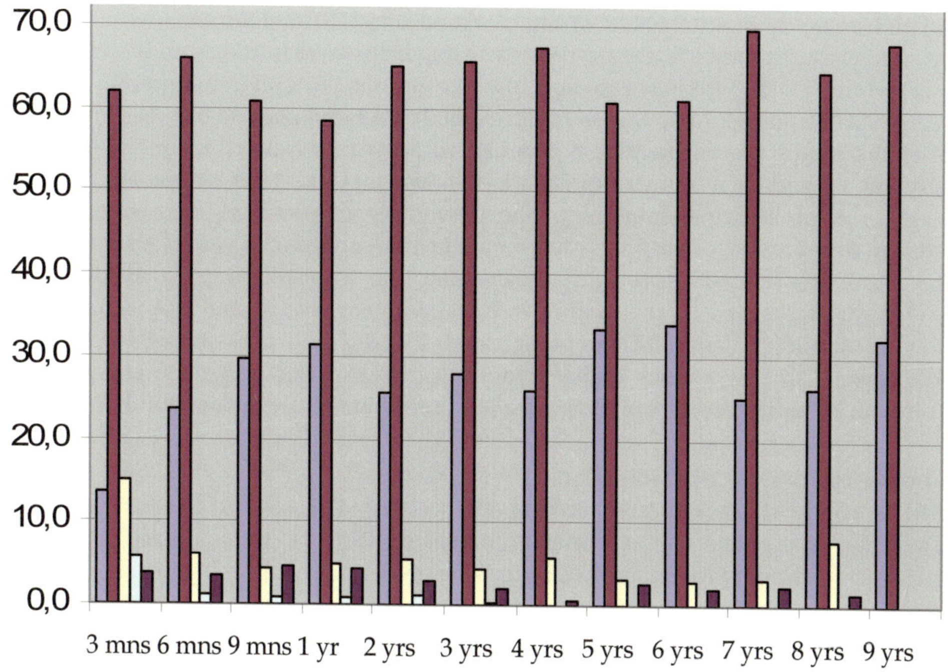

Fig. 1. Mothers thoughts about having a child with high genetic risk of T1D

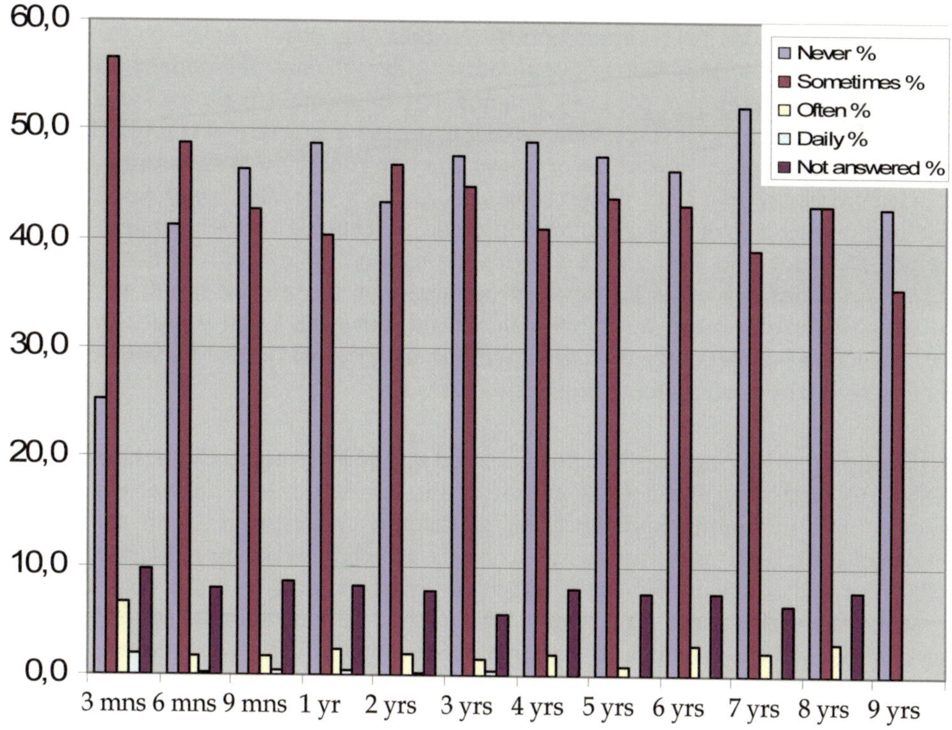

Fig. 2. Fathers thoughts about having a child with high genetic risk of T1D

3.4 The frequency of enterobius vermicularis among MIDIA children

During the last generation T1D has shown a strong increase in incidence in the Western part of the world. During the same period also the number of children suffering of allergic diseases has increased. In countries in Africa both T1D and allergic diseases are rare. The aim of this study was to examine if this had to do with the decrease in children having enterobius vermicularis (pinworm). Data has shown that intestinal worms are involved in development of intestinal immunity. The prevalence of pinworm has decreased in all European countries. While 40-60% was infected in 1947, only 5-23% has been shown positive in recent reports (Herrström et al., 1997). In MIDIA all who still participated in the project (N=943), was in the period January-June in 2010 invited to send in anal tape samples taken 3 following mornings. Of the 397 who participated, 18% did have pinworm egg on at least one of the tapes. This was a much higher frequency than expected, but more analysis will be performed, including analysis of the particular questionnaires developed for this project.

3.5 Lower respiratory tract infections

A MIDIA cohort study was most recently able to study 42 cases and 843 non-cases, which showed that self-reported "pneumonia, bronchitis or RS-virus" gave a hazard ration at 3.5, p=0.001 for developing for islet autoimmunity before 4 years of age.

4. Discussion

4.1 Data from the MIDIA project

The first nested case-control study in MIDIA on intestinal virus as triggers for Type 1 Diabetes did not support the hypothesis that faecal shedding of enteroviral RNA is a major predictor of advanced islet autoimmunity. Neither was there any association between human parechovirus and islet autoimmunity. Although also the rodent parechovirus, Ljungan virus, has been proposed as a potential environmental trigger for Type 1 Diabetes, the results from the MIDIA study indicate that Ljungan virus is rare in young children since it was not found neither in controls or cases. The two cohort studies performed in MIDIA do, however, show that both maternal weight and self reported lower respiratory tract infections predict risk of islet autoimmunity, and particularly in the youngest age group. The MIDIA study did not find any evidence supporting the notion that genetic risk information about newborns has a negative impact on the mental health of Norwegian mothers. All recruitment to the MIDIA study had, however, to be stopped in December 2007. The following part of the discussion will focus on the reason and the consequences for further research on environmental triggers of T1D.

4.1.1 Stopping of an ongoing T1D study based on the Norwegian Biotechnology Law

The MIDIA study had the needed approvals for research studies in Norway (from the Regional Ethic Committee and the Data Inspectorate) before recruitment started in the summer of 2001. Since all recruitment was based on special teaching of Norwegian public health care nurses given by the principal investigator and a study coordinator, the recruitment started in small scale. Most of the public health care nurses in Norway started after they had got the needed information and education to voluntary recruit to MIDIA as well as being responsible for most of the blood samples taken. From 2006 the recruitment covered the whole country. In June 2007, one of the mothers of a participating baby was, however, interviewed in the biggest newspaper in Norway. She here complained about not haven received good enough information about MIDIA before she and her husband had consented to participate. The Directorate for Health and Social Affairs then immediately decided that recruitment to MIDIA had to be stopped. Some days later it was, however, decided that new evaluation of the project had to take place according to the Norwegian Biotechnology Law, which tells that genotyping of children under the age of 18 years can only take place if there are a clear health benefit for a certain disease to get knowledge about genetics. During the fall of 2007 both the Biotechnology Board, the Ethical Committee for the Norwegian Medical Association, the National Committee for Medical Ethics as well as several experts contacted by the Directorate of Social and Health Affairs evaluated the MIDIA project. All these boards had earlier evaluated the MIDIA study; e.g. during the time of recruitment to the study. In addition the Health Department had clearly told that children who also had developed autoantibodies in MIDIA could get health insurance. The last aspect was based on the Biotechnology Law, which Norway has had since 1994, where it is clearly told that genetic risk for a disease cannot be used by the health insurance companies. The Directorate of Social and Health Affairs found, however, genotyping in MIDIA illegal December 10, 2007. A few days after the Norwegian Data Inspectorate said in newspapers that all data already collected from participants in MIDIA had to be thrown away. All ended luckily up with voting in the Norwegian Parliament in June 2008. As long as the Medical Regional Committee and the Norwegian Data Inspectorate approved the MIDIA study ones more, and all parents of children who already had been identified as high-risk children, gave a new informed consent , research in MIDIA could continue. In this respect Norway is different from Sweden, Finland, Germany and five states in USA were no similar Biotechnology Law Has given problems with genotyping of 350,000 children for the TEDDY study.

4.1.2 Ethics and data protection in human biomarker studies

The Norwegian Biotechnology Law tells: "Genetic testing of a child under the age of 18 years is not allowed if circumstances cannot be detected that can reduce or prevent health disadvantages for the child." Since the law came in 1994 it had only counted for clinical practice, the MIDIA project had been run for 6 ½ year before it was stopped December 10, 2007. In the work performed before the law got in use, science was never mentioned. Important questions in this context are:

1. Do important scientific T1D projects involving genotyping of children have to be performed elsewhere in the word? Should not Norway as one of the riches countries in the word has a certain responsibility?
2. Are not the parents able to give informed consent of behalf of their child?
3. How should health benefit be defined?
4. Is it not so that if clear health benefit has been shown, it is no longer research but part of general recommendation for public health or part of the health care system?

The year after recruitment to MIDIA was stopped funding was given from the Norwegian Research Council to the study "Nutritional Intervention to Prevent Type 1 Diabetes". The project was based on that the incidence of T1D is increasing, particularly in very young children. The hypothesis was that the Decrease of omega-3 fatty acids in the diet has contributed to this increase. One case-control study from Norway reported that children with T1D less often than the control children had a mother who had taken cod liver oil during pregnancy, while a newer study from Norway indicated a protective effect of cod liver oil during infancy (Stene et al., 2000; Stene & Joner, 2003). In the longitudinal, observational study, the Diabetes Autoimmunity Study in the Young (DAISY), conducted in

Denver, Colorado, between January 1994 and November 2006, 1770 children at increased genetic risk were followed. Islet autoimmunity was assessed in association with reported daily intake of polyunsaturated fatty acids. The data strongly indicated that dietary intake of omega-3 fatty acids is associated with reduced risk for autoimmunity in children at increased risk for T1D (Norris et al., 2007). We therefore proposed to conduct a prospective double blinded dietary intervention trial using high dosage of the omega-3 fatty acid DHA or "placebo" (containing the same amount of DHA found in the recommended daily dosage of cod liver oil). The reason for choosing 1,8 g DHA daily was to be able to be included in a multi-centre study since a pilot study in USA already have been performed as a feasibility study using exactly this dosage. But in USA they use plant oil as placebo (Chase et al, 2009). In Norway this cannot be given since mother of babies in Norway get recommended from their public health care nurse to give cod liver oil. But they are told to start with one tea spoon and to increase the daily intake to 5 ml within the child is 6 months. But at this stage babies start spotting. Indeed very few parents continue to give their infant cod liver oil. The Directorate for Health decided, however, that "Nutritional Intervention to Prevent Type 1 Diabetes" was illegal, and could therefore never be started based on the Norwegian Biotechnology Law.

4.1.3 Need for trans-national studies

Most recently two big NIH funded studies are going on. In the Type 1 Diabetes Genomics Consortium forces worldwide have been working together. All genotyping has been based on linkage studies (two siblings with Type 1 diabetes and parents without the disease is needed). Getting all who earlier was competing in identifying new T1D susceptibility genes to collaborate gave access to all available multiplex families. All genes that earlier was indicated to be of importance for T1D were confirmed, and 40 genes conferring susceptibility to T1D has now been identified (Barrett et al, 2009). In addition genome wide association studies have been performed by the same group (Welcome Trust Case Control Consortium, 2010).

In TEDDY (The Environmental Determinants for Type 1 Diabetes in the Young), another NIH funded study, centres in Denver, Colorado, Seattle, Washington, parts of Georgia and Florida, parts of Finland, Sweden and Germany have recruited and genotyped 350,000 new-borns and inform the parents about the high genetic risk. The protocol is the same everywhere, and all collected samples are sent to the coordinating centre in Florida. The follow-up is more intense than in MIDIA. Here all who participate, both scientists and parents know that it is an observational study where any intervention never can be given. The children Will be followed-up for 15 years.

5. Conclusions

The first nested case-control study in MIDIA on intestinal virus as triggers for Type 1 Diabetes did not support the hypothesis that faecal shedding of enteroviral RNA is a major predictor of advanced islet autoimmunity. Neither was there any association between human parechovirus and islet autoimmunity. Although also the rodent parechovirus, Ljungan virus, has been proposed as a potential environmental factor for Type 1 Diabetes, the results from the MIDIA study indicate that Ljungan virus is rare in young children since it was not found neither in controls or cases. The two cohort studies performed in MIDIA do, however, show that both maternal weight and self reported lower respiratory tract infections predict risk of islet autoimmunity, and particularly in the youngest age group. The MIDIA study did not find any evidence supporting the notion that genetic risk information about newborns has a negative impact on the mental health of Norwegian Mothers. Recruitment to MIDIA was stopped based on the Norwegian Biotechnology Law. It is therefore needed to extend international collaboration to identify the environmental triggers of type 1 diabetes. With the estimated increase of children with 50% having Type 1 Diabetes in 2020, and that the increase will be highest among children younger than 5 years (increase in prevalence with 70%) it is really important to extend collaborative efforts.

6. Acknowledgement

The MIDIA study was funded by the Norwegian Research Council (grants 135893/330, 155300/320, 156477/730, 166515/V50), The Norwegian Organisational for Help and Rehabilitation (EkstraStiftelsen), Norwegian Diabetes Association, New Generis (EU Grant Food-CT-2005-016320). The Norwegian Mother and Child Cohort Study Was supported by the Norwegian Ministry of Health, NIH-NIEHS (grant no. N01-ES-85433), NIH-NINDS (grant no. 1 UO1 NS 047537-01), and the Norwegian Research Council/FUGE (grant no. 151918/S10). I am very grateful for all the help I got from Trond Rasmussen in writing this book chapter.

7. References

Abed, Y. & Boivin, G. (2008). New Saffold cardioviruses in 3 children, Canada. *Emerg Infect Dis*, 14, 834-6.

Andreoletti, L. et al. (1997). Detection of coxsackie B virus RNA sequences in whole blood samples from adult patients at the onset of type I diabetes mellitus. *J Med Virol*, 52, 121-7.

Bach, J. F. (2002). The effect of infections on susceptibility to autoimmune and allergic diseases. *N Engl J Med*, 347, 911-20.

Bachlin A, Degremont A. (1997). Pinworm infection in kindergartens of Basel. *Schweiz Rundsch med Prax*,11, 1183-1185.

Barrett JC, Clayton DG, Concannon P, Akolkar B, Cooper JD et al. (2009). Genome-wide associationstudy and meta-analysis find over 40 loci affect risk of type 1 diabetes. *Nat Genet*, 41, 703-707.

Benson VS, Vanleeuwen Ja, Taylor J, McKinney PA, Van Til l. (2008). Food consumption and the risk of type 1 diabetes in children and youth: a population-based, case-control study in Prince Edward Island, Canada. *J Am Coll Nutr*, 27, 414-20.

Bingley PJ, Bonifacio E, Ziegler AG, Schatz DA, Atkinson MA, Eisenbarth GS. (2001). Proposed guidelines on screening for risk of type 1 diabetes. *Diabetes Carc*, 24, 398.

Blaser MJ. (1998). Helicobacters are indigenous to the human stomac; duodenal ulceration is due to changes in gastric microecology in modern era. *Gut*, 43, 721-727.

Blinkova, O. et al. (2009). Cardioviruses are genetically diverse and cause common enteric infections in South Asian children. *J Virol*, 83, 4631-41

Brantsæter AL, Haugen M, Rasmussen S, Alexander J, Samuelsen SO, Meltzer HM. (2007a). Urinary flavonoids and plasma carotenoids in the validation of fruit, vegetable and tea intake during pregnancy in the Norwegian Mother and Child Cohort Study (MoBa). *Public Health Nutrition*, 10, 274-283.

Brantsæter AL, Haugen M, Hagve T-A, Aksnes, Rasmussen SA, Julshamn K, Alexander J, Meltzer. HM. (2007b). Self-reported dietary supplement use is confirmed by biological markers in the Norwegian Mother and Child Cohort Study. *Ann Nutr Metab*, 51, 146-154.

Brantsæter AL, Haugen M, Alexander J, Meltzer HM. (2008). Validity of a new Food frequency questionnaire for pregnant women in the Norwegian Mother and Child Cohort Study. *Maternal and Child Nutrition*, 4, 14-27.

Brantsæter AL, Haugen M, Julshamn K, Alexander J, Meltzer HM. (2009). Evaluation of urinary iodine excretion as a biomarker for intake of milk and dairy products in pregnant women in the Norwegian Mother and Child Cohort Study (MoBa). *Eur J Clin Nutr*, 63, 347-54.

Carmichael SK, Johnson SB, Baughcum et al. (2003). Prospective assessment in newborns of diabetes autoimmunity (PANDA): Maternal understanding of infant diabetes risk. *Genetic in Medicine* 5, 77-83.

Chase HP, Williams RL, Dupont J. (1979). Increased prostaglandin synthesis in childhood diabetes mellitus. *J Pediatr*, 94, 185-9.

Chase HP, Lescheck E, Rafkin-Mervis L, Krause-Steinrauf H, Chritton S, Asare SM, Adams S, Skyler JS, Clare-Salzler M, And the Type 1 Diabetes TrialNet NIP Study Group. (2009). Nutritional Intervention to Prevent (NIP) Type 1 Diabetes. A Pilot Trial. ICAV: Infant, Child, & Adolescent Nutrition, E (Pub), 10.1177/1941406409333466, April 14, 98-107.

Chiu, C. Y. et al. (2008). Identification of cardioviruses related to Theiler's murine encephalomyelitis virus in human infections. *Proc Natl Acad Sci U S A*, 105, 14124-9.

Cinek O, Wilkinson E, Paltiel L, Saugstad OD, Magnus P, Rønningen KS. (2000). Screening for the IDDM high-risk genotype. A rapid microtitre plate method using serum as source of DNA. *Tissue Antigens*, 56, 344-9.

Cinek O, Witsø E, Jeansson S, Rasmussen T, Drevinek P, Wetlesen T, Vavrinec J, Grinde B, Rønningen KS. (2006). Longitudinal observation of enterovirus and adenovirus in stool samples from Norwegian infants with the highest genetic risk of type 1 diabetes. *J Clin Virol*, 35(1), 33-40.

Clements, G. B., Galbraith, D. N. & Taylor, K. W. (1995). Coxsackie B virus infection and onset of childhood diabetes. *Lancet*, 346, 221-3.

Comins, C. et al. (2008). Reovirus: viral therapy for cancer 'as nature intended'. *Clin Oncol (R Coll Radiol)* 20, 548-54.

Cooke, A. (2009). Infection and autoimmunity. *Blood Cells Mol Dis*, 42, 105-7.

Coulson, B. S. et al. (2002). Growth of rotaviruses in primary pancreatic cells. *J Virol*, 76, 9537-44.

Dahlquist GG, Blom LG, Persson LA, Sandström AI, Wall SG. (1990). Dietary factors and the risk of developing insulin dependent diabetes in childhood. *BMJ*, 300, 1302-6.

Dahlquist, GG., Blom, L., Lönnberg, G. (1991). The Swedish Childhood Diabetes Study-a multivariate analysis of risk determinants for diabetes in different age groups. *Diabetologia*, 34, 757-62

Dahlquist GG, Ivarsson S, Lindberg B, Forsgren M. (1995). Maternal enteroviral infection during pregnancy as a risk factor for childhood IDDM. A population-based case-control study. *Diabetes*, 44, 408-13.

Day, J. M. (2009). The diversity of the orthoreoviruses: molecular taxonomy and phylogentic divides. *Infect Genet Evol*, 9, 390-400.

Drexler, J. F. et al. (2008). Circulation of 3 lineages of a novel Saffold cardiovirus in humans. *Emerg Infect Dis*, 14, 1398-405.

Eizirik S, Freyer J, Siewert C Baron U, Olek S et al. (2009). The role of inflammation in insulitis and β-cell loss in type 1 diabetes. *Natr Rev Endocrinol*, 219-26.

Elfaitouri, A. et al. (2007). Recent enterovirus infection in type 1 diabetes: evidence with a novel IgM method. *J Med Virol*, 79, 1861-7.

Elfving, M. et al. (2008). Maternal enterovirus infection during pregnancy as a risk factor in offspring diagnosed with type 1 diabetes between 15 and 30 years of age. *Exp Diabetes Res*, 2008, 271958.

EURODIAB Substudy 2 Study Group. (1999). Vitamin D supplement in early childhood and risk for type 1 (insulin-dependent) diabetes mellitus. *Diabetologia*, 42, 51-4.

EURODIAB Substudy 2 Study Group. (2002). Rapid early growth is associated with increased risk of childhood type 1 diabetes in various European populations. *Diabetes Care*, 25, 1755-60.

Fourlanos S, Varney MD, Tait BD, Morrahan, Honeyman MC. (2008). The rising incidence of type 1 diabetes is accounted for by cases with lower-risk human leukocyte antigen genotypes. *Diabetes Care*, 31, 1546-9.

Frisk, G., Friman, G., Tuvemo, T., Fohlman, J. & Diderholm, H. (1992). Coxsackie B virus IgM in children at onset of type 1 (insulin-dependent) diabetes mellitus: evidence for IgM induction by a recent or current infection. *Diabetologia*, 35, 249-53.

Gibbon, C., Smith, T., Egger, P., Betts, P. & Phillips, D. (1997). Early infection and subsequent insulin dependent diabetes. *Arch Dis Child*, 77, 384-5.

Gillespie KM, Bain SC, Barnett AH, Bingley PJ, Christie MR et al. (2004). The rising incidence of childhood type 1 diabetes and reduced contribution of high-risk HLA haplotypes. *Lancet*, 364, 1699-1700.

Graves, P. M. et al. (2003). Prospective study of enteroviral infections and development of β-cell autoimmunity. Diabetes autoimmunity study in the young (DAISY). *Diabetes Res Clin Pract*, 59, 51-61.

Harvala, H. & Simmonds, P. (2009). Human parechoviruses: biology, epidemiology and clinical significance. *J Clin Virol*, 45, 1-9.

Herrström P, Friström A, Karlsson A, Högstedt B. (1997). Enterobius vermicularis and finger sucking in young Swedish children. *Scand J Prim Health Care*, 15(3), 146-8.

Herrström P, Henricson KA, Raberg A, Karlsson A, Hogstedt B. (2001). Allergic disease and the infestation of Enterobius vermicularis in Swedish chldren 4-10 years of age. *J Investg Allergol Clin Immunol*, 11, 157-160.

Hiemstra, H. S. et al. (2001). Cytomegalovirus in autoimmunity: T cell crossreactivity to viral antigen and autoantigen glutamic acid decarboxylase. *Proc Natl Acad Sci U S A*, 98, 3988-91.

Hilner, J.E., Perdue L.H., Sides E.G., Pierces J.J., Wagner A.M. et al. (2010). Designing and implementing samples and data collection for an international genetic study: the Type 1 Diabetes Genetic Consortium (T1DGC). *Clin Trials*, 7, S5-32.

Honeyman, M. C., Stone, N. L. & Harrison, L. C. (1998). T-cell epitopes in type 1 diabetes autoantigen tyrosine phosphatase IA-2: potential for mimicry with rotavirus and other environmental agents. *Mol Med*, 4, 231-9.

Honeyman, M. (2005). How robust is the evidence for viruses in the induction of type 1 diabetes? *Curr Opin Immunol* 17, 616-23.

Hood KK, Johnsen SB, Carmicael SK et al. (2005). Depressive symptoms in mothers of infants identified as genetically at risk for type 1 diabetes. *Diabetes Care*, 28, 1898-1903.

Horman A, Korpela H, Sutinen J, Wedel H, Hanninen M-L. (2004). Meta-analysis in assessment of the prevalence and annual incidence of Giardia spp. And Cryptosporium spp. infections in humans in the Nordic countries. *Inter J for Parasitol*, 34, 1337-1346.

Horwitz, M. S. et al. (1998). Diabetes induced by Coxsackie virus: initiation by bystander damage and not molecular mimicry. *Nat Med*, 4, 781-5.

Hyöty, H. et al. (1993). Decline of mumps antibodies in type 1 (insulin-dependent) diabetic children and a plateau in the rising incidence of type 1 diabetes after introduction of the mumps-measles-rubella vaccine in Finland. Childhood Diabetes in Finland Study Group. *Diabetologia*, 36, 1303-8.

Hyppönen E, Lärä E, Reunanen A, Järvelin MR, Virtanen SM. (2001). Intake of vitamin D and risk of type 1 diabetes: a birth-cohort study. Lancet, 358, 1500-3.

Hyttinen V, Kaprio J, Kinnunen L, Koskenvuo M, Tuomilehto J. (2003). Genetic liability of type 1 diabetes and the age of onset age among 22,650 young Finnish twin pairs: a nationwide follow-up study. *Diabetes*, 52, 1052-5.

Johnson SB, Baughcum AE, Carmicael SK, She JX, Schatz DA. (2004). Maternal anxiety associated with newborn genetic screening for type 1 diabetes. *Diabetes Care*, 27, 392-397.

Joner G & Søvik O. (1989). Increasing evidence of diabetes mellitus in Norwegian children 0-14 years of age 1973-1982. *Diabetologia*, 32, 79-83.

Joner G & Søvik O. (1991). The incidence of type 1 (insulin-dependent) diabetes mellitus 15-29 years in Norway 1978-1982. *Diabetologia*, 34, 271-4.

Jones, M. S., Lukashov, V. V., Ganac, R. D. & Schnurr, D. P. (2007). Discovery of a novel human picornavirus in a stool sample from a pediatric patient presenting with fever of unknown origin. *J Clin Microbiol*, 45, 2144-50.

Jones, P. D., Gibson, P. G. & Henry, R. L. (2000). The prevalence of asthma appears to be inversely related to the incidence of typhoid and tuberculosis; hypothesis to explain the variation in asthma prevalence around the world. *Med Hypotheses*, 55, 40-2.

Julier, C., Akolkar B., Concannon P., Motrahan G., Nierras, C., Pugliese, A. (2009). Type 1 Diabetes Consortium. The Type 1 Diabetes Consortium "Rapid Response" family-based candidate gene study; strategy, gene selection, and main outcome. *Genes Immun*, 10 (Suppl 1), 121-7.

Jun, H. S. & Yoon, J. W. (2003). A new look at viruses in type 1 diabetes. *Diabetes Metab Res Rev*, 19, 8-31.

Karjalainen J, Martin JM, Knip M, Ilonen J, Robinson BH, Savilahti E, Åkerblom HK, Dosch H. (1992). A bovine albumin peptide as a possible trigger of insulin-dependent diabetes mellitus. *N Eng J Med*, 327, 302-7.

Kerrush NJ, Campbell-Stokes PL, Gray A, Marriman TR, Robertson SP, Taylor BJ. (2007). Maternal psychological reactions to newborn screening for type 1 diabetes. *Pediatrics*, 120, 392-7.

Kimpimaki T, Kupila A, Hamalainen AM et. al. (2001). The first sign of β-cell autoimmunity appear in infancy in genetically susceptible children from the general population. The Finnish type 1 diabetes prediction and prevention study. *J of Clin Endocrinol and Metabolism*, 86, 4782-8.

Kiviniemi M, Hermann R, Nurmi J et al. (2007). A high-throughput population screening system for type 1 diabetes: An application for the TEDDY (The environmental determinants in the young) study. *Diabetes technology & therapeutics*, 9, 460-72.

Knekt P, Reunanen A, Marniemi J, Leino A, Aromaa A. (1999). Low vitamin E status is a potential risk factor for insulin-dependent diabetes mellitus. *J Intern Med*, 245, 99-102.

Knip M, Veijola R, Virtanen SM, Hyoty H, Vaarala O et al. (2005). Environmental triggers and determinants of type 1 diabetes. *Diabetes*, 54 (Suppl 2), 125-36.

Knip M & Siljander H. (2008). Autoimmune mechanisms in type 1 diabetes. *Autoimmun Rev*, 7, 550-7.

Krischer J. (2007). The environmental determinants of diabetes in the young (TEDDY) study; study design. *Pediatric Diabetes*, 8, 286-98.

Kyronseppa H. (1993). The occurence of human intestinale parasites in Finland. *Scand J Infect Dis*, 25, 671-673.

Lamb MM, Myers MA, Barriga K, Zimmet PZ, Rewers M, Norris JM. (2008). Maternal diet during pregnancy and islet autoimmunity in offspring. *Pediatric Diabetes*, 9, 135-41.

Lefebvre DE, Powell KL, Strom A, Scott FW. (2006). Dietary proteins as environmental modifiers of type 1 diabetes. *Annu Rev Nutr*, 26, 175-202.

Lernmark B, Elding-Larsson H, Hansson G, et al. (2004). Patient responses to participation in genetic screening for diabetes risk. *Pediatric Diabetes*, 5, 174-81.

Liang, Z., Kumar, A. S., Jones, M. S., Knowles, N. J. & Lipton, H. L. (2008). Phylogenetic analysis of the species Theilovirus; emerging murine and human pathogens. *J Virol*, 82, 11545-54.

Magnus P, Irgens LM, Haug K, Nystad W, Skjærven R, Stoltenberg C and the MoBa Study Group. (2006). Cohort profile: The Norwegian Mother and Child Cohort Study (MoBa). *Int J Epidemiol*, 35, 1146-50.

Malaty HM, Graham DY. (1994). Importance of childhood socioeconomic status on the current prevalence of Helicobacter pylori infections. *Gut*, 35, 742-5.

Menser, M. A., Forrest, J. M. & Bransby, R. D. (1978). Rubella infection and diabetes mellitus. *Lancet*, 1, 57-60.

Monetini L, Cavallo MG, Manfrini S, Stefanini L, Picarelli A, Di Tola M, et al. (2002). Antibodies to bovine β-casein in diabetes and other autoimmune diseases. *Horm Metab Res*, 34, 455-9.

Muinck EJD, Øien T, Storrø O, Johansen R, Stenseth NC, Rønningen KS, Rudi K. (2011). Diversity, transmission and presence of Escherichia coli in a cohort of mothers and their infants. *Environmental Microbiolog Reports*, published online Jan 5.

Mølbak AG, Christau B, Marner B, Borch-Johnsen K, Nerup J. (1994). Incidence of insulin-dependent diabetes mellitus in age groups over 30 years in Denmark. *Diabet Med*, 11, 650-5.

Niklasson, B., Nyholm, E., Feinstein, R. E., Samsioe, A. & Hornfeldt, B. (2006). Diabetes and myocarditis in voles and lemmings at cyclic peak densities-induced by Ljungan virus? *Oecologia*, 150, 1-7.

Norris JM & Scott FW. (1996). A meta-analysis of infant diet and insulin-dependent diabetes mellitus; do bias play a role? *Epidemiology*, 7, 87-92.

Norris JM, Barriga K, Klingensmith G, Hoffman M, Eisenbarth GS, Erlich HA, et al. (2003). Timing of initial cereal exposure in infancy and risk of islet autoimmunity. *JAMA*, 290, 1713-20.

Norris JM, Yin Xiang, Lamb MM, Barriga K, Seifert J, Hoffman M, Orton HD, Baron AE, Clare-Saltzler M, Chase HP, Szabo NJ, Erlich H, Eisenbarth GS, Rewers M. (2007). Omega-3 polyunsaturated fatty acid intake and islet autoimmunity in children at increased risk for type 1 diabetes. *JAMA*, 26, 1420-8.

Nygard k, Vold L, Robertson L, Lassen J. (2003). Are domestic Cryptosporium and Giardia infections in Norway underdiagnosed? *Tidsskr Nor Lægeforen*, 123, 3406-9.

Oikarinen, M. et al. (2008). Detection of enteroviruses in the intestine of type 1 diabetic patients. *Clin Exp Immunol*, 151, 71-5.

Osame, K. et al. (2007). Rapid-onset type 1 diabetes associated with cytomegalovirus infection and islet autoantibody synthesis. *Intern Med*, 46, 873-7.

Parslow, R. C., McKinney, P. A., Law, G. R. & Bodansky, H. J. (2001). Population mixing and childhood diabetes. *Int J Epidemiol*, 30, 533-8; discussion 538-9.

Patterson CC, Dahlquist GG, Gyurus E, Green A, Soltesz G, EURODIAB Study Group. (2009). Incidence trends for childhood type 1 diabetes I Europe during 1989-2003 and predicted new cases 2005-2020, a multicentre prospective registration study. *Lancet*, 373, 2027-33.

Petersen JS, Hejnaes KR, Moody A, Karlsen AE, Marshall MO, Hoier-Madsen M, et al. (1994). Detection of GAD65 antibodies in diabetes and other autoimmune diseases using a simple radioligand assay. *Diabetes*, 43, 459-6.

Pohl, D. (2009). Epstein-Barr virus and multiple sclerosis. *J Neurol Sci*, 286(1-2), 62-4.

Pundziute-Lycka, A., Urbonaite, B., Ostrauskas, R., Zalinkevicius, R. & Dahlquist, G. G. (2003). Incidence of type 1 diabetes in Lithuanians aged 0-39 years varies by the urban-rural setting, and the time change differs for men and women during 1991-2000. *Diabetes Care*, 26, 671-6.

Pundziute-Lycka A, Persson LA, Cedermark G, Jansson-Roth A, Nilsson U, Westin V, et al. (2004). Diet, growth, and the risk for type 1 diabetes in childhood: a matched case-referent study. *Diabetes Care*, 27, 2784-9.

Rasmussen T, Stene LC, Cinek O, Torjusen PA, Wetlesen T, Rønningen KS. (2009). Maternal body mass index before pregnancy and weight gain during pregnancy and risk of persistent diabetes associated autoantibodies in children with the high-risk HLA-genotype: The MIDIA study. *Diabetes Care*, 32(10), 1904-6.

Redendo MJ, Rewers M, Yu L, Garg S, Pilcher CC et al. (1999). Genetic determination of islet cell autoimmunity in monozygotic twin, dizygotic twin, and non-twin siblings of patients with type 1 diabetes: prospective twin study. *BMJ*, 318, 698-702.

Redendo MJ, Jeffrey J, Fain PR, Eisenbarth GS, Orban T. (2008). Concordance for islet autoimmunity among monozygotic twins. *N Engl J Med*, 359, 2849-50.

Rewers M, Bugawan TL, Norris JM et al. (1996). Newborn screening for HLA markers associated with IDDM: Diabetes Autoimmunity Study in the Young (DAISY). *Diabetologia*, 39, 807-12.

Richardson, S. J., Willcox, A., Bone, A. J., Foulis, A. K. & Morgan, N. G. (2009). The prevalence of enteroviral capsid protein vp1 immunostaining in pancreatic islets in human type 1 diabetes. *Diabetologia*, 52, 1143-51.

Richer, M. J. & Horwitz, M. S. (2008). Viral infections in the pathogenesis of autoimmune diseases: focus on type 1 diabetes. *Front Biosci*, 13, 4241-57.

Richer, M. J. & Horwitz, M. S. (2009). Coxsackievirus Infection as an Environmental Factor in the Etiology of Type 1 Diabetes. *Autoimmun Rev*, 8(7), 611-5.

Rosenbauer J, Herzig P, Giani G. (2008). Early infant feeding and risk of type 1 diabetes mellitus - a nationalwide population-based case-control study in pre-school children. *Diabetes Metab Res Rev*, 24, 211-22.

Round, J. L. & Mazmanian, S. K. (2009). The gut microbiota shapes intestinal immune responses during health and disease. *Nat Rev Immunol*, 9, 313-23.

Rønningen KS, Spurkland A, Iwe T, Vartdal F, Thorsby E. (1991). Distribution of HLA-DRB1, -DQA1 and -DQB1 alleles and DQA1-DQB1 genotypes among Norwegian patients with insulin-dependent diabetes mellitus. *Tissue Antigens*, 37, 105-111.

Rønningen KS, Atrazhev A, Luo L, Smith DK, Korbutt G, Rajotte RV, et al. (1998). Anti-BSA antibodies do not cross-react with the 69-kDa islet cell autoantigen ICA69. *J Autoimmun*, 11, 223-31.

Rønningen KS, Paltiel L, Meltzer HM, Nordhagen R, Lie KK, Hovengen R, Haugen M, Nystad W, Magnus P, Hoppin JA. (2006). The biobank of the Norwegian Mother and Child Cohort Study: a resource for the next 100 years. *Eur J Epidemiol*, 21(8), 619-25.

Samulsson U & Ludvigsson J. (2003). The consentrations of short-chain fatty acids and other microflora-associated characteristics in faeces from children with newly diagnosed type 1 diabetes and control children and their family mambers. *Diabetic Medicine*, 21, 64-67.

Sarugeri E, Dozio N, Meschi F, Pastore MR, Bonifacio E. (1999). Cellular and humoral immunity against cow's milk proteins in type 1 diabetes. *J Autoimmun*, 13, 365-73.

Schatz D, Muir A, Fuller K et al. (2000). Prospective assessment in newborn genetic screening program in the general population [Abstract]. *Diabetes*, 49, A69.

Sepp E, Jugle E, Vasar M, Naaber P, Bjørksten B, Mikelsaar M. (1997). Intestinal microflora of Estonian and Swedish infants. *Acta Paediatr*, 86, 956-61.

Serdula MK, Alexander MP, Scanlon KS, Bowman BA. (2001). What are preschool children eating? A review of dietary assessment. *Annu Rev Nutr*, 21, 475-98.

Stene LC, Ulriksen J, Magnus P, Joner G. (2000). Use of cod liver oil during pregnancy associated with lower risk of type I diabetes in the offspring. *Diabetologia*, 43, 1083-92.

Stene LC, Magnus P, Lie RT, Søvik O, Joner G, the Norwegian Childhood Diabetes Study Group. (2001). Birth weight and childhood onset type 1 diabetes: population based cohort study. *BMJ*, 322, 889-92.

Stene LC, Joner G, the Norwegian Childhood Diabetes Study Group. (2003). Use of cod liver oil during the first year of life is associated with lower risk of childhood-onset type 1 diabetes: a large, population based, case-control study. *Am J Clin Nutr*, 78, 1128-34.

Stene LC, Witsø E, Torjesen PA, Rasmussen T, Magnus P, Cinek O, Wetlesen T, Rønningen KS. (2007). Islet autoantibody development during follow-up of high-risk children from the general Norwegian population from three months of age: Design and early results from the MIDIA study. *J of Autoimmun*, 29, 44-51.

Stoll NR. (1947). This wormy world. *J Parasitol*, 33, 1-18.

Strachan, D. P. (1989). Hay fever, hygiene, and household size. *BMJ*, 299, 1259-60.

Tapia G, Cinek O, Witsø E, Kulich M, Rasmussen T, Grinde B, Rønningen KS. (2008). Longitudinal observation of parechovirus in stool samples from Norwegian infants. *J Med Virol*, 80(10), 1835-42.

Tapia G, Cinek O, Rasmussen T, Grinde B, Rønningen KS. (2010). No Ljungan virus RNA in stool samples from the Norwegian environmental triggers of type 1 diabetes (MIDIA) cohort study. *Diabetes Care*, 33(5), 1069-71.

Tapia G, Cinek O, Rasmussen T, Grinde B, Stene LC, Rønningen KS. (2011). Longitudinal study of parechovirus infection in infancy and risk of repeated positivity for multiple islet autoantibodies: The MIDIA study. *Pediatr Diabetes*, 12(1), 58-62.

Tapia G, Cinek O, Rasmussen T, Witsø E, Grinde B, Stene LC, Rønningen KS. (2011). Human enterovirus RNA in monthly fecal samples and islet autoimmunity in Norwegian children with high genetic risk for type 1 diabetes: the MIDIA study. *Diabetes Care*, 34(1), 151-5.

Tauriainen, S. et al. (2007). Human parechovirus 1 infections in young children-no association with type 1 diabetes. *J Med Virol*, 79, 457-62.

TEDDY study group. (2008). The environmental determinants in the young study. *Annals of the New York Academy of Sciences*, 1150, 1-13.

Toniolo, A., Onodera, T., Yoon, J. W. & Notkins, A. L. (1980). Induction of diabetes by cumulative environmental insults from viruses and chemicals. *Nature*, 288, 383-5.

Undlien DE, Friede T, Rammensee H-G, Joner G, Dahl-Jørgensen K, Søvik O, Akselsen HE, Knutsen I, Rønningen KS, Thorsby E. (1997). HLA-encoded genetic predisposition in IDDM. DR4 subtypes may be associated with different degrees of protection. *Diabetes*, 46, 143-9.

Uusitalo L, Knip M, Kenward MG, Alfthan G, Sundvall J, Aro A, Reunanen A, Åkerblom HK, Virtanen SM. (2005). Childhood diabetes in Finland study group. *J Pediatr Endocrinol Metab*, 18, 1409-16.

Uusitalo L, Nevalainen J, Niinisjø S, Alfthan G, Sundvall j, Korhonen T, Kenward MG, Oja H, Veijola R, Simell O, Ilonen J, Knip m, Virtanen SM. (2008). Serum alpha- and gammetocopherol concentration and risk of advanced β cell autoimmunity in children with HLA-conferred susceptibility to type 1 diabetes mellitus. *Diabetologia,* 51, 773-80.

van der Werf, N., Kroese, F. G., Rozing, J. & Hillebrands, J. L. (2007). Viral infections as potential triggers of type 1 diabetes. *Diabetes Metab Res Rev,* 23, 169-83.

Virtanen SM, Kenward MG, Erkkola M et al. (2006). Age at introduction of new food and advanced b-cell autoimmunity in young children withHLA-conferred susceptibility to type 1 diabetes. *Diabetologia,* 49, 1512-21.

Viskari, H. et al. (2005). Relationship between the incidence of type 1 diabetes and maternal enterovirus antibodies: time trends and geographical variation. *Diabetologia,* 48, 1280-7.

Vuorinen, T., Nikolakaros, G., Simell, O., Hyypia, T. & Vainionpaa, R. (1992). Mumps and Coxsackie B3 virus infection of human fetal pancreatic islet-like cell clusters. *Pancreas,* 7, 460-4.

Wetzel, J. D. et al. (2006). Reovirus delays diabetes onset but does not prevent insulitis in nonobese diabetic mice. *J Virol,* 80, 3078-82.

Wellcome Trust Case Control Consortium, Craddock, N., Hurles, M.E., Cardin N., Pearson, R.D., Plagnol, V. et al. (2010). Genome-wide association study of CNVs in 16,000 cases of eight common diseases and 3,000 shared controls. *Nature,* 464, 713-20.

Willett WC. (1998). Food-frequency methods. In: Willett WC, editor. Nutritional Epidemiology. Second edition ed. Oxford: *Oxford University Press,* 74-100.

Witsø E, Palacios G, Cinek O, Stene LC, Grinde B, Janowitz D, Lipkin WI, Rønningen KS. (2006). High prevalence of human enterovirus a infections in natural circulation of human enteroviruses. *J Clin Microbiol,* 44(11), 4095-100.

Witsø E, Palacios G, Rønningen KS, Cinek O, Janowitz D, Rewers M, Grinde B, Lipkin WI. (2007). Asymptomatic circulation of HEV71 in Norway. *Virus Res,* 123(1), 19-29.

Wolthers, K. C. et al. (2008). Human parechoviruses as an important viral cause of sepsislike illness and meningitis in young children. *Clin Infect Dis,* 47, 358-63.

Yazdanbakhsh, M., Kremsner, P. G. & van Ree, R. (2002). Allergy, parasites, and the hygiene hypothesis. *Science,* 296, 490-4.

Zazdanbakhsh M, van den Biggelaar AHJ, Maizels RM. (2001). Th2 responses without atopy: immunregulation in chronic helminth infections and reduced allergic disease. *Trends Immunol,* 22, 372-7.

Ziegler AG, Schmid S, Huber D, Hummel M, Bonifacio E. (2003). Early infant feeding and risk of developing type 1 diabetes-associated autoantibodies. *JAMA,* 290, 1721-8.

Ziegler AG, Pflueger M, Winkler C, Achenbach P, Akolkar B, Krischer JP, Bonifacio E. (2011). Accelerated progression from islet autoimmunity to diabetes is causing the escalating incidence of type 1 diabetes in young children. *J Autoimmun,* Mar 2.

Zoll, J. et al. (2009). Saffold virus, a human Theiler's-like cardiovirus, is ubiquitous and causes infection early in life. *PLoS Pathog,* 5, e1000416.

Øverby NC, Lillegaard IT, Johansson L, Andersen LF. (2004). High intake of added sugar among Norwegian children and adolescents. *Public Health Nutr,* 7, 285-93.

Aas KK, Tambs K, Kise MS, Magnus P, Rønningen KS. (2010). Genetic testing of newborns for type 1 diabetes susceptibility: a prospective cohort study on effects on maternal mental health. *BMC Med Genet*, 11, 112.

Part 5

Alternative Treatments for Diabetes

18

Potentials and Limitations of Bile Acids and Probiotics in Diabetes Mellitus

Momir Mikov[1,2], Hani Al-Salami[3] and Svetlana Golocorbin-Kon[1,2]

[1]*Department of Pharmacology, Toxicology and Clinical Pharmacology, Medical Faculty, Univeristy of Novi Sad*

[2]*Pharmacy Faculty, University of Montenegro, Podgorica*

[3]*Senior Lecturer, School of Pharmacy, Curtin University, Perth*

[1]*Serbia*

[2]*Montenegro*

[3]*Australia*

1. Introduction

Diabetes mellitus is a metabolic disorder classified as Type 1 (T1D) or Type 2 (T2D). T1D is an autoimmune disorder characterized by the destruction of the β-cells of the pancreas resulting in a partial or complete lack of insulin production and the inability of the body to control glucose homeostasis (Akerblom et al. 2002). T1D is also known as juvenile-onset diabetes because it manifests at a young age (Bruno et al. 2005). As it requires the patient to inject insulin to supplement the partial or complete lack of insulin production by the pancreas, it is also called insulin-dependent diabetes mellitus (IDDM). T2D, formerly known as noninsulin-dependent diabetes mellitus (NIDDM) or adult-onset diabetes, is a metabolic disorder with onset most common in middle age and later life (Campbell 1991). T2D may be controlled by diet and exercise and, unlike T1D, does not always require the use of insulin (Campbell 2004). However, the term "noninsulin-dependent" is a misnomer since many patients require insulin therapy at some time in the course of their disease. T2D is often associated with obesity, hypertension and insulin resistance and can result in the complete destruction of beta-cells of the pancreas leading to T1D (Campbell 2004; Weiss & Caprio 2006). The prevalence of T1D and T2D are on the rise worldwide, which has generated a strong drive towards developing preventative measures as well as cure. Recent data published by the International Diabetes Federation highlighted the severity of diabetes epidemic. Data show that the disease is currently affecting 246 million people worldwide, with 46% of all those affected in the 40-59 age group. Previous figures underestimated the scope of the problem, while even the most pessimistic predictions fell short of the current figure. It is predicted that the total number of people living with diabetes will increase to 380 million within twenty years if no new and substantially more effective drugs are produced (Moore et al. 2003a; Rosenbloom et al. 1999). On 2007, the health costs of diabetes have exceeded 200 billion dollars only in the US. This adds to the cost generated from higher rate of hospitalization, higher mortality rate, and impaired performance of workers with diabetes. This has generated a strong drive towards developing preventative measures as well as cure for the disease and its complications. Diabetes is a disease that incorporates various metabolic disturbances such as impaired glucose haemostasis, blood dyscrasias and hyperlipidemia. Major disturbances also include slower gut movement (gastroparesis) and microfloral overgrowth (especially of fermentation bacteria and yeasts due to the slightly more acidic gut contents) (Al-Salami et al. 2007; Husebye 2005). Improving diabetes complications, reducing prevalence and restoring normal physiological patterns should significantly optimise diabetes treatment and the quality of life for diabetic patients.

Side effects associated with diabetes therapy include hypoglycemia, toxin build up in the gut, and lactic acidosis. These remain major issues and cause of death especially in the presence of compromised liver and kidney functions. So despite strict glycemic control, the disease and its complications remain a growing health concern. Diabetic patients suffer complications due to disturbed physiological and biochemical processes associated with the disease including disturbed bile acids production and microfloral composition (Barbeau et al. 2006; Ogura et al. 1986; Peng & Hagopian 2007; Rozanova et al. 2002; Slivka et al. 1979a; Thomson 1983). Thus the use of bile acids and probiotics in diabetes treatment may improve glycemia as well the ameliorate complications. A major improvement would be the discovery of treatments for diabetes that avoid and even replace the absolute requirement for injected insulin. Recent studies in a rat model of Type 1 diabetes show that a multi-therapeutic approach incorporating bile acids and probiotics, as adjunct therapy, exerted better control over glycemia and resulted in ameliorating complications, than when each treatment was administered alone (Al-Salami et al. 2008a; Al-Salami et al. 2008b; Al-Salami et al. 2008e; Al-Salami et al. 2009b). Accordingly, improving diabetes complications, reducing prevalence and restoring normal physiological patterns should significantly optimise diabetes treatment and the quality of life of diabetic patients.

Bile has been used as a therapeutic agent since ancient times. The use of bear gall bladder in treating fever, liver diseases and eye infections has been an ancient phenomenon practiced by many civilizations including the Chinese. Recent studies have showed the therapeutic effects of bear bile in treating gallstones and liver diseases. Bear bile contains substantial amount of ursodeoxycholic acid (UDCA) and chenodeoxycholic acid (CDCA) (Bachrach & Hofmann 1982a; Bachrach & Hofmann 1982b), which recent reports have shown them to also be present in pig bile. Current Chinese medicine uses extracts from pig bile for constipation, jaundice, whooping cough and asthma. Pig bile has also been found to have anti-inflammatory, anticonvulsant and analgesic effects. The applications of bile acids to certain diseases as therapeutic agents have been greatly explored by the ancient Greeks in the sixth century B.C. The ancient Greeks proposed the *Doctrine of Four Humours* or *body fluids* which included yellow bile, black bile, blood and mucus or phlegm. Health is a result of a balanced mixture of the Four Humours (krasis) whereas disease is due to an excess of one of the Four Humours and an imbalance (dyskrasis) of the body fluids (Heaton 1971). Bile therapeutic applications have been explored further by Galen in the second century A.D., and bile was used to facilitate the excretion of stools as a laxative. In 1863 Hoppe-Seyler demonstrated even though bile salts are the major active component in bile, little bile acids is detected in the feces. He proposed bile acids be reabsorbed from the intestine and that bile salts are the major constituents and also proposed continuous recirculation of bile salts, now known as enterohepatic recycling. Heinrich Otto Wieland (1877-1957) won the Nobel Prize in chemistry in 1927 *for his investigations of the constitution of the bile acids and related substances.* In 1940, Roepke and Mason demonstrated that micelle formation was responsible for the solubilisation of non-polar lipids such as cholesterol and fat-soluble vitamins. Twenty years later it was proposed that bile salts were simultaneously absorbed into the ileal mucosa. Heaton and Morris confirmed that active transport of bile salts occurs but only in the ileum (Heaton 1971; Lowbeer et al. 1970).

Primary bile acids are synthesized in hepatocytes from endogenous or dietary cholesterol. They are then conjugated to glycine or taurine to form primary conjugated bile acids. In the small intestine, the conjugated bile acids are metabolised by the gut microflora into secondary bile acids before being reabsorbed in the process of enterohepatic recirculation (Ridlon et al. 2006). Approximately 90-95 % of bile acids secreted into the gut is reabsorbed from the intestine back into the circulation via bile acid transporters, while about 400-800 mg/day is excreted from the body in the faeces (Roberts et al. 2002). The bile acid transporters are mainly the sodium-dependent taurocholate cotransporting polypeptide (NTCP), sodium-independent organic anion transporting protein (OATP), the bile salt export pump (BSEP) (Ballatori et al. 2005a; Higgins & Gottesman 1992; Mao & Unadkat 2005), the organic cation transporter polypeptide (OCTP) and the apical sodium-dependent bile salt transporter (ASBT) (Bodo et al. 2003; Zelcer et al. 2003a; Zelcer et al. 2003b; Zollner et al. 2003). Conjugated bile acids are transported by ASBT, whereas unconjugated bile acids are transported by OATP and by passive diffusion. Conjugated bile acids are transported by intracellular transport mechanisms within hepatocytes to the canalicular poles and secreted into the canalicular lumen by BSEP (Asamoto et al. 2001; Mita et al. 2006).

Cholic acid is an important precursor for the synthesis of steroids and chenodeoxycholic acid, and of recently has been investigated and applied in biliary calculus (cholelith) therapy. To optimise the stability and minimise toxicity of cholic acid, a more stable semisynthetic analogue MKC has been designed and synthesized. This is done on cholic acid through replacing the hydroxyl group on carbon atom 12 with a ketone group. Generally, the hydroxyl groups on the carbon atoms, C7 and C12 are replaced by hydrogen to enhance stability and reduce side effects. However, despite bile acids being endogenous compounds, manufacturing stable analogues can be challenging. The challenges include:

1. The need for selective protection of 2 hydroxyl groups which is done by acylation.
2. The choice of a suitable reagent to transform the remaining hydroxyl groups as appropriate.

Although enzymatic dehydroxylation of cholic acid may easily overcome these challenges, chemical reactions involving suitable reagents is still favoured especially for industrial production (Mikov & Fawcett 2006a). 3 hydroxyl groups (C3, C7 and C12) are targeted for acylation. The type of reaction will depend on the type of the bond and its configurational arrangement in the molecule. C3-OH is equatorial thus can be removed through estrification while with C7 and C12 axial groups, oxidation is sufficient. In addition to exploring the potential effect of bile acids, they can also be used as absorption enhancers.

Today it is well known that bile is a complex fluid containing water, electrolytes and other organic molecules including bile salts, cholesterol, phospholipids and bilirubin that flows from the bile duct into the small intestine (Al-Salami et al. 2007). The main endogenous bile acids are primary (cholic and chenodeoxycholic acids) and secondary (deoxycholic and lithocholic acids). Approximately 1 L of bile is secreted by the liver daily. Bile has a pH of 7.8-8.6 and is nearly isotonic with blood. It is secreted from the liver into small ducts that join to form the common hepatic duct. Bile salts are anionic water-soluble products of cholesterol metabolism. Bile salts can form micelles 4-7 nm in diameters which contain fatty acids, monoglycerides and phospholipids. These micelles solubilise lipids and transport them across biological membranes (Hamada et al. 2006; Leng et al. 2003).

In the past, bile acids were considered to have three basic physiological functions (Kuhajda et al. 2006a; Kuhajda et al. 2006b; Mikov & Fawcett 2006b):

1. Elimination of excess cholesterol;
2. Facilitation of the digestion of dietary fats (emulsifying agents);
3. Facilitation of the absorption of fat soluble vitamins such as A, D and K.

However, recent studies have expanded the role of bile acids to include endocrine signalling to regulate glucose, lipid and their own homeostasis and influence energy expenditure and gut microfloral composition (48, 53, 88).

This chapter aims to explore the changes in gut physiology and metabolic pathways which are associated with diabetes. It also aims to identify current and potential applications of bile acids and probiotics in the prevention and treatment of the disease.

2. Glucose regulation and insulin secretion

Glucose is a major source of energy with the normal range (normoglycemia) being 3.5-7.8 mmol/l (Cubeddu & Hoffmann 2002). When the body is at absolute rest (the basal state), glucose consumption is equal to its production (Overkamp et al. 1997; Zisser et al. 2007). When glucose is absorbed into the circulation and the body has no immediate need for energy, glucose is stored in the liver and muscles as glycogen (Overkamp et al. 1997). In healthy individuals, glycogen synthesis (glyconeogenesis) in tissues is stimulated by insulin. When the amount of glucose in the blood gets low, glycogen breaks down in the liver to glucose (glycogenolysis). In healthy individuals, feedback processes ensure that glucose levels are under homeostatic control by balancing glyconeogenesis and glycogenolysis. The liver can also convert lactate to glucose via a process known as gluconeogenesis to further supply the required glucose to the blood when levels are low. Glyconeogenesis, glycogenolysis and gluconeogenesis are controlled by anabolic hormones released from the Islets of Langerhans in the pancreas such as glucagon (released from the α-cells) and insulin (released from the β-cells). These hormones bind to specific receptors to trigger a chain of reactions that control glucose homeostasis. GLUT-2 (mainly in beta-cells) and GLUT-4 (mainly in skeletal muscles) are the dominant glucose transporters. In general, insulin activates to become fully functional pores that are able to transport glucose molecules into tissues (Rosa et al. 2011; Stuart et al. 2009).

The pancreas produces large quantities of insulin which it stores in intracellular secretary granules (Al-Salami et al. 2007). Upon stimulation from rising levels of glucose, these granules release their insulin into the mesenteric veins (Juhl et al. 2002; Just et al. 2008). Insulin secretion is different in healthy and diabetic individuals. In healthy individuals, there are two phases of insulin secretion; first phase insulin secretion (FPIS) which starts immediately after the initial stimulus of raised glucose levels and second phase insulin secretion (SPIS) which starts shortly after FPIS, and has a shorter duration but greater magnitude. FPIS occurs from β-cells of the pancreas as a direct response to high influx of extracellular glucose. In T1D patients, FPIS and SPIS do not exist since there is a complete lack of insulin production while, in T2D patients, FPIS is impaired and further exposure to glucose results in a reduction in insulin secretion in SPIS due to the desensitization of β-cells to glucose.

3. Pathogenesis and risk factors of Type 1 diabetes

Recent studies have shown that the inflammation which leads to the destruction of β-cells is initiated in the gut (Devendra et al. 2004). It is likely to occur within the first three months of life (Notkins & Lernmark 2001) due to different diabetic-causing xenobiotics (diabetogenics) that include gluten (Akerblom et al. 2002), cow milk protein (Barbeau et al. 2007), viruses such as rubella (Vaarala 2006), and food-toxins such as alloxan, streptozotocin and N-nitroso compounds (Vaarala 2006; Ziegler et al. 2003). Although the pathogenesis of T1D remains unclear, the generally accepted explanation is that T1D is a chronic autoimmune disease triggered in genetically susceptible individuals by a primary insult initiated in the gut (Ghosh et al. 2004). T2D develops in adult life probably due to environmental factors (Moore et al. 2003b) that lead to tissue desensitization to insulin. Continuous stimulation of beta-cells through hyperglycemia or certain types of antidiabetic drugs such as sulphonylureas can lead to tissue exhaustion and eventual cessation of insulin production due to tissue damage which results in the development of T1D (Fajans 1987).

The associated-disturbances in the compositions of bile and gut microflora are reported in the literature. However whether the changes in bile and microfloral compositions are caused by diabetes, or diabetes develops as a result of disturbed bile and gut microflora, remains to be determined.

4. Diabetes-associated disturbances in bile acids and gut microflora

Disturbances in bile acids composition may result in tissue necrosis due to higher than normal concentrations of potent bile acids such as lithocholic acid compared with less potent bile acids such as chenodeoxycholic acid. Secondary bile acids are solely produced by the action of gut microflora on primary bile acids, and thus, microfloral composition is directly linked to secondary bile acid production and bile acid composition. This interaction between bile acid composition and the composition of gut microflora represents the base of the hypothesized link between bile acid, gut microflora and energy balance. However, even though the compositions of bile acids and gut microflora are reported to be different in diabetic patients (Duan et al. 2008; Gebel 2011; Morris 1989; Ogura et al. 1986; Slivka et al. 1979a; Thomson 1983), it is still not clear how these changes directly affect the development and progression of diabetes or its complications. These complications include cardiovascular, tissue necrosis and ulcerations, and metabolic disturbances.

The amino acid taurine, which is used by hepatocytes in bile acid conjugation and bile salts formation, has many other physiological functions including the regulation of intracellular osmolarity, cardiomyocytes functions, and as an antioxidant. Accordingly, a clear link between bile compositions, taurine concentrations and diabetes complications can be discussed. A hypoglycemic effect of taurine, directly or through synergizing the effect of insulin, has also been reported (Kulakowski & Maturo 1984). Conjugated bile acids includes glycine and taurine conjugates, both existing in constant ratio. Glycine conjugated bile acids are less soluble and are harder to excrete compared with taurine conjugated bile acids. This result in bile accumulation noticed in T1D subjects (Bennion & Grundy 1977). In T1D patients, who have increased lipid metabolism, the percentage of taurocholic acid in bile is decreased indicating an altered biosynthesis of taurine (Meinders et al. 1981c). In one study, diabetic patients showed altered taurine metabolism causing consequent cellular dysfunctions that resulted in worsening diabetic neuropathy, cardiomyopathy, platelet aggregation and endothelial dysfunction (Hansen 2001). In T1D rats, taurine concentrations were found different in various organs (Goodman & Shihabi 1990; Hansen 2001; Reibel et al. 1979). Taurine concentrations in kidney and liver were low, while they were higher in heart and skeletal muscle. One important diabetic complication, platelet hyperaggregation, has been normalized by the alteration of bile acids composition through the addition of taurine (Franconi et al. 1995). Another complication is T1D retinopathy which have shown significantly less taurine levels in the retina, compared with that in healthy rats (Vilchis & Salceda 1996). Diabetic nephropathy are other major complication of T1D. Taurine consumption has shown to reduce chronic diabetic nephropathy in T1D rats (Trachtman & Sturman 1996). Other diabetic complications can also be reduced or even prevented by the addition of taurine. These include high glucose induced apoptosis in human vascular endothelial cells (Di Wu et al. 1999) and impaired endothelium-dependent vasodilatation in diabetic mice.

Even though the composition of gut microflora has been reported to be different in T1D patients, it may be difficult to quantify or qualify such a difference. Gut microflora interacts closely with the body immune system and has shown to control the immune response to various inflammatory stimuli. The mechanism of action of probiotics could be one or more of the following. Firstly, by competitive exclusion, where gut microfloral bacteria resist colonization of other 'foreign' bacteria. Secondly, by barrier formation where the microflora forms a physical barrier reducing bacterial translocation by forming a wall surrounding the outside part of the gut enterocytes. Thirdly, gut bacteria can produce bacteriocins and change the pH to create a harsher environment for other invading bacteria to settle in the gut. Fourthly, gut microflora can influence the immune system through its effect on gut enterocytes (quorum sensing) and the innate and adaptive immune system (Gareau et al. 2010; Walker 2008a).

It is a common conception that the efficiency of the immune system is compromised in diabetic patients resulting in prolonged healing of infections and diabetic ulcers (Steed et al. 1996). This is also brought about by the higher rates of bacterial infections reported in diabetes and higher rate of antibiotic use (Goldberg & Krause 2009; Paccagnini et al. 2009). In one study, the effect of the probiotic bacteria, Lactobacillus plantarum (Lp) on infected diabetic ulcers, was examined. Topical application of Lp on diabetic ulcers for 30 days induced healing. This effect was observed in almost half of the treated diabetic patients. However, this was not significantly different from healthy treated control suggesting that probiotic treatment is effective in treating diabetic ulcers, but its effect does not vary between diabetic and non-diabetic individuals. It is therefore tempting to speculate that gut microfloral bacteria controls the innate immune responses towards normalizing harmful bacteria in an effort to protect its own environment and keep its own existence.

5. Animal models suitable for investigating bile acids and probiotics effects on Type 1 diabetes

During the process of drug development, various *in vivo, ex vivo, in situ* and *in silico* methods can be used. Each method has advantages and disadvantages, and so using more than one method can provide better confirmation of findings. *In silico* methods can provide an initial insight into a potential drug candidate with predicted high pharmacological activity and good stability, while *ex vivo* methods can provide more information about a drug's interaction with living tissue, and are more cost-effective compared with *in vivo* animal models (Qin et al. 2010). *In situ* methods can better predict drug absorption compared with *ex vivo* models but *in vivo* models can provide more comprehensive pharmacokinetic profiles and give a better understanding of drug-tissue interactions (Zanchi et al. 1998). I*n vivo* studies are usually carried out where drug therapeutic formulations are administered to animals in order to investigate short and long term safety, to explore various clinical effects and to study different physicochemical parameters before confirming suitability of the formulation to a disease condition(s). Various animal models are used to represent various diseases.

Although there is a surplus of animal models (spontaneous and induced) to study T1D, there is no ideal or standard model for studying the effect of bile acids and probiotics on T1D. Rats lack gall bladder which means bile is not stored before secretion but rather is secreted immediately after food intake. However, this does not seem to stop researches from using rats as an animal model of T1D (Al-Salami et al. 2008e). Rats, mice and hamsters have been used to study bile acids and probiotics applications in T1D, however, future research is needed, to compare the effect of bile acids and probiotics on T1D, using different animal models.

An ideal animal model should represent a specific medical condition in terms of disease development, pathophysiology, biological disturbances and short & long term complications.

If we are to create a better model of human T1D, we should carefully consider the disease effect on the following:

1. Relevant end points including primary, secondary and tertiary.
2. The relevant speed and stages of disease development and progression.
3. Disease complications, their progression and the relevant clinical end point(s).
4. Symptomatic/nonsymptomatic signs of the disease.
5. Feasibility of sample collections in terms of tissue site and sample volume.
6. The incidence in males vs. females.

The current therapeutics for T1D are inadequate, which necessitate further drug development and *in vivo* studies. Clinical translation of T1D pathophysiology and clinical manifestations, from animal to human, has been limited and rather difficult. This is because very little is known about T1D; the extent of heterogeneity, polymorphism, genetic distance, the exact site of initial immune response (gut or pancreas), and diabetogenic antigens. Creating a suitable animal model for T1D requires the ability to accurately translate the findings to human. These findings include therapeutic efficacy (prevention/treatment), safety and PK/PD profiles. There are various animal models for T1D, with the nonobese diabetic (NOD) mouse being the 'standard' one. Other models are induction models of rats, mice and hamsters using alloxan or streptozotocin to destroy pancreatic beta cells and induce T1D. The NOD mouse represents the best spontaneous model for a human autoimmune disease, in particular, T1D. NOD mouse model allows the investigation of various immunointerventions that can be used in human T1D. Similar to T1D in human, NOD mice have higher levels of macrophages, dendritic cells, CD4+ and B cells.

The induction of T1D in NOD mouse can be achieved through environmental conditions, mimicking the development of T1D in human. However, the development of T1D in NOD mouse takes place quickly and can produce a significant inflammatory condition that may over-respond to immunomanipulation and exaggerate the effect of a treatment. Also, the incidence of T1D is different between males and females in this model while the incidence is the same in males and females in human. This can further limit the applications and the findings of this animal model (Dieleman et al. 1997). Many therapeutics that showed good efficacy in this model failed to achieve similar results in T1D human subjects (Srinivasan & Ramarao 2007). Having said that and regardless of how different this model is, from the 'true' human TID, NOD mouse remains the most representative of human T1D. Interestingly, in a recently published study, the incidence of T1D was much higher, when the mice were maintained in a germ-free environment suggesting direct connection between gut microflora and the development of T1D (Li-Wen et al. 2007).

The suitable animal model for human T1D should ideally be easy to breed and handle, and can accommodate various medical conditions that may come about or be associated with T1D. Thus, extrapolation of its findings to human should be easily done, and with great accuracy and precision.

6. The therapeutic applications of bile acids and probiotics in Type 1 diabetes

In pathophysiology such as gall stone formations, inflammatory bowel disease and allergic reactions, the administration of probiotics significantly improves body physiology and reduces complications (Cary & Boullata 2010; Gourbeyre et al. 2011; Martin & Walker 2008; Morris et al. 2009; Stephani et al. 2011). In one study, the administration of bile acids and gliclazide to probiotic pre-treated diabetic animals showed efficacy and a significant reduction of diabetic complications (Al-Salami et al. 2008e; Al-Salami et al. 2008g).

The synthesis of bile acids is highly regulated by nuclear hormone receptors and other transcription factors, which ensure a constant supply of bile acids in a very changing metabolic environment. In healthy individuals, bile acids control their own haemostasis through feedback mechanisms involving phosphoenolpyruvate carboxykinase (PEPCK) and farnesoid X receptor alpha (FXR-alpha) nuclear receptors. Their direct effect on diabetes development remains debatable, but through the inhibition of PEPCK and FXR-alpha (via TGR5-D2 signalling pathways), bile acids also inhibits gluconeogenesis. Such mechanisms may seem to oppose that of insulin, which suggests direct effect on glucose haemostasis in healthy individuals. Inherited mutations that impair bile acid synthesis cause many human disorders including early childhood liver inflammation and failure. During the development of diabetes, bile acid synthesis is increased, the bile acid pool is expanded, and bile acid excretion is increased suggesting lack of adequate control over the feedback regulating bile acid haemostasis. Accordingly, several recent studies have investigated the role of and applications of bile acids in glucose haemostasis. Interestingly, where both factors, PEPCK and FXR-alpha fit remains under investigation. During the fasting state, hepatocytes produce more FXR-alpha suggesting that FXR-alpha production takes place in the absent of insulin (Zhang et al, 2004). In another study, when FXR-alpha was tested in diabetic animals, it was noticed to be lower than these in healthy, but when insulin was administered; it normalized such an effect (Duran-Sandoval et al, 2004). Overall, BAs have been reported to inhibit gluconeogenesis via downregulation of phosphoenolpyruvate carboxykinase (PEPCK) mRNA levels in a FXR-alpha-dependent and -independent manner (De Fabiani et al, 2003; Yamagata et al, 2004).

Apart from basic physiological functions like the elimination of cholesterol and the intestinal solubilisation (emulsification) of triacylglycerol, cholesterol and lipid, soluble vitamins, bile acids and their analogues are now recognized as having major therapeutic applications in the treatment of cholelithiasis, as transport promoters for other substances, in potentiating the action of other substances (analgesic, antiviral, hypoglycaemic) and as hypoglycaemic and hypolipidemic agents. In one study, lithocholic acid concentration was higher after diabetes development which resulted in gallstone formation (Chijiiwa 1990). This indicates that diabetes directly altered bile composition. However, the exact mechanism by which diabetes can alter bile acid composition remains unclear.

One hypothesis linking bile acid disturbance with the initiation of diabetes development, is through the over-production of lithocholic acid, brought about by disturbances in the gut microflora (De Leon et al. 1978; Kokk et al. 2005; Meinders et al. 1981a; Meinders et al. 1981b). Diabetes mellitus has been associated with unbalanced secretion of bile (cholelithiasis). In addition, many studies have linked changes in bile composition to the changes in the composition of the gut microflora (Kokk et al. 2005; Mikov et al. 2004; Mikov et al. 2005; Mikov et al. 2006; Mikov & Fawcett 2006b).

Potential therapeutic use of bile acids in T1D can be achieved through two main applications; as hypoglycaemic agents and as absorption-enhancing agent to insulin delivery.

Monoketocholic acid (MKC) (Figure 1) is a stable semisynthetic primary bile acid (cholic acid analogue) with low toxicity that has been shown to enhance the nasal absorption of insulin in rats (89). In addition, MKC has been shown to exert a effect in its own right when administered by the oral route in alloxan-induced T1D rats (Mikov et al. 2007).

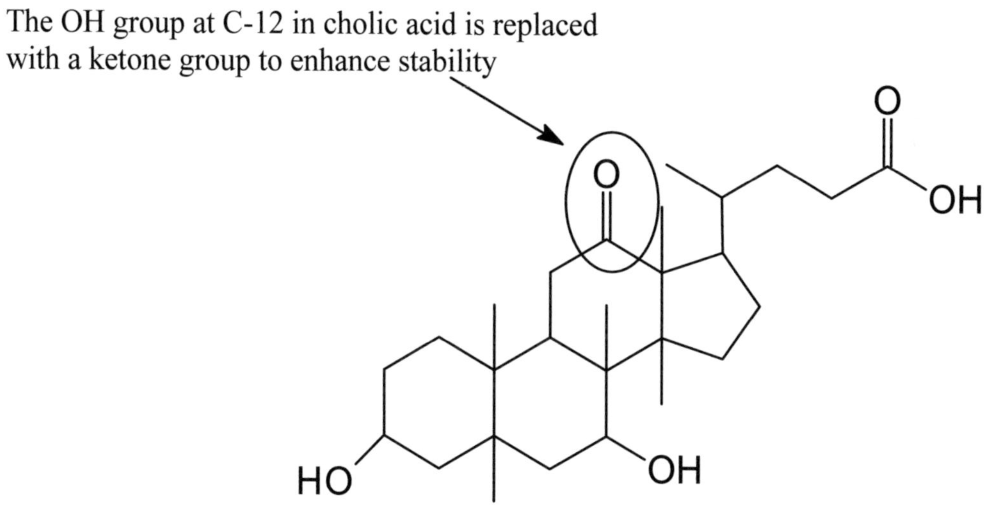

Fig. 1. The chemical structure of 12-monoketocholic acid (MKC).

Permeation enhancement through the tissue-solubilising effect of bile salts was found to be one of several mechanisms by which bile salts can facilitate drug absorption. Other mechanisms involve bile salts' effect on efflux and afflux protein transporters on the cell wall of various tissues including gut enterocytes, hepatocytes, nasal mucosa and others (Al-Salami et al. 2008c; Al-Salami et al. 2008d; Al-Salami et al. 2009a).

7. The interaction between protein transportors, bile acid composition and diabetes developement

Bile acids effect on T1D development and progression may also be through their effect on protein transporters, since many transporters have their expression and functionality altered in T1D (Al-Salami et al. 2008c). The exact mechanism associating the change in transporters, bile acids composition and diabetes development, is still unknown but there are few assumptions to explain such an interaction. The first assumption is that T1D starts on the first few months of life with a direct insult in the gut, initiating a disturbance in the gut microflora and a consequent disturbed bile flow. This results in an altered bile feedback mechanisms and a change in the expression of protein transporters responsible for bile enterohepatic recirculation. This results in an inflammatory condition that brings about T1D and beta cells destruction. The second assumption is that disturbance in protein transporters expression and functionality, caused by a genetic mutation, produces a disturbance in bile flow. This leads to disturbances in gut microflora initiating inflammation in the gut affecting beta cells and resulting in T1D. The third assumption is that the functionality of the immune system is altered (due to either an insult in the gut or genetic mutation). This alters the composition of gut microflora resulting in initiating of inflammation reaching the beta cells, as a case of mistaken identity. As a consequence of beta cell inflammation, bile acids synthesis and flow are disturbed resulting in exacerbation of the inflammation and worsening of symptoms. In all these assumptions, genetic susceptibility is expected, and contributes further to T1D development and progression. The above assumptions were based on the work of the authors as well as careful evaluation of the literature.

In recent publications, alterations in the functionality of some transporters have been linked to the development of diabetes; however, the exact mechanism remains not fully understood. Bile salts output in diabetic animals was extremely high compared with healthy, and the expression of Mdr2 was also high after STZ treatment (van Waarde et al. 2002). In another study, a mutation in Zinc transporter 8 (ZT8) located in beta cells, is implicated in the dysregulation of insulin transport and release, and an exacerbation of the inflammatory response leading to T1D. In this study, ZT8 was considered as an autoantigen resulting in the stimulation and production of beta cells autoantibodies and T1D development (Rungby 2010). Moreover, streptozotocin (STZ) had different but significant effect on the expression of Na/Cl/glucose cotransporters, and the administration of insulin reduced such an effect (Vidotti et al. 2008). Hyperglyemia itself directly reduced the activity of Mdr1 suggesting a clear association between pre-T1D hyperglycemia and disturbances in protein transporters (Tramonti et al. 2006). In another recent study, the effect of STZ on cation protein transporters was reported, interestingly, at different levels of protein synthesis; transcriptional and posttranscriptional depending on the type of the transporters affected (Grover et al. 2004). However, some studies suggest a diabetic influence is stronger on enzymatic activities than on protein transporters with the enzymatic influence being the cause of exacerbation of inflammation and development of the disease (Py et al. 2002). The impairment of protein transporters functionality, reported in the diabetic animals can take place either by reduced protein expression or reduced action. When glucose protein transporters in the blood brain barrier were studied under chronic hyperglycemia, their concentrations remain constant but functionality and glucose intake were impaired (Mooradian & Morin 1991). However, under acute hyperglycemia induced by STZ, their concentration decreased suggesting different response at different stages of the disease

(Matthaei et al. 1986). Accordingly, protein transporters have shown strong association with diabetes development and progression as well as diabetic complications.

8. The effect of co-administration of gliclazide on bile acids & probiotics

Gliclazide is used in Type 2 diabetes (T2D) to stimulate insulin production but it also has beneficial extrapancreatic effects which makes it potentially useful in T1D. In fact, some T2D patients continue to use gliclazide even after their diabetes progresses to T1D since it provides better glycemic control than insulin alone. Gliclazide has three main structural features, an aromatic ring, a sulphonylurea group and an azabicyclic ring (Figure 2).

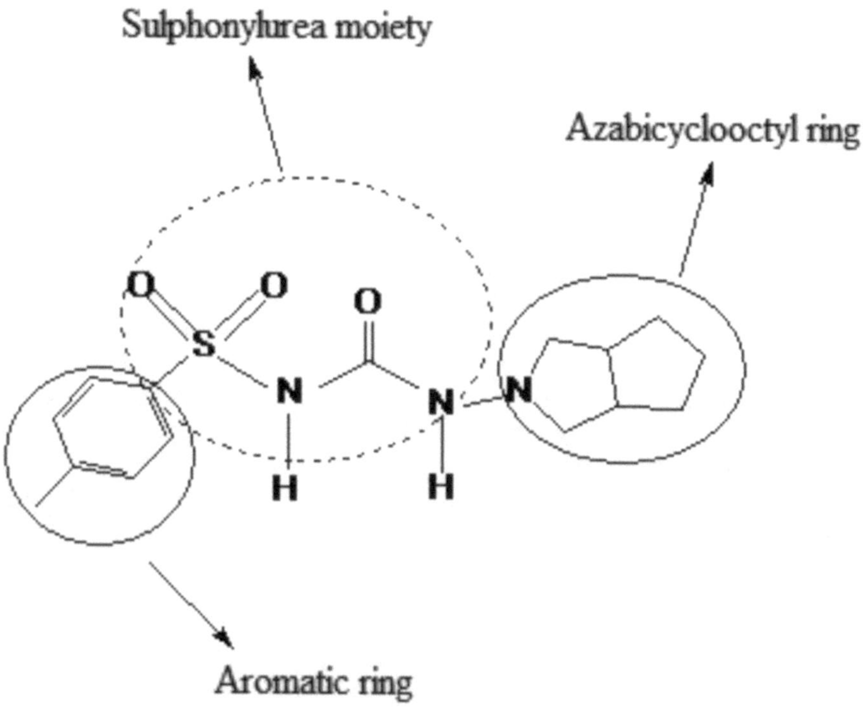

Fig. 2. The chemical structure of gliclazide with three main groups: aromatic ring, sulphonylurea moiety and azabicyclooctyle ring.

In a recent study investigating the applications of bile acids and probiotics in T1D, the bile acid analogue, MKC, was administered i.v. (four groups) and orally (four groups) to healthy, diabetic, probiotic pretreated healthy and probiotic pretreated diabetic rats. The pharmacokinetic parameters of MKC after i.v. administration were found to be similar in all four groups suggesting no significant differences in pharmacokinetic parameters between healthy and diabetic rats irrespective of probiotic pretreatment. C_{max} (maximum concentration), AUC (area under the curve) and F (bioavailability) values after oral administration to untreated healthy rats were also found similar to corresponding values in untreated diabetic rats suggesting similar mechanisms of absorption and systemic distribution of MKC. MKC also showed clear evidence of enterohepatic recycling with probiotic pretreatment delaying its absorption. This suggests different pharmacokinetic properties of the stable bile acid, MKC, in healthy rats compared with diabetic rats. This further supports the authors' previous findings showing that bile acid recirculation in diabetic animals is disturbed compared with healthy ones. When MKC was administered i.v. (to four groups) or orally (to four groups), there was no significant changes in blood glucose in any group of rats after the i.v. dose but, after oral administration to untreated diabetic rats, the elevated blood glucose level was significantly reduced from 23.6 ± 3.1 to 14.1 ± 2.4 mmol/l. Interestingly, diabetic rats pretreated with probiotics showed less weight loss, urine production and water consumption, and improvement in behaviour (curious, active) and survival rate than untreated diabetic rats. In a more recent study, the authors combined bile acid with an antidiabetic drug, gliclazide, and administered that to a rat model of T1D. Interestingly, and through unknown mechanism, the combination of MKC and gliclazide exerted a better hypoglycaemic effect to probiotic pretreated diabetic rats than MKC alone. In this study, pharmacokinetic parameters of i.v. MKC were not affected by the concomitant i.v. administration of gliclazide in either healthy or diabetic rats with and without probiotic pretreatment. Accordingly, even though exact mechanism of interaction, at the molecular level, between MKC and gliclazide is unknown, there is a clear synergistic effect between MKC, gliclazide and probiotic pretreatment in T1D resulting in a profound hypoglycaemic effect and sound reduction in the diabetic complications in those treated diabetic animals.

Overall, the authors confirmed that at the start of experiments, baseline blood glucose levels in each of the four groups (untreated and probiotic treated healthy and diabetic rats) were comparable. the authors also presented initial data supporting the effect of probiotics on the development of T1D. The administration of probiotics to healthy rats had no effect on blood glucose levels but the same treatment of diabetic rats reduced the elevated blood glucose levels by nearly 30% and improved clinical signs and symptoms. These findings present a clear synergistic effect between bile acids, probiotics and gliclazide. More importantly, it shows clearly that intervention by bile acids and probiotics exert a direct and significantly positive effect on glycemic control and the progression of diabetic complications. Even though the details of such effect remains unclear, multitherapeutic approach in treating diabetes showed better efficacy and continue to gain interest worldwide.

Having said that a likely explanation for the effect of probiotics is that they stimulate the GI mucosa to produce insulinotropic polypeptides (Cornell 1985) and glucagon-like peptide-1 (Raymond et al. 1981) and/or induce the gut microflora to release endotoxins which cause an increase in skeletal muscle glucose uptake (Raymond et al. 1980). Probiotic treatment alone was found to influence gliclazide permeation differently in health and diabetic animals (Al-Salami et al. 2008f) while the fact that administration of gliclazide following probiotic pretreatment did not further reduce glucose levels indicates the effect of probiotics is not due to stimulation of insulin release by residual pancreatic cells or to regeneration of functional pancreatic cells. Furthermore, i.v. administration of MKC to healthy and diabetic rats with and without probiotic pretreatment produced little effect. However, oral administration of MKC to diabetic rats produced a significant effect 3 hours after administration suggesting it arises from metabolic activation of MKC in the gut. The effect of oral MKC was not significant in probiotic pretreated diabetic rats that had lower blood glucose levels at the time of MKC administration possibly due to an interaction in the gut. The combination of gliclazide and MKC produced a greater effect in diabetic rats than MKC alone. This synergistic effect could be due to gliclazide enhancing the production and/or absorption of MKC active metabolites in the gut. The administration of gliclazide+MKC also produced the most significant reduction in blood glucose levels in probiotic pretreated diabetic rats (from 12.6 ± 2.0 to 10 ± 2.0 mmol/l, $p<0.01$). Overall, pretreatment with probiotics and subsequent oral administration of gliclazide+MKC resulted in the greatest effect in this model of T1D as well as in improved signs and symptoms in the animals. In healthy rats, neither probiotic treatment, nor oral administration of gliclazide, MKC or gliclazide+MKC had any effect on blood glucose levels. More interestingly, the authors hypothesized that the chronic treatment of diabetic rats with probiotics may have stimulated the metabolism of the stable bile acid, MKC, in a similar way as reported between cholic acid and *Lactobacilli* (Pigeon et al. 2002). The hypothesis of direct induction of probiotic treatment to bile acid metabolism may explain the therapeutic efficacy of probiotics in treating various disorders implementing a better role of bile acids in such therapeutic effects. Holding true, this should take us a step closer to understand better how probiotic administration exerted a hypoglycaemic effect, when administered alone, to T1D rats. This should also create a new approach to enhancing probiotic efficacy, through the concurrent administration with stable bile acids.

This multidrug therapy shows potential in T1D. This is illustrated by the reduction of blood glucose levels, improvement of diabetic symptoms, and the lower rate of diabetes development by alloxan when injected to rats pretreated with probiotics. Furthermore, the change in PK of gliclazide and MKC after probiotic pretreatment emphasizes the importance of not only investigating the use of probiotics in a disease state, but also investigating the influence of probiotics on drugs that could be used for such a disease. In addition, T1D clearly illustrates different gut biomorphology and response compared with healthy control which should be taken into account when discussing multidrug approach to the disease.

Gliclazide has been used for decades to treat T2D and thus future work should include applying the combination of probiotics, gliclazide and MKC on T2D rats then implications of the findings may be extrapolated to human subjects as appropriate. However, these findings should not be overplayed since variation in gliclazide pharmacokinetics is higher in human than rats (Palmer & Brogden 1993) which may limit further the applications of these findings in human.

One of the applications of the findings is the use of gliclazide, MKC and probiotics in T2D. T2D is characterized by hyperglycemia and hypercholesterolemia and thus bile acids have been used to lower cholesterol levels in diabetic patients (Goldfine 2008). Accordingly, the use of gliclazide, MKC and probiotics may improve glucose and cholesterol unbalance in T2D.

9. The effect of gut microflora and diet on inflammation

There is a great conclusion regarding the importance of gut microflora, made by Sir Henry Shaw (1818–1885): 'I have finally come to the conclusion that a good reliable set of bowels is worth more to a man than any quantity of brains'.

Many autoimmune and inflammatory diseases have shown positive response to probiotic and prebiotic treatments (Sherman et al. 2009; Tlaskalova-Hogenova et al. 2011). These diseases include acute gastroenteritis, antibiotic-associated diarrhoea and colitis, inflammatory bowel disease, type 1 diabetes, irritable bowel syndrome and necrotizing enterocolitis. The composition of the intestinal microflora may also affect mammalian physiology outside the gastrointestinal tract. Recent studies have shown significant changes in gut microfloral and bile acid compositions in T1D (Jaakkola et al. 2003; Siow et al. 1991; Slivka et al. 1979b; Uchida et al. 1979; Uchida et al. 1985). Thus, it is clear that our symbiotic microflora award many metabolic capabilities that our mammalian genomes lack (Zaneveld et al. 2008), and so therapeutics that target microfloral modulation may prove rewarding. When the newborn baby leaves the germ free uterus, she/he enters a highly contaminated extra-uterus environment. This requires the activation of her/his immune system to prevent infection. Over the period of the first year, the newborn's intestinal microflora develops and its composition becomes her/his gut microfloral fingerprint! Gut microflora has been shown to play a major rule in controlling the inflammatory response of the host immune system through direct and indirect bacteria-bacteria and bacteria-host interactions. These interactions include physical and metabolic functions of the gut microfloral bacteria, which protect the intestinal tract from foreign pathogenic bacteria, eliminate the presence of unwanted bacteria through producing bacteriocins and other chemicals, and inform the gut epithelium and the host immune system about whether a local inflammatory response is needed (Shi & Walker 2004; Walker 2008b). Gut microflora can control the host immune system through four main actions. The induction of IgA secretion to protect against infection, triggers localized inflammatory responses, neutralizing T-helper (Th) cell response and also contributing to the induction or inhibition of generalized mucosal immune responses. Recent studies have shown that in autoimmune diseases and gut inflammation disorders, there is a significant disturbances in the ratios of Th cells such as the increase in the Th-2/Th-1 ratio associated with inflammatory bowel diseases, which has been linked to exacerbation of the gut inflammation and the development of the disease. In recent studies, gut-associated dendritic cells in the lamina propria can extend their appendices reaching the gut mucosa and using their Toll-like receptors (TLR) 2 and 4, to sample bacterial metabolites (Rescigno et al. 2001; von & Nepom 2009a). This may result in dendritic cells releasing certain cytokines that stimulate the activation of naive Th-0 into active Th- cells such as 1, 2 and 3/1 (von & Nepom 2009b; Walker 2008b). Interestingly, some microfloral bacteria can actually cross enterocytic microfolds and interact with antigen presenting immune cells in mesenteric lymph nodes to activate naive plasma cells into IgA-producing B cells (Macpherson & Uhr 2004). IgA coats the intestinal mucosa and control further bacterial penetration thus protecting the host from potential pathogenic bacteria. Even more interestingly, gut microflora bacteria have shown ability to not only initiate an inflammatory response but also to control and inhibit such a response. Some microfloral bacteria or their metabolites can interact with the intracellular receptor TLR-9, to which the bacteria activates T cells through the production of potent anti-inflammatory cytokines such as IL-10 (Rachmilewitz et al. 2004). Microfloral bacteria can also produce small molecules that can enter intestinal epithelial cells to inhibit activation of nuclear factor kappa-light-chain-enhancer of activated beta-cells (NFkB) (Neish et al. 2000). Moreover, prolonged exposure to bacterial endotoxins, in particular, LPS (which interacts with TLR 2 and 4) can activate intracellular anti-inflammatory associated proteins that result in an overall anti-inflammatory effect (Otte & Podolsky 2004). Such gut bacterial-host interactions are critical in maintaining a balanced and effective immune response to various infections while maintaining control over prolonged or chronic inflammation and reducing the overstimulation of the host immune system.

Recent evidence suggests that a particular gut microfloral community may favour occurrence of the metabolic diseases. It is well know that the composition of gut microflora changes with diet and also as we age (Rebole et al. 2010; Respondek et al. 2008; Yen et al. 2011). In one study, a high fat diet was associated with higher endotoxaemia and a lowering of bifidobacterium species in mice cecum (Cani et al. 2008). In a follow up study, the administration of prebiotics, in particular, oligofructose, to mice given high fat diet, restored the reduced quantity of bifidobacterium. This also resulted in reducing metabolic endotoxaemia, the inflammatory tone and slowing the development of diabetes. In this study and compared with control mice on chow diet, high fat diet significantly reduced intestinal Gram negative and Gram positive gut bacteria, increased endotoxaemia and diabetes-associated inflammation. However, when diabetic mice on high fat diet were given oligofructose, metabolic normalization took place including the quantity of gut bifidobacteria. In these mice, multiple correlation analyses showed that endotoxaemia negatively correlated with bifidobacteria quantity. By the same token, bifidobacterium quantity significantly and positively correlated with improved glucose tolerance, glucose-induced insulin secretion and normalised inflammatory tone (decreased endotoxaemia and plasma and adipose tissue proinflammatory cytokines) (Cani et al. 2007). In general, the level of microfloral diversity and gut bifidobacteria in human, relate to health status and both decrease with age (Hopkins & Macfarlane 2002).

Compromised gut movement associated with diabetes can result in substantial bacterial and yeast overgrowth which is postulated to disturb bile acids composition and exacerbate the diabetes-associated inflammation (Cani et al. 2009; Fox et al. 2010). Diabetes inflammation and bile acids disturbances can cause chemical unbalance that has been linked to poor tissue sensitivity to insulin (Maki et al. 1995), rise in the levels of reactive radicals in the blood (Jain et al. 2002), poor enterohepatic recirculation and negatively affecting liver detoxification and performance (Oktar et al. 2001; Quraishy et al. 1996). Accordingly, future diabetes therapy should not only focus on rectifying glucose imbalance but also in targeting the disturbances in bile acids composition and the inflammation cascade initiated in the gut. This can be achieved through normalizing the composition of bile acids and microflora, gut immune-response and microflora-epithelial interactions towards maintaining normal biochemical reactions and healthy body physiology. Physiological features of human development including the innate and adaptive immunity, immune tolerance, bioavailability of nutrients, and intestinal barrier functions, are directly related to the composition and functionality of the human microflora. This includes the percentages of what is currently known as good and bad gut microflora. Good microflora includes two main species, Lactobacillius and Bifidobacteria. Microflora modifications may take place due to antibiotics consumption, prebiotic and probiotics administration and the use of drugs which affect gastric motility resulting in changes in gastric pH and gut-emptying rate. These modifications have been shown to be significantly profound in diabetic subjects resulting in the reduction of the percentage of good bacteria, the increase of the percentage of bad bacteria and yeasts and the consequent increase in the percentage of toxic bile salts such as lithocholic acid. This can also contribute to the higher incidence of gall stones and liver necrosis reported in diabetic patients. Accordingly, probiotics can introduce missing microbial components with known beneficial functions for the human host, while prebiotics can enhance the proliferation of beneficial microbes or probiotics, resulting in sustainable changes in the human microflora. Symbiotic relationship between probiotics and prebiotic administration is expected to exert a synergistic effect and in the right dose, may normalize and even reverse dysbiosis-associated complications.

10. The applications of probiotics in diabetes

Probiotics are dietary supplements containing bacteria which, when administered in adequate amounts, confer a health benefit on the host (FAO/WHO 2002). Combinations of different bacterial strains can be used (Bezkorovainy 2001) but a mixture of *Lactobacilli* and *Bifidobacteria* is a common choice (Karimi & Pena 2003). Probiotics have been shown to be beneficial in wide range of conditions including infections, allergies, metabolic disorders such as diabetes mellitus, ulcerative colitis and Crohn's disease (Altenhoefer et al. 2004; Rozanova et al. 2002; Ziegler et al. 2003).

There are reports in the literature that probiotic treatment can be useful in diabetes (Al-Salami et al. 2008b) but there is little explanation of the mechanisms involved. The initial site of diabetogenic cells has been hypothesized to be in the gut whereas pancreatic lymph nodes serve as the site of amplification of the autoimmune response (Jacobs et al. 1989). This autoimmune response may disturb the composition of the normal gut flora. Treatment with *Bifidobacteria* and *Lactobacilli* has been shown to normalize the composition of the gut flora in children with T1D (Rozanova et al. 2002). In addition, the administration of *Lactobacilli* to alloxan-induced diabetic mice prolonged their survival (Matsuzaki et al. 1997a) and administration to non-obese diabetic (NOD, a rodent model of T1D) mice inhibited diabetes development possibly by the regulation of the host immune response and reduction of nitric oxide production (Matsuzaki et al. 1997b). Furthermore, the administration of a mixture of *Bifidobacteria, Lactobacilli* and *Streptococci* to NOD mice was protective against T1D development postulated to be through induction of interleukins IL4 and IL10 (Calcinaro et al. 2005).

Slowing of peristalsis (gastroparesis) has been reported in T1D patients. This can result in a bigger population of bacteria in the gut and a subsequent rise in the concentration of secondary bile acids (Meinders et al. 1981a) such as lithocholic acid which is toxic at high concentrations and can induce gut inflammation and blood dyscrasias (Malavolti et al. 1989; Miyai et al. 1982). In addition, the disturbed bile acid composition in T1D (Meinders et al. 1981a) is strongly linked with autoimmune and liver diseases. The administration of *Lactobacilli* and *Bifidobacteria* may restore the bile acid composition (Kurdi et al. 2000; Kurdi et al. 2006). It is important to select the right probiotic species based on efficacy, stability in

Probiotic strain	pH tolerability	Bile tolerability
Lactobacillus rhamnosus	At pH < 2 (after 2 hours) reduction by 2 - 3 log CFU/ml At pH < 1 (after 2 hours), reduction by 6 – 8 log CFU/ml (Succi et al. 2005).	Good survival rate in 3% bile salts for up to 24 hours (Succi et al. 2005).
Lactobacillus acidophilus	At pH < 1 (after 1 hour), reduction by 1 log CFU/ml (Favaro-Trindade & Grosso 2002).	Good survival rate in 4% bile for up to 12 hours (Favaro-Trindade & Grosso 2002).
Bifidobacterium lactis	At pH < 1 (after 1 hour), reduction by 1 log CFU/ml (Favaro-Trindade & Grosso 2002).	Good survival rate in 4% bile for up to 12 hours (Favaro-Trindade & Grosso 2002).

Table 1. pH and bile tolerability of Lactobacillus rhamnosus, Lactobacillus acidophilus and Bifidobacterium lactis.

the gut (bile and pH tolerability) and long term safety. Lactobacillus rhamnosus, Lactobacillus acidophilus and Bifidobacterium lactis show good bile and pH tolerability under normal conditions of pH (1.5-8) and bile acid concentration (0.8 - 3 %) (Table 1), in addition to long term safety (Franz & Bode 1973; Hedenborg & Norman 1984; Hedenborg & Norman 1985).

11. Bile acids as absorption enhancers in Type 1 diabetes therapy

Bile acids and their derivatives can act as absorption enhancers where they are capable of promoting mucosal and systemic drug absorption. Bile acids and their derivatives can increase drug bioavailability, allowing therapeutic doses to be administered by several routes. Bile acids as therapeutic agents have the potential to produce beneficial effects in improving primary biliary cirrhosis and primary sclerosing cholangitis. Bile acids can also control endocrine signalling and enzymatic activities in various disorders. This includes inflammatory diseases (such as diabetes) and cholestatic liver disease in cystic fibrosis.

Permeation of a drug through a biological membranes by passive diffusion is influenced by the drug's solubility and molecular weight, the thickness of both, the mucous and the cytoplasmic membrane, while drug diffusibility is influenced by permeability, surface area and the concentration gradient (Higgins & Gottesman 1992; Maki et al. 2003; Mao & Unadkat 2005; Neubert et al. 1987).

Bile salts (conjugated bile acids) are known to increase the permeation of many drugs. They increase the permeability of the mucosal membrane by breaking down mucous and disrupting cells, thus widening the tight junctions between these cells. This enhances penetration of drugs via the paracellular route. Bile salts can also improve transcellular absorption by increasing drug solubility and dissolution rate. Bile salts can form micelles which increase the permeability of the mucosal membrane by overcoming resistance at the aqueous diffusion layer. They also enhance drug delivery by interacting with membrane lipids and proteins that affect membrane fluidity and the rate of drug trafficking.

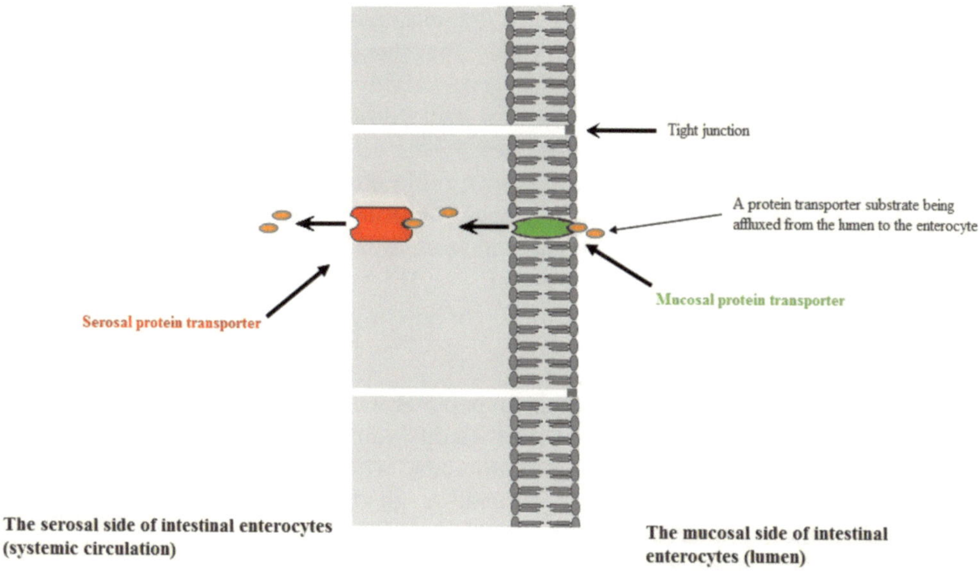

Fig. 3. Protein transporters in the mucosal and serosal sides of the gut enterocytes.

Recent studies suggest a bigger role for Mdr and Mrp transporters in the enterohepatic recirculation of bile acids (Asamoto et al. 2001). Mrp2 and Mrp3 recognize monovalent (those with a single charge) and divalent (those with a double charge) bile acids as their substrates (St-Pierre et al. 2000; St-Pierre et al. 2001; Zollner et al. 2003) while Mdr1 and Mdr3 recognise bile acid taurocholate, glutathione, bile salt glucuronide and sulfate conjugates (Ballatori et al. 2005a; Ballatori et al. 2005b). Mrp2 is located in the apical membrane of the bile canaliculus where it removes newly formed divalent bile acids into the bile duct. Mrp3 is located in the basolateral membrane of the ileal enterocytes where it removes monovalent bile acids from the gut lumen into the portal vein (Houten et al. 2006a). Figure 3 shows the locations of a mucosal and a serosal protein transporters (mucosal transporter is in green & serosal transporter is in red) expressed in enterocytes.

12. Oral absorption

Drug oral administration is the most convenient and popular route of drug delivery. However, some drugs have low bioavailability and slow absorption rate, thus limited efficacy. Bile salts have been shown to increase the absorption of intestinal insulin by masking its hydrophilic surface resulting in higher permeation through the ileal mucosa and into the systemic circulation, thus enhancing insulin bioavailability. In one study, insulin was formulated with different bile salts and administered orally to rabbits. Bile salts enhanced insulin permeation through the ileal mucosa and resulted in a significant effect which varied based on the type of bile salt used (Mesiha et al. 2002a). When insulin was administered with palmitic acid combined with bile salts, in the form of aqueous fatty acid solution, significant hypoglycaemic effects was observed in the treated diabetic animals. In an aqueous environment, insulin's hypoglycaemic effect was improved by the addition of glycocholate and, to a lesser extent, cholate. Accordingly, bile salts improved insulin's hypoglycaemic effect in the following descending order; sodium deoxycholate > sodium cholate > sodium glycocholate > sodium glycodeoxycholate > sodium taurodeoxycholate (Mesiha et al. 2002b). In general, there are few examples of known bile salt derivatives which are known absorption enhancers. Cholylsarcosine (CS) is an absorption enhancer as well as a non-toxic bile salt derivative. It has good stability and safety profile and is resistant to bacterial degradation in the gastrointestinal tract (Mesiha et al. 2002c; Mikov & Fawcett 2006b). Due to its stability, it does not form deoxycholic acid which can cause hepatotoxicity. Chenodeoxycholic acid and cholyltaurine were more effective than CS, but due to their susceptibility to bacterial degradation, they have poor safety profile. The applications of bile salts as absorption enhances is gaining more interest, especially with the ocular, transermal, nasal, buccal and rectal mucosal routes.

13. Occular absorption

Due to the normally high rates of lacrimation and tear wash-out, occular drug delivery has low efficiency and requires the drug to have high diffusibility through the anterior region of the eye Figure 4. However, when a drug is formulated with a suitable abortion enhancer, its permeation can be doubled or even tripled. A good example of bile salts occular applications is the administration of insulin. In one study that investigated the occular permeation of insulin, less than 1% of insulin reached the systemic circulation via the ocular route. The addition of some absorption enhancers may improve the permeation to around

4%. This still remains a limiting factor in insulin clinical applications (25). An estimated 80% of administered drug is eliminated through the nasal cavity after occular application (26). Another study (Yamamoto et al. 1989) determined the extent to which absorption promoters could enhance the absorption of insulin via the ocular route. When administered alone, occular insulin serum levels reached Cmax within 15 minutes of occular administration while when formulated with sodium glycocholate, sodium taurocholate and sodium deoxycholate (as absorption enhancers), insulin Cmax was reached within 5 minutes. When insulin was co-administered with sodium glycocholate, the amount of insulin permeating the eyes and reaching the systemic circulation increased from 1% to 5.5%. Sodium deoxycholate was found to be more effective and sodium taurocholate least effective at enhancing the occular absorption of insulin. This implies a good potential of bile acid applications in insulin occular delivery in T1D, when other routes as less desirable.

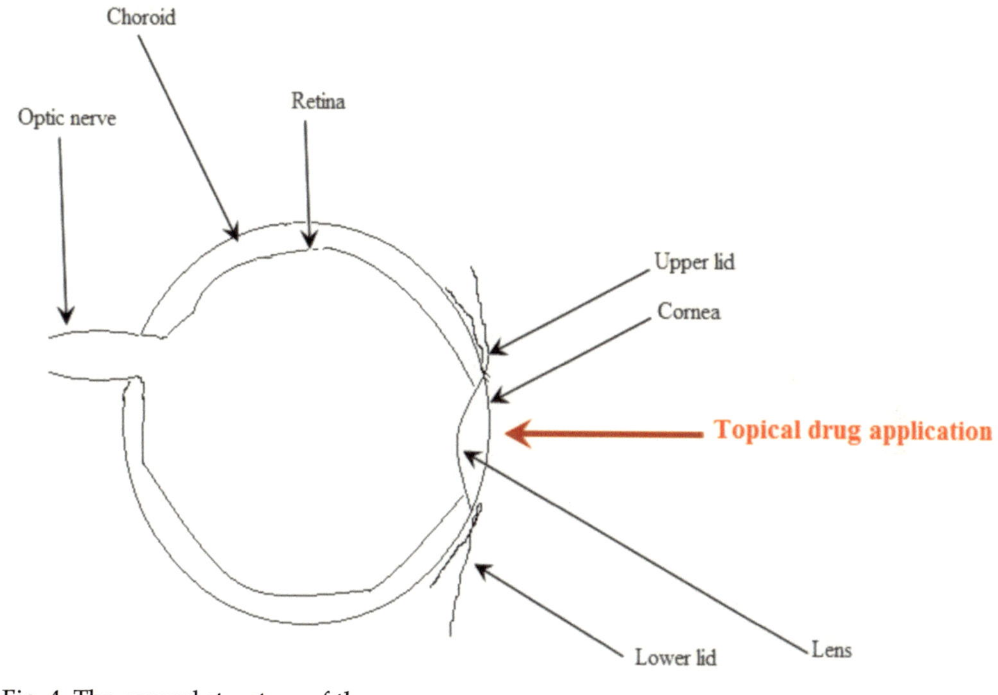

Fig. 4. The general structure of the eye.

14. Nasal absorption

The Nasal route is a convenient and popular method of drug administration as it is feasible and it has fast absorption rate. It also provides reasonable bioavailability as it bypasses first pass hepatic metabolism. However, pharmacologically active peptides such as hormones and proteins with molecular weights > 10 kDa do not have the ability to permeate the nasal mucosal layer without being significantly trapped, washed out (through the nasopharyngeal cavity), or degraded before reaching the systemic circulation. In order to optimise nasal drug delivery to drugs such as insulin, suitable permeation enhancers such as bile salts may be appropriate. For insulin to be delivered nasally, it has to permeate the nasal mucosa and into the systemic circulation (nasal vasculature). Large peptides such as insulin are not easily absorbed through the nasal mucosa when administered via a nasal spray (Hirai et al. 1978). Insulin must be transported between or through the apical and basal membranes of columnar cells, basal cells and capillary endothelial cells of blood vessels (Figure 5) (Gordon et al. 1985a; Li et al. 1992). However, it must first cross the mucous layer which varies in thickness averaging between 5 and 20 mm in depth. Mucociliary clearance washes out mucous and entrapped particles from the anterior to the posterior nasal cavity and down the oesophagus. Drugs administered through the nasal route must dissolve rapidly in the mucous before reaching the epithelium. The drug must then move between tight junctions, survive the intercellular matrix and diffuse between the basolateral cells to reach the subepithelial space through which it can enter the nasal vasculature (Junginger 1992). Bile salts exert their permeation enhancing effect through solubilising cellular proteins, membrane phospholipids and through limiting the effect of metabolizing enzymes. Although the exact mechanism by which bile salts solubilise cellular components without necessarily damaging tissues is unknown, bile salts enhance absorption of drugs across membranes. The solubilisation of membrane components may be related to the ability of bile acids to overcome nasal membrane barrier resistance (Shao et al. 1992a). In one study (Shao et al. 1992b), the effect of bile salts on the structure, integrity, configuration and strength of the nasal mucosa, was study. The effect was investigated through administering bile salts to animal's nasal cavity then measuring the levels of cellular proteins (in the cell membrane and the cytoplasm), DNA-metabolizing enzymes and other biomarkers. The study concluded that deoxycholate caused the greatest solubilising effect on the nasal mucosa while taurocholate caused the least effect. Another study (Gordon et al. 1985a) was carried out in human, to investigate the physicochemical properties of bile salts and their relations to the permeation effect in nasal drug delivery. As expected, the rate of absorption of drug molecules was directly correlated to the bile salt's lipophilicity and their permeation effect. The most effective permeation enhancer, through the nasal mucosa, was deoxycholate, followed by, chenodeoxycholate, cholate then finally ursodeoxycholate.

However, large or too frequent doses of bile salts have been found to cause significant damage to the nasal mucosa and subsequent nasal bleeding (Hersey & Jackson 1987a). Moreover, enhancing further the nasal absorption of an insulin-bile salt formulation, through the use of starch microspheres, has been investigated (Illum et al. 2001). Microspheres are non-toxic and biocompatible with rabbit nasal mucosa (Bjork et al. 1991). Illum *et al.* examined the effect of starch microspheres on the absorption enhancing efficiency of bile salts in formulations with insulin, after application in the nasal cavity of sheep. The enhancers were selected on the basis of their perceived or proven mechanism of action and worked predominantly by interacting with the lipid membrane. The microsphere formulation was placed in the anterior part of the nasal cavity where few cilia are present. The bioadhesive properties provide a high drug concentration in close contact with the epithelial surface for an extended time period. Generally, microspheres can assist the passage of small drug molecules but an absorption enhancer is necessary for polypeptides with molecular weights above 6000 Da. Bioadhesive starch microspheres synergistically increase the effect of absorption enhancers on the absorption of insulin across the nasal membrane in sheep. The bioadhesive starch microspheres were shown to increase synergistically the effect of the bile salts on the transport of the insulin across the nasal mucosa. So when bile salts were used in conjunction with bioadhesive starch microspheres, they increased the amount of absorption by a factor ranging from 1 to 5, compared to bile salts alone (Illum et al. 2001). Such maximization of insulin-bile salt mucosal permeation was successful to enhance insulin absorption through the nasal mucosa, and thus shows great potential in insulin nasal delivery.

The ability of a bile acid to enhance permeation is heavily dependent on its hydroxyl groups and the concentration of bile acid present in solution. Insulin absorption increases when the concentration of bile salt exceeds its aqueous critical mice concentration (CMC). The amount of insulin absorbed also increases with increasing hydrophobicity of the bile salt. The order of bile salts' ability to increase insulin absorption is DCA>CDCA>CA>UDCA (Gordon et al. 1985b). When sodium deoxycholate, the most hydrophobic bile salt, is co-administered with insulin, the absorbed insulin causes more than 30% reduction in blood glucose levels in diabetic subjects (Moses et al. 1983). When a bile salt possess poor hydrophobicity, its efficacy is significantly reduced. When the highly hydrophilic sodium ursodeoxycholate is formulated with insulin then administered to diabetic subjects, the bile salt showed no significant permeation enhancing effect on insulin, and almost no decrease in blood sugar was reported in the treated diabetic subjects. Bile salts may increase the absorption of insulin by forming micelles in which the insulin resides in high concentrations. Another proposed mechanism is that bile acids form reverse micelles which form channels across the nasal membrane through which insulin can move to reach the bloodstream (Gordon et al. 1985b). Bile salts may also bind and trap Ca^{2+} causing tight junctions to loosen and allowing insulin to pass. In addition, sodium lauryl sulphate (SLS) may enhance drug absorption via the nasal route by lyzing biological membranes. This involves lipid solubilisation and subsequent protein denaturation and dissolution (Donovan et al. 1990). Accordingly, SLS has a unique ability to enhance absorption efficiently and at low concentration.

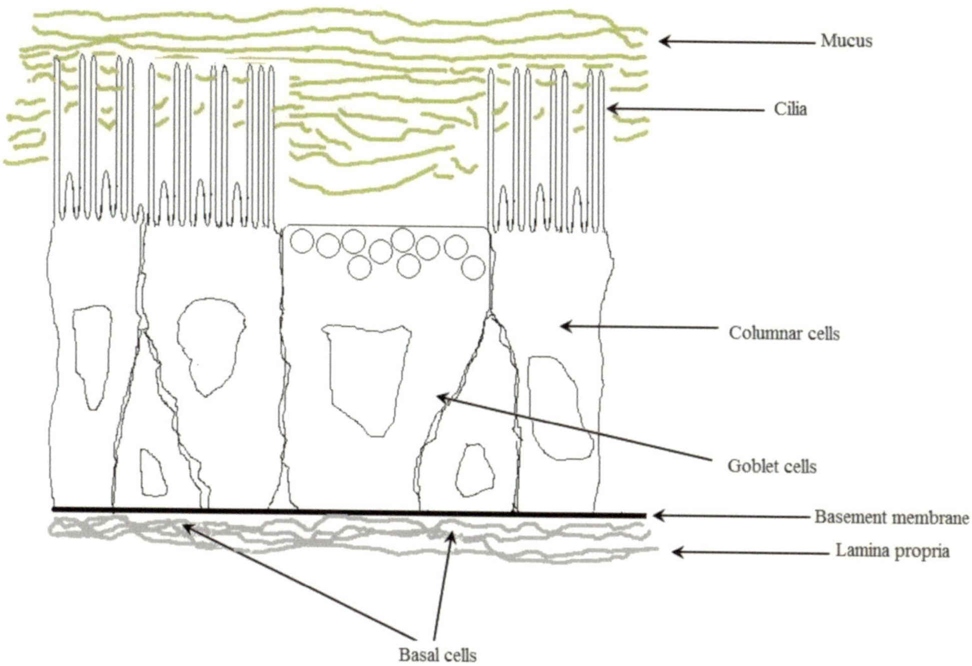

Fig. 5. The mucosal layer of the nasal cavity.

15. Rectal absorption

The rectum is the final part of the intestinal tract and about 4-5 inches long. It is the part of the gastrointestinal tract that extends from the colon in the lower left part of the abdomen to the anus. Its temperature is the same as the body temperature, constant at 37 °C. For insulin to be administered rectally, it needs to pass through the rectal epithelia, lamina propria and muscularis mucosa. The rectum has a rich vasculature making it a good site for drug administration.

For maximum absorption, insulin suppositories should not be inserted too high into the rectum since the superior rectal vein takes blood straight to the liver, where first pass effect is taking place. Inserting insulin to the lower part of the rectum will result in insulin permeation to the inferior or middle rectal veins which drain into the inferior vena cava bypassing the liver and avoiding first pass metabolism. However, reaching the higher part of the colon is not feasible thus rendering insulin rectal delivery ineffective. Enhancing insulin rectal absorption can be achieved using bile salts (Sayani & Chien 1996).

Bile acids have shown good efficacy in enhancing rectal absorption when complexed with or added to drug formulations. In human, INF-α, an antiviral, antineoplastic and immunoregulatory molecule, was not absorbed when administered rectally in a hydrophilic suppository, but when sodium ursodeoxycholate was incorporated into the suppository base, detectable levels were obtained (Lee et al. 1991; Lee 1991). By the same token, the effect of bile salts in insulin rectal absorption was investigated. Rectal administration with 5% sodium glycocholate produced a large increase in the effect of a 10 U/kg dose. Rectal and nasal administration reduced plasma glucose approximately half as effectively as intramuscular insulin in the presence of this bile salt (Aungst & Rogers 1988). This method of administration may be beneficial to those requiring only small doses of insulin or those uncomfortable with injection. Thus, it is clear that bile salts are effective promoters for rectal administration of insulin. The proposed mechanism of action involves enhanced membrane permeability, lipid solubilizing and the inhibition of proteolytic enzymes at the absorption site. However, rectal drug administration remains unfavorable and invasive and thus remains a major limitation for such a drug delivery system.

16. Pulmonary absorption

Pulmonary drug delivery is effective due to fast and convenient drug absorption. Lungs have rich vasculature and their blood output bypasses the liver metabolism, resulting in high drug bioavailability. It is commonly used to deliver anti-inflammatory therapeutics such as in asthma treatment. To maximize drug permeation through the lungs, reducing particle size may be appropriate. Particle size less than 5 μm ensures high absorbability but very low particle size (1 μm or less) makes particle-expulsion most likely and thus renders drug ineffective (Agu et al. 2001a; Agu et al. 2001b). Administration of insulin through inhalation may be effective but faces many challenges including mucous, mucociliary clearance, lung surfactants and proteases and peptidases at the alveolar surface (Heinemann et al. 2000). The addition of bile acids to insulin should minimise such challenges through enhancing mucus permeation and reducing enzymatic degradation. This is particularly interesting since current subcutaneous insulin injection causes wide range of side effects such as irritation and scarring as well as being highly unfavourable by patients due to its invasiveness and discomfort. In one study (45), the bioavailability of inhaled insulin was measured with and without the addition of bile acids. The bioavailability of inhaled insulin was 7.8% but, with the addition of a bile acid, absolute bioavailability reached 10.2% ($p < 0.05$). This was a small but significant increase which presents bile acids as permeation enhancers in pulmonary drug applications. Bile acids could have enhanced insulin effect through exerting their own hypoglycemic effect causing a further reduction in glucose levels after administration with insulin. The study also reported that the onset of the hypoglycemic effect after insulin inhalation with bile acids was more than ten times faster, then when insulin was injected SC alone. However, interpatient variation was large in terms of hypoglycemia, which was a disadvantage for such a method of insulin delivery. In other studies (Agu et al. 2001a; Agu et al. 2001b), insulin was administered via the lung with and without sodium glycocholate. The addition of 1% sodium glycocholate inhibited insulin degradation within the lung. Although neither the types of proteolytic enzymes involved in insulin hydrolysis nor the specific mode of stabilization by bile acids were investigated, sodium glycocholate was suggested to be an aminopeptidase inhibitor. Bile acids wide use in pulmonary drug formulation is limited by their safety profile. at the dose required to increase absorption, bile acids are non-toxic and relatively safe. However, when aspirated in large amounts, bile acids have been shown to cause pulmonary oedema and haemorrhage due to dissolution of pulmonary membranes (Kaneko et al. 1990).

17. Bile acids as hypoglycemic agents

Recent studies have shown that the semisynthetic bile acid analogue, 12-monoketocholic acid (MKC) exerted a significant hypoglycemic effect when administered alone to a rat model of T1D. When administered with insulin, MKC exerted a synergistic effect potentiating the hypoglycemic effect of insulin (Kuhajda et al. 2000; Mikov et al. 2008). MKC hypoglycemic effect was studied using various formulations including the oral, nasal, ocular and rectal applications. Then, the hypoglycemic effect was compared with that of insulin injected subcutaneously. The mixture of MKC and insulin also tested for hypoglycemic activity. Nasal administration of the insulin-MKC mixture resulted in a decrease of blood glucose concentration that reached 54% of that obtained after subcutaneous application of insulin. However, following nasal administration of the MKC, the decrease in blood glucose reached 36% of that obtained after subcutaneous application of insulin. The discovery of a link between bile acids and glucose regulation offers a new perspective in the design of hypoglycaemic drugs in treating diabetes (Miljkovic et al. 2000). The mechanisms by which, bile acids such as MKC exerts its hypoglycemic effect in T1D, was explored further. The hypoglycemic effect of bile acids on T1D rats could be explained through their effect on FXR and PPARs metabolic pathways (Houten et al. 2006b; Trauner et al. 2010). However such mechanisms remain to be fully characterized.

18. Safety of bile acids and probiotics

Many studies have been conducted to test the toxicity and safety of primary and secondary bile salts and their derivatives. Some bile salts have excellent safety profiles while others are not safe. Bile salts can be used as therapeutic agents, as absorption enhancers and as formulation excipients. Deoxycholic acid is used in manufacturing steroids and in vaccine production (e.g. influenza vaccine). However, its use is severely limited by its narrow safety profile. In relatively high doses, deoxycholic acid can cause hepatotoxicity and can damage the gastric mucosa. Cholylsarcosine (CS) is a stable bile salt derivative of deoxycholic acid. It resists bacterial activation to the more toxic bile acid, deoxycholic acid, and thus has a good safety profile. It is commonly used as an absorption enhancer in the treatment of primary biliary cirrhosis (Ricci et al. 1998). Deoxycholic acid salt is also used in the formulation of Amphotericin B, which is commonly used for treating fungal infections of the eyes (Samiy et al. 1996). However, due to its limited safety profile, Amphotericin B in doses as low as 1 μg has been shown to cause retinal damage despite the fact that the recommended dose is 5-10 μg (Souri & Green 1974). The administration of Amphotericin B deoxycholate may also result in cataract formation, opacity, retinal necrosis and retinal ganglion cell loss (Cannon et al. 2003).

When it comes to predicting the toxicity of bile salts, it seems that toxicity increases with their permeation ability. The more capable bile salts are to solubilizing membrane proteins, the more toxic they are (Shao et al. 1992a). In one study (Hersey & Jackson 1987b), bile acids damaged nasal epithelium causing nasal irritation, congestion and bleeding. The authors concluded that nasal applications of bile salts should be limited with infrequent dosing regimen.

Formulation of bile salts in inhalations can cause pulmonary oedema, when inhaled in large quantities. This is due to the solubilization and dissolution of the pulmonary membranes and pulmonary hemorrhage (Kaneko et al. 1990). However, such side effects are only caused by largely inhaled doses.

Probiotic administration has shown good safety profile in individuals with overall good health status, and may be suffering from mild infections or GI disorders (Luoto et al. 2010). Probiotic safety stems from the fact that many strains are of human origin and present in large numbers in human GIT (Rozanova & Voevodin 2008). Accordingly, the reported incidences of probiotics inducing bacterial infection and bacteremia are very low (Snydman 2008). The only major concern with probiotic administration is the potential of bacterial translocation resulting in the induction of antibiotic-resistance strains that may lead to pathogenesis and haemodyscrasia (Liong 2008; Snydman 2008). Having said that risks of infections caused by probiotic treatment is expected to be significant in immunocompromised patients (Marteau & Shanahan 2003; Rayes et al. 2005).

If the use of probiotics and bile acids is to become part of T1D therapy, their safety concerns may be overcome by thoroughly studying appropriate dosing and frequency, their short and long term effect on mucosal membranes and the variation of their effect in different populations.

19. Conclusion

Conjugated bile acids (bile salts) can form micelles that solubilise and transport lipids across biological membranes. Bile acids as absorption promoters have the potential to aid intestinal, ocular, nasal, pulmonary and rectal absorption of insulin. Bile acids are hypoglycemic agents on their own and thus can be used as adjunct therapy in treating T1D. However, in high concentrations, bile acids may damage tissue, so it is important to examine their safety profile thoroughly before application e.g. in buccal formulations as there is conflicting evidence on the morphological changes that occur in the buccal epithelium upon contact with bile acids. However, such an improvement in insulin absorption is still insufficient and subcutaneous injection remains the commonly used method. Nasal administration has certain advantages such as ease of use and high bioavailability. However, it does not allow transport of high molecular weight proteins and peptides. Bile acids have demonstrated the ability to enhance the nasal absorption of insulin and other drugs. One of the main disadvantages of the applications of bile acids as permeation enhancers is that the greater the bile acid is at promoting permeation of through mucosa, the more toxic it becomes. Accordingly, it is important to determine the mechanism of action by which bile acids enhance absorption in order to design absorption promoting agents that are not toxic or irritant. In addition, knowledge of the mechanism of action may allow prediction of the exact amount of a therapeutic substance that will reach the systemic circulation. The metabolism and deconjugation of bile acids are brought about by the gut microflora. Interestingly, gut microflora plays a major rule in energy balance and gut inflammation. Probiotics have shown hypoglycemic effect, when administered alone, thus, their use in T1D should be studied further.

Type 1 diabetes and its complications cannot be cured by the best most intensive insulin therapy (Shamoon et al. 1993). This clearly emphasizes the fact that the disease is more complex, interdependent, and challenging to treat than being a simple hyperglycemia. That is why, in our opinion, multidrug approach which integrates a comprehensive, targeted, and tailored treatment should guarantee the best outcome for diabetic patients.

20. Acknowledgement

This work has been supported by Ministry of Science and Technology of Serbia Research grant No 41012.

21. References

Agu, R.U., Jorissen, M., Willems, T., Augustijns, P., Kinget, R. & Verbeke, N. (2001a) In-vitro nasal drug delivery studies: comparison of derivatised, fibrillar and polymerised collagen matrix-based human nasal primary culture systems for nasal drug delivery studies. *Journal of Pharmacy and Pharmacology*, 53, 1447-1456.

Agu, R.U., Ugwoke, M.I., Armand, M., Kinget, R. & Verbeke, N. (2001b) The lung as a route for systemic delivery of therapeutic proteins and peptides. *Respiratory Research*, 2, 198-209.

Akerblom, H.K., Vaarala, O., Hyoty, H., Ilonen, J. & Knip, M. (2002) Environmental factors in the etiology of type 1 diabetes. 115, 18-29.

Al-Salami, H., Butt, G., Fawcett, J.P., Tucker, I.G., Golocorbin-Kon, S. & Mikov, M. (2008a) Probiotic treatment reduces blood glucose levels and increases systemic absorption of gliclazide in diabetic rats. *Eur.J.Drug Metab Pharmacokinet.*, 33, 101-106.

Al-Salami, H., Butt, G., Fawcett, J.P., Tucker, I.G., Golocorbin-Kon, S. & Mikov, M. (2008b) Probiotic treatment reduces blood glucose levels and increases systemic absorption of gliclazide in diabetic rats. *European Journal of Drug Metabolism and Pharmacokinetics*, 33, 101-106.

Al-Salami, H., Butt, G., Tucker, I., Fawcett, P.J., Golocorbin-Kon, S., Mikov, I. & Mikov, M. (2009a) Gliclazide reduces MKC intestinal transport in healthy but not diabetic rats. *European Journal of Drug Metabolism and Pharmacokinetics*, 34, 43-50.

Al-Salami, H., Butt, G., Tucker, I. & Mikov, M. (2008c) Influence of the semisynthetic bile acid (MKC) on the ileal permeation of gliclazide in healthy and diabetic rats. *Pharmacol.Rep.*, 60, 532-541.

Al-Salami, H., Butt, G., Tucker, I. & Mikov, M. (2008d) Influence of the semisynthetic bile acid MKC on the ileal permeation of gliclazide ex vivo in healthy and diabetic rats treated with probiotics. *Methods and Findings in Experimental and Clinical Pharmacology*, 30, 107-113.

Al-Salami, H., Butt, G., Tucker, I. & Mikov, M. (2008e) Probiotic treatment proceeded by a single dose of bile acid and gliclazide exert the most hypoglycemic effect in Type 1 diabetic rats. *Medical Hypothesis Research*, 4, 93-101.

Al-Salami, H., Butt, G., Tucker, I., Skrbic, R., Golocorbin-Kon, S. & Mikov, M. (2008f) Probiotic Pre-treatment Reduces Gliclazide Permeation (ex vivo) in Healthy Rats but Increases It in Diabetic Rats to the Level Seen in Untreated Healthy Rats. *Arch.Drug Inf.*, 1, 35-41.

Al-Salami, H., Butt, G., Tucker, I.G., Fawcett, J.P. & Mikov, M. (2009b) Probiotic treatment decreases the oral absorption of the semisynthetic bile acid, MKC, in healthy and diabetic rats. *The European journal of drug metabolism and pharmacokinetics.*

Al-Salami, H., Grant, B., Ian, T. & Mikov, M. (2008g) The influence of probiotics pre-treatment, on the ileal permeation of gliclazide, in healthy and diabetic rats. *The archives of drug information*, 1, 35-41.

Al-Salami, H., Kansara, H., King, J., Morar, B., Jayathilaka, B., Fawcett, P.J. & Mikov, M. (2007) Bile acids: a bitter sweet remedy for diabetes. *The New Zealand Pharmacy Journal*, 27, 17-20.

Altenhoefer, A., Oswald, S., Sonnenborn, U., Enders, C., Schulze, J., Hacker, J. & Oelschlaeger, T.A. (2004) The probiotic Escherichia coli strain Nissle 1917 interferes with invasion of human intestinal epithelial cells by different enteroinvasive bacterial pathogens. 40, 223-229.

Asamoto, Y., Tazuma, S., Ochi, H., Chayama, K. & Suzuki, H. (2001) Bile-salt hydrophobicity is a key factor regulating rat liver plasma-membrane communication: relation to bilayer structure, fluidity and transporter expression and function. 359, 605-610.

Aungst, B.J. & Rogers, N.J. (1988) Site Dependence of Absorption-Promoting Actions of Laureth-9, Na Salicylate, Na2Edta, and Aprotinin on Rectal, Nasal, and Buccal Insulin Delivery. *Pharmaceutical Research*, 5, 305-308.

Bachrach, W.H. & Hofmann, A.F. (1982a) Ursodeoxycholic Acid in the Treatment of Cholesterol Cholelithiasis .1. *Digestive Diseases and Sciences*, 27, 737-761.

Bachrach, W.H. & Hofmann, A.F. (1982b) Ursodeoxycholic Acid in the Treatment of Cholesterol Cholelithiasis .2. *Digestive Diseases and Sciences*, 27, 833-856.

Ballatori, N., Christian, W.V., Lee, J.Y., Dawson, P.A., Soroka, C.J., Boyer, J.L., Madejczyk, M.S. & Li, N. (2005a) OSTalpha-OSTbeta: a major basolateral bile acid and steroid transporter in human intestinal, renal, and biliary epithelia. 42, 1270-1279.

Ballatori, N., Hammond, C.L., Cunningham, J.B., Krance, S.M. & Marchan, R. (2005b) Molecular mechanisms of reduced glutathione transport: role of the MRP/CFTR/ABCC and OATP/SLC21A families of membrane proteins. 204, 238-255.

Barbeau, W.E., Bassaganya-Riera, J. & Hontecillas, R. (2006) Putting the pieces of the puzzle together - a series of hypotheses on the etiology and pathogenesis of type 1 diabetes. 68, 607-609.

Barbeau, W.E., Bassaganya-Riera, J. & Hontecillas, R. (2007) Putting the pieces of the puzzle together - a series of hypotheses on the etiology and pathogenesis of type 1 diabetes. 68, 607-619.

Bennion, L.J. & Grundy, S.M. (1977) Effects of diabetes mellitus on cholesterol metabolism in man. 296, 1365-1371.

Bezkorovainy, A. (2001) Probiotics: determinants of survival and growth in the gut. 73, 399S-405S.

Bjork, E., Bjurstrom, S. & Edman, P. (1991) Morphological Examination of Rabbit Nasal-Mucosa After Nasal Administration of Degradable Starch Microspheres. *International Journal of Pharmaceutics*, 75, 73-80.

Bodo, A., Bakos, E., Szeri, F., Varadi, A. & Sarkadi, B. (2003) Differential modulation of the human liver conjugate transporters MRP2 and MRP3 by bile acids and organic anions. 278, 23529-23537.

Bruno, G., Runzo, C., Cavallo-Perin, P., Merletti, F., Rivetti, M., Pinach, S., Novelli, G., Trovati, M., Cerutti, F. & Pagano, G. (2005) Incidence of type 1 and type 2 diabetes in adults aged 30-49 years: the population-based registry in the province of Turin, Italy. 28, 2613-2619.

Calcinaro, F., Dionisi, S., Marinaro, M., Candeloro, P., Bonato, V., Marzotti, S., Corneli, R.B., Ferretti, E., Gulino, A., Grasso, F., De Simone, C., Di Mario, U., Falorni, A., Boirivant, M. & Dotta, F. (2005) Oral probiotic administration induces interleukin-10 production and prevents spontaneous autoimmune diabetes in the non-obese diabetic mouse. *Diabetologia*, 48, 1565-1575.

Campbell, I.W. (1991) Management of type 2 diabetes mellitus with special reference to metformin therapy. 17, 191-196.

Campbell, I.W. (2004) Long-term glycaemic control with pioglitazone in patients with type 2 diabetes. 58, 192-200.

Cani, P.D., Bibiloni, R., Knauf, C., Neyrinck, A.M., Neyrinck, A.M., Delzenne, N.M. & Burcelin, R. (2008) Changes in gut microbiota control metabolic endotoxemia-induced inflammation in high-fat diet-induced obesity and diabetes in mice. *Diabetes*, 57, 1470-1481.

Cani, P.D., Neyrinck, A.M., Fava, F., Knauf, C., Burcelin, R.G., Tuohy, K.M., Gibson, G.R. & Delzenne, N.M. (2007) Selective increases of bifidobacteria in gut microflora improve high-fat-diet-induced diabetes in mice through a mechanism associated with endotoxaemia. *Diabetologia*, 50, 2374-2383.

Cani, P.D., Possemiers, S., Van de Wiele, T., Guiot, Y., Everard, A., Rottier, O., Geurts, L., Naslain, D., Neyrinck, A., Lambert, D.M., Muccioli, G.G. & Delzenne, N.M. (2009) Changes in gut microbiota control inflammation in obese mice through a mechanism involving GLP-2-driven improvement of gut permeability. *Gut*, 58, 1091-1103.

Cannon, J.P., Fiscella, R., Pattharachayakul, S., Garey, K.W., De Alba, F., Piscitelli, S., Edward, D.P. & Danziger, L.H. (2003) Comparative toxicity and concentrations of intravitreal amphotericin B formulations in a rabbit model. *Investigative Ophthalmology & Visual Science*, 44, 2112-2117.

Cary, V.A. & Boullata, J. (2010) What is the evidence for the use of probiotics in the treatment of inflammatory bowel disease? *J.Clin.Nurs.*, 19, 904-916.

Chijiiwa, K. (1990) The effects of ethinylestradiol, a glucose diet and streptozotocin induced diabetes mellitus on gallstone formation and biliary lipid composition in the hamster. *Jpn.J.Surg.*, 20, 567-576.

Cornell, R.P. (1985) Endogenous Gut-Derived Bacterial-Endotoxin Tonically Primes Pancreatic-Secretion of Insulin in Normal Rats. *Diabetes*, 34, 1253-1259.

Cubeddu, L.X. & Hoffmann, I.S. (2002) Insulin resistance and upper-normal glucose levels in hypertension: a review. *J.Hum.Hypertens.*, 16 Suppl 1, S52-S55.

De Leon, M., Ferenderes, R. & Carulli, N. (1978) Bile lipid composition and bile acid pool size in diabetes. 23, 710-716.

Devendra, D., Liu, E. & Eisenbarth, G.S. (2004) Type 1 diabetes: recent developments. 328, 750-754.

Di Wu, Q., Wang, J.H., Fennessy, F., Redmond, H.P. & Bouchier-Hayes, D. (1999) Taurine prevents high-glucose-induced human vascular endothelial cell apoptosis. *American Journal of Physiology-Cell Physiology*, 277, C1229-C1238.

Dieleman, L.A., Pena, A.S., Meuwissen, S.G. & van Rees, E.P. (1997) Role of animal models for the pathogenesis and treatment of inflammatory bowel disease. 223, 99-104.

Donovan, M.D., Flynn, G.L. & Amidon, G.L. (1990) The Molecular-Weight Dependence of Nasal Absorption - the Effect of Absorption Enhancers. *Pharmaceutical Research*, 7, 808-815.

Duan, F., Curtis, K.L. & March, J.C. (2008) Secretion of insulinotropic proteins by commensal bacteria: rewiring the gut to treat diabetes. *Appl.Environ.Microbiol.*, 74, 7437-7438.

Fajans, S. (1987) [Classification, pathogenesis and course of various types of diabetes mellitus]. 93, 139-144.

FAO/WHO. (2002) guidelines for the evaluation of probiotics in food.

Favaro-Trindade, C.S. & Grosso, C.R. (2002) Microencapsulation of L. acidophilus (La-05) and B. lactis (Bb-12) and evaluation of their survival at the pH values of the stomach and in bile. 19, 485-494.

Fox, J.G., Feng, Y., Theve, E.J., Raczynski, A.R., Fiala, J.L.A., Doernte, A.L., Williams, M., McFaline, J.L., Essigmann, J.M., Schauer, D.B., Tannenbaum, S.R., Dedon, P.C., Weinman, S.A., Lemon, S.M., Fry, R.C. & Rogers, A.B. (2010) Gut microbes define liver cancer risk in mice exposed to chemical and viral transgenic hepatocarcinogens. *Gut*, 59, 88-97.

Franconi, F., Bennardini, F., Mattana, A., Miceli, M., Ciuti, M., Mian, M., Gironi, A., Anichini, R. & Seghieri, G. (1995) Plasma and Platelet Taurine Are Reduced in Subjects with Insulin-Dependent Diabetes-Mellitus - Effects of Taurine Supplementation. *American Journal of Clinical Nutrition*, 61, 1115-1119.

Franz, B. & Bode, J.C. (1973) [Plasma bile acid concentration (PGK): fasting values, daily fluctuations and effect of intraduodenal bile acid administration in healthy subjects and patients with chronic liver diseases]. *Z Gastroenterol*, 11, 131-134.

Gareau, M.G., Sherman, P.M. & Walker, W.A. (2010) Probiotics and the gut microbiota in intestinal health and disease. *Nature Reviews Gastroenterology & Hepatology*, 7, 503-514.

Gebel, E. (2011) The host with the most. A human body's bacteria may offer clues to why diabetes develops. *Diabetes Forecast.*, 64, 36-39.

Ghosh, S., van Heel, D. & Playford, R.J. (2004) Probiotics in inflammatory bowel disease: is it all gut flora modulation? 53, 620-622.

Goldberg, E. & Krause, I. (2009) Infection and type 1 diabetes mellitus - a two edged sword? *Autoimmun.Rev.*, 8, 682-686.

Goldfine, A.B. (2008) Modulating LDL cholesterol and glucose in patients with type 2 diabetes mellitus: targeting the bile acid pathway. 23, 502-511.

Goodman, H.O. & Shihabi, Z.K. (1990) Supplemental Taurine in Diabetic Rats - Effects on Plasma-Glucose and Triglycerides. *Biochemical Medicine and Metabolic Biology*, 43, 1-9.

Gordon, G.S., Moses, A.C., Silver, R.D., Flier, J.S. & Carey, M.C. (1985a) Nasal Absorption of Insulin - Enhancement by Hydrophobic Bile-Salts. *Proceedings of the National Academy of Sciences of the United States of America*, 82, 7419-7423.

Gordon, G.S., Moses, A.C., Silver, R.D., Flier, J.S. & Carey, M.C. (1985b) Nasal absorption of insulin: enhancement by hydrophobic bile salts. 82, 7419-7423.

Gourbeyre, P., Denery, S. & Bodinier, M. (2011) Probiotics, prebiotics, and synbiotics: impact on the gut immune system and allergic reactions. *J.Leukoc.Biol.*, 89, 685-695.

Grover, B., Buckley, D., Buckley, A.R. & Cacini, W. (2004) Reduced expression of organic cation transporters rOCT1 and rOCT2 in experimental diabetes. *J.Pharmacol.Exp Ther.*, 308, 949-956.

Hamada, T., Goto, H., Yamahira, T., Sugawara, T., Imaizumi, K. & Ikeda, I. (2006) Solubility in and affinity for the bile salt micelle of plant sterols are important determinants of their intestinal absorption in rats. *Lipids*, 41, 551-556.

Hansen, S.H. (2001) The role of taurine in diabetes and the development of diabetic complications. *Diabetes Metab Res.Rev.*, 17, 330-346.

Heaton, K.W. (1971) Abnormal Bile Or Faulty Gall Bladder. *British Medical Journal*, 1, 289-&.

Hedenborg, G. & Norman, A. (1984) The nature of urinary bile acid conjugates in patients with extrahepatic cholestasis. 44, 725-733.

Hedenborg, G. & Norman, A. (1985) Fasting and postprandial serum bile acid concentration with special reference to variations in the conjugate profile. 45, 151-156.

Heinemann, L., Klappoth, W., Rave, K., Hompesch, B., Linkeschowa, R. & Heise, T. (2000) Intra-individual variability of the metabolic effect of inhaled insulin together with an absorption enhancer. *Diabetes Care*, 23, 1343-1347.

Hersey, S.J. & Jackson, R.T. (1987a) Effect of bile salts on nasal permeability in vitro. *J.Pharm.Sci.*, 76, 876-879.

Hersey, S.J. & Jackson, R.T. (1987b) Effect of bile salts on nasal permeability in vitro. *J.Pharm.Sci.*, 76, 876-879.

Higgins, C.F. & Gottesman, M.M. (1992) Is the multidrug transporter a flippase? 17, 18-21.

Hirai, S., Ikenaga, T. & Matsuzawa, T. (1978) Nasal Absorption of Insulin in Dogs. *Diabetes*, 27, 296-299.

Hopkins, M.J. & Macfarlane, G.T. (2002) Changes in predominant bacterial populations in human faeces with age and with Clostridium difficile infection. *Journal of Medical Microbiology*, 51, 448-454.

Houten, S., Watanabe, M. & Auwerx, J. (2006a) Endocrine functions of bile acids. 25, 1419-1425.

Houten, S.M., Watanabe, M. & Auwerx, J. (2006b) Endocrine functions of bile acids. *Embo Journal*, 25, 1419-1425.

Husebye, E. (2005) The pathogenesis of gastrointestinal bacterial overgrowth. *Chemotherapy*, 51 Suppl 1, 1-22.

Illum, L., Fisher, A.N., Jabbal-Gill, I. & Davis, S.S. (2001) Bioadhesive starch microspheres and absorption enhancing agents act synergistically to enhance the nasal absorption of polypeptides. *International Journal of Pharmaceutics*, 222, 109-119.

Jaakkola, I., Jalkanen, S. & Hanninen, A. (2003) Diabetogenic T cells are primed both in pancreatic and gut-associated lymph nodes in NOD mice. *Eur J Immunol*, 33, 3255-3264.

Jacobs, D.B., Hayes, G.R. & Lockwood, D.H. (1989) In vitro effects of sulfonylurea on glucose transport and translocation of glucose transporters in adipocytes from streptozocin-induced diabetic rats. 38, 205-211.

Jain, S.K., Kannan, K., Lim, G., Mcvie, R. & Bocchini, J.A. (2002) Hyperketonemia increases tumor necrosis factor-alpha secretion in cultured U937 monocytes and type 1 diabetic patients and is apparently mediated by oxidative stress and cAMP deficiency. *Diabetes*, 51, 2287-2293.

Juhl, C., Grofte, T., Butler, P.C., Veldhuis, J.D., Schmitz, O. & Porksen, N. (2002) Effects of fasting on physiologically pulsatile insulin release in healthy humans. *Diabetes*, 51 Suppl 1, S255-S257.

Junginger, H.E. (1992) Formulation Aspects on Dermatological Preparations and Transdermal Drug Delivery Systems. *Acta Pharmaceutica Nordica*, 4, 117.

Just, T., Pau, H.W., Engel, U. & Hummel, T. (2008) Cephalic phase insulin release in healthy humans after taste stimulation? *Appetite*, 51, 622-627.

Kaneko, T., Sato, T., Katsuya, H. & Miyauchi, Y. (1990) Surfactant Therapy for Pulmonary-Edema Due to Intratracheally Injected Bile-Acid. *Critical Care Medicine*, 18, 77-83.

Karimi, O. & Pena, A.S. (2003) Probiotics: Isolated bacteria strain or mixtures of different strains? Two different approaches in the use of probiotics as therapeutics. 39, 565-597.

Kokk, K., Verajankorva, E., Laato, M., Wu, X.K., Tapfer, H. & Pollanen, P. (2005) Expression of insulin receptor substrates 1-3, glucose transporters GLUT-1-4, signal regulatory protein 1alpha, phosphatidylinositol 3-kinase and protein kinase B at the protein level in the human testis. 80, 91-96.

Kuhajda, K., Kandrac, J., Kevresan, S., Mikov, M. & Fawcett, J.P. (2006a) Structure and origin of bile acids: an overview. 31, 135-143.

Kuhajda, K., Kevresan, S., Kandrac, J., Fawcett, J.P. & Mikov, M. (2006b) Chemical and metabolic transformations of selected bile acids. 31, 179-235.

Kuhajda, K., Kevresan, S., Mikov, M., Sabo, A. & D., M. (2000) Influence of 3a,7a-dihydroxy-12-keto-5ß-cholanate on blood glucose level in rats. 8, 304-308.

Kulakowski, E.C. & Maturo, J. (1984) Hypoglycemic Properties of Taurine - Not Mediated by Enhanced Insulin Release. *Biochemical Pharmacology*, 33, 2835-2838.

Kurdi, P., Kawanishi, K., Mizutani, K. & Yokota, A. (2006) Mechanism of growth inhibition by free bile acids in lactobacilli and bifidobacteria. 188, 1979-1986.

Kurdi, P., van Veen, H.W., Tanaka, H., Mierau, I., Konings, W.N., Tannock, G.W., Tomita, F. & Yokota, A. (2000) Cholic acid is accumulated spontaneously, driven by membrane deltapH, in many lactobacilli. 182, 6525-6528.

Lee, V.H.L. (1991) Trends in Peptide and Protein Drug Delivery. *Biopharm-the Technology & Business of Biopharmaceuticals*, 4, 22-25.

Lee, V.H.L., Yamamoto, A. & Kompella, U.B. (1991) Mucosal Penetration Enhancers for Facilitation of Peptide and Protein Drug Absorption. *Critical Reviews in Therapeutic Drug Carrier Systems*, 8, 91-192.

Leng, J., Egelhaaf, S.U. & Cates, M.E. (2003) Kinetics of the micelle-to-vesicle transition: aqueous lecithin-bile salt mixtures. *Biophys.J.*, 85, 1624-1646.

Li, Y.P., Shao, Z.Z. & Mitra, A.K. (1992) Dissociation of Insulin Oligomers by Bile-Salt Micelles and Its Effect on Alpha-Chymotrypsin-Mediated Proteolytic Degradation. *Pharmaceutical Research*, 9, 864-869.

Li-Wen, H., Bi-Zhou, L., Xue-Zhong, L., Xiu-Feng, H. & Ling, B. (2007) Synthesis, structure and characterization of [Cu(2,2 '-bpy)(2)][{Cu(2,2 '-bpy)(2)}(2)W12O40(H-2)]center dot 4H(2)O. *Chinese Journal of Structural Chemistry*, 26, 1435-1440.

Liong, M.T. (2008) Safety of probiotics: translocation and infection. *Nutr.Rev.*, 66, 192-202.

Lowbeer, T.S., Heaton, K.W. & Read, A.E. (1970) Gallbladder Inertia in Adult Coeliac Disease. *Gut*, 11, 1057-&.

Luoto, R., Laitinen, K., Nermes, M. & Isolauri, E. (2010) Impact of maternal probiotic-supplemented dietary counselling on pregnancy outcome and prenatal and postnatal growth: a double-blind, placebo-controlled study. *Br J Nutr*, 103, 1792-1799.

Macpherson, A.J. & Uhr, T. (2004) Induction of protective IgA by intestinal dendritic cells carrying commensal bacteria. *Science*, 303, 1662-1665.

Maki, M., Huupponen, T., Holm, K. & Hallstrom, O. (1995) Seroconversion of Reticulin Autoantibodies Predicts Celiac-Disease in Insulin-Dependent Diabetes-Mellitus. *Gut*, 36, 239-242.

Maki, N., Hafkemeyer, P. & Dey, S. (2003) Allosteric modulation of human P-glycoprotein. Inhibition of transport by preventing substrate translocation and dissociation. 278, 18132-18139.

Malavolti, M., Fromm, H., Ceryak, S. & Shehan, K.L. (1989) Interaction of Potentially Toxic Bile-Acids with Human-Plasma Proteins - Binding of Lithocholic (3-Alpha-Hydroxy-5-Beta-Cholan-24-Oic) Acid to Lipoproteins and Albumin. *Lipids*, 24, 673-676.

Mao, Q. & Unadkat, J.D. (2005) Role of the breast cancer resistance protein (ABCG2) in drug transport. 2005/09/09, E118-E133.

Marteau, P. & Shanahan, F. (2003) Basic aspects and pharmacology of probiotics: an overview of pharmacokinetics, mechanisms of action and side-effects. *Best.Pract.Res.Clin.Gastroenterol.*, 17, 725-740.

Martin, C.R. & Walker, W.A. (2008) Probiotics: role in pathophysiology and prevention in necrotizing enterocolitis. *Semin.Perinatol.*, 32, 127-137.

Matsuzaki, T., Nagata, Y., Kado, S., Uchida, K., Hashimoto, S. & Yokokura, T. (1997a) Effect of oral administration of Lactobacillus casei on alloxan-induced diabetes in mice. 105, 637-642.

Matsuzaki, T., Nagata, Y., Kado, S., Uchida, K., Kato, I., Hashimoto, S. & Yokokura, T. (1997b) Prevention of onset in an insulin-dependent diabetes mellitus model, NOD mice, by oral feeding of Lactobacillus casei. 105, 643-649.

Matthaei, S., Horuk, R. & Olefsky, J.M. (1986) Blood-brain glucose transfer in diabetes mellitus. Decreased number of glucose transporters at blood-brain barrier. *Diabetes*, 35, 1181-1184.

Meinders, A.E., Henegouwen, V.B., Willekens, F.L.A., Schwerzel, A.L., Ruben, B.A. & Huybregts, A.W.M. (1981a) Biliary lipid and bile acid composition in insulin-dependent diabetes mellitus. 26, 402-408.

Meinders, A.E., Van Berge Henegouwen, G.P., Willekens, F.L., Schwerzel, A.L., Ruben, A. & Huybregts, A.W. (1981b) Biliary lipid and bile acid composition in insulin-dependent diabetes mellitus. Arguments for increased intestinal bacterial bile acid degradation. 26, 402-408.

Meinders, A.E., Vanbergehenegouwen, G.P., Willekens, F.L.A., Schwerzel, A.L., Ruben, A. & Huybregts, A.W.M. (1981c) Biliary Lipid and Bile-Acid Composition in Insulin-Dependent Diabetes-Mellitus - Arguments for Increased Intestinal Bacterial Bile-Acid Degradation. *Digestive Diseases and Sciences*, 26, 402-408.

Mesiha, M.S., Ponnapula, S. & Plakogiannis, F. (2002a) Oral absorption of insulin encapsulated in artificial chyles of bile salts, palmitic acid and alpha-tocopherol dispersions. 249, 1-5.

Mesiha, M.S., Ponnapula, S. & Plakogiannis, F. (2002b) Oral absorption of insulin encapsulated in artificial chyles of bile salts, palmitic acid and alpha-tocopherol dispersions. *International Journal of Pharmaceutics*, 249, 1-5.

Mesiha, M.S., Ponnapula, S. & Plakogiannis, F. (2002c) Oral absorption of insulin encapsulated in artificial chyles of bile salts, palmitic acid and alpha-tocopherol dispersions. *International Journal of Pharmaceutics*, 249, 1-5.

Mikov, M., Al-Salami, H., Golocorbin-Kon, S., Skrbic, R., Raskovic, A. & Fawcett, J.P. (2008) The influence of 3 alpha,7 alpha-dihydroxy-12-keto-5 beta-cholanate on gliclazide pharmacokinetics and glucose levels in a rat model of diabetes. *European Journal of Drug Metabolism and Pharmacokinetics*, 33, 137-142.

Mikov, M., Boni, N.S., Al-Salami, H., Kuhajda, K., Kevresan, S., Golocorbin-Kon, S. & Fawcett, J.P. (2007) Bioavailability and hypoglycemic activity of the semisynthetic bile acid salt, sodium 3alpha,7alpha-dihydroxy-12-oxo-5beta-cholanate, in healthy and diabetic rats. *Eur.J.Drug Metab Pharmacokinet.*, 32, 7-12.

Mikov, M. & Fawcett, J.P. (2006a) Bile acids - Chemistry, biosynthesis, analysis, chemical & metabolic transformations and pharmacology. *European Journal of Drug Metabolism and Pharmacokinetics*, 31, 133-134.

Mikov, M. & Fawcett, J.P. (2006b) Chemistry, biosynthesis, analysis, chemical & metabolic transformations and pharmacology. 31, 133-134.

Mikov, M., Fawcett, J.P., Kuhajda, K. & Kevresan, S. (2006) Pharmacology of bile acids and their derivatives: absorption promoters and therapeutic agents. 31, 237-251.

Mikov, M., Raskovic, A., Jakovljevic, E., Dudvarski, D. & Fawcett, J.P. (2005) Influence of the bile salt sodium 3alfa,7alfa-dihydroxy-12-oxo-5beta-cholanate on ampicillin pharmacokinetics in rats. 5, 197-200.

Mikov, M., Raskovic, A., Kuhajda, K., Kevresan, S. & Potsides, C.Y. (2004) Therapeutic perspective of bile acids-Toxicity and interaction. 1, S-1.

Miljkovic, D., Kuhajda, K., Mikov, M., Kevresan, S. & A., S. (2000) US patent No. 6060465 on bile acids and their derivatives as glycoregulatory agents. *US*.

Mita, S., Suzuki, H., Akita, H., Hayashi, H., Onuki, R., Hofmann, A.F. & Sugiyama, Y. (2006) Inhibition of bile acid transport across Na+/taurocholate cotransporting polypeptide (SLC10A1) and bile salt export pump (ABCB 11)-coexpressing LLC-PK1 cells by cholestasis-inducing drugs. 34, 1575-1581.

Miyai, K., Javitt, N.B., Gochman, N., Jones, H.M. & Baker, D. (1982) Hepatotoxicity of Bile-Acids in Rabbits - Ursodeoxycholic Acid Is Less Toxic Than Chenodeoxycholic Acid. *Laboratory Investigation*, 46, 428-437.

Mooradian, A.D. & Morin, A.M. (1991) Brain uptake of glucose in diabetes mellitus: the role of glucose transporters. *Am.J.Med.Sci.*, 301, 173-177.

Moore, P.A., Zgibor, J.C. & Dasanayake, A.P. (2003a) Diabetes: a growing epidemic of all ages. *J Am Dent Assoc*, 134 Spec No, 11S-15S.

Moore, P.A., Zgibor, J.C. & Dasanayake, A.P. (2003b) Diabetes: a growing epidemic of all ages. *J Am Dent Assoc*, 134 Spec No, 11S-15S.

Morris, J.A. (1989) A possible role for bacteria in the pathogenesis of insulin dependent diabetes mellitus. *Med.Hypotheses*, 29, 231-235.

Morris, J.D., Diamond, K.A. & Balart, L.A. (2009) Do probiotics have a role in the management of inflammatory bowel disease? *J.La State Med.Soc.*, 161, 155-159.

Moses, A.C., Gordon, G.S., Carey, M.C. & Flier, J.S. (1983) Insulin Administered Intranasally As An Insulin-Bile Salt Aerosol - Effectiveness and Reproducibility in Normal and Diabetic Subjects. *Diabetes*, 32, 1040-1047.

Neish, A.S., Gewirtz, A.T., Zeng, H., Young, A.N., Hobert, M.E., Karmali, V., Rao, A.S. & Madara, J.L. (2000) Prokaryotic regulation of epithelial responses by inhibition of IkappaB-alpha ubiquitination. *Science*, 289, 1560-1563.

Neubert, R., Furst, W. & Wurschi, B. (1987) [Drug permeation through artificial lipoid membranes. 20. The effectiveness of multiple-lamellar liposomes for evaluating drug transport]. *Pharmazie*, 42, 102-103.

Notkins, A.L. & Lernmark, A. (2001) Autoimmune type 1 diabetes: resolved and unresolved issues. 108, 1247-1252.

Ogura, Y., Ito, T. & Ogura, M. (1986) Effect of diabetes and of 7 alpha-hydroxycholesterol infusion on the profile of bile acids secreted by the isolated rat livers. *Biol.Chem.Hoppe Seyler*, 367, 1095-1099.

Oktar, B.K., Gulpinar, M.A., Ercan, F., Cingi, A., Alican, I. & Yegen, B.C. (2001) Beneficial effects of glycocholic acid (GCA) on gut mucosal damage in bile duct ligated rats. *Inflammation*, 25, 311-318.

Otte, J.M. & Podolsky, D.K. (2004) Functional modulation of enterocytes by gram-positive and gram-negative microorganisms. *Am.J.Physiol Gastrointest.Liver Physiol*, 286, G613-G626.

Overkamp, D., Gautier, J.F., Renn, W., Pickert, A., Scheen, A.J., Schmulling, R.M., Eggstein, M. & Lefebvre, P.J. (1997) Glucose turnover in humans in the basal state and after intravenous glucose: a comparison of two models. *Am.J.Physiol*, 273, E284-E296.

Paccagnini, D., Sieswerda, L., Rosu, V., Masala, S., Pacifico, A., Gazouli, M., Ikonomopoulos, J., Ahmed, N., Zanetti, S. & Sechi, L.A. (2009) Linking chronic infection and autoimmune diseases: Mycobacterium avium subspecies paratuberculosis, SLC11A1 polymorphisms and type-1 diabetes mellitus. *PLoS One*, 4, e7109.

Palmer, K.J. & Brogden, R.N. (1993) Gliclazide. An update of its pharmacological properties and therapeutic efficacy in non-insulin-dependent diabetes mellitus. 46, 92-125.

Peng, H. & Hagopian, W. (2007) Environmental factors in the development of Type 1 diabetes.

Pigeon, R.M., Cuesta, E.P. & Gililliand, S.E. (2002) Binding of free bile acids by cells of yogurt starter culture bacteria. 85, 2705-2710.

Py, G., Lambert, K., Milhavet, O., Eydoux, N., Prefaut, C. & Mercier, J. (2002) Effects of streptozotocin-induced diabetes on markers of skeletal muscle metabolism and monocarboxylate transporter 1 to monocarboxylate transporter 4 transporters. *Metabolism*, 51, 807-813.

Qin, X., Yuan, F., Zhou, D. & Huang, Y. (2010) Oral characteristics of bergenin and the effect of absorption enhancers in situ, in vitro and in vivo. *Arzneimittelforschung.*, 60, 198-204.

Quraishy, M.S., Chescoe, D., Mullervy, J., Coates, M., Hinton, R.H. & Bailey, M.E. (1996) Influence of the gut microflora and of biliary constituents on morphological changes in the small intestine in obstructive jaundice. *HPB Surg*, 10, 11-20.

Rachmilewitz, D., Katakura, K., Karmeli, F., Hayashi, T., Reinus, C., Rudensky, B., Akira, S., Takeda, K., Lee, J., Takabayashi, K. & Raz, E. (2004) Toll-like receptor 9 signaling mediates the anti-inflammatory effects of probiotics in murine experimental colitis. *Gastroenterology*, 126, 520-528.

Rayes, N., Seehofer, D., Theruvath, T., Schiller, R.A., Langrehr, J.M., Jonas, S., Bengmark, S. & Neuhaus, P. (2005) Supply of pre- and probiotics reduces bacterial infection rates after liver transplantation--a randomized, double-blind trial. *Am.J.Transplant.*, 5, 125-130.

Raymond, R.M., Harkema, J.M. & Emerson, T.E. (1980) Direct Effects of Escherichia-Coli Endotoxin in Promoting Skeletal-Muscle Glucose-Uptake in the Dog. *Circulatory Shock*, 7, 218-219.

Raymond, R.M., Harkema, J.M. & Emerson, T.E. (1981) Direct Effects of Gram-Negative Endotoxin on Skeletal-Muscle Glucose-Uptake. *American Journal of Physiology*, 240, H342-H347.

Rebole, A., Ortiz, L.T., Rodriguez, M.L., Alzueta, C., Trevino, J. & Velasco, S. (2010) Effects of inulin and enzyme complex, individually or in combination, on growth performance, intestinal microflora, cecal fermentation characteristics, and jejunal histomorphology in broiler chickens fed a wheat- and barley-based diet. *Poult.Sci.*, 89, 276-286.

Reibel, D.K., Shaffer, J.E., Kocsis, J.J. & Neely, J.R. (1979) Changes in Taurine Content in Heart and Other Organs of Diabetic Rats. *Journal of Molecular and Cellular Cardiology*, 11, 827-830.

Rescigno, M., Urbano, M., Valzasina, B., Francolini, M., Rotta, G., Bonasio, R., Granucci, F., Kraehenbuhl, J.P. & Ricciardi-Castagnoli, P. (2001) Dendritic cells express tight junction proteins and penetrate gut epithelial monolayers to sample bacteria. *Nat.Immunol.*, 2, 361-367.

Respondek, F., Goachet, A.G. & Julliand, V. (2008) Effects of dietary short-chain fructooligosaccharides on the intestinal microflora of horses subjected to a sudden change in diet. *J.Anim Sci.*, 86, 316-323.

Ricci, P., Hofmann, A.F., Hagey, L.R., Jorgensen, R.A., Dickson, E.R. & Lindor, K.D. (1998) Adjuvant cholylsarcosine during ursodeoxycholic acid treatment of primary biliary cirrhosis. *Digestive Diseases and Sciences*, 43, 1292-1295.

Ridlon, J.M., Kang, D.J. & Hylemon, P.B. (2006) Bile salt biotransformations by human intestinal bacteria. 47, 241-259.

Roberts, M.S., Magnusson, B.M., Burczynski, F.J. & Weiss, M. (2002) Enterohepatic circulation: physiological, pharmacokinetic and clinical implications. 41, 751-790.

Rosa, S.C., Rufino, A.T., Judas, F., Tenreiro, C., Lopes, M.C. & Mendes, A.F. (2011) Expression and function of the insulin receptor in normal and osteoarthritic human chondrocytes: modulation of anabolic gene expression, glucose transport and GLUT-1 content by insulin. *Osteoarthritis.Cartilage.*

Rosenbloom, A.L., Joe, J.R., Young, R.S. & Winter, W.E. (1999) Emerging epidemic of type 2 diabetes in youth. *Diabetes Care*, 22, 345-354.

Rozanova, G.N. & Voevodin, D.A. (2008) [A case of an effective application of probiotics in the complex therapy of severe type 1 diabetes mellitus and intestinal disbacteriosis]. *Klin.Med (Mosk)*, 86, 67-68.

Rozanova, G.N., Voevodin, D.A., Stenina, M.A. & Kushnareva, M.V. (2002) Pathogenetic role of dysbacteriosis in the development of complications of type 1 diabetes mellitus in children. 133, 164-166.

Rungby, J. (2010) Zinc, zinc transporters and diabetes. *Diabetologia*, 53, 1549-1551.

Samiy, N., Ng, E.W.M., Ruoff, K., Baker, A.S. & Damico, D.J. (1996) Pneumococcal endophthalmitis in the rat: Clinical and histological characterization. *Investigative Ophthalmology & Visual Science*, 37, 3556.

Sayani, A.P. & Chien, Y.W. (1996) Systemic delivery of peptides and proteins across absorptive mucosae. *Critical Reviews in Therapeutic Drug Carrier Systems*, 13, 85-184.

Shamoon, H., Duffy, H., Fleischer, N., Engel, S., Saenger, P., Strelzyn, M., Litwak, M., Wylierosett, J., Farkash, A., Geiger, D., Engel, H., Fleischman, J., Pompi, D., Ginsberg, N., Glover, M., Brisman, M., Walker, E., Thomashunis, A., Gonzalez, J., Genuth, S., Brown, E., Dahms, W., Pugsley, P., Mayer, L., Kerr, D., Landau, B., Singerman, L., Rice, T., Novak, M., Smithbrewer, S., Mcconnell, J., Drotar, D., Woods, D., Katirgi, B., Litvene, M., Brown, C., Lusk, M., Campbell, R., Lackaye, M., Richardson, M., Levy, B., Chang, S., Heinheinemann, M., Barron, S., Astor, L., Lebeck, D., Brillon, D., Diamond, B., Vasilasdwoskin, A., Laurenzi, B., Foldi, N., Rubin, M., Flynn, T., Reppucci, V., Heise, C., Sanchez, A., Whitehouse, F., Kruger, D., Kahkonen, D., Fachnie, J., Fisk, J., Carey, J., Cox, M., Ahmad, B., Angus, E., Campbell, H., Fields, D., Croswell, M., Basha, K., Chung, P., Schoenherr, A., Mobley, M., Marchiori, K., Francis, J., Kelly, J., Etzwiler, D., Callahan, P., Hollander, P., Castle, G., Bergenstal, R., Spencer, M., Nelson, J., Bezecny, L., Roethke, C., Orban, M., Ulrich, C., Gill, L., Morgan, K., Laechelt, J., Taylor, F., Freking, D., Towey, A., Lieppman, M., Rakes, S., Mangum, J., Cooper, N., Upham, P., Jacobson, A., Crowell, S., Wolfsdorf, J., Beaser, R., Ganda, O., Rosenzweig, J., Stewart, C., Halford, B., Friedlander, E., Tarsy, D., Arrigg, P., Sharuk, G., Shah, S., Wu, G., Cavallerano, J., Poole, R., Silver, P., Cavicchi, R., Fleming, D., Marcus, J., Griffiths, C., Cappella, N., Nathan, D., Larkin, M., Godine, J., Lynch, J., Norman, D., Mckitrick, C., Haggen, C., Delahanty, L., Anderson, E., Lou, P., Taylor, C., Cros, D., Folino, K., Brink, S., Abbott, K., Sicotte, K., Service, F.J., Schmidt, A., Rizza, R., Zimmerman, B., Schwenk, W., Mortenson, J., Ziegler, G., Lucas, A., Hanson, N., Sellnow, S., Pach, J., Stein, D., Eickhoff, B., Woodwick, R., Tackmann, R., Trautmann, J., Rostvold, J., Link, T., Dyck, P., Daube, J., Colligan, R., Windebank, A., King, J., Colwell, J., Wood, D., Mayfield, R., Picket, J., Chitwood, M., Billings, D., Dabney, Y., Buse, J., King, L., Vale, S., Thompson, T., Bohm, B., Lyons, T., Hermayer, K., Rice, A., Molitch, M., Schaefer, B., Johnson, C., Lyons, J., Metzger, B., Cohen, B., Nishida, T., Parque, K., Yusim, V., Moore, M., Jampol, L., Dineen, K.,

Stahl, J., Richine, L., Weinberg, D., Loose, I., Kushner, M., Morrison, A., Jalbert, A., Tildesley, H., Leung, S., Begg, I., Johnson, D., Lalani, S., Kennedy, T., Meadows, G., Kolterman, O., Lorenzi, G., Jones, K., Goldbaum, M., Swenson, M., Lyon, R., Giotta, M., Kadlec, K., Reed, R., Kirsch, L., Goodman, J., Cahill, S., Clark, T., Abram, R., Sayner, L., Ochabski, R., Gloria, R., Birchler, G., Grant, J., Grasse, B., Christle, L., Abreu, B., Grant, I., Heaton, R., Zeitler, R., Sivitz, W., Bayless, M., Schrott, H., Olson, N., Tindal, B., Snetselaar, L., Mueller, D., Dudler, A., Swartzendruber, J., Hoffman, R., Macindoe, J., Kramer, J., Weingeist, T., Kimura, A., Stone, E., Grout, T., Fountain, C., Karakas, S., Vogel, C., Montague, P., Keyser, D., Mennen, S., Doggett, C., Rose, G., Devet, K., Muhle, P., Kowarski, A., Ostrowski, D., Levin, P., Chalew, S. & Hylton, J. (1993) The Effect of Intensive Treatment of Diabetes on the Development and Progression of Long-Term Complications in Insulin-Dependent Diabetes-Mellitus. *New England Journal of Medicine*, 329, 977-986.

Shao, Z., Krishnamoorthy, R. & Mitra, A.K. (1992a) Cyclodextrins As Nasal Absorption Promoters of Insulin - Mechanistic Evaluations. *Pharmaceutical Research*, 9, 1157-1163.

Shao, Z., Krishnamoorthy, R. & Mitra, A.K. (1992b) Cyclodextrins As Nasal Absorption Promoters of Insulin - Mechanistic Evaluations. *Pharmaceutical Research*, 9, 1157-1163.

Sherman, P.M., Cabana, M., Gibson, G.R., Koletzko, B.V., Neu, J., Veereman-Wauters, G., Ziegler, E.E. & Walker, W.A. (2009) Potential roles and clinical utility of prebiotics in newborns, infants, and children: proceedings from a global prebiotic summit meeting, New York City, June 27-28, 2008. *J.Pediatr.*, 155, S61-S70.

Shi, H.N. & Walker, A. (2004) Bacterial colonization and the development of intestinal defences. *Can.J.Gastroenterol.*, 18, 493-500.

Siow, Y., Schurr, A. & Vitale, G.C. (1991) Diabetes-induced bile acid composition changes in rat bile determined by high performance liquid chromatography. *Life Sci.*, 49, 1301-1308.

Slivka, O.I., Zelinskii, B.A. & Zelinskii, S.T. (1979a) [Bile acids in the bile in diabetes mellitus]. *Probl.Endokrinol.(Mosk)*, 25, 16-19.

Slivka, O.I., Zelinskii, B.A. & Zelinskii, S.T. (1979b) [Bile acids in the bile in diabetes mellitus]. 25, 16-19.

Snydman, D.R. (2008) The safety of probiotics. *Clin.Infect.Dis.*, 46 Suppl 2, S104-S111.

Souri, E.N. & Green, W.R. (1974) Intravitreal Amphotericin-B Toxicity. *American Journal of Ophthalmology*, 78, 77-81.

Srinivasan, K. & Ramarao, P. (2007) Animal models in type 2 diabetes research: an overview. 125, 451-472.

St-Pierre, M.V., Kullak-Ublick, G.A., Hagenbuch, B. & Meier, P.J. (2001) Transport of bile acids in hepatic and non-hepatic tissues. 204, 1673-1686.

St-Pierre, M.V., Serrano, M.A., Macias, R.I., Dubs, U., Hoechli, M., Lauper, U., Meier, P.J. & Marin, J.J. (2000) Expression of members of the multidrug resistance protein family in human term placenta. 279, R1495-R1503.

Steed, D.L., Donohoe, D., Webster, M.W. & Lindsley, L. (1996) Effect of extensive debridement and treatment on the healing of diabetic foot ulcers. Diabetic Ulcer Study Group. *J.Am.Coll.Surg.*, 183, 61-64.

Stephani, J., Radulovic, K. & Niess, J.H. (2011) Gut microbiota, probiotics and inflammatory bowel disease. *Arch.Immunol.Ther.Exp (Warsz.)*, 59, 161-177.

Stuart, C.A., Howell, M.E., Zhang, Y. & Yin, D. (2009) Insulin-stimulated translocation of glucose transporter (GLUT) 12 parallels that of GLUT4 in normal muscle. *J.Clin.Endocrinol Metab*, 94, 3535-3542.

Succi, M., Tremonte, P., Reale, A., Sorrentino, E., Grazia, L., Pacifico, S. & Coppola, R. (2005) Bile salt and acid tolerance of Lactobacillus rhamnosus strains isolated from Parmigiano Reggiano cheese. 244, 129-137.

Thomson, A.B. (1983) Uptake of bile acids into rat intestine. Effect of diabetes mellitus. *Diabetes*, 32, 900-907.

Tlaskalova-Hogenova, H., Stepankova, R., Kozakova, H., Hudcovic, T., Vannucci, L., Tuckova, L., Rossmann, P., Hrncir, T., Kverka, M., Zakostelska, Z., Klimesova, K., Pribylova, J., Bartova, J., Sanchez, D., Fundova, P., Borovska, D., Srutkova, D., Zidek, Z., Schwarzer, M., Drastich, P. & Funda, D.P. (2011) The role of gut microbiota (commensal bacteria) and the mucosal barrier in the pathogenesis of inflammatory and autoimmune diseases and cancer: contribution of germ-free and gnotobiotic animal models of human diseases. *Cell Mol.Immunol.*, 8, 110-120.

Trachtman, H. & Sturman, J.A. (1996) Taurine: A therapeutic agent in experimental kidney disease. *Amino Acids*, 11, 1-13.

Tramonti, G., Xie, P., Wallner, E.I., Danesh, F.R. & Kanwar, Y.S. (2006) Expression and functional characteristics of tubular transporters: P-glycoprotein, PEPT1, and PEPT2 in renal mass reduction and diabetes. *Am.J.Physiol Renal Physiol*, 291, F972-F980.

Trauner, M., Claudel, T., Fickert, P., Moustafa, T. & Wagner, M. (2010) Bile Acids as Regulators of Hepatic Lipid and Glucose Metabolism. *Digestive Diseases*, 28, 220-224.

Uchida, K., Makino, S. & Akiyoshi, T. (1985) Altered bile acid metabolism in nonobese, spontaneously diabetic (NOD) mice. 34, 79-83.

Uchida, K., Takase, H., Kadowaki, M., Nomura, Y., Matsubara, T. & Takeuchi, N. (1979) Altered bile acid metabolism in alloxan diabetic rats. 29, 553-562.

Vaarala, O. (2006) Is it dietary insulin? 1079, 350-359.

van Waarde, W.M., Verkade, H.J., Wolters, H., Havinga, R., Baller, J., Bloks, V., Muller, M., Sauer, P.J. & Kuipers, F. (2002) Differential effects of streptozotocin-induced diabetes on expression of hepatic ABC-transporters in rats. *Gastroenterology*, 122, 1842-1852.

Vidotti, D.B., Arnoni, C.P., Maquigussa, E. & Boim, M.A. (2008) Effect of long-term type 1 diabetes on renal sodium and water transporters in rats. *Am.J.Nephrol.*, 28, 107-114.

Vilchis, C. & Salceda, R. (1996) Effect of diabetes on levels and uptake of putative amino acid neurotransmitters in rat retina and retinal pigment epithelium. *Neurochemical Research*, 21, 1167-1171.

von, H.M. & Nepom, G.T. (2009a) Animal models of human type 1 diabetes. *Nat.Immunol.*, 10, 129-132.

von, H.M. & Nepom, G.T. (2009b) Animal models of human type 1 diabetes. *Nat.Immunol.*, 10, 129-132.

Walker, W.A. (2008a) Mechanisms of action of probiotics. *Clinical Infectious Diseases*, 46, S87-S91.

Walker, W.A. (2008b) Mechanisms of action of probiotics. *Clinical Infectious Diseases*, 46, S87-S91.

Weiss, R. & Caprio, S. (2006) Development of type 2 diabetes in children and adolescents. 97, 263-269.

Yamamoto, A., Luo, A.M., Doddakashi, S. & Lee, V.H.L. (1989) The Ocular Route for Systemic Insulin Delivery in the Albino Rabbit. *Journal of Pharmacology and Experimental Therapeutics*, 249, 249-255.

Yen, C.H., Tseng, Y.H., Kuo, Y.W., Lee, M.C. & Chen, H.L. (2011) Long-term supplementation of isomalto-oligosaccharides improved colonic microflora profile, bowel function, and blood cholesterol levels in constipated elderly people--a placebo-controlled, diet-controlled trial. *Nutrition*, 27, 445-450.

Zanchi, A., Stergiopulos, N., Brunner, H.R. & Hayoz, D. (1998) Differences in the mechanical properties of the rat carotid artery in vivo, in situ, and in vitro. *Hypertension*, 32, 180-185.

Zaneveld, J., Turnbaugh, P.J., Lozupone, C., Ley, R.E., Hamady, M., Gordon, J.I. & Knight, R. (2008) Host-bacterial coevolution and the search for new drug targets. *Curr Opin Chem Biol*, 12, 109-114.

Zelcer, N., Reid, G., Wielinga, P., Kuil, A., van der Heijden, I., Schuetz, J.D. & Borst, P. (2003a) Steroid and bile acid conjugates are substrates of human multidrug-resistance protein (MRP) 4 (ATP-binding cassette C4). 371, 361-367.

Zelcer, N., Saeki, T., Bot, I., Kuil, A. & Borst, P. (2003b) Transport of bile acids in multidrug-resistance-protein 3-overexpressing cells co-transfected with the ileal Na+-dependent bile-acid transporter. 369, 23-30.

Ziegler, A.G., Schmid, S., Huber, D., Hummel, M. & Bonifacio, E. (2003) Early infant feeding and risk of developing type 1 diabetes-associated autoantibodies. 290, 1721-1728.

Zisser, H.C., Bevier, W.C. & Jovanovic, L. (2007) Restoring euglycemia in the basal state using continuous glucose monitoring in subjects with type 1 diabetes mellitus. *Diabetes Technol.Ther.*, 9, 509-515.

Zollner, G., Fickert, P., Fuchsbichler, A., Silbert, D., Wagner, M., Arbeiter, S., Gonzalez, F.J., Marschall, H.U., Zatloukal, K., Denk, H. & Trauner, M. (2003) Role of nuclear bile acid receptor, FXR, in adaptive ABC transporter regulation by cholic and ursodeoxycholic acid in mouse liver, kidney and intestine. 39, 480-488.

19

Role of Vitamin D in the Pathogenesis and Therapy of Type 1 Diabetes Mellitus

Agustin Busta, Bianca Alfonso and Leonid Poretsky
Albert Einstein College of Medicine, Beth Israel Medical Center New York U.S.A.

1. Introduction

This chapter will review the role of vitamin D in the pathogenesis and treatment of type 1 diabetes mellitus.
We will discuss the mechanisms through which vitamin D might affect pancreatic function. We will summarize the results of in-vitro and animal studies and will conclude with a review of the relevant clinical trials.

2. Definition

Type 1 diabetes mellitus is an autoimmune disease in which the pancreas is unable to respond to secretagogue stimulation with appropriate insulin secretion. Hyperglycemia develops when more than 70-90% of the insulin-producing beta cells are destroyed. An autoimmune destructive process, which plays a central role in the development of type 1 diabetes mellitus, is facilitated by the subject's own genetic susceptibility and by non-genetic factors. Non-genetic factors include viral infections, toxic chemicals, and others. Vitamin D deficiency is a non-genetic factor that appears to be associated with an increased risk of developing type 1 diabetes mellitus.
Type 1 diabetes mellitus complications are classified into acute and chronic. The acute complications include life-threatening conditions like severe hypoglycemia or diabetic ketoacidosis (DKA). Chronic diabetic complications can be divided into microvascular complications (retinopathy, neuropathy and nephropathy) and macrovascular complications (cardiovascular, cerebrovascular and peripheral vascular disease). Severe microvascular and macrovascular complications can lead to renal failure (the most common cause of hemodialysis in the US), blindness or lower extremity amputations.
Overall, uncontrolled diabetes mellitus in patients over 50 years of age reduces life expectancy in males and females by 7.5 and 8.2 years respectively (Franco et al.,2007).

3. Epidemiology

In 2010, about 215,000 people younger than 20 years of age had diabetes (type 1 or type 2) in the United States.– A 2011 Centers for Disease Control and Prevention (CDC) report estimates that nearly 26 million Americans have diabetes.– Diabetes affects 8.3% of

Americans of all ages and 11.3% of adults aged 20 years and older, according to the National Diabetes Fact Sheet for 2011. About 27% of those with diabetes (approximately 7 million Americans) do not know they have the disease. 1 in every 400 children and adolescents has type 1 diabetes.

Type 1 diabetes mellitus continues to be highly prevalent in many countries, with an overall annual increase estimated at 3% (International Diabetes Federation [IDF] 2010). Worldwide, it is more common in males than in females, with a ratio of 1.5.

The 4th edition of the IDF Diabetes Atlas, released in 2009 at the 20th World Diabetes Congress, estimated that in 2010, 285 million people would have diabetes (6.4% of world's adult population). The same forum predicts that by 2030, 438 million people will have diabetes world-wide. Type 1 diabetes in children is estimated at 480,000 patients worldwide in 2010, and the number of newly diagnosed cases per year is 75,800 (IDF 2010).

3.1 Natural history

The natural history of type 1 diabetes is characterized by an autoimmune destruction of the beta cells in the islands of Langerhans in the pancreas. The autoimmune process has cellular and humoral components, leading to the destruction of the beta cells and a decreased insulin secretion. As beta-cell mass declines, insulin secretion decreases until the available insulin no longer is adequate to maintain normal blood glucose levels. After 70-90% of the beta cells are destroyed, hyperglycemia develops and diabetes may be diagnosed.

The natural history of type 1 diabetes has 4 stages: genetic susceptibility, autoimmune process, pre-diabetes and diabetes.

The rate of beta cell destruction is variable. In some patients years will go by before the onset of diabetes, while other patients may never develop beta cell insufficiency, perhaps due to the regaining of tolerance. Most patients with type 1 diabetes mellitus have one or more susceptible human leukocyte antigen (HLA) class II, and over 90% have beta cell autoantibodies present. The appearance of circulating islet cell autoantibodies is the first detectable sign of this immune process.

4. Pathogenesis of type 1 diabetes mellitus

4.1 Genetic component

Genetics has an important role in the etiology of type 1 diabetes. However, extra-genetic components influence the penetrance of diabetes susceptibility genes. If data are obtained at a single point in time, the risk of type 1 diabetes mellitus between monozygotic twins can be as low as 30%, but if the monozygotic twins are followed long-term, the cumulative incidence of diabetes reaches 65% (Redondo et al., 2008). In the same cohort of monozygotic twins, the rate of persistent autoantibody positivity, type 1 diabetes mellitus, or both, reached 78% (Redondo et al., 2008).

To better understand the genetic susceptibility to diabetes, candidate gene studies were conducted in order to identify genes that are associated with autoimmune type 1 diabetes.

Human leukocyte antigen (HLA) associations have been long recognized in many autoimmune diseases. In type 1 diabetes mellitus, the HLA on chromosome 6p21 is well described and is considered to play an important role in more than 50% of the familial cases in Caucasians (Noble et al., 1996). HLA DR4-DQ8 or DR3-DQ2 haplotypes are detected in up to 90% of patients with type 1 diabetes mellitus (Devendra & Eisenbarth, 2003). The combination of these 2 types, DR4-DQ8/DR3-DQ2, carries the highest risk and type 1 diabetes mellitus occurs at a very early age in this population. First-degree relatives of the patients who carry the highest risk haplotype combination also have a higher risk of developing diabetes mellitus as compared to the relatives of diabetes patients who do not have this haplotype and who develop type 1 diabetes mellitus later in life (Gillespie et al., 2002).

Another HLA haplotype (DR15-DQ6) might have protective properties, and is found in a much larger percentage in the general population (20%) as compared to less than 1% in patients with type 1 diabetes mellitus (Eisenbarth & Gottlieb, 2004).

HLA haplotypes appear to have an association with islet autoantibodies. Glutamic acid decarboxylase (GAD) antibodies are more frequent in patients with HLA DR3-DQ2, whereas insulin auto-antibodies (IAA) and protein tyrosine phosphatase-like protein antibodies (IA-2 antibodies) are more frequent in patients with HLA DR4-DQ8. Patients that do not have these haplotypes are less likely to develop islet autoantibodies (Achenbach et al., 2005).

Another key genetic factor is the insulin gene (INS), with different forms of the promoter region conferring either protection or increased susceptibility to autoimmune diabetes mellitus (Bennett et al., 1995). The insulin gene contributes 10% to the genetic susceptibility in developing autoimmune diabetes (Bell et al., 1984). The risk of developing diabetes depends on the expression of the insulin protein in the thymus which can cause a defective central tolerance to the insulin molecule. The degree of immune tolerance may be reflected by the less common presence of insulin autoantibodies (IAA) in patients or relatives who have the protective INS class I/III or III/III genotypes (Vafiadis et al., 1997).

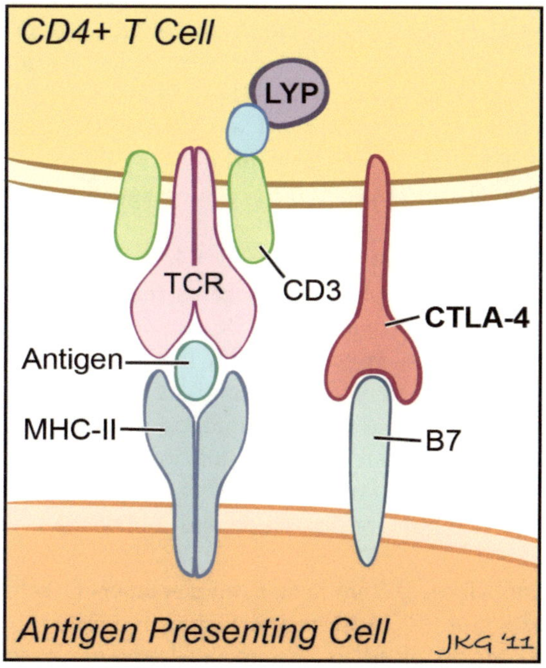

Fig. 1. Antigen Presenting Cell. The activation of the T-cell by various stimuli (antigens), is brought by major histocompatibility complex (MHC-HLA II). This figure shows also, inhibitors of T-cell activation: cytotoxic T lymphocyte antigen 4 (CTLA-4) and lymphoid tyrosine phosphatase (LYP).

T cells are recognized to be a major part of the immune process in diabetes mellitus, and several genes involved in T cell regulation are associated with type 1 diabetes mellitus. Two genes encoding factors that are suppressive to the T cell activation appear to have a close association with autoimmune diabetes: lymphoid tyrosine phosphatase locus (LYP/PTPN22) (Smyth et al., 2004), and cytotoxic T lymphocyte antigen 4 (CTLA-4) (Ueda et al., 2003) (Figure 1), located on chromosome 2q33.

The CTLA-4, which is a T-Lymphocyte receptor, is expressed after T-cell activation (Greenwald et al., 2005). It turns off T-cell responses by inhibiting the production of interleukine-2. CTLA-4 polymorphism in humans has been associated with an increased risk of autoimmune disease, including type 1 diabetes mellitus (Gough et al., 2005).

Another gene linked to an increased risk for type 1 diabetes is the gene for the intercellular adhesion molecule (ICAM-1) (Nejentsev et al., 2003). A recent genome-wide association study described over 40 loci associated with an increased risk for type 1 diabetes (Barrett et al., 2009).

4.2 Autoimmune process

One of the best animal models for type 1 diabetes mellitus is the nonobese diabetic mouse (NOD). NOD mouse develops type 1 diabetes mellitus spontaneously, over the course of a few months, allowing the investigators to study this process stage by stage. Many reports describe in detail the genetics, the immune process, the influence of the environment and most importantly, the potential therapies to prevent, delay or reverse the destructive process that leads to type 1 diabetes mellitus in this model. Delovitch and Singh (Delovitch & Singh, 1997) reviewed the use of NOD mouse in the studies of type 1 diabetes mellitus. In NOD mice, the first step is the infiltration of the peri-islet regions of the pancreatic islets by dendritic cells (DC) and macrophages, followed by T cells (CD4+ and CD8+). This stage is known as peri-insulitis, occurring around 3-4 weeks of age. It is followed by a slower, progressive T cell destruction of the beta cells (insulitis), by 4-6 months of age (Delovitch & Singh, 1997). Thus, the T cells and the dendritic cells are key players in the immune process leading to type 1 diabetes mellitus.

The dendritic cells (DC) are antigen-presenting cells which originate from the bone marrow. They become active once they capture and process the antigens. After infiltrating the pancreas and undergoing antigenic maturation, DC secrete IL-12 and present the processed antigen (on their surface and in association with the major histocompatibility complex [MHC] class II) to other cells of the immune system (i.e. T cells) (see Fig 1).

T cells are categorized mainly based on their immune actions, achieved via the different cytokines they secrete. Cytokines are classified into two types: type 1 cytokines, which activate the cellular immunity and suppress the humoral immune response, and type 2 cytokines, which activate the humoral immunity and inhibit the cellular immune process (Rabinovitch, 1998).

Th1 cells are preferentially formed from their T cell precursors (T helper 0) under the direct influence of mature DC and IL-12 (Banchereau & Steinman, 1998).

T helper 1 cells (Th1) are involved in cell-mediated immune responses (inflammation, cytotoxicity, delayed hypersensitivity) and produce type 1 cytokines: tumor necrosis factor β (TNFβ), interferon γ (IFNγ), and interleukin 2 (IL-2). T helper 2 cells (Th2) are important in humoral immunity (activate B cells and antibody production, down regulating Th 1 cells) and secrete type 2 cytokines: interleukins 4, 5, 6, 9 and 10 (Rabinovitch, 1998) (Fig. 2).

The Th2 cells are protective for the beta cells. They have an inhibitory effect on the Th1 cells, which are destructive to the pancreatic beta cells. In the NOD mouse, it appears that the immunologic self-tolerance to pancreatic beta cells is lost. The disruption of the equilibrium between Th1 and Th2 cells in the thymus and in the periphery is believed to play a crucial role in the pathogenesis of autoimmune diabetes mellitus (Delovitch & Singh, 1997). Once Th1 cells are produced they will secrete interferon γ (IFN γ) and IL-2, leading to the activation of macrophages and cytotoxic T cells, which are destructive to the pancreatic beta cells (Adorini, 2001). The same Th1 cells will stimulate the IgG2a autoantibodies against the islet beta cells autoantigens (Delovitch & Singh, 1997). Autoimmune diabetes can be transferred from a diabetic NOD mouse to an unaffected mouse via T cells (Bendelac et al., 1987). NOD mice develop a spontaneous loss of T-cell tolerance to glutamic acid decarboxylase antibodies (GAD), leading to autoimmune diabetes (Kaufman et al., 1993). In NOD mice, there is an increased resistance to apoptosis in immunocytes (Leijon et al., 1995, Penha-Goncalves et al., 1995).

Immune responses to several beta-cell proteins have been described (auto-antigens). Exposure to glutamic acid decarboxylase (GAD65 and GAD67) led to an increased T cell proliferation as early as 4 weeks of life in NOD mice, coinciding with the onset of insulitis (Tisch 1993). Some of the other beta-cell antigens elicited an increased immune response after a few more weeks, but there were other beta-cell antigens that did not trigger an immune reaction (for example, amylin) (Tisch 1993). The same study showed that intrathymic injections of GAD65 had a protective effect from autoimmune diabetes in NOD mice (delaying the onset of disease and decreasing the frequency) (Tisch etal., 1993)

GAD65- reactive T cells were proven to have the ability to transfer diabetes to NOD/SCID (severe combined immunodeficiency) mice (Zekzer et al., 1998). To further support the central role of GAD antigen in autoimmune diabetes, the beta-cell-specific suppression of GAD expression in antisense GAD transgenic NOD mice was demonstrated to prevent the production of diabetogenic T cells and the onset of diabetes (Yoon et al., 1999)

In humans, the pancreas becomes infiltrated with mononuclear cells. Autoantibodies to insulin (IAA), glutamic acid decarboxylase (GAD) and insulinoma associated-2 antibody (IA-2) are demonstrated years before the clinical symptoms of diabetes. (Kulmala et al., 1998) T cell responses to several islet cells antigens (insulin, GAD, IA-2) have been reported in IDDM (MacCuish et al., 1975). The presence of autoantibodies alone does not explain the development of diabetes, since it is recognized now that children born to type 1 diabetic mother with high antibody titers transferred through the umbilical cord do not develop diabetes more often than expected. An interesting case was published by Martin et al in 2001, describing a case of type 1 diabetes mellitus occurring in a patient that had a hereditary B-cell defect (Martin et al., 2001).

4.3 Environmental component

The environment is implicated in the pathogenesis of type 1 diabetes mellitus by many studies.

Environmental factors have an important role in initiating an immune process that ultimately leads to pancreatic beta cell destruction and clinically apparent diabetes mellitus. Many environmental factors have been proposed, including viruses (rubella, mumps or coxsackievirus B4), toxic substances and cytotoxins. Nutritional status and diet have also been implicated as potential players in type 1 diabetes pathogenesis: vitamin D deficiency, early protein diet exposure or exposure to cow's milk in infancy.

Viruses are among the main culprits studied. Before the eradication of rubella in most countries, congenital rubella was strongly associated with the development of type 1 diabetes mellitus (Menser et al., 1978). A recent meta analysis of observational studies has shown an association between type 1 diabetes and enterovirus infection (Yeung 2011).

While some theories implicate viral infections in the pathogenesis of type 1 diabetes, a recent hypothesis argues that a decreased exposure to microbes may contribute to the current increase in autoimmune disease. This theory is known as "the hygiene hypothesis" (Gale, 2002).

It is a known fact that the incidence of autoimmune diabetes follows a geographical pattern, with many studies reporting an association between type 1 diabetes and vitamin D status. A few large ecological studies describe a pattern of geographical variation, with an increased incidence of type 1 diabetes in the areas located north of the equator. Furthermore, seasons appear to also influence the incidence of type 1 diabetes, with the highest incidence during winter and the lowest during summer. The month of birth during springtime is associated with a higher risk of type 1 diabetes (Kahn et al., 2009), a finding that could be explained by possible low circulating vitamin D levels in both mother and fetus through the winter months of the pregnancy.

In order to develop more information about environmental factors that play a role in the pathogenesis of diabetes, an international initiative (the Environmental Determinants of Diabetes in the Young) will be following thousands of infants with an increased genetic risk from birth until adolescence and will gather data about infectious agents, dietary or other environmental factors.

Typically, the treatment for type 1 diabetes mellitus involves insulin therapy, but in the last few years new therapies have been approved as well (for example, Symlin). For newly diagnosed patients with autoimmune diabetes, combination therapy has been suggested in an attempt to minimize beta cell destruction and prolong pancreatic function. The new therapeutic options include: immunotherapy, vaccines, drugs that influence T cell action, anti-inflammatory drugs (for example, one time use of anti-IL-1R drug), or long-term treatment with B cell components to induce regulatory T cells (oral or nasal insulin, insulin peptide therapy, GAD-Alum or the proinsulin DNA vaccines). Glucagon-like peptide 1-related drugs (GLP-1) could be also considered as a therapeutic option because they promote peritubular pancreatic cell growth (Von Herrath, 2010).

5. Vitamin D

Although initially described as a "vitamin", vitamin D is now recognized to be a hormone, synthesized in the human body and exerting its action on other organs via a nuclear receptor (vitamin D receptor, VDR).

Even though vitamin D can be obtained from the diet in small quantities, the main source of vitamin D is the skin. Under the direct influence of ultra violet B light (UVB light), 7-dehydrocholesterol (DHC) (provitamin D3) is converted into pre-vitamin D3, which is then further converted into cholecalciferol (vitamin D3) via thermal isomerization. Interestingly, if pre-vitamin D3 continues to be exposed to UVB, it will be converted into biologically inactive metabolites (tachysterol and lumisterol), preventing a potential UVB- induced vitamin D intoxication (Holick, 1999) The other source of vitamin D is the diet, which contains cholecalciferol (vitamin D3), originating from animal sources, and ergocalciferol (vitamin D2), deriving from plants (Holick, 1999).

Regardless of their source, once they enter into the circulation, forms of inactive vitamin D3 or D2 bind to the vitamin D-binding protein (DBP) and are transported to the liver. The inactive vitamin D is activated through a 2-step hydroxylation process via two hydroxylases that belong to the cytochrome P450- dependent steroid hydroxylases (CYP450). In the liver, vitamin D undergoes the first hydroxylation at C-25 via some of the CYP 450 vitamin D 25-hydroxylases, forming calcidiol (25-hydroxyvitamin D) (Prosser & Jones, 2004). This is the major circulating form of vitamin D. At the level of the proximal renal tubule, 25-OH vitamin D is further hydroxylated to calcitriol (1,25 dihydroxyvitamin D, the active form of vitamin D) by the 1α-hydroxylase (1α(OH)ase, CYP27B1) (Prosser & Jones, 2004).

Both calcidiol and calcitriol are inactivated via the 25-hydroxyvitamin D3-24-hydroxylase (CYP24), forming the inactive metabolite 24,25- dihydroxyvitamin D (Holick, 1999).

1α-hydroxylase has been described in many extrarenal tissues: macrophages, monocytes, and placenta, rendering these cells capable of synthesizing 1α-,25$(OH)_2D_3$from 25(OH)vitamin D (Weisman et al., 1979, Bhalla et al., 1983, Stoffels et al., 2007, Adams et al., 1983). The activity of 1α-hydroxylase in the immune cells is not under the regulation of parathyroid hormone and 1α-,25$(OH)_2D_3$, but rather under immune cytokine regulation. A defect in the up-regulation of 1α-hydroxylase after immune stimulation is described in NOD mouse (Overbergh et al., 2000). Extrarenal distribution of 1α-hydroxylase becomes important in understanding the extra-skeletal effects of vitamin D.

VDR is part of the nuclear receptor super family of ligand-activated transcription factors, which also includes glucocorticoid, thyroid hormone and estrogen receptors. The gene for VDR is located on chromosome 12q12-14, and shows great polymorphism (Haussler et al., 1998). After 1,25 $(OH)_2D_3$ binds to VDR, it induces conformational changes that facilitate heterodimerization with the retinoid X receptor and the recruitment of nuclear receptor coactivator proteins, which then act on the chromatin. The specific DNA sequence that is ultimately affected by the vitamin D is known as the vitamin D responsive element (VDRE) (Carlberg & Polly, 1998).

The discovery of the vitamin D receptor (VDR) on the immune cells (Strugnell & DeLuca, 1997), led to the hypothesis that vitamin D could affect the autoimmune processes. However, in VDR deficient mice models, there is no increase in autoimmune diseases (Mathieu et al., 2001)

The protective effects of vitamin D in several autoimmune diseases have been described in animal models (experimental autoimmune encephalomyelitis (Lemire, 1995), murine models of human multiple sclerosis and murine models of rheumatoid arthritis (Cantorna et al., 1996). In other autoimmune diseases, like psoriasis, vitamin D analogues are the mainstay of treatment today.

The extraskeletal effects of 1α-,25$(OH)_2D_3$ can usually be observed only at very high concentrations (10^{-10}mol/l), higher than physiological levels needed for calcium balance (concentrations that could probably be achieved in specific target tissues via the macrophages' 1α-hydroxylase) (Mathieu et al., 2005). Thus a risk of hypercalcemia and other side effects of 1α-25$(OH)_2D_3$ could occur if it were used for its anti-autoimmune properties. Numerous vitamin D analogs have been developed to exert extraskeletal effects, with less pronounced action on the calcium metabolism. Most of these analogs are used for laboratory research purposes, but some are part of standard treatment for certain autoimmune diseases (for example, calcipotriol for psoriasis).

There are several theories that attempt to explain the link between Vitamin D and autoimmune diabetes. This relationship appears to be complex, with actions at multiples levels: genetic, autoimmune and also direct action on the pancreatic beta cells.

6. Vitamin D and type 1 diabetes

Animal studies and clinical trials in patients with new onset of type 1 diabetes show that the replacement of vitamin D may arrest the deterioration of pancreatic function and improve C-peptide levels.

There is strong epidemiologic data showing that the population in countries with a high prevalence of type 1 diabetes mellitus is commonly vitamin D deficient. Vitamin D supplementation during pregnancy decreased the risk of the development of type 1 diabetes mellitus for offspring (Fronczak et al., 2003). Supplementation of vitamin D at an early age also decreases the risk for developing type 1 diabetes (Hypponen et al., 2001)

The vitamin D receptor (VDR) has been described on almost every tissue in the human body, including the cells of the immune system, as discussed earlier.

The VDR gene is located on chromosome 12, and has a few allelic variants. It has been reported that some of these allelic variations of the VDR gene are linked to an increased risk of type 1 diabetes mellitus in the German and the Indian Asian population (Pani et al., 2000, Chang et al., 2000). On the other hand, the same association was not found in another population sample (British, Portuguese and Finnish origin) (Guo et al., 2006, Lemos, 2008, Turpeinen, 2002).

An interaction between specific VDR polymorphisms and predisposing HLA DRB1 0301 allele was described in North Indian patients (Israni et al., 2009) and is associated with an increased risk of developing type 1 diabetes mellitus.

As discussed earlier, the last step in the activation of vitamin D is facilitated by the key enzyme 1α-hydroxylase, encoded by the CYP27B1 gene on the chromosome 12q13.1-q13.3. Polymorphism in this gene is described as being associated with an increased risk of type 1 diabetes mellitus (Lopez et al., 2004, Bailey et al., 2007). The polymorphism in the CYP27B1 gene could potentially lead to the reduced expression of 1α-hydroxylase, less production of the active $1\alpha,25\ (OH)_2\ D_3$, and ultimately, to the increased risk of type 1 diabetes.

6.1 Vitamin D and type 1 diabetes: The effects on the immune processes

Vitamin D interacts with most immune cells and affects their cytokine production. Overall, vitamin D has a protective effect on the pancreatic beta cells (Figure 2).

DCs are affected by $1\alpha,25\ (OH)_2D_3$ in many ways. DCs mature after they engulf the antigen, increasing the expression of MHC-II molecules on their surface and secreting IL-12. Studies show that vitamin D analogs suppress the expression of MHC-II molecules (Griffin 2000) The cytokine secretion by DC is affected as well: the IL-12 is inhibited (D'Ambrosio 1998), while IL-10 production is increased (Penna 2000). Furthermore, DC apoptosis is promoted by exposure to vitamin D (Penna 2000).

If DC are exposed to $1\alpha,25\ (OH)_2\ D_3$, they do not mature at a subsequent exposure to an antigen, becoming tolerogenic (Griffin et al., 2001). After being treated with a vitamin D analog, the DC do not simply remain immature, but instead are transformed into tolerogenic DC with special endocytic properties (Ferreira et al., 2009). Adorini et al published a paper describing how 1α,25$(OH)_2$ D_3 can change the dendritic cells into a tolerogenic phenotype which is thought to induce T regulatory cells and inhibit autoimmune diseases, like type 1 diabetes (Adorini, 2003) (Fig 2).

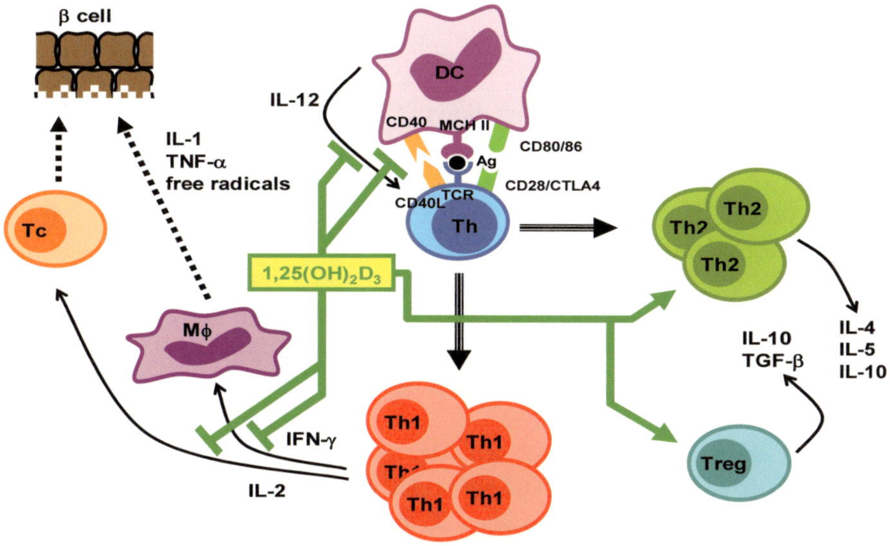

Fig. 2. The immunomodulatory effects of 1α,25(OH)2D3. At the level of the antigen-presenting cell (such as dendritic cells; DCs), 1α,25(OH)2D3 inhibits the surface expression of MHC class II-complexed antigen and of co-stimulatory molecules, in addition to production of the cytokine IL-12, thereby indirectly shifting the polarization of T cells from a Th1 towards a Th2 phenotype. In addition, 1α,25(OH)2D3 has immunomodulatory effects directly at the level of the T cell, by inhibiting the production of the Th1 cytokines IL-2 and IFN-γ and stimulating the production of Th2 cytokines. Moreover, 1α,25(OH)2D3 favors the induction of regulatory T cells. Both Th2 and Tregs can inhibit Th1 cells through the production of counteracting or inhibitory cytokines. Together, these immunomodulatory effects of 1α,25(OH)2D3 can lead to the protection of target tissues, such as β cells, in autoimmune diseases and transplantation. CD40L, CD40 ligand; Mf, macrophage; Tc, cytotoxic T cell; TGF- β, transforming growth factor β; Th1,T helper type 1; TNF-α, tumor necrosis factor α; Treg, regulatory T cell. This figure was published in Trends in Endocrinology and Metabolism Vol.16 No.6 August 2005. Vitamin D and type 1 diabetes mellitus: state of art. Chantal Mathieu and Klaus Badenhoop. Copyright @ Elsevier 2005. Used with permission.

Descriptions of the VDR on T lymphocytes lead to the subsequent investigation of vitamin D actions on these immune cells. Interestingly, 1α-hydroxylase is not expressed in the T cells, and vitamin D activated in the macrophages acts on the T cells, suggesting an autocrine action of 1α,25 dihydroxyvitamin D_3.

Rigby and his team proved that cytokine production by T cells is influenced by vitamin D analogs: IL-2 and IFN γ are inhibited (Rigby et al., 1987), while production of some of the type 2 cytokines (IL-4, 5, and 10) is enhanced (Boonstra et al., 2001)

Inhibition of mitogen-stimulated T-cell cultures by vitamin D has been also reported (Rigby et al., 1984)

On the other hand, suppressor T cells are stimulated by vitamin D, leading to the inhibition of T-cell mediated immunity (Mathieu et al., 1994).

While inhibiting the IL-12 production from the DC, vitamin D is able to shift the differentiation of T naïve cells into Th0 cells and further into Th2 cells (IL-12 is an important cytokine that preferentially promotes the Th1 cell formation from the Th0 cells) (Willheim et al., 1999).

A recent study reported the direct modulation of CD4+ T cell function by active vitamin D, describing the inhibition of IL-17, IL-21, IFNγ, and the induction of T reg cells expressing CTLA-4 and FoxP3. If the T cells are grown in an environment rich in IL-2 and vitamin D, they express the highest levels of CTLA-4 and FoxP3, and are able to suppress the proliferation of the resting CD4+ T cells (Jeffery et al., 2009).

VDR is normally expressed on the B cells only upon their activation. Chen reported that 1α,25 $(OH)_2D_3$ decreased B cell proliferation and immunoglobulin production and induced cell death (Chen et al., 2007).

Vitamin D inhibits the production of inflammatory interleukins: IL-12, IL-2, interferon γ, tumor necrosis factor (TNF)-α, and TNF-β ,while the production of anti-inflammatory cytokines (IL-4, IL-10, TGF-β) is stimulated. This may disrupt the production of Th1 cells, which are destructive for the pancreatic beta cells, with a resultant beneficial effect on the beta cells (Lemire, 1995, van Etten & Mathieu 2005).

6.2 Vitamin D and type 1 diabetes: Direct effects on pancreatic cells

1α,25 $(OH)_2$ D_3 appears to have a direct protective effect against pancreatic beta cell destruction by reducing the expression of MHC class I molecules (Hahn et al, 1997). In addition, vitamin D appears to increase islet cell expression of the A20 protein, which has antiapoptotic function (Riachy et al., 2002) (Fig 2). Vitamin D also decreases the expression of Fas, which is a transmembrane cell surface receptor mediator, involved in pancreatic beta cell apoptosis (Riachy et al., 2006).

7. Animal studies – vitamin D and type 1 diabetes

Insulitis can be inhibited by the administration of high doses of vitamin D in NOD mice (Mathieu et al., 1992), and 1α,25$(OH)_2D_3$ can prevent autoimmune diabetes in these animals (Mathieu et al., 1994). In both spontaneously developing and cyclophosphamide induced models of diabetes mellitus, vitamin D protects against autoimmune diabetes in NOD mice through restoration of the deficient suppressor cell function (Mathieu et al., 1995). VDR ligands enhance CD4+CD25+ regulatory T cells; these cells may play a role in protecting against insulitis in NOD mice (Adorini, 2003).

The loss of balance between the Th1 cells and Th2 cells, with the overproduction of the Th1 cells, appears to be central in the autoimmune diabetes pathogenesis. In NOD mice, the exposure to GAD65 leads to T cell proliferation and antibody production (Kaufman et al., 1993), at the same time as insulitis develops. 1,25 dihydroxyvitamin D_3 administration leads to a local immune shift of the balance between the Th1 cells and Th2 cells, favoring the increase in IL-4 production and the decrease in the γ interferon secretion.

Overbergh et al demonstrated that in NOD mice the immune shift between Th1/Th2 cells occurs in the periphery and is not limited to the pancreas (Overbergh et al., 2000). Furthermore, this change in the immune milieu occurs only in the autoantigen-specific immune response (exposure to GAD65, insulin B-chain, heat shock protein 65), and is not observed in the immune response associated with other antigens (ovalbumin, tetanus toxins, etc).

The recurrence of autoimmune diabetes mellitus after islet cell transplant was prevented in NOD mice by treatment with vitamin D analogs in combination with cyclosporine A (Casteels et al., 1998). Further, the administration of a nonhypercalcemic vitamin D analog in combination with an immunosuppressant (cyclosporine A) prevented progression to overt diabetes mellitus, even after the insulitis developed (Casteels et al., 1998). This effect, however, could not be reproduced when the vitamin D analog was administered without the addition of cyclosporine.

The NOD mice have an increased resistance to apoptosis in their immune cells. 1,25-dihydroxyvitamin D3 restores apoptosis in NOD mice in the thymus, leading to the increased destruction of autoimmune effector cells (Casteels et al., 1998).

In the BB rat, another animal model for autoimmune diabetes mellitus, 1,25-dihydroxyvitamin D did not lead to any significant difference in the incidence of diabetes when given from weaning to 120 days (Mathieu et al., 1997). This finding illustrates the issue of potentially different disease mechanisms in various animals and the difficulty of applying research findings from one animal model to another, or to humans.

8. Clinical studies – vitamin D and type 1 diabetes

The data available from human studies is scant and controversial.

A few ecological studies support the theory that vitamin D is a major player in the autoimmune disease pathogenesis, including type 1 diabetes mellitus.

A study in Northern Europe described the seasonal pattern of disease onset for autoimmune diabetes mellitus (Karvonen et al., 1998). The Diabetes Epidemiology Research International Group reported in 1988 an increased incidence of autoimmune diabetes with lower average yearly temperatures, which, in turn, was strongly associated with increasing latitude distances from the equator. This variation is thought to be due to the decreased exposure of the skin to the UV radiation.

In a very large worldwide study, Mohr et al analyzed the data from the Diabetes Mondial Project Group and found that in children younger than 14 years of age, the incidence rates of type 1 diabetes mellitus were significantly increased at higher latitudes and with low UVB exposure. Incidence rates of type 1 diabetes mellitus approached zero in the region with high UVB irradiance (Mohr et al., 2008).

Several European studies reported a decreased risk of diabetes in infants supplemented with high doses of vitamin D. The EURODIAB substudy 2 study group in seven European centers reported that vitamin D supplementation in infancy decreased the risk of autoimmune diabetes in a fairly consistent manner (Dalquist et al., 1999). Hypponen et al published the results of a birth-cohort study in northern Finland that included all pregnant women who were due to give birth in 1966, and recorded the frequency and the dosing of the vitamin D supplementation in the first year of life, as well as the presence of suspected rickets. 30 years later, the authors found that there was a lower incidence of diabetes mellitus in children who took any dose of vitamin D as compared with children that did not take any vitamin D supplementation. Even more so, the risk was lower in children that took the highest dose (2000 IU daily) as compared to the lower dose of vitamin D. Children with suspected rickets had a 3 fold increased risk of developing insulin-dependent diabetes mellitus (Hypponen et al., 2001). The risk of developing islet auto-antibodies in the children of mothers that took vitamin D during pregnancy was decreased in the Diabetes Autoimmunity Study in the Young (DAISY) (Fronczak et al., 2003). It is unclear from these studies if the protective effect is due to the supplementation with extra doses of vitamin D or prevention of vitamin D deficiency.

Two new interventional trials have been published in the last 2 years supporting the beneficial effect of vitamin D on the development of autoimmune diabetes.

A pilot study looking at patients with adult-onset latent autoimmune diabetes (LADA) demonstrated that supplementation with 1,25 dihydroxyvitamin D3 for 1 year resulted in beta cell preservation, as assessed by C-peptide levels (Li et al., 2009).

Aljabri et al conducted a prospective study in which patients with vitamin D deficiency were assigned to receive 4000 IU of vitamin D3 daily and had vitamin D 25 (OH) levels and hemoglobin A1c measured at baseline and at 12 weeks. The results revealed that the patients who achieved higher circulating levels of vitamin D 25 (OH) had a lower hemoglobin A1c (Aljabri et al., 2010).

Other studies, however, did not find similar results. A study which examined the effects of supplementation with cod liver oil during the first year of life, found that the infants who were supplemented had a decreased risk of developing childhood-onset type 1 diabetes. However, this decreased risk of type 1 diabetes mellitus was not observed in the infants if the cod liver oil was supplemented during pregnancy or if the vitamin D preparations were supplemented during the first year of the infant's life. Since cod liver oil has a high content of vitamin D along with the long-chain n-3 fatty acids (eicosapentaenoic and docosahexaenoic), it is not clear if these effects are due to the high vitamin D content of the cod liver oil or due to the fatty acids (Stene et al., 2003).

Pittoco et al reported the results of an interventional trial in children with newly diagnosed type 1 diabetes, in which the patients were administered calcitriol or nicotinamide in order to preserve beta-cell function. Even though there was a decrease in the insulin requirements at 3 and 6 months in the calcitriol treated group, at the end of the first year there was no difference between the C-peptide levels or hemoglobin A1c between the two groups (Pitocco et al., 2006).

Bizzarri et al investigated whether supplementation with calcitriol in recent onset autoimmune diabetes has a protective effect on the pancreatic beta cells and found that, at the doses used in the study, calcitriol did not confer protection against the autoimmune destruction of the beta cells (Bizzarri et al., 2010). In Germany, Walter et al supplemented newly diagnosed adult patients with 1,25(OH)2D3 for 18 months. At the end of the study there was no difference in the areas under the curve (AUC) for C-peptide, peak C-peptide, or fasting C-peptide after a mixed meal tolerance test between the treatment and the placebo groups (Walter et al., 2010).

9. Conclusion

In conclusion, the data on the role of vitamin D in the pathogenesis of autoimmune diabetes mellitus is inconclusive. More studies, particularly, interventional trials, with vitamin D or vitamin D nonhypercalcemic analogs need to be performed before the interaction between autoimmunity, diabetes mellitus and vitamin D is completely understood.

10. Acknowledgements

We would like to thank Barbara Pietrzyk-Busta, RN, MA for her invaluable assistance in the preparation and editing of this manuscript, and to Jill Gregory, CMI, FAMI for designing an illustration of Figure 1.

11. References

Adams JS, Singer FR, Gacad MA, Sharma OP, Hayes MJ, Vouros P & Holick M (1995). Isolation and structural identification of 1,25-dihydroxyvitamin D3 produced by cultured alveolar macrophages in sarcoidosis. J Clin Endocrinol Metab, 60:960-966.

Adams JS, Sharma OP, Gacad MA & Singer FR (1983). Metabolism of 25-hydroxyvitamin D3 by cultured pulmonary alveolar macrophages in sarcoidosis. J Clin Invest, 72:1856–1860.

Adorini L (2003) Tolerogenic dendritic cells induced by vitamin D receptor ligands enhance regulatory T cells inhibiting autoimmune diabetes. Ann N Y Acad Sci, 987:258–261.

Adorini L (2001). Interleukin 12 and autoimmune diabetes. Nat Genet 27(2):131–132.

Aljabri KS, Bokhari SA & Khan MJ. (2010). Glycemic changes after vitamin D supplementation in patients with type 1 diabetes mellitus and vitamin D deficiency. Ann Saudi Med, 30(6):454-458.

Achenbach P, Bonifacio E, Koczwara K & Ziegler AG (2005). Natural history of type 1 diabetes. Diabetes,54(Suppl2):S25-S31.

Banchereau J & Steinman RM. (1998). Dendritic cells and the control of immunity. Nature 392(6673):245–252.

Bailey R , Cooper JD, Zeitels L,Smyth DJ, Yang JH, Walker NM, Hypponen E, Dunger DB, Ramos-Lopez E, Badenhoop K, Nejentsev S & Todd JA (2007). Association of the Vitamin D metabolism gene CYP27B1 with type 1 diabetes. Diabetes,56(10):2616-2621.

Barrett JC, Clayton DG, Concannon P, Akolkar B, Cooper JD, Erlich HA, Julier C, Morahan G, Nerup J, Nierras C, Plagnol V, Pociot F, Schuilenburg H, Smyth DJ, Stevens H, Todd JA, Walker NM & Rich SS (2009). Genome-wide association study and a meta-analysis find that over 40 loci affect risk of type 1 diabetes. Nature Genetics. 41(6):703-707.

Bhalla AK, Amento EP, Clemens TL, Holick MF & Krane SM. (1983). Specific high-affinity receptors for 1,25 dihydroxyvitamin D3 in human peripheral mononuclear cells: Presence in monocytes and induction in T lymphocytes following activation. J Clin Endocrinol Metab 57(6):1308-1310.

Bendelac A, Carnaud C, Boitard C & Bach JF. (1987). Syngeneic transfer of autoimmune diabetes from diabetic NOD mice to healthy neonates. Requirement for both L3T4+ and Lyt-2+ T cells. J Exp Med 166:823-832.

Bennett ST, Lucassen AM, Gough SC, Powell EE, Undlien DE, Pritchard LE, Merriman ME, Kawaguchi Y, Dronsfield MJ & Pociot F (1995). Susceptibility to human type 1 diabetes at IDDM2 is determined by tandem repeat variation at the insulin gene mini satellite locus. Nat Genet, 9:284-292.

Bell GI, Horita S & Kharam JH (1994). A polymorphic locus near the insulin gene is associated with insulin-dependent diabetes mellitus. Diabetes ,33:176-83.

Benoist C & Mathis D. 1997. Cell death mediators in autoimmune diabetes—No shortage of suspects. Cell 89(1):1-3.

Bizzarri C, Pitocco D, Napoli N, Di Stasi E, Maggi D, Manfrini S, Suraci C, Cavallo MG, Cappa M, Ghirlanda G, Pozzilli P & IMDIAB Group. 2010. No protective effect of calcitriol on beta-cell function in recent-onset type 1 diabetes .Diabetes Care 33:1962-1963.

Boonstra A, Barrat FJ, Crain C, Heath VL, Savelkoul HF & O'Garra A. 1alpha,25-Dihydroxyvitamin D3 has a direct effect on naïve CD4+ T cells to enhance the development of Th2 cells. J Immunol 2001;167(9):4974-4980.

Bonifacio E & Ziegler AG (2010). Advances in the prediction and natural history of type 1 diabetes. Endocrinol Metab Clin N Am 39: 513–525.

Cantorna MT, Hayes CE & DeLuca HF (1996). 1,25-dihydroxyvitamin D3 reversibly blocks the progressions of relapsing encephalomyelitis, a model of multiple sclerosis. Proc Natl Acad Sci USA 93(15):7861–7864.

Cantorna MT, Hayes CE & DeLuca HF (1998). 1,25-dihydroxyvitamin D3 prevents and ameliorates symptoms in two experimental models of human arthritis. J Nutr 128(1):68–72.

Carlberg C & Polly P (1998). Gene regulation by vitamin D3. Crit. Rev. Eukaryot. Gene Expr. 8, 19–42.

Casteels K, Waer M, Bouillon R, Depovere J, Bouillon R & Mathieu C (1998). 1,25-dihydroxy-vitamin D3 restores sensitivity to cyclophosphamide-induced apoptosis in non-obese diabetic (NOD) mice and protects against diabetes. Clin Exp Immunol 112:181–187.

Casteels KM, Waer M, Laureys J, Valckx D, Depovere J, Bouillon R & Mathieu C (1998). Prevention of autoimmune destruction of syngeneic islet grafts in spontaneously diabetic nonobese diabetic mice by a combination of a vitamin D3 analog and cyclosporine. Transplantation 65:1225–1232.

Chang TJ, Lei HH, Yeh JI, Chiu KC, Lee KC, Chen MC, Tai TY & Chuang LM (2000). Vitamin D receptor gene polymorphisms influence susceptibility to type 1 diabetes mellitus in the Taiwanese population. Clin Endocrinol (Oxf ,52(5):575–580.

Casteels KM, Mathieu C, Ware M, Valckx D, Overbergh L, Laureys JM & Bouillon R (1998). Prevention of type 1 diabetes in nonobese diabetic mice by late intervention with nonhyperclcemic analogs of 1,25-dihydroxyvitamin D3 in combination with a short induction course of cyclosporine A. Endocrinology. 139:95-102.

Chen S, Sims GP, Chen XX, Gu YY, Chen S & Lipsky PE (2007). Modulatory effects of 1,25-dihydroxyvitamin D3on human B cell differentiation. J Immunol,179(3):1634–1647.

Clemes DL & Mahan KJ (2010). Alcoholic pancreatitis: lessons from the liver. World J Gastroenterol, 16(11):1314-1320.

Dalquist G et al (1999). The EURODIAB Substudy 2 Study Group. Vitamin D supplement in early childhood and risk for type 1 (insulin-dependent) diabetes mellitus. Diabetologia 42:51–54.

Delovitch TL & Singh B (1997). The nonobese diabetic mouse as a model of autoimmune diabetes: Immune dysregulation gets the NOD. Immunity 7(6):727–738.

Devendra D & Eisenbarth GS (2003). Immunologic endocrine disorders. J Allergy Clin Immunol ,111:S624-S636.

D'Ambrosio D, Cippitelli M, Cocciolo MG, Mazzeo D, Lucia PD, Lang R, Sinigaglia F & Panina-Bordignon P (1998). Inhibition of IL12 production by 1,25-dihydroxyvitamin D3: involvement of NF-□B down regulation by 1,25-dihydroxy vitamin D3. J Clin Invest 101:252–262.

Diabetes Epidemiology Research International Group (1988). Geographic patterns of childhood insulin-dependent diabetes mellitus. Diabetes 37(8):1113–1119.

Eisenbarth GS & Gottlieb PA (2004). Autoimmune polyendocrine syndromes. N Engl J Med, 350:2068-2079.

Ferreira GB, van Etten E, Lage K, Hansen DA, Moreau Y, Workman CT, Waer M, Verstuyf A, Waelkens E, Overbergh L & Mathieu C (2009). Proteome analysis demonstrates profound alterations in human dendritici cell nature by TX527, an analogue of vitamin D. Proteomics , 9(14):3752-3764.

Franco OH, Steyerberg EW, Hu FB, Mackenbach J, Nusselder W (2007). Associations of diabetes mellitus with total life expectancy and life expectancy with and without cardiovascular disease. Arch Intern Med.;167:1145-1151.

Fronczak CM, Baron AE, Chase HP Ross C, Brady HL, Hoffman M, Eisenbarth GS, Rewers & Norris JM (2003) In utero dietary exposures and risk of islet autoimmunity in children. Diabetes Care 26:3237–3242.

Gamble DR & Taylor KW (1969). Seasonal incidence of diabetes mellitus. Br Med J 3:631-633.

Gamble DR, Kinsley ML, Fitzgerald MG Bolton R & Taylor KW (1969). Viral antibodies in diabetes mellitus. Br Med J 3:627-630.

Gale EA (2002). A missing link in the hygiene hypothesis? Diabetologia, 45:588-94.

Guo SW, Magnuson VL, Schiller JJ, Wang X, Wu Y & Ghosh S (2006). Meta-analysis of vitamin D receptor polymorphism and type 1 diabetes: a HuGE review of genetic association studies. Am J Epidemiol,164(8):711-724.

Gillespie KM (2006). Type 1 diabetes: pathogenesis and prevention. CMAJ,175(2):165-170.

Gillespie KM, Gale EAM & Bingley PJ (2002). High familial risk and genetic susceptibility in early onset childhood diabetes. Diabetes ,51:210-214.

Giulietti A, Gysemans C, Stoffels K, VAN Etten E, Decallonne B, Overbergh L, Bouillon R & Mathieu C (2004) Vitamin D deficiency in early life accelerates type 1 diabetes in non-obese diabetic mice. Diabetologia 47:451-462.

Gough SC, Walker LS & Sansom DM (2005): CTLA4 gene polymorphism and autoimmunity. Immunol, 204:102-115.

Griffin MD, Lutz WH, Phan VA, Bachman LA, McKean DJ & Kumar R (2000). Potent inhibition of dendritic cell differentiation and maturation by vitamin D analogs. Biochem Biphys Res Commun, 270(3):701-708.

Griffin MD, Lutz W, Phan VA, Bachman LA, McKean DJ & Kumar R (2001). Dendritic cell modulation by 1alpha,25 dihydroxyvitamin D3 and its analogs: A vitamin D receptor-dependent pathway that promotes a persistent state of immaturity in vitro and in vivo. Proc Natl Acad Sci USA 98:6800–6805.

Gregori S, Giarratana N, Smiroldo S, Uskokovic M & Adorini L (2002). A 1alpha,25-dihydroxyvitamin D(3) analog enhances regulatory T-cells and arrests autoimmune diabetes in NOD mice. Diabetes 51:1367–1374.

Greenwald RJ, Freeman GJ & Sharpe AH (2005). The B7 family revisited. Annu Rev Immunol 2005;23:515-548.

Hahn HJ Kuttler B, Mathieu C & Bouillon R (1997). 1,25 dihydroxyvitamin D3 reduces MHC antigen expression on pancreatic beta-cells in vitro. Transplant Proc,29(4):2156-2157.

Haussler MR, Whitfield GK, Haussler CA, Hsieh JC, Thompson PD, Selznick SH, Dominguez CE & Jurutka PW (1998). The nuclear vitamin D receptor: biological and molecular regulatory properties revealed. J Bone Miner Res 13:325–349.

Helfand RF, Gary HE Jr, Freeman CY, Anderson LJ & Pallansch MA (1995). Serologic evidence of an association between enteroviruses and the onset of type 1 diabetes mellitus. Pittsburgh Diabetes Reseacrh Group. J Infect Dis 172:1206-1211.

Hypponen E, Laara E, Reunanen A, Jarvelin MR & Virtanen SM (2001). Intake of vitamin D and risk of type 1 diabetes: a birth-cohort study. Lancet,358: 1500–1503.

Holick MF (1999). Vitamin D: photobiology, metabolism, mechanism of action, and clinical applications. In: Favus M, editor. Primer on the metaboilic bone diseases and disorders of mineral metabolism. Philadelphia: Lippincott Williams and Wilkins, pp92-98.

IDF. International Diabetes Federation World Atlas of Diabetes. 2006.

Israni N, Goswami R, Kumar A & Rani R (2009). Interaction of vitamin D receptor with HLA DRB1 0301 in type 1 diabetes patients from North India. PLoS One , 4(12):e8023.

Jeffery LE, Burke F, Mura M, Zheng Y, Qureshi OS, Hewison , Walker LS, Lammas DA, Raza K & Sansom DM (2009). 1,25-Dihydroxyvitamin D3 and IL-2 combine to inhibit T cell production of inflammatory cytokines and promote development of regulatory T cells expressing CTLA-4 and FoxP3. J Immunol;183(9):5458-5467.

Kahn HS, Morgan TM, Case LD, Dabelea D, Mayer-Davis EJ, Lawrence JM, Marcovina SM & Imperatore G (2009). Association of type 1 diabetes with month of birth among US youth: the SEARCH for diabetes in Youth study. Diabetes Care, 32(11):2010-2015.

Karvonen M, Jantti V, Muntoni S, Stabilini M, Stabilini L, Muntoni S & Tuomilehto J (1998) Comparison of the seasonal pattern in the clinical onset of IDDM in Finland and Sardinia. Diabetes Care 21:1101–1109.

Kaufman DL, Clare-Salzler M, Tian J, Forsthuber T, Ting GST, Robinson P, Atkinson MA, Sercarz EE, Tobin AJ & Lehmann PV (1993). Spontaneous loss of T-cell tolerance to glutamic acid decarboxylase in murine insulin-dependent diabetes. Nature 366:69–72.

Kulmala P, Savola K, Peteren JS, Vähäsalo P, Karjalainen J, Löppönen T, Dyrberg T, Akerblom HK & Knip M. The Childhood Diabetes in Finland Study Group (1998). Prediction of insulin-dependent diabetes mellitus in siblings of children with diabetes. A population-based study. J Clin Invest 101:327-336.

Lampeter E, Signore A, Gale E & Pozzilli P (1989). Lessons from the NOD mouse for the pathogenesis and immunotherapy of human type I (insulin-dependent) dia- betes mellitus. Diabetologia 32:703–708, 1989.

Lemire JM (1995). Immunomodulatory actions of 1,25 dihydroxyvitamin D3. J Steroid Biochem Mol Biol, 53(1–6): 599–602.

Lemire JM (1995). 1, 25 dihydroxylase vitamin D3 prevents the in vivo induction of murine experimental autoimmune encephalomyelitis. J Clin Invest 87(3): 1103-1107.

Lemos MC (2008). Lack of association of vitamin D receptor gene polymorphism with susceptibility to type 1 diabtes mellitus in the Portughese population Hum Immunol, 69(2):134-138.

Leijon K, Hammarström B & Holmberg D (1994). NOD mice display enhanced immune responses and prolonged survival of lymphoid cells. Int Immunol 6:339–345.

Li X, Liao L, Yan X, Huang G, Lin J, Lei M, Wang X & Zhou Z (2009). Protective effects of 1-α-hydroxyvitamin D3 on residual β-cell function in patients with adult-onset latent autoimmune diabetes (LADA). Diabetes Metab Res Rev. 25(5): 411–416.

Lopez, ER, O Zwermann, M Segni, G Meyer, M Reincke, J Seissler, J Herwig, KH Usadel, & K Badenhoop (2004). A promoter polymorphism of the CYP27B1 gene is associated with Addison's disease, Hashimoto's thyroiditis, Graves' disease and type 1 diabetes mellitus in Germans. Eur. J. Endocrinol. 151, 193–197.

Lopez ER, Regulla K, Pani MA, Krause M, Usadel KH & Badenhoop K (2004). CYP27B1 polymorphism variants are associated with type 1 diabetes mellitus in Germans. J. Steroid Biochem. Mol. Biol. 89–90, 155–157.

Mathieu C, Laureys J, Sobis H, Vandeputte M, Waer M & Bouillon R (1992). 1,25-Dihydroxyvitamin D3 prevents insulitis in NOD mice. Diabetes 41:1491–1495.

Mathieu C, Waer M, Laureys J, Rutgeerts O & Bouillon R (1994). Prevention of autoimmune diabetes in NOD mice by 1, 25 dihydroxyvitamin D3. Diabetologia, 37:552–558.

Mathieu C, Waer M, Casteels K, Laureys J & Bouillon R (1995). Prevention of type I diabetes in NOD mice by nonhypercalcemic doses of a new structural analog of 1,25-dihydroxyvitamin D3, KH1060. Endocrinology 136:866–872.

Mathieu C, Casteels K & Bouillon R (1997). Vitamin D and diabetes. In: Feldman D, Glorieux F, Pike J (eds) Vitamin D. Academic, San Diego, pp 1183–1196.

Mathieu C, Van Etten E, Gysemans C, Decallonne B, Kato S, Laureys J, Depovere J, Valckx D, Verstuyf A & Bouillon R (2001). In vitro and in vivo analysis of the immune system of vitamin D receptor-knock out mice. J. Bone Miner. Res. 16, 2057–2065.

Mathieu C, Gysemans C, Giulietti A & Bouillon R (2005). Vitamin D and diabetes. Diabetologia. 48:1247-1257.

MacCuish AC, Jordan J, Campbell CJ, Duncan LJ & Irvine WJ (1975). Cell-mediated immunity in diabetes mellitus: lymphocyte transformation by insulin and insulin fragments by insulin and insulin fragments in insulin-treated and newly-diagnosed diabetics. Diabetes 24:36-43.

Makino S, Kunimoto K, Muraoka Y, Katakiri K & Tochino Y (1980). Breeding of a non-obese, diabetic starin of mice. Exp Anim, 29:1-8.

Martin S, Wolf-Eichbaum D, Duinkerken G, Scherbaum WA, Kolb H, Noordzij JG, & Roep OP (2001). Development of type 1 diabetes despite severe hereditary B-lymphocyte deficiency. N Engl J Med 345:1036-1040.

Mohr SB, Garland CF, Gorham ED & Garland FC (2008). The association between ultraviolet B irradiance, vitamin D status and incidence rates of type 1 diabetes in 51 regions worldwide. Diabetologia, 51(8);1391-1398.

Menser MA, Forrest JM & Bransby RD (1978). Rubella infection and diabetes melliyus. Lancet i:57-60.

Nakayama M, Abiru N,Moriyama H, Babaya N, Liu E, Miao L, Yu L, Wegmann DR, Hutton JC, Elliott JF & Eisenbarth GS (2005). Prime role for an insulin epitope in the development of type 1 diabetes in NOD mice. Nature, 435:220.

Nejentsev S, Guja C, McCormack R, , Cooper J, Howson S, Nutland S, Rance H,Neil Walker N, Undlien D, Ronningen KS, Tuomilehto-Wolf E, Tuomilehto J, Ionescu-Tirgoviste C, Gale EAM, Bingley PJ , Gillespie KM, Savage DA , Carson JD, Patterson CC, Maxwell AP & Todd JA (2003). Association of intercellular adhesion molecule-1 gene with type 1 diabetes. Lancet, 362:1723-4.

Noble JA, Valdes AM, Cook M, Klitz W, Thomson G & Erlich HA (1996). The role of HLA class II genes in insulin-dependent diabetes mellitus: molecular analysis of 180 Caucasian, multiplex families. Am J Hum Genet 59:1134–1148.

Overbergh L, Decallonne B, Valckx D, Verstuyf A, Depovere J, Laureys J, Rutgeerts O, Saint-Arnaud R, Bouillon R & C Mathieu (2000). Identification and immune regulation of 25-hydroxyvitamin D-1-alpha-hydroxylase in murine macrophages. Clin Exp Immunol 120: 139–146.

Overbergh L, Decallonne B, Waer M, Rutgeerts O, Valkx D, Casteels KM, Laureys J, Bouillon R & Mathieu C (2000). 1alpha,25- dihydroxyvitamin D3 induces an autoantigen-specific T-helper 1/T-helper 2 immune shift in NOD mice immunized with GAD65 (p524-543). Diabetes 49:1301–1307.

Pani MA, Knapp M, Donner H, Braun J, Baur M & Usadel K (2000). Vitamin D receptor allele combinations influence genetic susceptibility to type 1 diabetes in Germans. Diabetes,49(3):504–507.

Penna G & Adorini L (2000). 1 Alpha,25-dihydroxyvitamin D3 inhibits differentiation, maturation, activation, and survival of dendritic cells leading to impaired alloreactive T cell activation. J Immunol, 164(5):2405–2411.

Penha-Goncalves C, Leijon K, Persson L & Holmberg D (1995). Type I diabetes and the control of dexamethasone-induced apoptosis in mice maps to the same region on chromosome 6. Genomics 28:398–404.

Prosser DE & Jones G (2004). Enzymes involved in the activation and inactivation of vitamin D. Trends Biochem Sci,29:664-673.

Pitocco D, Crinò A, Di Stasio E, Manfrini S, Guglielmi C, Spera S, Anguissola GB, Visalli N, Suraci C, Matteoli MC, Patera I P, Cavallo MG, Bizzarri C & Pozzilli P on behalf of the IMDIAB Group (2006). The effects of calcitriol and nicotinamide on residual pancreatic beta-cell function in patients with recent-onset type 1 diabetes (IMDIAB XI). Diabet Med, 23(8):920–923.

Rabinovitch A (1998). An update on cytokines in the pathogenesis of insulin-dependent diabetes mellitus. Diabetes Metab Rev 14(2):129–151.

Redondo MJ, Jeffrey J, Fain PR, Eisenbarth GS & Orban T (2008). Concordance for islet autoimmunity among monozygotic twins. NEJM, 359;26:2849-2850.

Riachy R, Vandewalle B, Kerr Conte, Riachy J, Moerman E, Sacchetti P, Lukowiak B, Gmyr V, Bouckenooghe T, Dubois M, Pattou F (2002). 1,25 dihydroxy vitamin D protects RINm5F and human islet cells against cytokine-induced apoptosis: implications of the antiapoptoctic protein A20. Endocrinology 2002;143(12):4809-4819.

Riachy R, Vandewalle B, Moerman E, Belaich S, Lukowiak B, Gmyr V, Muharram G, Kerr Conte J & Pattou F (2006). 1,25 dihydroxy vitamin D protects human pancreatic islets against cytokine-induced apoptosis via down-regulation of the Fas receptor . Apoptosis, 11(2):151-159.

Rigby WF, Denome S & Fanger MW (1987). Regulation of lymphokine production and human T lymphocyte activation by 1,25-dihydroxyvitamin D3. Specific inhibition at the level of messenger RNA. J Clin Invest, 79(6):1659-1664.

Rigby WF, Stacy T & Fanger MW (1984). Inhibition of T lymphocyte mitogenesis by 1,25-dihydroxyvitamin D3 (calcitriol). J Clin Invest, 74(4):1451-1455.

Stene LC, Joner G & Norwegian Childhood Diabetes Study Group (2003). Norwegian Childhood Diabetes Study Group.Use of cod liver oil during the first year of life is associated with lower risk of childhood-onset type 1 diabetes: a large, population-based, case-control study. Am J Clin Nutr, 78: 1128–1134.

Smyth D, Cooper JD, Collins JE, Heward JM, Franklyn JA, Howson JMM, Vella A, Nutland S, Rance HE, Maier L, Barratt BJ, Guja C, Ionescu-Tîrgoviste C, Savage DA, Dunger DB, Widmer B, Strachan DP, Ring SM, Walker N, Clayton DG, Twells RCJ, Gough SCL & Todd JA (2004). Replication of an association between the lymphoid tyrosine phosphatase locus (LYP/PTPN22) with type 1 diabetes, and evidence for its role as a general autoimmunity locus. Diabetes, 53:3020-2023.

Stoffels K, Overbergh L, Bouillon R & Mathieu C (2007). Immune regulation of 1 alpha-hydroxylase in murine peritoneal macrophages: unraveling the IFNgamma pathway. J Steroid biochem Mol Biol, 103:567-571.

Strandell E, Eizirik DL & Sandler S (1994). Reversal of beta-cell suppression in vitro in pancreatic islets isolated from nonobese diabetic mice during the phase preceding insulin-dependent diabtes mellitus. J Clin Invest, 85:1944-1950.

Strugnell SA & DeLuca HF (1997). The vitamin D receptor - structure and transcriptional activation. Proc Soc Exp Biol Med 215:223-228.

Tisch R, Yang XD, Singer SM, Liblau RS, Fugger L & McDevitt HO (1993). Immune response to glutamic acid decarboxylase correlates with insulitis in nonobese diabetic mice. Nature 366:72–75.

Turpeinen H (2003).Vitamin D receptor polymorphism: no association with type 1 diabtes in the Finnish population. Eur J Endocrinol, 149(6):591-596.

Ueda H, Howson JM, Esposito L, Heward J, Snook H, Chamberlain G, Rainbow DB, Hunter KM, Smith AN, Di Genova G, Herr MH, Dahlman I, Payne F, Smyth D, Lowe C, Twells RC, Howlett S, Healy B, Nutland S, Rance HE, Everett V, Smink LJ, Lam AC, Cordell HJ, Walker NM, Bordin C, Hulme J, Motzo C, Cucca F, Hess JF, Metzker ML, Rogers J, Gregory S, Allahabadia A, Nithiyananthan R, Tuomilehto-Wolf E, Tuomilehto J, Bingley P, Gillespie KM, Undlien DE, Rønningen KS, Guja C, Ionescu-Tîrgovişte C, Savage DA, Maxwell AP, Carson DJ, Patterson CC, Franklyn JA, Clayton DG, Peterson LB, Wicker LS, Todd JA & Gough SC (2003) Association of the T-cell regulatory gene CTLA4 with susceptibility to autoimmune disease. Nature , 423:506-511.

Van Etten E & Mathieu C (2005). Immunoregulation by 1,25-dihydroxyvitamin D3: basic concepts J Steroid Biochem Mol Biol , 97(1-2):93-101.

Vafiadis P, Bennett ST, Todd JA, Nadeau J, Grabs R, Goodyer CG, Wickramasinghe S, Colle E & Polychronakos C (1997). Insulin expression in human thymus is modulated by INS VNTR alleles at the IDDM2 locus. Nat Genet 15:289–292.

Walter M Kaupper T, Adler K, Foersch J, Bonifacio E & Ziegler AG (2010). No effect of the 1alpha,25-dihydroxyvitamin D3 on beta-cell residual function and insulin requirement in adults with new onset type 1 diabetes. Diabetes Care 33:1443-1448.

Weisman Y, Harell A, Edelstein S, et al. (1979) 1 alpha, 25-hydroxyvitamin D3 and 24,25-dihydroxyvitamin D3 in vitro synthesis by human decidua and placenta. Nature 281:317-319.

Yeung WG , Rawlinson WD, Craig ME (2011). Enterovirus infecction and type 1 diabetes mellitus:systemic review and meta-analysis of observational molecular studies BMJ, 342:d35.

Willheim M, Thien R, Schrattbauer K, Bajna E, Holub M, Gruber R, Baier K, Pietschmann P, Reinisch W, scheiner O, Peterlik M (1999). Regulatory effects of 1alpha,25-dihydroxyvitamin D3 on the cytokine production of human peripheral blood lymphocytes. J Clin Endocrinol Metab, 84(10):3739-3744.

Von Herrath M (2010). Combination therapies for type 1 diabetes: why not now? Immunotherapy, 2(3):289–291.

Yoon J-W, Yoon C-S, Lim H-W, Huang Q, Kang Y, Pyun K, Hirasawa K, Sherwin R &

Jun H-S (1999). Control of autoimmune diabetes in NOD mice by GAD expression or suppression in β cells. Science 284:1183–1187.

Zekzer D, Wong FS, Ayalon O, Millet I, Altieri M, Shintani S, Solimena M & Sherwin RS (1998) GAD-reactive CD4+ Th1 cells induce diabetes in NOD/SCID mice. J Clin Invest 101:68–73.

20

Honey and Type 1 Diabetes Mellitus

Mamdouh Abdulrhman[1], Mohamed El Hefnawy[2],
Rasha Ali[1] and Ahmad Abou El-Goud[1]
[1]*Pediatric Department, Faculty of Medicine, Ain Shams University, Abbasia - Cairo*
[2]*National Institute of Diabetes, Cairo*
Egypt

1. Introduction

Type 1 diabetes mellitus is by far the most common metabolic and endocrinal disease in children (Peters & Schriger, 1997). The major dietary component responsible for fluctuations in blood glucose levels is carbohydrate. The amount, source (Jenkins et al., 1981; Gannon et al., 1989) and type (Brand et al., 1985) of carbohydrate appear to have profound influence on postprandial glucose levels. The chronic hyperglycemia of diabetes is associated with long-term damage, dysfunction and failure of various organs especially the eyes, kidneys, nerves, heart and blood vessels (American Diabetes Association, 2001).

The glycemic effect of any foodstuff is defined as its effect on blood glucose level postprandially. Both the glycemic index (GI) and the peak incremental index (PII) are used to assess the glycemic effect of different food stuffs (Jenkins et al., 1981). Jennie et al (2003) who studied the use of low glycemic index diets in the management of diabetes found that diets with low glycemic indices (GI), compared with conventional or high-GI diets, improved overall glycemic control in individuals with diabetes, as assessed by glycemic index, peak incremental index, reduced HbA1c and fructosamine. They concluded that using low-GI foods in place of conventional or high-GI foods has a clinically useful effect on postprandial hyperglycemia similar to that offered by pharmacological agents that target postprandial hyperglycemia. Similarly, the American Diabetes Association (2002) stated that the use of low-GI foods may reduce postprandial hyperglycemia.

Honey is the substance made when the nectar and sweet deposits from plants are gathered, modified and stored in the honeycomb by honey bees. It is composed primarily of the sugars glucose and fructose; its third greatest component is water. Honey also contains numerous other types of sugars, as well as acids, proteins and minerals (White et al., 1962; White, 1980; White, 1975). The water content of honey ranges between 15 to 20% (average 17.2%). Glucose and fructose, the major constituents of honey, account for about 85% of the honey solids. Besides, about 25 different sugars have been detected. The principal oligosaccharides in blossom honeys are disaccharides: sucrose, maltose, turanose, erlose. Trace amounts of tetra and pentasaccharides have also been isolated (Bogdanov, 2010). The protein and amino acid content of honey varies from 0.05 to 0.3 %. The honey proteins are mainly enzymes (White, 1975). Honey also contains varying amounts of mineral substances ranging from 0.02 to 1.03 g/100 g (White, 1975). Among honey benefits are its anti-inflammatory (Al Waili & Boni, 2003), anti- oxidant (Frankel et al., 1998; Gheldof & Engeseth, 2002; Gross et al., 2004) and anti-microbial effects (Molan, 1992; Steinberg et al., 1996; Molan, 1997; Theunissen et al., 2001). Further-more, several studies have shown that honey produced an attenuated postprandial glycemic response when compared with sucrose in both patients with diabetes and normal subjects (Ionescu-Tirgoviste et al., 1983; Shambaugh et al., 1990; Samanta et al., 1985; Al Waili, 2004; Agrawal et al., 2007).

C-peptide is considered to be a good marker of insulin secretion and has no biologic activity of its own (Ido et al., 1997). Measurement of C-peptide, however, provides a fully validated means of quantifying endogenous insulin secretion. C-peptide is co-secreted with insulin by the pancreatic cells as a by-product of the enzymatic cleavage of proinsulin to insulin. Consequently, serum C-peptide level can be used as a true indicator of any change in the insulin level, which is the main determinant of plasma glucose level.

Several studies were performed in healthy and in type 2 diabetic patients to evaluate the effects of honey on the insulin and C-peptide levels, and the results were controversial (Bornet et al., 1985; Elliott et al., 2002; Watford, 2002; Al-Waili, 2003).

2. Aim of the study

The aim of this work was to compare the effects of honey, sucrose and glucose on plasma glucose and C-peptide levels in children and adolescents with type 1 diabetes mellitus.

3. Subjects and methods

3.1 Subjects

Twenty patients with type 1 diabetes mellitus, aged 3–18 (mean 10.95 years) and ten healthy non-diabetic children and adolescents, aged 1–17 (mean 8.5 years) were studied. All subjects were within 68–118% and 77–125% of their ideal body weight and height, respectively. The mean BMI of patients and controls were 22.60 and 23.15, respectively. All patients with diabetes had a mean glycosylated hemoglobin of 9.9% (range = 7–15%). The sex ratio in patients and controls was 1:1. The patients were recruited from the regular attendants of the children clinic of the National Institute of Diabetes in Cairo, Egypt. The study was approved by the local ethical committee, and an informed written consent was obtained from at least one parent of each subject before the study. All patients were receiving three insulin injections per day, each consisting of a mixture of a medium-acting insulin (isophane NPH) and a short-acting soluble insulin (human Actrapid).

3.2 Methods

All patients were primarily diagnosed with type 1 insulin-dependent diabetes mellitus by measuring the serum level of C-peptide on presentation [the patient was considered suffering from insulin-dependent diabetes mellitus type 1 if the C-peptide level was below 0.4 ng/dl (Connors, 2000)]. All subjects were subjected to the following:

1. Anthropometric measures including weight in kg and height in cm which were plotted against percentiles for age and sex.
2. Oral sugar tolerance tests using glucose, sucrose and honey in three separate sittings: After an overnight fast (8 h) and omission of the morning insulin dose, a calculated amount of each sugar (amount = weight of subject in kg X 1.75 with a maximum of 75 g) (William & Ruchi, 2005) was diluted in 200 ml water and then ingested over 5 min in a

random order, on separate mornings 1 week apart. The honey dose for each patient was calculated based on the fact that each 100 gm of the honey used in this study contained 77.3 gm sugars. So if a patient weighs for example 20 kg, he/she should receive 20 x 1.75 = 35 gm sugar which will be present in (35 x 100) ÷ 77.3 = 45.3 gm honey. Venous blood was sampled just before ingestion and then every 30 min postprandial for 2 h thereafter. Samples were left to clot, centrifuged and glucose assay was performed chemically on the Synchron CX5 autoanalyzer (Beckman instruments Inc.)[1].

3. Measurement of fasting and postprandial serum C- peptide level: Venous blood samples were withdrawn from each subject at 0 (fasting) and 2 h postprandial after ingestion of each individual sugar. The samples were then centrifuged and serum was stored in aliquots at - 20°C. At the end of the study, samples were calibrated for C-peptide using the biosource c-pep-easia[2], which is a solid phase enzyme amplified sensitivity immunoassay performed on a microtiter plate. A fixed amount of C-peptide labeled with horseradish peroxidase (HRP) competes with unlabeled C-peptide present in the calibrators controls and samples for a limited number of binding sites on a specific antibody. After 2 h incubation at room temperature, the microtiter plates were washed to stop the competition reaction. The chromogenic solution (TMB-H2O2) was added and incubated for 30 min. The reaction was stopped with the addition of stop solution, and the microtiter plate was then read at the appropriate wave length. The amount of substrate turnover was determined colorimetrically by measuring the absorbance which was inversely proportionate to the C-peptide concentration. A calibration curve was plotted and C-peptide concentration in samples was determined by interpolation from the calibration curve.
4. Calculation of glycemic and peak incremental indices (see example figure 3.1):

$$\text{Glycemic index of the food (Jenkins, 1987)} = \frac{\text{Area under glycemic curve of test food}}{\text{Area under glycemic curve of glucose}}$$

- Area under curve (AUC) refers to the area included between the baseline and incremental blood glucose points when connected by straight lines. The area under each incremental glucose curve is calculated using the trapezoid rule (note: only areas above the baseline are used).
- Peak incremental index (PII) (Samanta et al., 1985) is defined as the ratio of the maximal increment of plasma glucose produced by sugar to that produced by glucose

$$\text{Peak incremental index} = \frac{\text{Maximal increment produced by the sugar tested}}{\text{Maximal increment produced by glucose}}$$

Maximal increment is the difference between the peak point and the fasting point.

3.3 Statistical analysis

Standard computer program SPSS for Windows, release 13.0 (SPSS Inc., USA) was used for data entry and analysis. All numeric variables were expressed as mean ± standard deviation (SD). Comparison of different variables in various groups was done using student t-test and Mann–Whitney test for normal and non-parametric variables, respectively. Wilcoxon signed

[1] Beckman: 2005, kraemerBLW, Brew, CA 92621, USA.

[2] Biosource Europe S.A – Rue de lindustrie, 8-B-1400-Nivelles-Belgium.

rank tests were used to compare multiple readings of the same variables. Chi-square ($\chi 2$) test was used to compare frequency of qualitative variables among the different groups (Daniel, 1995).

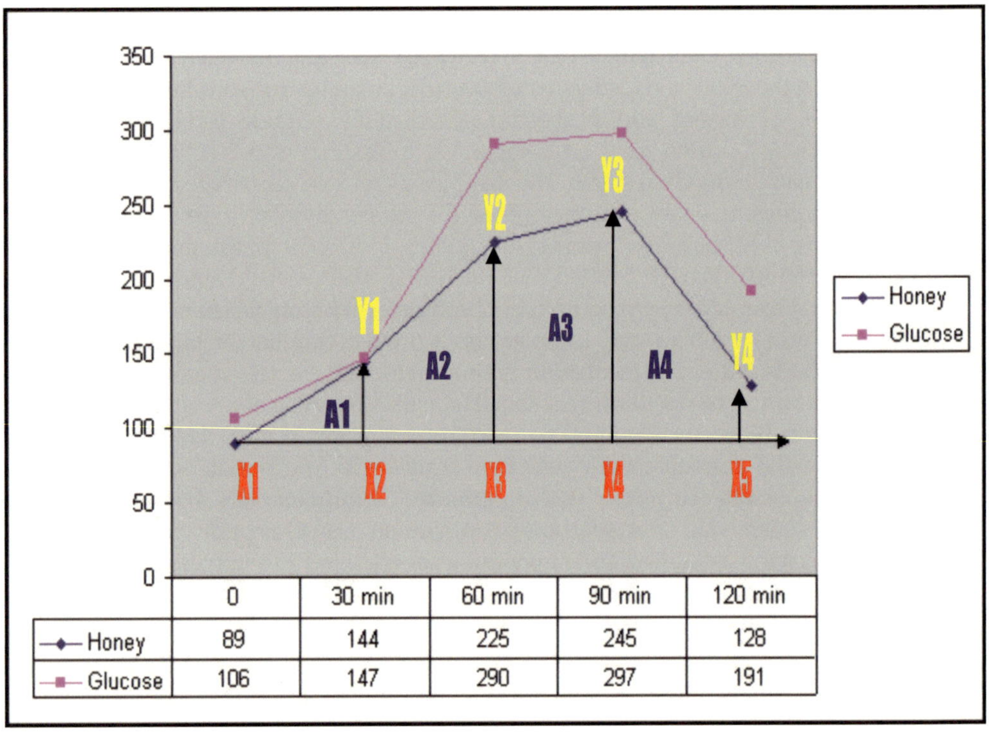

Fig. 3.1 Oral glucose tolerance curve of one of our patients

For calculation of the area under honey curve (AUC) $=A_1+A_2+A_3+A_4$

A_1 is a triangle = 1/2 base x height = $1/2(X_2 - X_1) \times (Y_1 - X_2) = ½(30) \times (144 - 89) = 15 \times 55 = 825$

A_2 is a trapezoid = 1/2 sum of the parallel sides (heights) x base

$$= 1/2[(Y_1 - X_2) + (Y_2 - X_3)] \times (X_4 - X_5) = 1/2[(144 - 89) + (225 - 89)] \times 30 = 1/2(55 + 136) \times 30 = 1/2(191) \times 30 = 95.5 \times 30 = 2865$$

A_3 is a trapezoid = 1/2 sum of the parallel sides (heights) x base

$$= 1/2[(Y_2 - X_3) + (Y_3 - X_4)] \times (X_4 - X_3) = 1/2[(225 - 89) + (245 - 89)] \times 30 = 1/2(136 + 156) \times 30 = 1/2(292) \times 30 = 146 \times 30 = 4380$$

A_4 is a trapezoid = 1/2 sum of the parallel sides (heights) x base

$$= 1/2[(Y_3 - X_4) + (Y_4 - X_5)] \times (X_3 - X_2) = 1/2[(245 - 89) + (128 - 89)] \times 30 = 1/2(156 + 39) \times 30 = 1/2(195) \times 30 = 97.5 \times 30 = 2925$$

$$AUC = A_1 + A_2 + A_3 + A_4 = 825 + 2865 + 4380 + 2925 = 10995$$

4. Results

No significant difference was found between patients (diabetics) and controls (non-diabetics) as regards the age and anthropometric measures (table 4.1). The mean age of subjects in the diabetic and non- diabetic groups was 11.3 and 8.5 years, respectively, with no statistically significant difference between groups (P > 0.05). The mean weight %, height % and body mass index did not also differ significantly between diabetics and non-diabetics (93.6%, 99.2%, 22.6 versus 94%, 98.2%, 23.1, respectively; P > 0.05). The mean plasma glucose level at 0 (fasting) and 30 min postprandial (i.e. 30 min after intake of glucose, sucrose or honey) did not differ significantly between subjects in both groups (diabetics and non-diabetics) (Tables 4.2 - 4.5) (P > 0.05). In non-diabetics (control), as shown in tables 4.2 and 4.3, the mean plasma glucose level 60, 90 and 120 min after intake of honey became significantly lower than after either glucose or sucrose (P< 0.05). Similarly, as shown in tables 4.4 and 4.5, there was a statistically significant decrease of plasma glucose in diabetics at 60, 90 and 120 min after honey intake, when compared with either glucose or sucrose (P< 0.05). The glycemic index (GI) and the peak incremental index (PII) of either sucrose or honey did not differ significantly between patients and controls (P > 0.05). On the other hand, both the GI and PII of honey were significantly lower when compared with sucrose in patients and controls. In non-diabetics, the glycemic index (GI) of honey was 0.69 compared to 1.32 for sucrose, with statistically significant difference (P< 0.05). In diabetics, the GI of honey was also significantly lower than that of sucrose (o.61 versus 1.19, respectively; P< 0.001) (table 4.6; figure 4.1). The PII of honey in non-diabetics was 0.61, compared to 1.25 for sucrose (P< 0.05). In diabetics, the PII of honey was also significantly lower than that of sucrose (0.60 versus 1.10, respectively; P< 0.001) (table 4.7; figure 4.2).

The mean (±SD) fasting C-peptide of patients and controls were 0.15 (±0.13) and 1.91 (±0.77) ng/ml, respectively (P< 0.001). All diabetic patients had a basal C-peptide level less than 0.7 ng/ml. In diabetics, although honey intake resulted in increase in the mean level of C-peptide, yet this increase was not statistically significant when compared with either glucose or sucrose (P> 0.05) (Table 4.8; figure 4.3). On the other hand, in non-diabetics, honey produced a statistically significant higher C-peptide level, when compared with either glucose or sucrose (P< 0.05) (Table 4.8; figure 4.4).

Variable	Diabetics	Non-diabetics	P
Age (yr)	11.30 ± 4.80	8.50 ± 5.38	>0.05
Weight %	93.60 ± 13.82	94.00 ± 14.28	>0.05
Height %	99.20 ± 13.01	98.20 ± 11.14	>0.05
BMI	22.59 ± 5.50	23.14 ± 2.90	>0.05

P > 0.05 is non significant
BMI: Body Mass Index

Table 4.1 Age and anthropometric measures in diabetics and non-diabetic controls (mean ± SD)

Time (min)	Glucose	Honey	P
0	75.20 ± 17.45	72.30 ± 9.09	> 0.05
30	86.00 ± 19.88	83.30 ± 9.52	> 0.05
60	102.90 ± 24.47	88.80 ± 10.04	< 0.05
90	103.60 ± 21.24	88.50 ± 8.64	< 0.05
120	91.10 ± 20.74	81.00 ± 8.30	< 0.05

Table 4.2 Mean plasma glucose (±SD) (mg/dl) in non-diabetics (control) following equivalent amount of glucose or honey ($P < 0.05$ is significant)

Time (min)	Sucrose	Honey	P
0	68.50 ± 12.59	72.30 ± 9.09	> 0.05
30	83.80 ± 13.56	83.30 ± 9.52	> 0.05
60	101.60 ± 11.45	88.80 ± 10.04	< 0.05
90	105.40 ± 18.03	88.50 ± 8.64	< 0.05
120	93.60 ± 17.25	81.00 ± 8.30	< 0.05

Table 4.3 Mean plasma glucose (±SD) (mg/dl) in non-diabetics (control) following equivalent amount of sucrose or honey ($P < 0.05$ is significant)

Time (min)	Glucose	Honey	P
0	206.05 ± 95.79	208.10 ± 92.76	> 0.05
30	257.55 ± 92.79	247.75 ± 99.44	> 0.05
60	339.80 ± 96.86	285.50 ± 86.29	< 0.05
90	328.05 ± 99.75	272.25 ± 85.33	< 0.05
120	297.90 ± 106.86	236.75 ± 76.80	< 0.05

Table 4.4 Mean plasma glucose (±SD) (mg/dl) in diabetics following equivalent amount of glucose or honey ($P < 0.05$ is significant)

Time (min)	Sucrose	Honey	P
0	198.30 ± 77.762	208.10 ± 92.76	> 0.05
30	268.25 ± 78.78	247.75 ± 99.44	> 0.05
60	320.35 ± 67.17	285.50 ± 86.29	< 0.05
90	323.65 ± 71.27	272.25 ± 85.33	< 0.05
120	310.15 ± 92.63	236.75 ± 76.80	< 0.05

Table 4.5 Mean plasma glucose (±SD) (mg/dl) in diabetics following equivalent amount of sucrose or honey ($P < 0.05$ is significant)

	Sucrose	Honey	
	GI	GI	P
Non- diabetics	1.32 (0.85–1.92)	0.69 (0.43–1.43)	< 0.05
Diabetics	1.19 (0.31–3.08)	0.61 (0.15–1.92)	< 0.001

Table 4.6 Glycemic index (GI) mean (range) of sucrose and honey (glycemic index of glucose = 1) ($P < 0.05$ is significant; $P < 0.001$ is highly significant)

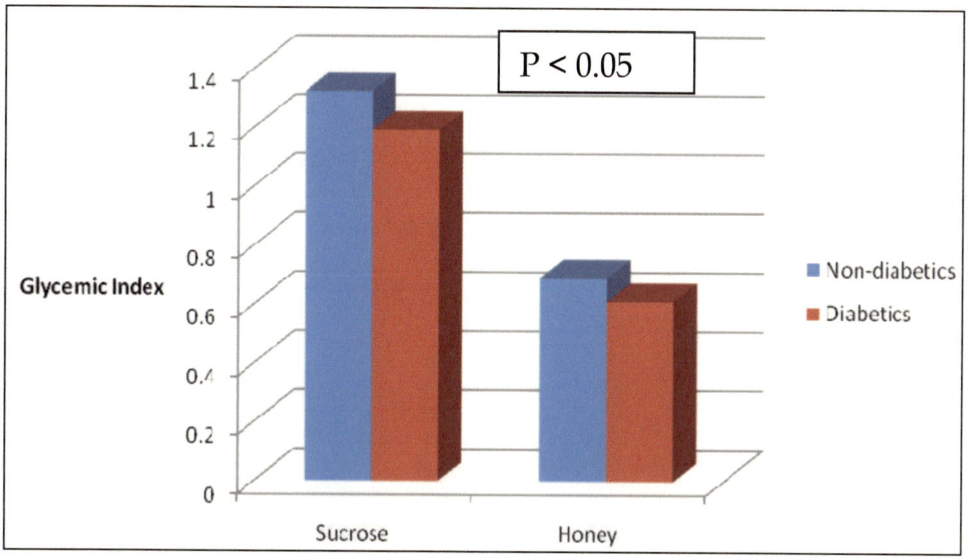

Fig. 4.1 Glycemic index of sucrose and honey

	Sucrose	Honey	P
	PII	PII	
Non- diabetics	1.25 (0.50–1.82)	0.61 (0.30–1.10)	< 0.05
Diabetics	1.10 (0.65–2.98)	0.60 (0.20–1.60)	< 0.001

Table 4.7 Peak incremental index (PII) mean (range) of sucrose and honey (peak incremental index of glucose = 1) ($P < 0.05$ is significant; $P < 0.001$ is highly significant)

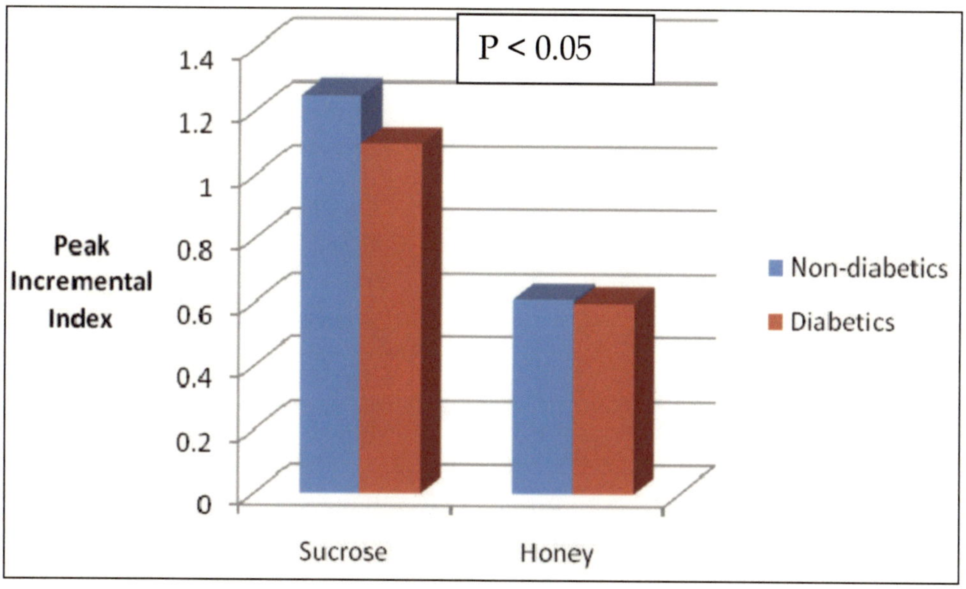

Fig. 4.2 Peak incremental index of sucrose and honey

Group	C-peptide (ng/ml)			P
	After glucose	After sucrose	After honey	
Non-diabetics	3.96 ± 0.84	3.99 ± 1.10	5.50 ± 1.15	P < 0.05
Diabetics	0.29 ± 0.53	0.32 ± 0.53	0.47 ± 1.09	P > 0.05

Table 4.8 Mean C-peptide (±SD) (ng/ml) following equivalent amount of glucose, sucrose or honey in non-diabetics and diabetics (P < 0.05 is significant)

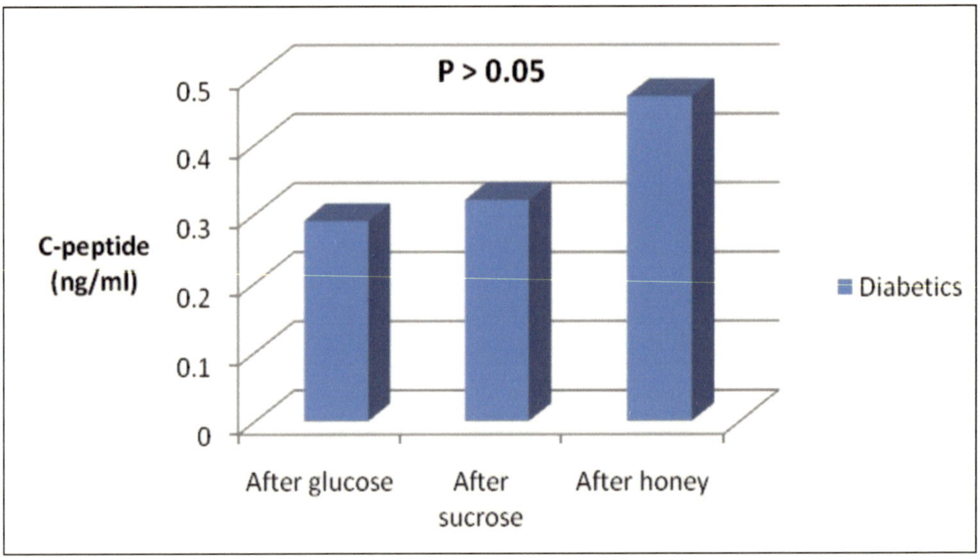

Fig. 4.3 C-peptide following equivalent amount of glucose, sucrose or honey in diabetics

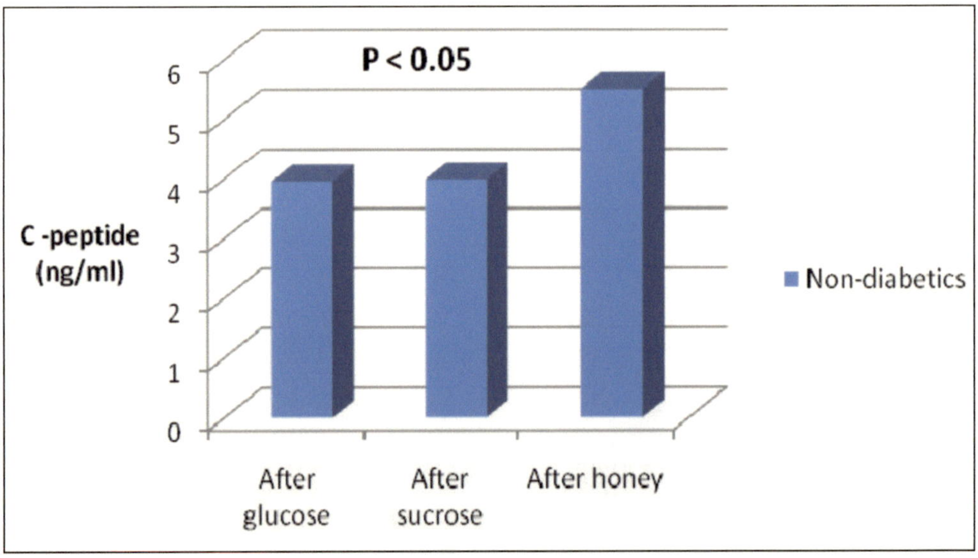

Fig. 4.4 C-peptide following equivalent amount of glucose, sucrose or honey in non-diabetics

5. Discussion

As shown in many studies, sustained hyperglycemia is a risk factor for both micro vascular and macro vascular (as cardiovascular) complications in type 2 diabetes mellitus (Laakso & Lehto, 1997; Bretzel et al., 1998 as cited from Oizumi et al., 2007), while postprandial hyperglycemia has also been considered a risk factor for cardiovascular complications (Tominaga et al., 1999; Risso et al., 2001; Chiasson et al., 2002; Hanefeld et al., 2004; Nakagami et al., 2004 as cited from Oizumi et al., 2007). Many experimental and epidemiological studies have shown that increased postprandial plasma glucose levels may have equally or even more harmful effects than fasting hyperglycemia (Tominaga et al., 1999; Risso et al., 2001; Nakagami et al., 2004 as cited from Oizumi et al., 2007), and the reduction of postprandial plasma glucose levels delays the development of cardiovascular complications (Chiasson et al., 2002; Hanefeld et al., 2004 as cited from Oizumi et al., 2007).

Jenkins (1987) defined the glycemic index as the ratio between the blood glucose areas produced after ingestion of a studied sugar compared to the blood glucose area produced after glucose ingestion itself. He stated that the glycemic response to food affects the insulin response which in turn is also potentiated by other non-glucose dependent factors in this food (Ostman et al., 2001). On the other hand, FAO/WHO (1998) defined the glycemic index as the incremental blood glucose area (0–2 h) following ingestion of 50 g of available carbohydrates (no fibers or resistant starch included), expressed as a percentage of the corresponding area following an equivalent amount of carbohydrate from a standard reference product. Samnata et al (1985) defined the peak incremental index of a certain sugar as the ratio between the maximal increments of the glucose level after ingestion of the sugar compared to the maximal increment produced after ingestion of glucose. He also mentioned that both the glycemic and the peak incremental indices are closely related, highly dependent and positively correlated to the plasma glucose produced after ingestion of any given sugar. Therefore, any change in the plasma glucose level after ingestion of a certain sugar will markedly affect both the glycemic index and the peak incremental index. Hence, the glycemic and the peak incremental indices measure how fast and how much a food raises blood glucose levels. Foods with higher index values raise blood sugar more rapidly than foods with lower index values do in case of the glycemic index and much more in case of peak incremental index.

In our study, no statistically significant differences were found between diabetic patients and non-diabetic controls regarding the glycemic and the peak incremental indices of the studied sugars. Similarly, Samnata et al (1985), who studied the glycemic effect of glucose, sucrose and honey in 12 normal volunteers, eight patients with insulin-dependent diabetes mellitus (IDDM) and six patients with non-insulin-dependent diabetes mellitus (NIDDM), found no significant differences between the normal volunteers and diabetic patients regarding the glycemic and peak incremental indices of both sugars. Since the glycemic index (GI) is the ratio between the area under curve (AUC) of the studied sugar and the AUC of glucose, and the peak incremental index (PII) is the ratio between the maximal blood glucose increment of the studied sugar and that of glucose; it may be expected that both GI and PII will be the same in both diabetics and non-diabetics. Our study showed that honey has statistically significant lower glycemic and peak incremental indices than sucrose and glucose in both patients and controls (< 1 with honey, 1 with glucose being the reference sugar and >1 with sucrose). In agreement, Kaye et al (2002), who published the international table of glycemic index and glycemic load values, found that the GI of honey (0.55 ± 0.05) was lower than that of sucrose (1.10 ± 0.21). Also, Shambaugh et al (1990) found that sucrose caused higher blood sugar readings than honey in normal volunteers. In the study of

Samnata et al (1985), honey ingestion in both diabetics (IDDM) and non-diabetics also resulted in a significantly lower PII compared to the glucose and sucrose. In the study done by Al-Waili (2004), honey compared with dextrose and sucrose caused a lower elevation of plasma glucose levels (PGL) in both diabetics (IDDM) and normal subjects. In an attempt to explain his results, he stated that the mild reduction of plasma glucose levels obtained by honey might be a result of the fructose content of honey which requires metabolic transformation in the liver, a slow process conferring relatively low-GI on these sugars (Jenkins et al., 1981; Wolever et al., 1991). Also, Watford (2002) demonstrated that very small amounts of fructose, which is the main component of honey, could increase hepatic glucose uptake and glycogen storage, as well as reduce peripheral glycemia which could be beneficial in diabetic patients. In the study performed by Agrawal et al (2007), honey was found to produce an attenuated postprandial glycemic response especially in subjects with glucose intolerance. They referred these results to the possibility that the glucose component of honey might be poorly absorbed from the gut epithelium. Also, Tirgoviste et al (1983) studied blood glucose and plasma insulin responses to various carbohydrates in type 2 diabetes, and they found that the increase in plasma glucose was significantly higher after administration of more refined carbohydrates such as glucose than after the complex ones such as honey. Meanwhile, Oizumi et al (2007) and Arai et al (2004) found that consumption of a palatinose (a disaccharide found in honey)-based balanced formula suppressed postprandial hyperglycemia, glycemic and peak incremental indices and produced beneficial effects on the metabolic syndrome–related parameters (namely, the lipid profile and visceral fat accumulation) in diabetic patients. They stated the reason of this observation to be due to the fact that although palatinose is completely absorbed, yet it has the specific characteristics of delayed digestion and absorption as reported by Dahlquist et al (1963) and Lina et al (2002).

Our results showed that honey, compared to glucose and sucrose, caused a significant elevation in the C-peptide levels in non-diabetic subjects. Meanwhile, in diabetic patients, the plasma C-peptide levels did not differ significantly between the three types of sugars. To our knowledge, no similar work was done to study the effects of honey on C-peptide levels in type 1 diabetes mellitus. However, several studies were performed in healthy and in type 2 diabetic patients to evaluate the effects of honey on the insulin and C-peptide levels, and the results were controversial. In the study of Al Waili (2003), inhalation of honey solution, when compared with hyperosmolar dextrose and hypoosmolar distilled water, resulted in a significant elevation of plasma insulin and C-peptide in both normal individuals and in patients with type 2 diabetes mellitus. However, in 2004, the same author found that honey ingestion, when compared with sucrose, caused a greater elevation of insulin and C-peptide in type 2 diabetic patients, while in healthy subjects dextrose ingestion caused a significant elevation of plasma insulin and C-peptide when compared with honey. The author hypothesized that honey may have the ability to stimulate insulin production and secretion from the pancreas than do sucrose in type 2 diabetes mellitus. On the other hand, Bornet et al (1985) reported no significant changes in plasma insulin levels after honey ingestion compared to sucrose in type 2 diabetics. Liljeberg et al (1999) found that high-GI foods induced a greater elevation of blood insulin than did low glycemic index meals (like honey). Elliott et al (2002) tried to explore whether fructose consumption might be a contributing factor to the development of obesity and the accompanying metabolic abnormalities observed in the insulin resistance syndrome and they found that honey intake caused a significant lowering of plasma insulin and C-peptide in normal subjects when compared to sucrose and dextrose. They related their findings to the fructose content of honey which does not stimulate insulin secretion from pancreatic beta cells and that consumption of foods and beverages containing fructose produced a smaller postprandial insulin excursions than did consumption of glucose-containing carbohydrates (Glinsmann & Bowman, 1993). Also, Watford et al (2002) stated that very small amounts of fructose, which is the main component of honey, could increase hepatic glucose uptake and glycogen storage, as well as reduce peripheral glycemia and thus insulin levels. Ionescu-Tirgoviste et al (1983) studied the blood glucose and plasma insulin responses to some simple carbohydrates (glucose, fructose, lactose) and some complex ones (apples, potatoes, bread, rice, carrots and honey) in 32 type 2 (non-insulin-dependent) diabetic patients, and they found that increases in plasma insulin were significantly higher after the more refined carbohydrates (glucose, fructose and lactose) than after the more complex ones (apples, potatoes, rice, carrots and honey, P less than 0.01).

We hypothesize that honey might have a direct stimulatory effect on the healthy beta cells of pancreas; an effect which may be related to the non-sugar part of honey. This hypothesis is based on the finding that honey caused significant postprandial increase in the C-peptide level despite its lower glycemic and peak incremental indices when compared to either glucose or sucrose. On the other hand, the lack of significant increase in C-peptide levels among diabetic patients might be due to the minimal residual function of the patient's pancreatic beta cells, which is beyond their capacity of further postprandial response. This proposal is backed up by the findings of Pozzan et al (1997) who investigated the relation between the fasting C-peptide level and the ability to respond to a particular stimulus, and they reported that there is a positive significant correlation between the basal value (BV) and the peak value (PV) of C-peptide in insulin dependent diabetic patients and that positive responses need a minimal basal level of 0.74 ng/ml. In all our studied patients, the basal C-peptide level was less than 0.7 ng/ml. Also other authors found significant correlations between the basal and the maximum C-peptide values after a stimulus. However, they reported different basal values which can respond to stimulation. Such values were 0.09 (Clarson et al., 1987), 0.18 (Eff et al., 1989) and 0.39 ng/ml (Faber & Binder, 1977). The variation in these levels was probably due to the different ages and different diabetes duration of the studied populations (Pozzan et al., 1997).

6. Conclusions and recommendations

1. Honey has a lower glycemic and peak incremental indices compared to glucose and sucrose in both type 1 diabetic patients and non-diabetics. Therefore, we recommend using honey as a sugar substitute in type 1 diabetic patients.
2. In spite of its significantly lower glycemic and peak incremental indices, honey caused significant post- prandial rise of plasma C-peptide levels when compared to glucose and sucrose in non-diabetics; indicating that honey may have a direct stimulatory effect on the healthy beta cells of pancreas. On the other hand, C-peptide levels were not significantly elevated after honey ingestion when compared with either glucose or sucrose in type 1 diabetic patients. Whether or not ingestion of honey in larger doses or/and for an extended period of time would have a significant positive effect on the diseased beta cells, needs further studies.

7. References

Agrawal, O.; Pachauri, A.; Yadav, H.; Urmila, J.; Goswamy, H.; Chapperwal, A.; Bisen, P. & Prasad, G. (2007). Subjects with impaired glucose tolerance exhibit a high degree of tolerance to honey. J Med Food 10(3):473–478

Al Waili, N. (2004). Natural honey lowers plasma glucose, C-reactive protein, homocysteine, and blood lipids in healthy, diabetic, and hyperlipidemic subjects: comparison with dextrose and sucrose. J Med Food 7(1):100–107

Al Waili, N. & Boni, N. (2003). Natural honey lowers plasma prostaglandin concentrations in normal individuals. J Med Food 6(2):129–133

Al-Waili, N. (2003). Intrapulmonary administrations of natural honey solution, hyperosmolar dextrose or hyperosmolar distill water to normal individuals and to patients with type 2 diabetes mellitus or hypertension: their effects on blood glucose level, plasma insulin and C-peptide, blood pressure and peak expiratory flow rate. Eur J Med Res 8(7):295–303

American Diabetes Association. (2001). Report of the expert committee on the diagnosis and classification of diabetes mellitus (committee report).Diabetes care 24, (Suppl.1)

American Diabetes Association (2002). Evidence-based nutrition principles and recommendations for the treatment and prevention of diabetes and related complications. Diabetes Care 25:202–212

Arai, H.; Mizuno, A.; Matsuo, K.; Fukaya, M.; Sasaki, H.; Arima, H.; Matsuura, M.; Taketani, Y.; Doi, T. & Takeda, E. (2004). Effect of a novel palatinose-based liquid balanced formula (MHN-01) on glucose and lipid metabolism in male Sprague-Dawley rats after short- and long-term ingestion. Metabolism 53:977–983

Bogdanov, S. (December 2010). Book of Honey, Chapter 5, Honey Composition, Bee Product Science, available from www.bee-hexagon.net

Bornet, F.; Haardt, M.; Costagliola, D.; Blayo, A. & Slama, G. (1985). Sucrose or honey at breakfast has no additional acute hyper-glycemic effect over an isoglucidic amount of bread in type 2 diabetic patients. Diabetologia 28(4):213–217

Brand, J.; Nicholson, P.; Thorburn, A. & Truswell, A. (1985). Food processing and the glycemic index. Am J Clin Nutr. Dec; 42(6):1192-6

Bretzel, R.; Voigt, K. & Schatz, H. (1998). The United Kingdom Prospective Diabetes Study (UKPDS) implications for the pharmacotherapy of type 2 diabetes mellitus. Exp Clin Endocrinol diabetes 106: 369-372

Chiasson, J.; Josse, R.; Gomis, R.; Hanefeld, M.; Karasik, A. & Laakso, M. (2002). STOP-NIDDM Trial Research Group. Acarbose for prevention of type 2 diabetes mellitus: the STOP- NIDDM trial. Lancet 259: 2072-2077

Clarson, C.; Daneman, D.; Drash, A.; Beckert, D. & Ehelich, R. (1987). Residual B-cell function in children with IDDM; reproducibility of testing and factors influencing insulin secretory reserve. Diabetes Care 10(1):33–38 515

Connors, T. (September 2000). Interpreting your C-peptide values; diabetes health, available from http://www.diabeteshealth.com.html. Updated 2000/09, accessed Jan 2008

Dahlquist, A.; Auricchio, S.; Semenza, G. & Prader, A. (1963). Human intestinal disaccharidases and hereditary disaccharide intolerance: the hydrolysis of sucrose, isomaltose, palatinose (isomaltulose), and 1, 6-a-oligosaccharide (isomalto-oligosaccharide) preparation. J Clin Invest 42:556–562

Daniel, W. (1995). Biostatistics: a foundation for analysis in the health sciences, 6th edn. Wiley, New York

Eff, C.; Fabet, O. & Deckert, T. (1989). Persistent insulin secretion assessed by plasma C-peptide estimation in long-term juvenile diabetes with a low insulin requirement. Diabetologia 32:305- 311

Elliott, S.; Keim, N. & Stern, J. (2002). Fructose, weight gain and the insulin. Am J Clin Nutr 76:911–922

Faber, O. & Binder, C. (1977). B-cell function and blood glucose control in insulin dependent diabetes within the first month of insulin treatment. Diabetologia 13:263–268

FAO/WHO. (1998). Carbohydrates in human nutrition (Paper No. 66). Food and Agricultural Organization and Geneva, World Health Organization, Rome

Frankel, S.; Robinson, G. & Berenbaum, M. (1998). Antioxidant capacity and correlated characteristics of 14 unifloral honeys. J Apic Res 37(1):27–31

Gannon, M.; Nuttall, F.; Westphal, S.; Neil, B. & Seaquist, E. (1989). Effects of dose of ingested glucose on plasma metabolite and hormone responses in type II diabetic subjects. Diabetes Care12:544-552

Gheldof, N. & Engeseth, N. (2002). Antioxidant capacity of honeys from various floral sources based on the determination of oxygen radical absorbance capacity and inhibition of in vitro lipoprotein oxidation in human serum samples. J Agric Food Chem 50(10):3050–3055

Glinsmann, W. & Bowman, B. (1993). The public health significance of crystalline fructose, glucose tolerance. Am J Clin Nutr 77(3):612–621 506

Gross, H.; Polagruto, J.; Zhu, Q.; Kim, S.; Schramm, D. & Keen, C. (2004). Effect of honey consumption on plasma antioxidant status in human subjects. Abstracts of Papers of the American Chemical Society, 227: U29

Hanefeld, M.; Cagatay, M.; Petrowitsch, T.; Neuser, D.; Petzinna, D. & Rupp, M. (2004). Acarbose reduces the risk of myocardial infarction in type 2 diabetic patients: meta-analysis of seven long- term studies. Eur Heart J 25:10-16

Ido, Y.; Vindigni, A. & Chang, K. (1997). Prevention of vascular and neural dysfunction in diabetic rats by C-peptide. Science 277(5325):563–566

Ionescu-Tirgoviste, C.; Popa, E.; Sintu, E.; Mihalache, N.; Cheta, D. & Mincu, I. (1983). Blood glucose and plasma insulin responses to various carbohydrates in type 2 non-insulin-dependent diabetes. Diabetologia 24:80–84

Jenkins, D. (1987). The glycemic index and the dietary treatment of hypertriglyceridemia and diabetes. J Am Coll Nutr 61:11–17

Jenkins, D.; Wolever, T.; Taylor, R.; Barker, H.; Fielden, H.; Baldwin, J.; et al (1981). Glycemic index of foods: a physiological basis for carbohydrate exchange. Am J Clin Nutr 34(3):362– 366

Jennie, B.; Hayne, S.; Petocz, P. & Stephen, C. (2003). Low-glycemic index diets in the management of diabetes. Diabetes Care 26:2261–2267

Kaye, F.; Holt, S. & Janette, C. (2002). International table of glycemic index and glycemic load values. Am J Clin Nutr 76:5n56

Laakso, M. & Lehto, S. (1997). Epidemiology of macrovascular disease in diabetes. J Diabetes Rev 5: 294-315

Liljeberg, H.; Akerberg, A. & Bjorck, I. (1999). Effect of the glycemic index and content of indigestible carbohydrates of cereal-based breakfast meals on glucose tolerance at lunch in healthy subjects. Am J Clin Nutr 69:647–655 503

Lina, B.; Jonker, D. & Kozianowski, G. (2002). Isomaltulose (palatinose): a review of biological and toxicological studies. Food Chem Toxicol 40:1375–1381

Molan, P. (1992). The antibacterial activity of honey. 1. The nature of the antibacterial activity. Bee World 73(1):5–28 (2. Variation in the potency of the antibacterial activity. Bee World 73(2): 59–76)

Molan, P. (1997). Honey as an antimicrobial agent. In: Mizrahi A, Lensky Y (eds) Bee products: properties, applications and api-therapy. Plenum, London, pp 27–37

Nakagami, T. & the DECODA Study Group. (2004). Hyperglycemia and mortality from all causes and from cardiovascular disease in five populations of Asian origin. Diabetologia 47: 385-394

Oizumi, T.; Daimon, M.; Jimbu, Y.; Kameda, W.; Arawaka, N.; Yamaguchi, H.; Ohnuma, H.; Sasaki, H. & Kato, T. (2007). A palatinose- based formula improves glucose tolerance, serum free fatty acid levels and body fat composition. Tohoku J Exp Med 212:91–99

Ostman, E.; Liljeberg, H.; Elmstahl, H. & Bjorck, I. (2001). Inconsistency between glycemic and insulinemic responses to regular and fermented milk products. Am J Clin Nutr 74(1):96–100

Peters, A. & Schriger, D. (1997). Impact of new diagnostic criteria on the diagnosis of diabetes (abstract). Diabetes 46 (Suppl.1):7A

Pozzan, R.; Dimetz, T.; Gazolla, H. & Gomes, M. (1997). Discriminative capacity of fasting C-peptide levels in a functional test according to different criteria of responser to a stimulus; a study of Brazilian insulin-dependent diabetic patients. Braz J Med Biol Res 30(10):1169–1174 511

Risso, A.; Mercuri, F.; Quagliaro, L.; Damante, G. & Ceriello, A. (2001). Intermittent high glucose enhances apoptosis in human umbilical vein endothelial cells in culture. Am J Physiol Endocrinol Metab 281: E924-E930

Samanta, A.; Burden, A. & Jones, G. (1985). Plasma glucose responses to glucose, sucrose, and honey in patients with diabetes mellitus: an analysis of glycemic and peak incremental indices. Diabet Med 2:371–373

Shambaugh, P.; Worthington, V. & Herbert, J. (1990). Differential effects of honey, sucrose, and fructose on blood sugar levels. J Manip Physiol Ther 13:322–325

Steinberg, D.; Kaine, G. & Gedalia, I. (1996). Antibacterial effect of propolis and honey on oral bacteria. Am J Dent 9(6):236–239

Theunissen, F.; Grobler, S. & Gedalia, I. (2001). The antifungal action of three South African honeys on Candida albicans. Apidologie 32(4):371–379

Tominaga, M.; Eguchi, H.; Manaka, H.; Igarashi, K.; Kato, T. & Sekikawa, A. (1999). Impaired glucose tolerance is a risk factor for cardiovascular disease, but not impaired fasting glucose. The Funagata Diabetes Study. Diabetes Care 22: 920-924

Watford, M. (2002). Small amounts of dietary fructose dramatically increase hepatic glucose uptake. Nutr Rev 60(8):253–257

White, JW Jr. (1980). Detection of honey adulteration by carbohydrate analysis. JAOAC 63(1):11–18

White, JW Jr.; et al. (1962). Composition of American honeys. Tech. Bull. 1261. Agricultural Research Service, USDA, Washington DC

White, J. (1975). Composition of honey. In Crane, E (ed.) Honey. A Comprehensive survey, Heinemann Edition; London, pp 157-206

William, C. & Ruchi, M. (2005). Glucose tolerance test, available from http://www.medicinenet.com/glucose_tolerance_test/article.htm. 2005.medicinenet

Wolever, T.; Jenkins, D.; Jenkins, A. & Josse, R. (1991). The glycemic index: methodology and clinical implications. Am J Clin Nutr 54(5):846–854

21

Fatty Acid Supply in Pregnant Women with Type 1 Diabetes Mellitus

Éva Szabó, Tamás Marosvölgyi and Tamás Decsi
University of Pécs, Department of Pediatrics, Pécs
Hungary

1. Introduction

Long-chain polyunsaturated fatty acids (LCPUFAs) play an important role in the human body in building up cell membranes and in regulating their fluidity. The most important fatty acids are the essential n-3 fatty acid, alpha-linolenic acid (C18:3n-3, ALA) and the essential n-6 fatty acid, linoleic acid (C18:2n-6, LA), and their most important metabolites, docosahexaenoic acid (C22:6n-3, DHA) and arachidonic acid (C20:4n-6, AA). LCPUFAs are precursors of different eicosanoids, and their availability may be disturbed in several diseases. As insulin is one of the most potent activators of Δ-6 desaturase enzyme, type 1 diabetes mellitus (T1DM) is characterised by the diminished levels of n-3 LCPUFAs (Decsi et al., 2002, 2007; Szabó et al., 2010b).

2. Role of polyunsaturated fatty acids

Polyunsaturated fatty acids (PUFAs) are components of the lipid bilayer of cell membranes, where they also regulate membrane fluidity. Cell membranes containing more saturated fatty acids and cholesterol are more rigid, while PUFAs increase their fluidity as well as the number of receptors and their affinity to their substrates, like hormones and growth factors (Das, 2006).

PUFAs are also precursors of several second messengers. From the n-6 group, especially from AA proinflammatory eicosanoids are synthesized, while the n-3 fatty acids, especially eicosapentaenoic acid (C20:5n-3, EPA) are precursors of antiinflammatory eicosanoids.

The n-6 essential fatty acid (EFA), LA plays an important role in the maintenance of the epidermal water barrier (Koletzko & Rodriguez-Palmero, 1999), preventing thereby the transepidermal water loss and epidermal damage (Yen et al., 2008). There are data indicating that LA also lowers plasma total cholesterol levels (Nikkari et al., 1983). In an animal study the n-3 EFA, ALA lowered serum and liver triacylglycerol levels, while it increased serum HDL-cholesterol levels (Murano et al., 2007).

AA and DHA play an important role in the maturation of the developing nervous system: during the third trimester and in the first months of life there is an increased incorporation into the fetal/neonatal brain and retinal membranes (Farquharson et al., 1992; Martinez & Mougan, 1998).

Fish oil, containing EPA and DHA, may be beneficial not only during infancy, but also during adulthood. It may prevent the development of macula degeneration (Chua et al.,

2006), may lower the risk of developing dementia and Alzheimer-disease (Morris et al., 2003; Schaefer et al., 2006) and may be beneficial in bipolar depression (Noaghiul & Hibbeln, 2003). N-3 LCPUFAs play also an important role in the prevention of cardiovascular diseases: fish oil supplementation increased HDL-cholesterol levels, while decreased triacylglycerol levels (Laidlaw & Holub, 2003), reduced the progression of atherosclerosis (Erkkilä et al., 2004), the risk of coronary heart disease (Iso et al., 2006; Mozaffarian et al., 2005), fatal myocardial infarction (Yuan et al., 2001), sudden cardial death (Albert et al., 1998), incidence of atrial fibrillation (Mozaffarian et al., 2004) and the risk of stroke (Mozaffarian et al., 2005). In a longitudinal, observational study, fish oil supplementation reduced the risk of developing islet autoimmunity in children at increased genetic risk for T1DM (Norris et al, 2007).

Trans isomeric fatty acids increase serum lipoprotein(a), LDL-cholesterol, triacylglycerol (Katan et al., 1995) and total cholesterol levels (Louheranta et al., 1999), as well as significantly decrease the levels of HDL-cholesterol (Dyerberg et al., 2004; Louheranta et al., 1999; Sun et al., 2007); in summary, they increase the risk of cardiovascular diseases (Sun et al., 2007). In an animal study rats fed with *trans* fatty acid diet (similar to saturated fatty acid diet) had high levels of fasting plasma insulin and decreased adipocyte insulin sensitivity (Ibrahim et al., 2005). In contrast, in a human study *trans* fatty acid diet did not alter insulin sensitivity (Louheranta et al., 1999).

2.1 Biochemistry of fatty acids

The physiologically most important PUFAs contain 2-6 double bonds and have a chain length of 18, 20 or 22 carbon atom. The methyl end of the molecule is called the omega end. On the basis of the distance of the first double bond from the carbon atom at the omega end, three different groups of fatty acids can be distinguished: omega-3 (n-3), omega-6 (n-6) and omega-9 (n-9) fatty acids.

The human body is unable to establish double bond in the n-3 and n-6 position, so we have to ingest the EFAs, the n-3 ALA and n-6 LA with our diet. The most important dietary sources of these fatty acids are vegetables and vegetable oils.

From the essential n-6 LA, after $\triangle$-6 desaturation γ-linolenic acid (C18:3n-6, GLA) and after elongation dihomo-γ-linolenic acid (C20:3n-6, DHGLA) is synthesised. After a $\triangle$-6 desaturational step, the most important metabolite, AA is produced (Fig. 1).

The metabolism of the n-3 group is a longer, more complicated process. After elongation, $\triangle$-5 and $\triangle$-6 desaturation eicosapentaenoic acid (C20:5n-3, EPA) is formed. After chain elongation docosapentaenoic acid (C22:5n-3, DPA) is synthesised. The most important n-3 metabolite, DHA is produced after $\triangle$-6 desaturation and peroxisomal β-oxidation (Fig. 1).

Although the same enzymes are involved into the metabolism of the n-3 and n-6 group, these fatty acids cannot be transformed into each other, because the molecule can only be activated from the carboxyl end. In the metabolism, the elongation is a quicker, while desaturation is a slower step, so these desaturational steps determine the speed of metabolism (i.e. these are the rate-limiting steps).

In the nature, PUFAs can be found predominantly as cis isomers, while *trans* fatty acids are produced in the stomach of ruminants and during the partial hydrogenation of vegetable oils. Cis double bond bends the molecule, while *trans* double bond straightens the fatty acid, so it is similar to saturated fatty acids. From this difference arise their different physiological effects: *trans* isomers are similar to saturated fatty acids, while cis isomers have more beneficial effects. As cis and *trans* fatty acids use the same enzymes during their metabolism, several studies have indicated, that *trans* fatty acids may disturb the metabolism of the physiologically important n-3 and n-6 fatty acids (Szabó et al, 2007, 2010a; Vidgren et al., 1998).

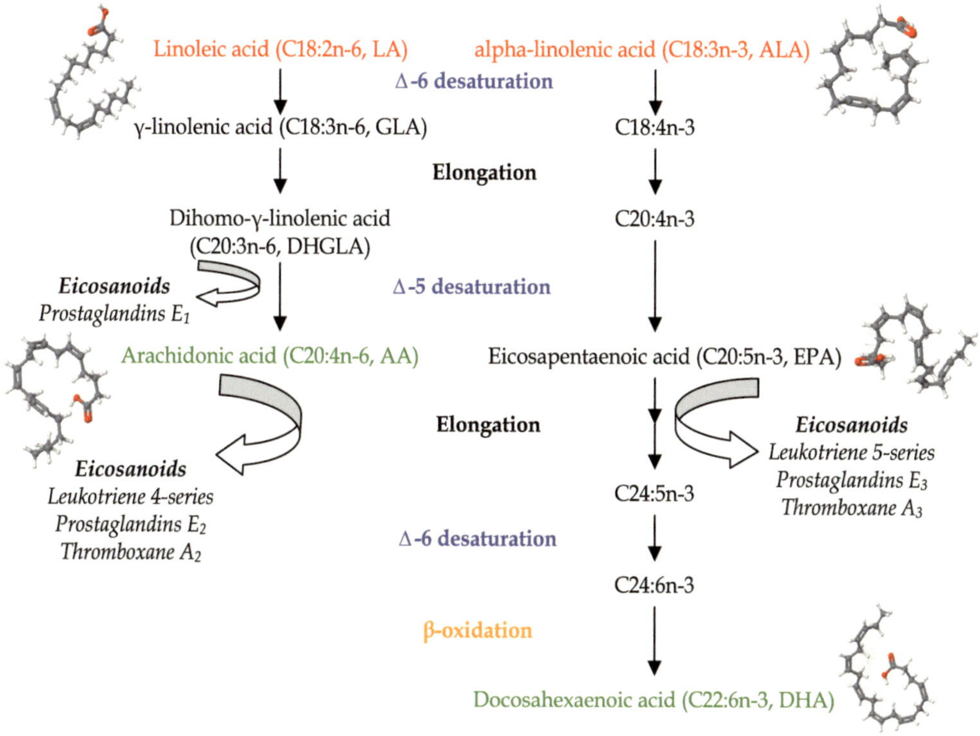

Fig. 1. Metabolism of n-6 and n-3 fatty acids
figure modified from http://www.lpi.oregonstate.edu; source of fatty acid figures: http://www.3dchem.com/index.asp

2.2 Dietary sources of fatty acids

The n-3 EFA, ALA is found in the highest quantity in linseed oil, and considerable amounts are found in hempseed oil (20%) as well (Erasmus, 1993); however, from the dietary point of view its most important sources are walnut and rapeseed oils (Beare-Rogers et al., 2001). The n-6 EFA, LA can be found in the highest proportion in primrose (81%; Erasmus, 1993) and grapeseed oils, but its most important dietary sources are sunflower, corn and pumpkin seed oils (Table 1; Beare-Rogers et al., 2001). Compared to vegetable sources, animal lipid sources contain smaller quantities of ALA and LA (Table 2).

Flesh of herbivorous animals is very rich in the most important n-6 metabolite, AA (Table 2). On the other hand, haslets of terrestrial animals, like liver and kidney contains DHA also in relative high concentrations.

The most important n-3 LCPUFAs, EPA and DHA can be found in fatty sea fishes (Table 3). The DHA content of sea fishes may vary according to season, area of catching and to age and gender of the fish (Racine & Deckelbaum, 2007). Marine fish contains higher levels of n-3 PUFAs, EPA and DHA, while lower n-6 PUFAs, LA and AA compared to freshwater species. In a Chinese study, the edible meat of cultured freshwater fish contained more n-3

PUFAs, EPA and DHA, than the meat of wild freshwater fish (Li et al., 2011). Fatty acid composition of fishes living in the Mediterranean Sea showed seasonal variation (mackerel: lowest in winter-14.44%, highest in spring-38.27%; European eel: lowest in autumn-7.88%, highest in spring-9.46%; Soriguer et al., 1997).

	LA	ALA
Corn oil*	39.4-65.6	0.5-1.5
Grapeseed oil*	58-78	<1.0
Linseed oil*	17-30	47-55
Olive oil*	3.5-20.0	0.0-1.5
Palm kernel oil*	6.5-12	<0.5
Pumpkin seed oil#	42-57	0-15
Rapeseed oil*	11-23	5-13
Sesame oil*	41.5-47.9	0.3-0.4
Soya bean oil	49.8-57.1	5.5-9.5
Sunflower oil (high LA content)*	65.7	–
Walnut oil*	52.9	10.4

* data modified from Beare-Rogers et al., 2001
# data modified from Erasmus, 1993

Table 1. Fatty acid composition (g fatty acid/100 g fat) of selected vegetable sources, fats and oils

	LA	ALA	AA	DHA
Chicken flesh	26.5	1.1	1.7	0.6
Duck flesh	13.9	1.5	–	–
Heart (beef)	20.9	10.5	0.5	–
Kidney (lamb)	9.7	3.4	6.4	1.5
Kidney (veal)	13.4	1.7	7.8	0.7
Lamb	6.2	0.7	0.7	–
Liver (chicken)	14.0	4.2	0.3	2.0
Liver (pork)	13.6	17.2	1.3	1.0
Milk (cow)	2.6	1.6	–	–
Rabbit	20.2	5.2	–	–
Turkey flesh	24.2	1.3	2.3	0.5
Veal	9.4	0.6	2.3	–
Venison	14.6	3.3	4.7	–

Table 2. Fatty acid composition (g fatty acid/100 g fat) of selected terrestrial animal lipid sources (data modified from Beare-Rogers et al., 2001)

	LA	ALA	AA	DHA
*High fat fishes (>8%)**				
Blue fish, mature (31.3%)*	2.2	n.d.	4.2	13.8
Horse mackerel (12.8%) *	1.1	n.d.	1.4	6.6
Rainbow trout (9.0%)#	5.4	1.4	0.8	10.8
Sardine (11.3%)*	2.2	1.4	2.6	14.7
Striped mullet (11.0%)*	2.7	0.73	3.1	11.7
*Medium fat fishes (4-8%)**				
Anchovy (7.1%)*	2.8	1.4	2.4	16.2
Atlantic mackerel (6.1%)*	2.1	0.68	2.8	25.3
Crucian carp, wild (6.02%)$	11.4	4.0	3.6	5.0
Mackerel (7.45%)#	1.9	2.3	1.7	15.9
Silver carp (5.36%)$	2.4	4.4	4.9	15.5
White herring (6.88%)$	1.2	3.6	2.8	11.8
*Low fat fishes (2-4%)**				
Anchovy (3.49%)#	1.5	2.2	1.4	25.5
Crucian carp, cultured (3.60%)$	17.0	2.6	4.0	6.7
Swordfish (1.93%)#	0.7	1.0	1.1	9.3
Tuna (1.16%)#	2.3	1.3	1.8	16.9

data modified from: * Tanakol et al., 1999 [Black & Marmara Sea]; # Soriguer et al., 1997 [Atlantic Ocean & Mediterranean Sea]; $Li et al., 2011 [East China Sea & Quiantang River]

Table 3. Fat content and fatty acid composition (g fatty acid/100 g fat) of selected sea fishes

2.3 Fatty acids during pregnancy

LCPUFAs play an important role in the maturation of the developing nervous system. AA and DHA are accreted in large amounts into the fetal nervous system: into the cortex and retinal cell membranes during the third trimester of pregnancy and in the first months of life (Farquharson et al., 1992; Martinez & Mougan, 1998). DHA can be predominantly found in the grey matter and retina (Horrocks & Yeo, 1999), while the highest AA content is in the amygdala (Brenna & Diau, 2007). In a primate study (Diau et al., 2005), the highest DHA content was found in globus pallidus (15.8%), while the lowest in the optic nerve (4.5%). AA content was the highest in the amygdale (13.7%) and the lowest in the optic tract (6.8%). Grey matter was richer is both AA and DHA, but there was a discontinuity between grey and white matter DHA concentration, while this great difference wasn't seen in AA concentrations.

The human body has the enzymes needed to synthesise LCPUFAs from their parent essential fatty acids, but the synthesis is a very slow, limited process. In vivo human studies showed that from ALA only a little part is metabolised into EPA and DHA: when supplementing ALA in low dose (<100 mg) only 1.5-7.0% EPA and max. 0.3% DHA were synthesised, while supplementing ALA in high dose (>100 mg) resulted in the synthesis of 0.2-9.0% EPA and 3.8-10.4% DHA. Hence, rise of EPA by 20-100% can be seen in a dose-dependent manner after the administration of ALA. In contrast, the change in DHA values is rather negligible in healthy adults. Similarly, LA supplementation has little effect on AA supply, only ~0.1% of dietary LA is converted to AA in healthy adults (Plourde & Cunnane, 2007).

As AA and DHA play a key role in the fetal and neonatal brain and visual development, several authors investigated whether the fetus and/or the infant is capable to synthesise AA and DHA from LA and ALA, respectively. In an experimental study (Salem et al., 1996), in vivo conversion of EFAs in newborns was investigated. After the administration of deuterium-labeled LA and ALA, deuterium-labeled AA, EPA and DHA appeared in the neonatal blood. However, this capacity can hardly cover the LCPUFA requirement of the developing brain. Two groups of infants with sudden and unexpected death were studied (at the age of 2 to 48 weeks) and significantly higher AA and DHA values were found in erythrocyte and brain cortex lipids in breastfed infants than in infants fed formula that contained only LA and ALA, and the accretion of DHA was correlated with the length of breastfeeding (Makrides et al., 1994).

Since LCPUFA synthesis in the human organism is limited, the most important source of AA and DHA is diet. During pregnancy maternal diet covers the fetal requirements of these fatty acids, while after delivery either maternal diet (breastfeeding) or the independent diet of the infant (formula feeding). In an animal study (Diau et al., 2005), baboon neonates were fed either breastmilk or formula with or without AA and DHA. DHA supplementation restored the DHA supply in the grey matter to breastfed levels, while dietary AA had little effect on brain AA content. In other words: AA seems to be less sensitive to dietary manipulation than DHA.

Maternal diet and metabolism as well as maternal stores are the sources of fetal fatty acid supply. As the ability of the fetus to synthesise LCPUFAs is limited, placenta plays an important role in transferring AA and DHA from mother to the fetus. Several research groups (Berghaus et al., 1998; Gil-Sanchez et al., 2010; Ortega-Senovilla et al., 2009) investigated the differences in maternal and fetal (newborn) blood fatty acid composition and found a higher proportion of LCPUFAs, while lower proportion of the EFAs in the fetal circulation than in the mothers. This phenomenon is called "biomagnification" and may be related to the ability of the placenta to selectively transport LCPUFAs to the fetus. In an in vivo study (Larqué et al., 2003), pregnant women undergoing elective caesarean section received 4 h before delivery an oral dose of ^{13}C-labeled palmitic acid, oleic acid, LA and DHA. Venous blood was taken from the mothers every hour, and cord blood and placental tissues were also collected at delivery. All four fatty acids appeared in the placental tissues and cord blood triacylglycerol (TG) and non-esterified fatty acid (NEFA) lipids, and there was a preferential sequestration of DHA into the placenta. In a recent study (Gil-Sanchez et al., 2010), it was also shown that all labeled fatty acids were enriched in maternal plasma, as well as placental and cord blood lipids. This was the first study that showed a higher ratio of ^{13}C-labeled DHA in cord to maternal plasma. Unesterified fatty acids are transferred to the fetal circulation by both passive diffusion and through a complex, saturable, protein-mediated transport (Koletzko et al., 2007a). There are several fatty acid transfer proteins in the placenta, like fatty acid binding protein (FABP), that preferentially binds LCPUFAs, fatty acid translocase (FAT) and fatty acid transporter protein (FATP) located on both sides of trophoblast cells transporting fatty acids bidirectionally (Cetin et al., 2009). The plasma membrane FABP is located exclusively on the maternal side of membranes and might be involved in the preferential uptake of LCPUFAs by these cells (Koletzko et al., 2007a).

Fish or fish oil intake during pregnancy and lactation improves maternal fatty acid supply and, hence, may enhance fetal DHA concentrations. The increased DHA intake during pregnancy resulted in better visual and neural development in infants at the age of 18 months (Bouwstra et al., 2006), 3.5 years (Williams et al., 2001) and 4 years (Helland et al., 2003), while other studies failed to corroborate these findings (Bakker et al., 2003; Ghys et al., 2002). Because of the beneficial fetal/neonatal effects of n-3 LCPUFAs, for pregnant and lactating women, at least 200 mg/day DHA intake is recommended (Koletzko et al., 2007b).

3. Effect of type 1 diabetes mellitus on fatty acid supply

T1DM disturbs not only the carbohydrate, but also the lipid metabolism. The most extensively studied experimental animal model of T1DM is the alloxane or streptozotocin-induced diabetic rat or mouse. The results of animal studies are quite unequivocal: in diabetic animals significantly higher LA contents were found in liver, renal cortex and heart lipids (Ramsammy et al., 1993), in liver microsomes and erythrocyte membranes (Shin et al., 1995) as well as in plasma, liver and skeletal muscle phospholipids (Mohan & Das, 2001), while its most important metabolite, AA was significantly decreased in diabetic animals. These results can be explained with the diminished activity of Δ-5 (Ramsammy et al., 1993) and Δ-6 desaturase enzymes in T1DM (Ramsammy et al., 1993; Shin et al., 1995). On the basis of these animal studies, insulin is considered as the most potent activator of both Δ-5 and Δ-6 desaturase enzymes (Brenner, 2003).

Human studies are even less unambiguous than animal observations. Some studies found significantly higher LA values in diabetic patients (Decsi et al., 2002, 2007; Tilvis & Miettinen, 1985), while others found no significant differences (Ruiz-Gutierrez et al., 1993; Seigneur et al., 1994). On the other hand, most studies report significantly lower AA (Decsi et al., 2002; Ruiz-Gutierrez et al., 1993) and DHA values (Decsi et al., 2002; Ruiz-Gutierrez et al., 1993; Tilvis & Miettinen, 1985) in diabetic patients than in controls. In one study (Tilvis et al., 1986), diabetic patients treated with continuous insulin infusion therapy had significantly lower LA, and significantly higher AA and DHA values both in plasma and erythrocyte membrane lipids than patients with conventional insulin therapy. These results suggest that better diabetic control may improve the activity of Δ-6 desaturase enzyme.

After a longer period, hyperglycaemia and hypoinsulinemia may lead to several complications in diabetic patients. Several studies investigated the relationship between disturbed fatty acid status in diabetic patients and a number of complications, like diabetic neuropathy, nephropathy and retinopathy. These relationships and the potential role of n-3 fatty acid supplementation in diabetic patients are reviewed elsewhere (Szabó et al., 2010b).

3.1 Fatty acid supply during pregnancy in women with type 1 diabetes mellitus: Maternal effects

T1DM disturbs the fatty acid supply, therefore maternal LCPUFA stores may be compromised compared to healthy pregnant women. Disturbed fatty acid supply and metabolism may influence the course of pregnancy and delivery and may lead both to maternal and fetal complications. Nevertheless, we found only two human studies investigating the fatty acid supply during pregnancy in women with T1DM and four studies investigating fatty acid supply in cord blood lipids of newborns born from mothers with T1DM (Table 4).

Ghebremeskel et al. (Ghebremeskel et al., 2002) induced diabetes with streptozotocin in pregnant rats and investigated the liver fatty acid composition. They found significantly higher essential fatty acid values (ALA and LA) as well as n-3 and n-6 LCPUFA values (AA, EPA, DPA and DHA) in the TG and NEFA fractions. In an earlier study (Chen CH et al.,

1965), only LA was determined and no significant differences were found in plasma NEFA fraction between diabetic and control mothers.

Author	Number	Change in EFAs	Change in LCPUFAs
T1DM: maternal effects			
Chen CH et al., 1965	n = 3	pl. NEFA: LA ↔	no data
Min et al., 2005a	n = 32	pl. TG, CPG: LA, ALA ↔ RBC PC, PE: LA, ALA ↔	pl. CPG: DHA ↓ RBC PC: DPA, DHA ↓ RBC PE: DHA ↓
T1DM: fetal effects			
Chen CH et al., 1965	n = 4	pl. NEFA: LA ↔	no data
Ghebremeskel et al., 2004	n = 31	pl. CPG: LA, ALA ↑ pl. TG: LA, ALA ↓ pl. STE: LA, ALA ↔	pl. CPG: AA, DPA, DHA ↓ pl. TG: DHGLA ↓ pl. STE: AA, DHA ↓
Min et al., 2005a	n = 26	pl. TG: ALA ↓ pl. CPG: LA, ALA ↔ RBC PC, PE: LA, ALA ↔	pl. TG: DHGLA, DPA, DHA ↓ pl. CPG: AA, DHA ↓ RBC PC: AA, DHA ↔ RBC PE: DHA ↓
Winkler et al., 2008*	a.) n = 23 b.) n = 25	a.) RBC PC, PE: LA, ALA ↔ b.) RBC PE: LA, ALA ↑ RBC PC: LA, ALA ↔	a.) RBC PC: DPA ↓ RBC PE: AA, DHA ↔ b.) RBC PE: DHA ↓ RBC PC: AA, DHA ↔

* a.) = age of 3 months; b.) = age of 12 months
Abbreviations: AA: arachidonic acid, ALA: alpha-linolenic acid, CPG: choline phosphoglycerol, DHA: docosahexaenoic acid, DHGLA: dihomo-gamma-linolenic acid, DPA: docosapentaenoic acid, EFAs: essential fatty acids, EPA: eicosapentaenoic acid, LA: linoleic acid, LCPUFAs: long-chain polyunsaturated fatty acids, NEFA: non-esterified fatty acid, PC: phosphatidylcholine, PE: phosphatidylethanolamine, pl.: plasma, PL: phospholipid, RBC: erythrocyte, SM: sphyngomyeline, STE: sterol esther, T1DM: type 1 diabetes mellitus, TG: triacylglycerol

Table 4. Change in essential fatty acid and long-chain polyunsaturated fatty acid values compared to controls in pregnant women with type 1 diabetes mellitus and newborns from mothers with type 1 diabetes mellitus

Plasma and erythrocyte membrane fatty acid composition was studied in women with and without T1DM at midgestation (Min et al., 2005a). In the maternal plasma only choline phosphoglyceride (CPG) DHA was found to be decreased in diabetic patients, while in the erythrocyte membrane lipids more pronounced differences were found. Both the phosphatidylcholine (PC) fraction and in the phosphatidylethanolamine (PE) fraction significantly lower DHA values were found in mothers with T1DM than in healthy pregnant women. The authors hypothesised that this difference might be due to the synergistic effect of diabetes and pregnancy.

3.2 Fatty acid supply in newborns of mothers with type 1 diabetes mellitus: Fetal effects

AA and DHA play an important role in the maturation of the fetal nervous system. Although the developing fetus can synthesise AA and DHA from their precursors, this synthesis is rather slow and can't meet the requirements of the fetus. As T1DM disturbs the fatty acid supply of pregnant women, newborns of mothers with diabetes may have inadequate in utero n-3 and n-6 LCPUFA supply. In contrast to the lack of data on maternal fatty acid supply, cord blood lipids in neonates of mothers with T1DM were published from several studies.

Chen CH et al. (Chen CH et al., 1965) found no differences between cord blood LA values between newborns of diabetic and control mothers. Cord blood of newborns from mothers with T1DM and healthy controls was analysed in detail in an English study (Ghebremeskel et al., 2004). In the plasma CPG fraction there were significantly higher LA and ALA values in cord blood of neonates from diabetic mothers, while their long-chain metabolites, AA and DHA were lower in both plasma CPG and sterin esther (STE) fractions, which may reflect impaired placental transfer of the n-3 and n-6 LCPUFAs. The authors speculated that the effect of T1DM and pregnancy-induced metabolic changes together with the Western diet might have resulted in decreased AA and DHA levels in pregnant women with T1DM.

In another study, cord blood samples of newborns of mothers with T1DM contained significantly lower ALA, DPA and DHA in the plasma TG fraction and significantly lower AA and DHA in the plasma CPG fraction (Min et al., 2005a). However, only DHA values were decreased in the erythrocyte PE fraction in the cord blood of the T1DM group.

In the BABYDIET study, newborns with increased genetic and familiar risk for T1DM were investigated (Winkler et al., 2008). Erythrocyte membrane PC and PE were determined in infants of mothers with and without T1DM at the age of 3 and 12 months. No differences were found in the values of the most important LCPUFAs, AA and DHA in the PC fraction, while significantly lower DPA values were found in the infants of diabetic mothers at the age of 3 months, than in those of the healthy controls. In contrast, comparing only the exclusively breastfed infants of mothers with and without T1DM, no differences were found in the values of n-3 and n-6 PUFAs. At the age of 12 months, infants from mothers with T1DM had significantly higher essential fatty acid (ALA and LA) values, but DHA values were decreased in the PE fraction.

As newborns of mothers with diabetes may have diminished AA and DHA supply, the neurodevelopment of these infants may also be affected. In an experimental animal study (Zhao et al., 2009), diabetes was induced in rats who were divided into two groups, one with good and one with poor diabetic control and were fed either with AA or control diet. After one week the animals were mated and the neurodevelopment of the pups was investigated. Maternal dietary AA supplementation through pregnancy and lactation resulted in improved sensorimotor and developmental performances of the offspring of both healthy controls and poorly controlled diabetic dams. Maternal AA supplementation also improved the AA supply of the offspring's liver, but not in the brain.

Maternal diabetes may disturb fetal fatty acid supply, however, from the epidemiological point of view the longer term effects are more important. Offspring of diabetic mothers may develop different malformations such as spina bifida, at birth they might be macrosomic and develop hypoglycaemia. The potential role of fatty acids in hyperglycaemia-induced teratogenesis was studied in an experimental animal model (Goldman et al., 1985). Diabetic pregnant rats without insulin treatment received subcutaneous AA injection during the period of organogenesis and although maternal glucose concentration didn't change, there was a significant decrease in the incidence of neural tube defects (from 11% to 3.8%), micrognathia (from 7% to 0.8%) and cleft palate (from 11% to 4%). These data suggest that beside good diabetes control also AA supplementation in diabetes might reduce the teratogenetic effect of hyperglycaemia.

4. Effect of gestational diabetes mellitus on fatty acid supply

Gestational diabetes mellitus (GDM) affecting 2-10% of pregnant women in the United States (National Diabetes Statistics, 2011) is associated with insulin resistance during pregnancy. Its prevalence is rising worldwide. Analysing the GDM screening results between 1994-2002 in Colorado state (Dabelea et al., 2005), the prevalence of GDM was increasing from 1994-1996 to 2000-2002 in all ethnic groups: Hispanic (2.8% to 5.1%), African American (2.5% to 4.6%), Asian (6.3% to 8.6%) and non-Hispanic white (1.9% to 3.4%). Women with GDM are at risk to develop type 2 diabetes mellitus either immediately after delivery (5-10%) or later, in 10-20 years (35-60%).

The risk factors of developing GDM during pregnancy are higher pre-pregnancy BMI, smoking, increasing maternal age and GDM during previous pregnancy. Western diet contains high fat intake with high n-6/n-3 fatty acid ratio, refined sugar, fried and snack foods with high *trans* fatty acid content; all these factors may play an important role in developing impaired glucose tolerance and, hence, GDM. Maternal high fat diet during pregnancy decreased EPA and DHA values in liver in newborn pups as well as in suckling pups born from both diabetic and control mothers (Ghebremeskel et al., 1999). In the Project Viva (Radesky et al., 2008), pregnant women with maternal age above 40 years (OR: 11.3), pre-pregnancy BMI above 30 kg/m^2 (OR: 3.44), GDM during prior pregnancy (OR: 58.3) and Hispanic ethnicity (OR: 3.19) had increased risk of developing GDM. However, dietary pattern during early pregnancy had no association with developing GDM.

4.1 Fatty acid supply during pregnancy in women with gestational diabetes mellitus: Maternal effects

As type 2 diabetes mellitus and obesity disturbs fatty acid supply, GDM may also have an effect on fatty acid metabolism in pregnant women. While only two studies were found investigating the effect of T1DM on maternal blood fatty acid composition, GDM was investigated in a number of studies. We found nine studies investigating the fatty acid supply during pregnancy in women with GDM and five studies investigating the fatty acid supply of newborns from mothers with GDM (Table 5).

In an early study (Chen CH et al., 1965), no difference was seen in LA values of mothers with GDM and controls at delivery. When in 2000 the diet and blood samples of pregnant women with GDM during the third trimester were analysed (Wijendran et al., 2000) women with GDM had significantly higher AA, EPA and DHA intakes than controls. Maternal erythrocyte PL contained more DHA, while other fatty acids didn't differ. The authors also determined the effect of fatty acid supply on plasma PL in these women at the 27-30th, 33-35th and 36-39th weeks of pregnancy (Wijendran et al., 1999). Although there were no significant differences in the LA and AA values between the two groups, values of DHGLA and C22:5n-6 were significantly lower at each investigated time points. In contrast, among the n-3 fatty acids, ALA and DPA were significantly lower, while DHA was significantly higher in women with GDM than in healthy controls. Wijendran et al. provided three possible explanations for the lower ALA and higher DHA values: 1. either increased desaturation and elongation of ALA to DHA may be responsible for these alterations, or 2. increased selective oxidation of ALA or 3. enhanced release of DHA into plasma PL. Both in controls and mothers with GDM, the n-3 and n-6 LCPUFAs decreased as the result of the physiologic adaptation in pregnant women to the increased fetal n-3 and n-6 LCPUFA requirement during the third trimester. The authors also investigated the correlations

Author	Number	Change in EFAs	Change in LCPUFAs
GDM: maternal effects			
Chen CH et al., 1965	n = 8	pl. NEFA: LA ↔	no data
Chen X et al., 2010	n = 49	pl.: LA, ALA ↑	pl.: AA, EPA, DHA ↑
Min et al., 2004	n = 53	pl. CPG: ALA ↓ RBC PC: ALA ↓ RBC PE: ALA ↑	pl. CPG: AA ↑ RBC PC: DHGLA, AA, EPA, DPA, DHA ↓ RBC PE: DHGLA, DPA, DHA ↓
Min et al., 2005b	n = 40	pl. TG: LA, ALA ↔ pl. CPG: ALA ↓ RBC PC, PE: LA, ALA ↔	pl. TG: AA, DHA ↔ pl. CPG: AA ↑ RBC PC: AA ↓ RBC PE: AA, DHA ↔
Min et al., 2006	n = 12	pl. TG: LA, ALA ↔ pl. PC: ALA ↓ pl. SM: LA ↔ RBC PC, PE: LA, ALA ↔ RBC SM: LA ↔	pl. TG: AA, DHA ↔ pl. PC: DHA ↑ pl. SM: AA, DHA ↔ RBC PC: AA ↓ RBC PE: AA ↓ RBC SM: AA, DHA ↔
Ortega-Senovilla et al., 2009	n = 15	pl.: LA, ALA ↔	pl.: AA, DHA ↔
Thomas et al., 2004	n = 44	pl. CPG: ALA ↓ pl. TG: LA ↑ pl. STE: ALA ↓	pl. CPG: AA ↑ pl. TG: DHA ↑ pl. STE: AA ↑
Wijendran et al., 1999	n = 15	pl. PL: ALA ↓	pl. PL: DHGLA, DPA ↓, DHA ↑
Wijendran et al., 2000	n = 13	RBC PL: ALA ↓	RBC PL: DHA ↑
GDM: fetal effects			
Chen CH et al., 1965	n = 9	pl. NEFA: LA ↔	no data
Min et al., 2005b	n = 40	pl. TG: LA, ALA ↓ pl. CPG: LA, ALA ↔ RBC PC, PE: LA, ALA ↔	pl. TG: AA, DHA ↔ pl. CPG: DHA ↓ RBC PC: DHA ↓ RBC PE: AA, DHA ↔
Ortega-Senovilla et al., 2009*	n = 15	a.) pl.: LA, ALA ↔ b.) pl.: LA, ALA ↔	a.) pl.: AA, DHA ↔ b.) pl.: AA, DHA ↓
Thomas et al., 2005	n = 37	pl. TG: ALA ↓ pl. CPG, STE: LA, ALA ↔	pl. CPG: DHGLA, DHA ↓ pl. STE: DHGLA ↓ pl. TG: AA, DHA ↔
Wijendran et al., 2000	n = 13	RBC PL: LA, ALA ↔	RBC PL: AA, DHA ↓

* a.) = umbilical vein; b.) = umbilical artery. Abbreviations: see Table 4.

Table 5. Change in essential fatty acid and long-chain polyunsaturated fatty acid values compared to controls in mothers with gestational diabetes mellitus and infants born from mothers with gestational diabetes mellitus (GDM)

between, on the one hand, maternal fatty acids and on the other hand, HbA_{1c} and prepregnancy BMI. Though there was an inverse association between plasma HbA_{1c} and plasma PL AA also in the controls, this association was more pronounced in women with GDM. Similarly, positive correlation was found between mean fasting plasma insulin and plasma PL AA values. These correlations may indicate impairment in the transport of AA to the fetus. Prepregnancy BMI was correlated inversely to maternal DHA and positively to maternal AA values in the diabetic group. These findings suggest that maternal alterations in plasma PL DHA values may be more pronounced in obese women with GDM.

An English research group (Thomas et al., 2006) investigated the diet of pregnant women with and without GDM during the third trimester, and reported several differences. Diabetic women ingested less fat than controls, and the ratios of fatty acids in the diet were also different: diabetic women had lower saturated, monounsaturated and *trans* fatty acid intake, but higher PUFA intake. Interestingly, the distribution of PUFAs was largely similar in the two groups, only one fatty acid differed between the two groups: mothers with GDM ingested more DHA. They also investigated the effect of ethnicity on dietary fatty acid intake. Afro-Caribbean mothers with GDM had lower total fat, saturated, monounsaturated, *trans* fatty acid and PUFA intake than Caucasian mothers. The diet of the Afro-Caribbean GDM group contained lower LA, AA, n-6 PUFA and ALA values, while higher EPA and DHA compared to Caucasian mothers with GDM.

The same authors also compared the plasma fatty acid supply of these women at diagnosis (Thomas et al., 2004). Women with GDM had significantly higher LA values in the plasma TG fraction, higher AA values in the plasma CPG and STE fraction and higher DHA values in the plasma TG fraction than healthy controls, while ALA was significantly lower in plasma STE in women with GDM. These alterations may be explained by the high glucose concentration that led to the mobilisation of LA, ALA, AA and DHA from adipose tissue and liver. When comparing the fatty acid supply of both plasma and erythrocyte membrane lipids in these women at diagnosis (Min et al., 2004), in plasma CPG higher AA and lower ALA values were found in the mothers with GDM, while values of DHGLA, AA, C22:4n-6 as well as ALA, EPA, DPA and DHA was significantly lower in erythrocyte CPG lipids in the diabetic than in the control group. This discrepancy between plasma and erythrocyte membrane lipid composition may arise as an effect of GDM causing reduction of incorporation of these fatty acids into red blood cells and other tissues. As erythrocyte membrane lipid composition is very similar to that of the vascular endothelium, these alterations in erythrocyte membrane lipids may indicate that endothelium may be also affected in GDM.

In another study carried out in London, significantly lower ALA and higher AA in plasma CPG fraction was found in diabetic mothers than in healthy controls at delivery (Min et al., 2005b). However, AA was significantly lower in erythrocyte membrane PC fraction.

Min et al. carried out a pilot study in Korea, where the habitual diet contains higher n-3 fatty acid and lower total fat intake than the typical Western-type diet (Min et al., 2006). Women with GDM had lower ALA and higher DHA in plasma PC fractions at delivery, while values of AA was lower in erythrocyte PC and PE fractions in women with GDM than in controls. Comparing the AA and DHA values in GDM patients and controls living in Korea or in the UK, in both study groups lower AA and DHA values were found in erythrocyte PC lipids of the GDM groups than in the controls. However, Korean women (both diabetic and control) had higher DHA values than British women. This finding suggests that the reduction of erythrocyte membrane AA and DHA values in women with GDM might be attributed to effects of the disease itself regardless of ethnicity, obesity or diet. In contrast, there were no

significant differences in the fatty acid composition of plasma lipids between mothers with GDM and controls at delivery in an Italian study (Ortega-Senovilla et al., 2009).
As part of a prospective cohort study, a nested case-control study was carried out by Chen X et al. (Chen X et al., 2010) to investigate the differences in fatty acid status of women with impaired glucose tolerance, GDM and controls. In contrast to earlier studies (Wijendran et al., 2000; Thomas et al., 2006), this population had higher saturated fatty acid intake, while dietary LA, DHA and PUFA intakes were significantly lower in the diabetic group than in controls. At study entry (16th week) women who developed impaired glucose tolerance later, had higher plasma EPA absolute values; however, the percentage of PUFAs didn't differ significantly among the three groups. During the third trimester, mothers with GDM had higher AA, DHA and PUFA absolute concentrations, while women with impaired glucose tolerance had higher LA, ALA, EPA and DHA absolute values. Similarly to study entry, PUFA percents didn't differ among the groups. These data showed that not only GDM disturbs fatty acid supply of pregnant women, but impaired glucose tolerance as well. The authors also investigated the effect of BMI and found significantly higher concentrations of saturated and monounsaturated fatty acids and PUFAs in women with impaired glucose tolerance and BMI higher than 25 kg/m^2 at study entry than in normal weighted women with impaired glucose tolerance. During the third trimester, overweight and obese women with GDM had the highest fatty acid absolute concentration. These results indicate that the disturbance in the fatty acid metabolism is more pronounced when beyond the mild hyperglycaemia obesity is also present. Results of this study raised the possibility that reducing pregravid weight and modifying diet (increasing PUFAs and reducing saturated fatty acids) may reduce circulating free fatty acids, therefore decreasing insulin resistance and inflammation and lower future maternal risk of type 2 diabetes mellitus.

4.2 Fatty acid supply in newborns of mothers with gestational diabetes mellitus: Fetal effects

Macrosomia and lipid abnormalities are common complications associated with maternal diabetes during pregnancy. Offspring of diabetic mothers are prone to develop obesity, type 2 diabetes mellitus and cardiovascular diseases during adulthood. In an animal study (Soulimane-Mokhtari et al., 2008), diabetic and control rats were fed a control diet or diet rich in EPA and DHA. During pregnancy of the diabetic rats, VLDL- and LDL-cholesterol were significantly decreased in the intervention group. Moreover, similar changes were seen in the macrosomic offspring: maternal fish oil diet significantly decreased VLDL- and LDL-cholesterol. As n-3 LCPUFA supplementation during pregnancy restored tissue lipase activities to normal range and ameliorated long-term prognosis of macrosomia, n-3 fatty acid supplementation may be beneficial for mothers with GDM.
Maternal diabetes during pregnancy (characterised by hyperglycaemia, hyperlipidaemia, hyperlipoproteinaemia and altered T-cell function) may result in metabolic programming of the offspring causing obesity, impaired glucose tolerance, hyperlipidaemia and hyperlipoproteinaemia during adulthood (Khan, 2007). In Chinese children of mothers with GDM, significantly higher systolic and diastolic blood pressures and lower HDL-cholesterol levels were seen than in controls at the age of 8 years. High umbilical cord insulin was an independent risk factor of both abnormal glucose tolerance and obesity; hence, in utero hyperinsulinaemia and hyperglycaemia may have long-term effects on developing type 2

diabetes and metabolic syndrome (Tam et al., 2008). Type 2 diabetes was diagnosed at younger ages if the patients were exposed to maternal diabetes intrauterine, whereas this difference wasn't seen in the onset of type 1 diabetes (Pettitt et al., 2008). This finding suggests, that intrauterine hyperglycaemia predisposes to an earlier onset of type 2 diabetes, while type 1 diabetes is little influenced by the intrauterine milieu.

In the pioneer study published in 1965 by Chen CH et al. (Chen CH et al., 1965) newborns of mothers with GDM were also analysed and no differences were found in LA values between the diabetic and control groups. Wijendran et al. analysed not only the maternal diet and fatty acid composition of maternal erythrocyte PL, but also the fatty acid composition of cord blood erythrocyte membrane lipids (Wijendran et al., 2000). Though in the maternal blood only DHA differed between mothers with GDM and controls, in the cord blood several differences were found. Values of AA and n-6 PUFAs as well as DHA and n-3 PUFAs were significantly lower in the GDM group than in controls. The DHA sufficiency index calculated from DHA divided with C22:5n-6 was also decreased. This impaired AA and DHA supply in cord blood suggested the impaired fetal accretion of these LCPUFAs in pregnancy with GDM. The authors also correlated maternal and fetal fatty acids both in the GDM group and controls. Though in controls significant positive correlations were found between maternal plasma PL AA and DHA and cord blood plasma PL AA and DHA, these correlations were lost in the GDM group. In controls also an enrichment of AA and DHA in fetal erythrocyte was found, while in the GDM group fetal DHA was lower than maternal, and no difference in AA values were found. These alterations raised the possibility that placental transfer of maternal LCPUFAs during the third trimester may be altered in GDM. Maternal HbA_{1c} was also significantly and inversely correlated to fetal AA and DHA values. Although mothers had their HbA_{1c} values between 4-6%, these values were significantly higher than in controls suggesting a moderate impairment of glucose control. This altered glucose control may also have a negative impact on fetal LCPUFA accretion.

Min et al. (Min et al., 2005b) investigated cord blood samples of newborns from mothers with and without GDM in London and found significantly decreased ALA, LA, DHA and AA values in the plasma TG fraction. In contrast, in the plasma CPG fraction only DHA values were significantly lower in the diabetic group. Similarly, in the PC fraction of erythrocyte membrane lipids significantly decreased DHA values were found. This altered cord blood fatty acid supply may suggest the compromised placental fatty acid transport and/or fetal lipid metabolism.

In another English study (Thomas et al., 2005) also significantly lower DHA values were found in the cord blood plasma CPG lipids in the diabetic group. DHGLA was also decreased in plasma CPG and STE fractions. Values of LA, ALA and AA were not significantly different between the two groups in the plasma TG, CPG and STE fractions, but values of AA were reduced. Although mothers with GDM consumed more DHA, their neonates had reduced levels of both DHA and AA, suggesting that mothers with GDM have impaired placental transfer of LCPUFAs. Mead acid, which is considered as an indicator of shortage of EFAs, was increased in the plasma CPG and TG fractions. The elevated Mead acid values in the cord plasma TG and CPG fraction suggested fetal EFA deficiency.

In a recent study (Ortega-Senovilla et al., 2009) umbilical arterial and venous plasma fatty acid composition was analysed in women with GDM and controls who underwent elective caesarean section. While there were no significant differences in umbilical venous blood fatty acids between the two groups, in the umbilical arterial blood significantly lower AA, n-6 PUFA, DHA and n-3 PUFA values were found. Umbilical arterial and venous blood of both

GDM and control groups had lower LA and higher AA and DHA than their mothers. As umbilical venous blood comes from placental capillaries, these higher proportions of AA and DHA in umbilical venous than in maternal blood may indicate that the placental transfer remained unimpaired. However, the decreased n-3 and n-6 LCPUFA values might indicate enhanced utilization of these fatty acids.

4.3 Differences between fatty acid supply in pregnant women with type 1 diabetes mellitus and with gestational diabetes

We found ten studies about fatty acid supply of pregnant women with either T1DM or GDM. Five different research groups performed human investigations: Chen CH et al. from Cleveland, Chen X et al. from New Jersey, Min et al. from London (Min, Thomas), Ortega-Senovilla et al. from Madrid, finally Wijendran et al. from Hartford.

To the best of our knowledge, only one study investigated the LCPUFA supply in pregnant women with T1DM. In this study no differences were found in n-3 and n-6 EFA values, while the most important n-3 metabolite, DHA was lower in all lipid fractions. In GDM most of the studies found decreased or unchanged ALA values, while LA values remained in most cases stable. In case of LCPUFAs, the results are less unambiguous and there was a difference between plasma and erythrocyte LCPUFA values. In general we can say, that plasma LCPUFAs in most cases were higher in mothers with GDM than in controls or it remained unchanged. In contrast, in erythrocyte membrane lipids LCPUFAs were either lower or unchanged in women with GDM compared to healthy controls except for one study (Wijendran et al., 2000).

Although we found only one study about fatty acid supply of pregnant women with T1DM, it seems, that diabetes had no influence on the EFA supply in mothers. In contrast, GDM may diminish EFA supply during pregnancy. T1DM significantly lowered the LCPUFA values in both plasma and erythrocyte membrane lipids, while there was a discrepancy in the effect of GDM: in plasma lipids it rather increased while in erythrocyte membrane lipids decreased the availability of LCPUFAs.

4.4 Differences between fatty acid supply in neonates from mothers with type 1 diabetes mellitus and with gestational diabetes

There were seven human studies investigating the fatty acid supply in cord blood or blood from infants born from mother with either T1DM or GDM. Four different research groups have data about blood lipid fatty acid composition of these offspring: Min et al. from London (Ghebremeskel, Min, Thomas), Ortega-Senovilla et al. from Madrid, Wijendran et al. from Hartford, finally Winkler et al., from Munich.

In contrast to maternal data, four studies investigated the fatty acid composition of newborns or infants of mothers with T1DM. Findings of EFA values are rather unequivocal: values of LA and ALA are either higher or lower or remained unchanged in the T1DM group. However, result are more clear in the case of LCPUFAs, all three studies found significantly lower AA and/or DHA values in plasma lipids, while erythrocyte membrane DHA values were either lower or similar to AA values, they remained unchanged in the offspring of T1DM mothers.

Looking at the results about the effect of GDM, in most cases EFA values remained stable, while LCPUFAs, predominantly DHA was significantly lower in the GDM group. In cord blood there was no deviation between plasma and erythrocyte LCPUFA values: AA and

DHA were either lower or no significantly different in the offspring of GDM mothers than in controls.

To sum it up: T1DM has no clear effect on EFA status of the offspring, while GDM might lower it. In contrast, both T1DM and GDM lowered the availability of LCPUFAs in newborns and infants of diabetic mothers.

5. Conclusion

Data reviewed here indicate that both T1DM and GDM disturb the fatty acid supply in pregnant women and their offspring. Both types of diabetes during pregnancy may result in lower values of n-3 and n-6 LCPUFA in maternal erythrocyte lipids as well as in cord blood plasma and erythrocyte lipids. Therefore incorporation of fatty sea fishes rich in n-3 fatty acids into the diet (e.g. in the form of two 200 g pieces weekly) or other ways of n-3 LCPUFA supplementation during pregnancy may be beneficial.

6. References

Albert, CM., Hennekens, CH., O'Donnell, CJ., Ajani, UA., Carey, VJ., Willett, WC., Ruskin, JN. & Manson, JE. (1998). Fish consumption and risk of sudden cardiac death. *JAMA: The Journal of the American Medical Association,* Vol.279, No.1, (January 1998), pp. 23-28, ISSN 0098-7484

Bakker, EC., Ghys, AJ., Kester, AD., Vles, JS., Dubas, JS., Blanco, CE. & Hornstra, G. (2003). Long-chain polyunsaturated fatty acids at birth and cognitive function at 7 y of age. *European Journal of Clinical Nutrition,* Vol.57, No.1, (January 2003), pp. 89-95, ISSN 0954-3007

Beare-Rogers, J., Dieffenbacher, A. & Holm, JV. (2001). Lexicon of lipid nutrition (IUPAC Technical Report). *Pure and Applied Chemistry,* Vol.73, No.4, (April 2001), pp. 685-744, ISSN 0033-4545

Berghaus, TM., Demmelmair, H. & Koletzko, B. (1998). Fatty acid composition of lipid classes in maternal and cord plasma at birth. *European Journal of Pediatrics,* Vol.157, No.9, (September 1998), pp. 763-768, ISSN 0340-6199

Bouwstra, H., Dijck-Brouwer, J., Decsi, T., Boehm, G., Boersma, ER., Muskiet, FA. & Hadders-Algra, M. (2006). Neurologic condition of healthy term infants at 18 months: positive association with venous umbilical DHA status and negative association with umbilical trans-fatty acids. *Pediatric Research,* Vol.60, No.3, (September 2006), pp. 334-339, ISSN 0031-3998

Brenna, JT. & Diau, GY. (2007). The influence of dietary docosahexaenoic acid and arachidonic acid on central nervous system polyunsaturated fatty acid composition. *Prostaglandins, Leukotrienes, and Essential Fatty Acids,* Vol.77, No.5-6, (November-December 2007), pp. 247-250, ISSN 0952-3278

Brenner, RR. (2003). Hormonal modulation of delta6 and delta5 desaturases: case of diabetes. *Prostaglandins, Leukotrienes, and Essential Fatty Acids,* Vol.68, No.2, (February 2003), pp. 151-162, ISSN 0952-3278

Cetin, I., Alvino, G. & Cardellicchio, M. (2009). Long chain fatty acids and dietary fats in fetal nutrition. *The Journal of Physiology,* Vol.587, No.14, (July 2009), pp. 3441-3451, ISSN 0022-3751

Chen, CH., Adam, PA., Laskowski, DE., McCann, ML. & Schwartz, R. (1965). The plasma free fatty acid composition and blood glucose of normal and diabetic pregnant women and of their newborns. *Pediatrics,* Vol.36, No.6, (December 1965), pp. 843-855, ISSN 0031-4005

Chen, X., Scholl, TO., Leskiw, M., Savaille, J. & Stein, TP. (2010). Differences in maternal circulating fatty acid composition and dietary fat intake in women with gestational diabetes mellitus or mild gestational hyperglycemia. *Diabetes Care,* Vol.33, No.9, (September 2010), pp. 2049-2054, ISSN 0149-5992

Chua, B., Flood, V., Rochtchina, E., Wang, JJ., Smith, W. & Mitchell P. (2006). Dietary fatty acids and the 5-year incidence of age-related maculopathy. *Archives of Ophthalmology,* Vol.124, No.7, (July 2006), pp. 981-986, ISSN 0003-9950

Dabelea, D., Snell-Bergeon, JK., Hartsfield, CL., Bischoff, KJ., Hamman, RF., McDuffie, RS. & Kaiser Permanente of Colorado GDM Screening Program. (2005). Increasing prevalence of gestational diabetes mellitus (GDM) over time and by birth cohort: Kaiser Permanente of Colorado GDM Screening Program. *Diabetes Care,* Vol.28, No.3, (March 2005), pp. 579-584, ISSN 0149-5992

Das, UN. (2006). Essential Fatty acids - a review. *Current Pharmaceutical Biotechnology,* Vol.7, No.6, (December 2006), pp. 467-482, ISSN 1389-2010

Decsi, T., Minda, H., Hermann, R., Kozári, A., Erhardt, E., Burus, I., Molnár, S. & Soltész, G. (2002). Polyunsaturated fatty acids in plasma and erythrocyte membrane lipids of diabetic children. *Prostaglandins, Leukotrienes, and Essential Fatty Acids,* Vol.67, No.4, (October 2002), pp. 203-210, ISSN 0952-3278

Decsi, T., Szabó, É., Burus, I., Marosvölgyi, T., Kozári, A., Erhardt, É. & Soltész, G. (2007). Low contribution of n-3 polyunsaturated fatty acids to plasma and erythrocyte membrane lipids in diabetic young adults. *Prostaglandins, Leukotrienes, and Essential Fatty Acids,* Vol.76, No.3, (March 2007), pp. 159-164, ISSN 0952-3278

Diau, GY., Hsieh, AT., Sarkadi-Nagy, EA., Wijendran, V., Nathanielsz, PW. & Brenna, JT. (2005). The influence of long chain polyunsaturate supplementation on docosahexaenoic acid and arachidonic acid in baboon neonate central nervous system. *BMC Medicine,* Vol.23, No.3, (June 2005), pp. 11-22, ISSN 1741-7015

Dyerberg, J., Eskesen, DC., Andersen, PW., Astrup, A., Buemann, B., Christensen, JH., Clausen, P., Rasmussen, BF., Schmidt, EB., Tholstrup, T., Toft, E., Toubro, S. & Stender, S. (2004). Effects of trans- and n-3 unsaturated fatty acids on cardiovascular risk markers in healthy males. An 8 weeks dietary intervention study. *European Journal of Clinical Nutrition,* Vol.58, No.7, (July 2004), pp. 1062-1070, ISSN 0954-3007

Erasmus, U. (1993). *Fats that Heal, Fats that Kill,* (1st Edition) Alive Books, ISBN 978-0-920470-38-1, Vancouver, Canada

Erkkilä, AT., Lichtenstein, AH., Mozaffarian, D. & Herrington, DM. (2004). Fish intake is associated with a reduced progression of coronary artery atherosclerosis in postmenopausal women with coronary artery disease. *The American Journal of Clinical Nutrition,* Vol.80, No.3, (December 2004), pp. 626-632, ISSN 0002-9165

Farquharson, J., Cockburn, F., Patrick, WA., Jamieson, EC. & Logan, RW. (1992). Infant cerebral cortex phospholipid fatty-acid composition and diet. *Lancet,* Vol.340, No.8823, (October 1992), pp. 810-813, ISSN 0140-6736

Ghebremeskel, K., Bitsanis, D., Koukkou, E., Lowy, C., Poston, L. & Crawford, MA. (1999). Maternal diet high in fat reduces docosahexaenoic acid in liver lipids of newborn and sucking rat pups. *The British Journal of Nutrition,* Vol.81, No.5, (May 1999), pp. 395-404, ISSN 0007-1145

Ghebremeskel, K., Bitsanis, D., Koukkou, E., Lowy, C., Poston, L. & Crawford, MA. (2002). Liver triacylglycerols and free fatty acids in streptozotocin-induced diabetic rats have atypical n-6 and n-3 pattern. *Comparative Biochemistry and Physiology, Toxicology & Pharmacology,* Vol.132, No.3, (July 2002), pp. 349-354, ISSN 1532-0456

Ghebremeskel, K., Thomas, B., Lowy, C., Min, Y. & Crawford, MA. (2004). Type 1 diabetes compromises plasma arachidonic and docosahexaenoic acids in newborn babies. *Lipids,* Vol.39, No.4, (April 2004), pp. 335-342, ISSN 0024-4201

Ghys, A., Bakker, E., Hornstra, G. & van den Hout, M. (2002). Red blood cell and plasma phospholipid arachidonic and docosahexaenoic acid levels at birth and cognitive development at 4 years of age. *Early Human Development,* Vol.69, No.1-2, (October 2002), pp. 83-90, ISSN 0378-3782

Gil-Sánchez, A., Larqué, E., Demmelmair, H., Acien, MI., Faber, FL., Parrilla, JJ. & Koletzko, B. (2010). Maternal-fetal in vivo transfer of [13C]docosahexaenoic and other fatty acids across the human placenta 12 h after maternal oral intake. *The American Journal of Clinical Nutrition,* Vol.92, No.1, (July 2010), pp. 115-122, ISSN 0002-9165

Goldman, AS., Baker, L., Piddington, R., Marx, B., Herold, R. & Egler, J. (1985). Hyperglycemia-induced teratogenesis is mediated by a functional deficiency of arachidonic acid. *Proceedings of the National Academy of Sciences of the United States of America,* Vol.82, No.23, (December 1985), pp. 8227-8231, ISSN 0027-8424

Helland, IB., Smith, L., Saarem, K., Saugstad, OD. & Drevon, CA. (2003). Maternal supplementation with very-long-chain n-3 fatty acids during pregnancy and lactation augments children's IQ at 4 years of age. *Pediatrics,* Vol.111, No.1, (January 2003), pp. e39-44, ISSN 0031-4005

Horrocks, LA. & Yeo, YK. (1999). Health benefits of docosahexaenoic acid (DHA). *Pharmacological Research: the Official Journal of the Italian Pharmacological Society,* Vol.40, No.3, (September 1999), pp. 211-225, ISSN 1043-6618

Ibrahim, A., Natrajan, S. & Ghafoorunissa, R. (2005). Dietary trans-fatty acids alter adipocyte plasma membrane fatty acid composition and insulin sensitivity in rats. *Metabolism: Clinical and Experimental,* Vol.54, No.2, (February 2005), pp. 240-246, ISSN 0026-0495

Iso, H., Kobayashi, M., Ishihara, J., Sasaki, S., Okada, K., Kita, Y., Kokubo, Y., Tsugane, S. & JPHC Study Group. (2006). Intake of fish and n3 fatty acids and risk of coronary heart disease among Japanese: the Japan Public Health Center-Based (JPHC) Study Cohort I. *Circulation*, Vol.113, No.2, (January 2006), pp. 195-202, ISSN 0009-7322

Katan, MB., Zock, PL. & Mensink, RP. (1995). Trans fatty acids and their effects on lipoproteins in humans. *Annual Review of Nutrition*, Vol.15, (July 1995), pp. 473-493, ISSN 0199-9885

Khan, NA. (2007). Role of lipids and fatty acids in macrosomic offspring of diabetic pregnancy. *Cell Biochemistry and Biophysics*, Vol.48, No.2-3, (July 2007), pp. 79-88, ISSN 1085-9195

Koletzko, B. & Rodriguez-Palmero, M. (1999). Polyunsaturated fatty acids in human milk and their role in early infant development. *Journal of Mammary Gland Biology and Neoplasia*, Vol.4, No.3, (July 1999), pp. 269-284, ISSN 1083-3021

Koletzko, B., Larqué, E. & Demmelmair, H. (2007a). Placental transfer of long-chain polyunsaturated fatty acids (LC-PUFA). *Journal of Perinatal Medicine*, Vol.35, No.Suppl 1, (February 2007), pp. S5-11, ISSN 0300-5577

Koletzko, B., Cetin, I., Brenna, JT., Perinatal Lipid Intake Working Group; Child Health Foundation; Diabetic Pregnancy Study Group; European Association of Perinatal Medicine; European Society for Clinical Nutrition and Metabolism; European Society for Paediatric Gastroenterology, Hepatology and Nutrition, Committee on Nutrition; International Federation of Placenta Associations; & International Society for the Study of Fatty Acids and Lipids. (2007b). Dietary fat intakes for pregnant and lactating women. *The British Journal of Nutrition*, Vol.98, No.5, (November 2007), pp. 873-877, ISSN 0007-1145

Laidlaw, M. & Holub, BJ. (2003). Effects of supplementation with fish oil-derived n-3 fatty acids and gamma-linolenic acid on circulating plasma lipids and fatty acid profiles in women. *The American Journal of Clinical Nutrition*, Vol.77, No.1, (January 2003), pp. 37-42, ISSN 0002-9165

Larqué, E., Demmelmair, H., Berger, B., Hasbargen, U. & Koletzko, B. (2003). In vivo investigation of the placental transfer of (13)C-labeled fatty acids in humans. *Journal of Lipid Research*, Vol.44, No.1, (January 2003), pp. 49-55, ISSN 0022-2275

Li, G., Sinclair, AJ. & Li, D. (2011). Comparison of lipid content and fatty acid composition in the edible meat of wild and cultured freshwater and marine fish and shrimps from China. *Journal of Agricultural and Food Chemistry*, Vol.59, No.5, (March 2011), pp. 1871-1881, ISSN 0021-8561

Louheranta, AM., Turpeinen, AK., Vidgren, HM., Schwab, US. & Uusitupa, MI. (1999). A high-trans fatty acid diet and insulin sensitivity in young healthy women. *Metabolism: Clinical and Experimental*, Vol.48, No.7, (July 1999), pp. 870-875, ISSN 0026-0495

Makrides, M., Neumann, MA., Byard, RW., Simmer, K. & Gibson, RA. (1994). Fatty acid composition of brain, retina, and erythrocytes in breast- and formula-fed infants. *The American Journal of Clinical Nutrition*, Vol.60, No.2, (August 1994), pp. 189-194, ISSN 0002-9165

Martínez, M. & Mougan, I. (1998). Fatty acid composition of human brain phospholipids during normal development. *Journal of Neurochemistry*, Vol.71, No.6, (December 1998), pp. 2528- 2533, ISSN 0022-3042

Min, Y., Ghebremeskel, K., Lowy, C., Thomas, B. & Crawford, MA. (2004). Adverse effect of obesity on red cell membrane arachidonic and docosahexaenoic acids in gestational diabetes. *Diabetologia,* Vol.47, No.1, (January 2004), pp. 75-81, ISSN 0012-186X

Min, Y., Lowy, C., Ghebremeskel, K., Thomas, B., Offley-Shore, B. & Crawford, M. (2005a). Unfavorable effect of type 1 and type 2 diabetes on maternal and fetal essential fatty acid status: a potential marker of fetal insulin resistance. *The American Journal of Clinical Nutrition,* Vol.82, No.6, (December 2005), pp. 1162-1168, ISSN 0002-9165

Min, Y., Lowy, C., Ghebremeskel, K., Thomas, B., Bitsanis, D. & Crawford, MA. (2005b). Fetal erythrocyte membrane lipids modification: preliminary observation of an early sign of compromised insulin sensitivity in offspring of gestational diabetic women. *Diabetic Medicine: a Journal of the British Diabetic Association,* Vol.22, No.7, (July 2005), pp. 914-920, ISSN 0742-3071

Min, Y., Nam, JH., Ghebremeskel, K., Kim, A. & Crawford, M. (2006). A distinctive fatty acid profile in circulating lipids of Korean gestational diabetics: a pilot study. *Diabetes Research and Clinical Practice,* Vol.73, No.2, (August 2006), pp. 178-183, ISSN 0168-8227

Mohan, IK. & Das, UN. (2001). Prevention of chemically induced diabetes mellitus in experimental animals by polyunsaturated fatty acids. *Nutrition,* Vol.17, No.2, (February 2001), pp. 126-151, ISSN 0899-9007

Morris, MC., Evans, DA., Bienias, JL., Tangney, CC., Bennett, DA., Wilson, RS., Aggarwal, N. & Schneider, J. (2003). Consumption of fish and n-3 fatty acids and risk of incident Alzheimer disease. *Archives of Neurology,* Vol.60, No.7, (July 2003), pp. 940-946, ISSN 0003-9942

Mozaffarian, D., Psaty, BM., Rimm, EB., Lemaitre, RN., Burke, GL., Lyles, MF., Lefkowitz, D. & Siscovick, DS. (2004). Fish intake and risk of incident atrial fibrillation. *Circulation,* Vol.110, No.4, (July 2004), pp. 368-373, ISSN 0009-7322

Mozaffarian, D., Ascherio, A., Hu, FB., Stampfer, MJ., Willett, WC., Siscovick, DS. & Rimm, EB. (2005). Interplay between different polyunsaturated fatty acids and risk of coronary heart disease in men. *Circulation,* Vol.111, No.2, (January 2005), pp. 157-164, ISSN 0009-7322

Murano, Y., Funabashi, T., Sekine, S., Aoyama, T. & Takeuchi, H. (2007). Effect of dietary lard containing higher alpha-linolenic acid on plasma triacylglycerol in rats. *Journal of Oleo Science,* Vol.56, No.7, (July 2007), pp. 361-367, ISSN 1345-8957

National Diabetes Statistics, 2011, Available from http://diabetes.niddk.nih.gov/dm/pubs/statistics/

Nikkari, T., Räsänen, L., Viikari, J., Akerblom, HK., Vuori, I., Pyörälä, K., Uhari, M., Dahl, M., Lähde, PL., Pesonen, E. & Suoninen, P. (1983). Serum fatty acids in 8-year-old Finnish boys: correlations with qualitative dietary data and other serum lipids. *The American Journal of Clinical Nutrition,* Vol.37, No.5, (May 1983), pp. 848-854, ISSN 0002-9165

Noaghiul, S. & Hibbeln, JR. (2003). Cross-national comparisons of seafood consumption and rates of bipolar disorders. *The American Journal of Psychiatry,* Vol.160, No.12, (December 2003), pp. 2222-2227, ISSN 0002-953X

Norris, JM., Yin, X., Lamb, MM., Barriga, K., Seifert, J., Hoffman, M., Orton, HD., Barón, AE., Clare-Salzler, M., Chase, HP., Szabo, NJ., Erlich, H., Eisenbarth, GS. & Rewers, M. (2007). Omega-3 polyunsaturated fatty acid intake and islet autoimmunity in children at increased risk for type 1 diabetes. *JAMA : the Journal of the American Medical Association*, Vol.298, No.12, (September 2007), pp. 1420-1428, ISSN 0098-7484

Ortega-Senovilla, H., Alvino, G., Taricco, E., Cetin, I. & Herrera, E. (2009). Gestational diabetes mellitus upsets the proportion of fatty acids in umbilical arterial but not venous plasma. *Diabetes Care,* Vol.32, No.1, (January 2009), pp. 120-122, ISSN 0149-5992

Pettitt, DJ., Lawrence, JM., Beyer, J., Hillier, TA., Liese, AD., Mayer-Davis, B., Loots, B., Imperatore, G., Liu, L., Dolan, LM., Linder, B. & Dabelea, D. (2008). Association between maternal diabetes in utero and age at offspring's diagnosis of type 2 diabetes. *Diabetes Care,* Vol.31, No.11, (November 2008), pp. 2126-2130, ISSN 0149-5992

Plourde, M. & Cunnane, SC. (2007). Extremely limited synthesis of long chain polyunsaturates in adults: implications for their dietary essentiality and use as supplements. *Applied Physiology, Nutrition, and Metabolism,* Vol.32, No.4, (August 2007), pp. 619-634, ISSN 1715-5312

Racine, RA. & Deckelbaum, RJ. (2007). Sources of the very-long-chain unsaturated omega-3 fatty acids: eicosapentaenoic acid and docosahexaenoic acid. *Current Opinion in Clinical Nutrition & Metabolic Care,* Vol.10, No.2, (March 2007), pp. 123-128, ISSN 1363-1950

Radesky, JS., Oken, E., Rifas-Shiman, SL., Kleinman, KP., Rich-Edwards, JW. & Gillman, MW. (2008). Diet during early pregnancy and development of gestational diabetes. *Paediatric and Perinatal Epidemiology,* Vol.22, No.1, (January 2008), pp. 47-59, ISSN 0269-5022

Ramsammy, LS., Haynes, B., Josepovitz, C. & Kaloyanides, GJ. (1993). Mechanism of decreased arachidonic acid in the renal cortex of rats with diabetes mellitus. *Lipids,* Vol.28, No.5, (May 1993), pp. 433-439, ISSN 0024-4201

Ruiz-Gutierrez, V., Stiefel, P., Villar, J., García-Donas, MA., Acosta, D. & Carneado, J. (1993). Cell membrane fatty acid composition in type 1 (insulin-dependent) diabetic patients: relationship with sodium transport abnormalities and metabolic control. *Diabetologia,* Vol. 36, No.9, (September 1993), pp. 850-856, ISSN 0012-186X

Salem, N. Jr., Wegher, B., Mena P. & Uauy, R. (1996). Arachidonic and docosahexaenoic acids are biosynthesized from their 18-carbon precursors in human infants. *Proceedings of the National Academy of Sciences of the United States of America,* Vol.93, No.1, (January 1996), pp. 49-54, ISSN 0027-8424

Schaefer, EJ., Bongard, V., Beiser, AS., Lamon-Fava, S., Robins, SJ., Au, R., Tucker, KL., Kyle, DJ., Wilson, PW. & Wolf, PA. (2006). Plasma phosphatidylcholine docosahexaenoic acid content and risk of dementia and Alzheimer disease: the Framingham Heart Study. *Archives of Neurology,* Vol.63, No.11, (November 2006), pp. 1545-1550, ISSN 0003-9942

Seigneur, M., Freyburger, G., Gin, H., Claverie, M., Lardeau, D., Lacape, G., Le Moigne, F., Crockett, R. & Boisseau, MR. (1994). Serum fatty acid profiles in type I and type II diabetes: metabolic alterations of fatty acids of the main serum lipids. *Diabetes Research and Clinical Practice*, Vol.23, No.3, (April 1994), pp. 169-177, ISSN 0168-8227

Shin, CS., Lee, MK., Park, KS., Kim, SY., Cho, BY., Lee, HK., Koh, CS. & Min, HK. (1995). Insulin restores fatty acid composition earlier in liver microsomes than erythrocyte membranes in streptozotocin-induced diabetic rats. *Diabetes Research and Clinical Practice*, Vol.29, No.2, (August 1995), pp. 93-98, ISSN 0168-8227

Soriguer, F., Serna, S., Valverde, E., Hernando, J., Martín-Reyes, A., Soriguer, M., Pareja, A., Tinahones, F. & Esteva, I. (1997). Lipid, protein, and calorie content of different Atlantic and Mediterranean fish, shellfish, and molluscs commonly eaten in the south of Spain. *European Journal of Epidemiology*, Vol.13, No.4, (June 1997), pp. 451-563, ISSN 0393-2990

Soulimane-Mokhtari, NA., Guermouche, B., Saker, M., Merzouk, S., Merzouk, H., Hichami, A., Madani, S., Khan, NA. & Prost, J. (2008). Serum lipoprotein composition, lecithin cholesterol acyltransferase and tissue lipase activities in pregnant diabetic rats and their offspring receiving enriched n-3 PUFA diet. *General Physiology and Biophysics*, Vol.27, No.1, (March 2008), pp. 3-11, ISSN 0231-5882

Sun, Q., Ma, J., Campos, H., Hankinson, SE., Manson, JE., Stampfer, MJ., Rexrode, KM., Willett, WC. & Hu, FB. (2007). A prospective study of trans fatty acids in erythrocytes and risk of coronary heart disease. *Circulation*, Vol.115, No.14, (April 2007), pp. 1858-1865, ISSN 0009-7322

Szabó, É., Boehm, G., Beermann, C., Weyermann, M., Brenner, H., Rothenbacher, D. & Decsi, T. (2007). trans Octadecenoic acid and trans octadecadienoic acid are inversely related to long-chain polyunsaturates in human milk: results of a large birth cohort study. *The American Journal of Clinical Nutrition*, Vol.85, No.5, (May 2007), pp. 1320-1326, ISSN 0002-9165

Szabó, É., Boehm, G., Beermann, C., Weyermann, M., Brenner, H., Rothenbacher, D. & Decsi, T. (2010a). Fatty acid profile comparisons in human milk sampled from the same mothers at the sixth week and the sixth month of lactation. *Journal of Pediatric Gastroenterology and Nutrition*, Vol.50, No.3, (March 2010), pp. 316-320. ISSN 0277-2116

Szabó, É., Soltész, Gy. & Decsi, T. (2010b). Long-chain polyunsaturated fatty acid supply in diabetes mellitus, In: *Handbook of Type 1 Diabetes Mellitus*, L. Aucoin, T. Prideux (Ed.), pp. 265-295, Nova Science Publishers Inc., ISBN: 978-1-60741-311-0, New York, USA

Tam, WH., Ma, RC., Yang, X., Ko, GT., Tong, PC., Cockram, CS., Sahota, DS., Rogers, MS. & Chan, JC. (2008). Glucose intolerance and cardiometabolic risk in children exposed to maternal gestational diabetes mellitus in utero. *Pediatrics*, Vol.122, No.6, (December 2008), pp. 1229-1234, ISSN 0031-4005

Tanakol, R., Yazici, Z., Sener, E. & Sencer, E. (1999). Fatty acid composition of 19 species of fish from the Black Sea and the Marmara Sea. *Lipids*, Vol.34, No.3, (March 1999), pp. 291-297, ISSN 0024-4201

Thomas, B., Ghebremeskel, K., Lowy, C., Min, Y. & Crawford, MA. (2004). Plasma AA and DHA levels are not compromised in newly diagnosed gestational diabetic women. *European Journal of Clinical Nutrition,* Vol.58, No.11, (November 2004), pp. 1492-1497, ISSN 0954-3007

Thomas, B., Ghebremeskel, K., Lowy, C., Offley-Shore, B. & Crawford, MA. (2005). Plasma fatty acids of neonates born to mothers with and without gestational diabetes. *Prostaglandins, Leukotrienes, and Essential Fatty Acids,* Vol.72, No.5, (May 2005), pp. 335-341, ISSN 0952-3278

Thomas, B., Ghebremeskel, K., Lowy, C., Crawford, M. & Offley-Shore, B. (2006). Nutrient intake of women with and without gestational diabetes with a specific focus on fatty acids. *Nutrition,* Vol.22, No.3, (March 2006), pp. 230-236, ISSN 0899-9007

Tilvis, RS. & Miettinen, TA. (1985). Fatty acid compositions of serum lipids, erythrocytes, and platelets in insulin-dependent diabetic women. *The Journal of Clinical Endocrinology and Metabolism,* Vol.61, No.4, (October 1985), pp. 741-745, ISSN 0021-972X

Tilvis, RS., Helve, E. & Miettinen, TA. (1986). Improvement of diabetic control by continuous subcutaneous insulin infusion therapy changes fatty acid composition of serum lipids and erythrocytes in type 1 (insulin-dependent) diabetes. *Diabetologia,* Vol.29, No.10, (October 1986), pp. 690-694, ISSN 0012-186X

Vidgren, HM., Louheranta, AM., Agren, JJ., Schwab, US. & Uusitupa, MI. (1998). Divergent incorporation of dietary trans fatty acids in different serum lipid fractions. *Lipids,* Vol.33, No.10, (October 1998), pp. 955-962, ISSN 0024-4201

Wijendran, V., Bendel, RB., Couch, SC., Philipson, EH., Thomsen, K., Zhang, X. & Lammi-Keefe, CJ. (1999). Maternal plasma phospholipid polyunsaturated fatty acids in pregnancy with and without gestational diabetes mellitus: relations with maternal factors. *The American Journal of Clinical Nutrition,* Vol.70, No.1, (July 1999), pp. 53-61, ISSN 0002-9165

Wijendran, V., Bendel, RB., Couch, SC., Philipson, EH., Cheruku, S. & Lammi-Keefe, CJ. (2000). Fetal erythrocyte phospholipid polyunsaturated fatty acids are altered in pregnancy complicated with gestational diabetes mellitus. *Lipids,* Vol.35, No.8, (August 2000), pp. 927-931, ISSN 0024-4201

Williams, C., Birch, EE., Emmett, PM., Northstone, K. & Avon Longitudinal Study of Pregnancy and Childhood Study Team. (2001). Stereoacuity at age 3.5 y in children born full-term is associated with prenatal and postnatal dietary factors: a report from a population-based cohort study. *The American Journal of Clinical Nutrition,* Vol.73, No.2, (February 2001), pp. 316-322, ISSN 0002-9165

Winkler, C., Hummel, S., Pflüger, M., Ziegler, AG., Geppert, J., Demmelmair, H. & Koletzko, B. (2008). The effect of maternal T1DM on the fatty acid composition of erythrocyte phosphatidylcholine and phosphatidylethanolamine in infants during early life. *European Journal of Nutrition,* Vol.47, No.3, (April 2008), pp. 145-152, ISSN 1436-6207

Yen, CH., Dai, YS., Yang, YH., Wang, LC., Lee, JH. & Chiang, BL. (2008). Linoleic acid metabolite levels and transepidermal water loss in children with atopic dermatitis. *Annals of Allergy, Asthma & Immunology : Official Publication of the American College of*

Allergy, Asthma, & Immunology, Vol.100, No.1, (January 2008), pp. 66-73, ISSN 1081-1206

Yuan, JM., Ross, RK., Gao, YT. & Yu, MC. (2001). Fish and shellfish consumption in relation to death from myocardial infarction among men in Shanghai, China. *American Journal of Epidemiology*, Vol.154, No.9, (November 2001), pp. 809-816, ISSN 0002-9262

Zhao, J., Del Bigio, MR. & Weiler, HA. (2009). Maternal arachidonic acid supplementation improves neurodevelopment of offspring from healthy and diabetic rats. *Prostaglandins, Leukotrienes, and Essential Fatty Acids*, Vol.81, No.5-6, (November-December 2009), pp. 349-356, ISSN 0952-3278

Therapeutic Modelling of Type 1 Diabetes

Nilam Nilam[1], Seyed M. Moghadas[2] and Pappur N. Shivakumar[3]
[1]*Department of Mathematics, Delhi Technological University, Delhi*
[2]*Centre for Disease Modelling, York University, Toronto, Ontario*
[3]*Department of Mathematics, University of Manitoba, Winnipeg, Manitoba*
[1]*India*
[2,3]*Canada*

1. Introduction

In this Chapter, we are mainly concerned with mathematical modelling (using differential equations) of controlled continuous subcutaneous infusion of insulin in Type 1 diabetes using pumps. It occurs mainly in children where controlling levels of sugar is entirely dependent on external infusion of insulin. Type I diabetes is a result of loss of beta-cell functions in the body due to an autoimmune reaction There is vast literature concerning continuous infusion of insulin where feedback is intermittent and the dosage is adhoc. Other ways of combating Type I diabetes include transplantation of insulin producing tissues or introducing artificial beta cells. We mathematically model the sugar concentration in the body and use it to dovetail a previously medically prescribed sugar concentration curve. The modelling, for the first time, aids the continuous infusion of insulin based upon individuals requirements in terms of the curve of decay of sugar concentration in a prescribed time. For each individual, depending on many personal factors like obesity, age, kidney functions, etc., a prescription is made of the desirable curve of sugar concentration from its highest level to the desired lowest level in a given period of time. This fine tunes the delivery of insulin as it takes away much guesswork of amounts of insulin given intermittently or continuously. Devices attached to continuous monitoring device will infuse insulin continuously and as per prescribed curve of reduction of sugar concentration. Thus, the pumps delivery takes into consideration the time profile of the insulin release, with the release stopping after the prescribed values are attained. The amount released in a dual wave shaped insulin bolus combining [8] both the usual normal and square wave methods. The therapy described will be the forerunner of intense clinical research work.Mathematical models with numerical simulations and analysis based on experimental data can be more effective in terms of costs and an extraordinary amount of time dealing with diverse physiological situations. This is particularly so in view of the complexities of the functions in the human body and incomplete existing knowledge.
This chapter provides an overview of mathematical modelling of type 1 diabetes, with particular focus on pump therapy as a management strategy for continuous subcutaneous insulin infusion. Previous models describing the mechanism of glucose metabolism have mostly focused on type 2 diabetes, most notably the classical minimal model for explaining the profile of glucose concentration over time.[4,5] Here we summarize the conclusions of

these studies for management of diabetes, and attempt to lay out a framework for further development of these models to include pump therapy. These models are often formulated as a system of differential equations that describes the profile of insulin release and the dynamics of glucose concentration over specified period of time. In addition to providing background on existing modelling frameworks, the practical implications of their outputs are discussed.

The main goals are (a) formulation of the model using the pump mechanism (b) defining the parameters (c) profiling the insulin release (d) simulating using estimated parameter values and (e) modelling extensions to include obesity as it had been well established that obesity promotes insulin resistance through the inappropriate inactivation of a process called gluconeogenesis, where the liver creates glucose for fuel. The model consists of blood glucose concentration, remote insulin action and amount of insulin. The model predictions include insulin secreted, if any, in pancreas, role of other organs, tissue uptake etc. This chapter closes with future direction in mathematical modelling of type 1 diabetes for optimal usage of external insulin and measuring insulin dependency with an insight into the role of obesity in developing diabetes.

2. Diabetes

2.1 What is diabetes?

Diabetes is a global problem with devastating human, social and economic impact. Diabetes is a growing epidemic threatening to overwhelm global healthcare services, wipe out some indigenous populations and undermine economies worldwide, especially in developing countries. Today more than 250 million people worldwide are living with diabetes and by 2025, this total is expected to increase to over 380 million people. Approximately 24 million people are diabetics in United States which is about 8 percent of the total population. The number of people with diabetes is increasing due to population growth, aging, urbanization, and increasing prevalence of obesity and physical inactivity. Diabetes is a highly prevalent disease in India where more than 35 million people suffer from diabetes. Alarmingly, as much as 13 million cases remains undiagnosed which leads to long term complications. The prevalence of diabetes is greater amongst the urban South Asian population (12-15%) compared to urban population in the West (6%).[9] That is why Diabetes has been one of the most important subjects for biomedical research for many years.

Diabetes Mellitus, commonly referred to as Diabetes, means sweet urine. Consistently elevated levels of blood glucose lead to spillage to glucose into urine, hence the term sweet urine. When the blood sugar level consistently runs too high in our blood stream, the condition is named as Diabetes. In patients with Diabetes Mellitus, the absence or insufficient production of insulin by the liver causes hyperglycemia. Diabetes Mellitus is a syndrome characterized by chronic hyperglycemia resulting from absence or relative impairment in insulin secretion and/or insulin action. It can also be referred to as a condition characterized by the disturbances of carbohydrate, protein and fat metabolism, the way our bodies use digested food for growth and energy. The chronic hyperglycemia of diabetes is associated with long term damage, dysfunction and failure of various organs, especially the eyes, kidneys, nerves, heart and blood vessels.[7] Diabetes is the most common endocrine disorder. It is a chronic medical condition meaning it can last a lifetime which can be controlled but can not be cured completely.

Human body functions best at a certain level of sugar in the blood stream. Blood sugar levels are tightly controlled by insulin, the principal hormone that makes it possible for many cells (primarily muscle and fat cells) to use glucose from the blood. It is manufactured by the beta cells of the pancreatic islets of Langerhans, a small section of the pancreas. Secretion of insulin primarily occurs in response to increased concentration of glucose in the blood. Insulin helps the glucose from food get into the body cells. If body does not make enough insulin or if the insulin does not work the way it should, glucose can not get into the cells. It stays in the blood instead and blood glucose level gets too high causing to have Diabetes. Deficiency of insulin or its action plays a central role in all forms of diabetes. There are three major forms of diabetes:[18]

2.1.1 Type 1 diabetes

Type 1 diabetes is one of the most challenging medical disorder because of the demands it imposes on day-to-day life. It was formerly known as insulin dependent diabetes mellitus (IDDM) or juvenile onset diabetes mellitus.

In this type of diabetes, the pancreas undergoes an autoimmune attack by the body itself and is rendered incapable of making insulin. It is an autoimmune disorder, in which body's own immune system attacks the beta cells in the islets of Langerhans of the pancreas destroying them or damaging them sufficiently to reduce insulin production. The pancreas then produces little or no insulin. At present, scientists do not know exactly what causes the body's immune system to attack the beta cells, but it is believed that autoimmune, genetic, and environmental factors, possibly viruses, are involved. It develops most often in children and young adults, but can appear at any age.Type 1 diabetes, which predominately affects youth, is rising alarmingly worldwide, at a rate of 3% per year. Some 70,000 children worldwide are expected to develop type 1 diabetes annually. If not diagnosed and treated with insulin, a person with type 1 diabetes can lapse into a life-threatening diabetic coma, also known as diabetic ketoacidosis.

2.1.2 Type 2 diabetes

Type 2 diabetes, formerly called adult-onset diabetes or non-insulin- dependent diabetes mellitus (NIDDM), is the most common form of diabetes. Type 2 diabetes is responsible for 90 -95% of diabetes cases and is increasing at alarming rates globally as a result of increased urbanization, high rates of obesity, sedentary lifestyles and stress. Type 2 diabetes is increasingly being diagnosed in children and adolescents though it can occur at any age. Millions of people don't even know they have it because it can arise with minimal outward signs or symptoms. It is diagnosed with insulin resistance in which the pancreas is producing enough insulin but for unknown reasons, the body can not use the insulin effectively. This leads to a situation similar to type 1 diabetes in which the pancreas can't secrete enough insulin because of which glucose builds up in the blood and the body cannot make efficient use of its main source of fuel. This form of diabetes is associated with obesity, older age, a family history of diabetes, a history of gestational diabetes, certain medications, impaired glucose metabolism, psychological factors, and physical inactivity. Type 2 diabetes can be controlled with exercise, diet and lifestyle modifications.[6] This type of diabetes may develop microvascular complications, which may lead to retinopathy, nephropathy and peripheral and autonomic nephropathies, and macrovascular complications include atherosclerotic coronary and peripheral arterial disease.

2.1.3 Gestational diabetes

This type of diabetes develops just before or during the pregnancy. Though the patient may have diabetes before the onset of the pregnancy, it is termed gestational only if it is first identified after the pregnancy has occurred. Gestational diabetes is caused by the hormones of pregnancy which is produced when the placenta supports the growing fetus. These hormones may interfere with the mother's ability to produce and use her own insulin. Usually this form of diabetes goes away after the delivery but women who have had gestational diabetes have a 20 to 50 percent chance of developing type 2 diabetes within 5 to 10 years especially those who require insulin during pregnancy and those who are overweight. Untreated Gestational Diabetes Mellitus (GDM) can lead to fetal macrosomia, hypoglycemia, hypocalcemia and hyperbilirubinemia. Also chances of cesarean delivery and chronic hypertension increases in women with GDM.

2.2 History and causes of diabetes

Diabetes is not a newly born disease, it has been with human race from long back but, we came to knew about it in 1552 B.C. Since after than, many of Greek as well French **physicians** had worked on it and threw some light on the nature of disease, organs responsible for it etc. Diabetes was recognized and categorized with complete details and its types, Type 1and Type 2 in 1959. In 1870s, a French physician had discovered a link between Diabetes and diet intake, and then diabetic diet was formulated with inclusion of milk, oats and other fiber containing foods in 1900-1915. Dr. Frederick Banting, Prof. Macleod and Dr. Collip discovered the function of **insulin**, its nature, along with its use started at the University of Toronto from 1920 -1923, who were awarded a Noble prize. In 1922, 14 year old Leonard Thompson becomes the first human to receive insulin. In the decade of 1940, it has been discovered that different organs like kidney and skin are also affected if diabetes is creeping from a long term. A major turn in this **research** was in 1955, when the oral hypogycemic drugs had been manufactured. Paul E. Lacy, a JDRF - funded researcher at Washington University School of Medicine performs the first successful islets transplantation in diabetic animal models in 1976. The first experimental insulin pump was developed in 1979 which leads to further refined pumps to provide the infusion of insulin in a way which closely mimics the glucose response of human islets. Since then, scientists are trying their best to produce results with the most impact.

Diabetes and its complications occur among Americans of all ages and ethnicities but the elderly and certain racial/ethnic groups are more commonly affected. In comparison of non - Hispanic whites, African Americans and Hispanics/Latino Americans are about two times more likely to be affected by the disease. It has been found that one tribe in Arizona has the highest rate of diabetes in the world, with about 50 percent of the adults between the ages of 30 and 64 with the disease. Population of type 2 diabetes sufferers has officially reached epidemic proportions.

Diabetes mellitus is developed when pancreatic tissue responsible for the production of insulin is absent because it is destroyed by disease such as chronic pancreatitis, trauma or surgical removal of pancreas. It can also result from other hormonal disturbances such as excessive growth hormone production (acromegaly, in which a pituitary gland tumor at the base of the brain causes excessive production of growth hormone leading to hyperglycemia) and Cushing's syndrome, in which the adrenal glands produce an excess of cortisol which promotes blood sugar elevation. Several other factors that make it more likely that a person develop diabetes are as follows:

- Age-older than 45 years
- Obesity
- Family history of diabetes in a first degree relative (parent or sibling)
- History with gestational diabetes mellitus
- Hispanic, Native American, African American, Asian American or Pacific Islander descent
- Hypertension (>140/90 mm Hg) or dyslipidemia (high-density lipoprotein HDL cholesterol <35mg/dl or triglyceride level >250mg/dl)

2.3 Symptoms and diagnosis of diabetes mellitus

Diabetes mellitus (DM) has diverse intial presentations. The early symptoms of diabetes are related to elevated blood sugar levels in the body and loss of glucose in the urine. It usually presents with symptomatic hyperglycemia. Common sign and symptoms may include any of the following:

- Being very thirsty
- Urinating often
- Feeling very hungry or tired
- Losing weight without trying
- Repeated or slow healing infections
- Having dry, itchy skin
- Extreme fatigue
- Blurred vision
- Tingling or loss of feeling in the hands or feet

2.4 Biological terms commonly used in diabetes

Insulin: An anabolic hormone, produced by the beta cells of the islets of Langerhans of pancreas in response of elevated blood sugar level in the body. It helps to control the blood sugar level in the desirable range.

Glucose: Glucose is a simple sugar present in everyone's body. It is an essential nutrient that provides energy for the proper functioning of the body cells. After meals, food is digested in the stomach and intestines. The glucose in digested food is absorbed by the intestinal cells into the blood stream and is carried by the blood to all the cells in the body. Glucose needs insulin to enter into the body as it can not get into the cells alone.

Glucagon: Glucagon is a hormone synthesized and secreted from alpha cells of the pancreatic islets used for carbohydrate metabolism. Its secretion increases rapidly when the sugar level is too low in the body. It maintains the level of glucose in the blood by binding to specific receptors on hepatocytes causing the liver to release its intracellular stores of glucose. As these stores become depleted, glucagon then encourages the liver to synthesize glucose by gluconeogenesis which will be released to prevent the development of hypoglycemia, low sugar level.

Insulin Resistance: Sometimes the cells throughout the body become resistant to the insulin produced by the pancreas due to which it becomes difficult for the sugar to enter the cells. This condition is known as insulin resistance.

Diabetic Ketoacidosis: It is a condition in which the cells of muscle, liver and other body parts are unable to take up glucose for producing energy due to the absence of insulin. It is a

state of absolute or relative **insulin deficiency** aggravated by hyperglycemia, dehydration, and acidosis-producing derangements in intermediary metabolism. To avoid starvation the body begins to break down fat for energy. Fatty acids and ketone bodies are released due to the break down of fat causing chemical imbalance (metabolic imbalance) called Diabetic Ketoacidosis. Moderate or large amounts of **ketones** in urine are dangerous. They upset the chemical balance of the blood.
Chronic hyperglycemia: Chronic hyperglycemia means elevated blood sugar level in the blood.

2.5 Treatment therapies for diabetes

Type 1 Diabetes is very serious, with a sudden and dramatic onset, usually in youth. Type 1 diabetes is an autoimmune condition, where the body attacks its own insulin producing cells. The body's immune cells, or white blood cells, include B cells and T cells. B cells make antibodies and present 'antigens' to T cells, allowing them to recognize, and kill invaders. People with Type 1 diabetes must maintain an insulin-monitoring and insulin-injecting regimen for the rest of their lives as the islets of Langerhans are destroyed in this type of diabetes. Treatment for type 1 diabetes includes taking insulin shots or insulin pump to deliver insulin in the body, making wise food choices, exercising regularly and controlling blood pressure and cholesterol.
Type 2 diabetes can be treated successfully with diet, physical activity and medication, if necessary.[23] Physical activity can help to control blood sugar levels and increases body's sensitivity to insulin.[6] Also, it helps delays or stop heart diseases, a leading complication of diabetes. Diet plays an extremely important role in controlling this type of diabetes. Being overweight can increase the chances of developing type 2 diabetes. Usually GDM in pregnant women disappears itself after delivery.

2.6 Mathematical model

The first approach to measure the insulin sensitivity *in vivo* was introduced by Himsworth and Ker [24] and the first mathematical model to estimate the glucose disappearance and insulin sensitivity was proposed by Bolie. In this model, he assumed that glucose disappearance is a linear function of both glucose and insulin. The insulin secretion and disappearance is proportional to glucose and plasma insulin concentration respectively.
The main objective here is to prescribe a more accurate, but less simple, method of arranging the palatable composition of a diabetic diet.
The modified coupled differential equations for the plasma glucose and insulin concentration [1-14, 16-22], when the normal fasting level of plasma glucose is 70 - 120 mg/dl, are given as follows

$$\frac{dg}{dt} = -l_1 h\bar{g} + l_2(g_0 - g)U(g_0 - g) + l_3 F(t) \tag{1}$$

$$\frac{dh}{dt} = l_4(g - g_0)U(g - g_0) - l_5 h_0 + l_6 I(t) \tag{2}$$

where, g(t) - plasma glucose concentration, h(t) - insulin concentration, l_i - sensitivity constants, i = 1,2,3,4,5,6, F(t) - food source input for plasma glucose, I(t) – insulin input and $U(g_0 - g)$ is unit step function.

The insulin input I(t) will be given through injection at subcutaneous level at periodic intervals, which leaks its contents into the system over a period of time. Therefore, I(t) may be defined as

$$I(t)=\frac{\rho t}{\bar{t}-t_0}+b$$

At t = t_0, I(t) = 0

$$\Rightarrow b=-\frac{\rho\, t_0}{\bar{t}-t_0} \qquad \therefore I(t)=\frac{\rho(t-t_0)}{\bar{t}-t_0} \qquad =\lambda+\mu\, t \tag{3}$$

where, $\lambda=-\frac{\rho t_0}{\bar{t}-t_0}$, $\mu=\frac{\rho}{\bar{t}-t_0}$, ρ - quantity of injection, t_0 – time of injection, $\bar{t}$ -time lag to maximum.

Food input source term, F(t), is the source for food input to the plasma glucose level, the contents of which are reduced in a simple exponential manner. Therefore, F(t) may be modeled as

$$F(t)=\begin{cases} Se^{-\alpha(t-t_0)}, & t>t_0 \\ 0, & t\le t_0 \end{cases} \tag{4}$$

where, S - quantity constant of meal, α - delay parameter.

For $t \ge t_0$, in non – diabetic case, $F(t)\ne 0$ and $I(t)=0$ and for diabetic case, $F(t)\ne 0$, $I(t)\ne 0$.

A mathematical model for the dynamics of glucose concentration in patients with type 1 diabetes using CSII [15] therapy as an external source of insulin has been developed by us. We attempt to model the effect of an external source of insulin release, as a prescribed function of time, on glucose levels. The model is then used to assess the optimal insulin release profile, and the threshold amount required to bring the level of glucose to within a normal physiological range.

To model the pump's delivery of insulin, we take into account three major factors: (i) the total amount of insulin released over a specific period; (ii) the time profile of insulin release, f(t); and (iii) the glucose threshold concentration Gc, below which the pump stops releasing insulin. The amount of insulin (TDD) is proportional to the total amount of glucose, whose concentration is assessed by the sensor in the pump's controller. This amount is released by the pump in a dual wave shaped insulin bolus which allows the patient to combine both normal and square wave techniques. The body characteristics of the patient determine how much insulin is needed to maintain the glucose level within the normal physiological range after each meal. The dual wave shape also provides a rapid increase in insulin plasma concentration, and sustained high circulating insulin levels while a meal is being consumed. Here, we extend the minimal model to incorporate the above factors, which leads to the following differential equations:

$$\frac{dG}{dt} = -XG + l_1(G_b - G)^+, \tag{5}$$

$$\frac{dX}{dt} = -p_1 X + p_2(I - I_b), \tag{6}$$

$$\frac{dI}{dt} = -l_2(G - G_c)^+ f(t) - l_3(I - I_b), \tag{7}$$

where G is the blood glucose concentration, X is an auxiliary function representing remote insulin action, and I is the insulin plasma concentration. A description of the model parameters and their values are given in Table 1.
The important part of this extension is the first term of (7) which models all three factors mentioned above. This term contributes to the insulin plasma when the glucose concentration exceeds the threshold Gc, and is defined as

$$l_2(G - G_c)^+ = \begin{cases} l_2(G(t) - G_c) f(t) & if\ G(t) > G_c \\ 0 & if\ G(t) < G_c \end{cases} \tag{8}$$

The function models the profile of insulin release from the pump, and the coefficient represents a scaling factor determining TDD of insulin released by the pump. In the next section, we discuss different profiles of insulin release and compare their effects on the optimal control of glucose concentration. The newer generation of pumps can be programmed to release insulin using three different bolus techniques.
A normal bolus can be used if small amounts of carbohydrates are consumed or if a correction to the blood glucose level outside the physiological range needs to be made. A square wave profile is helpful when eating foods that are high in both fat/protein and carbohydrate (fat and protein delay the absorption of carbohydrates). If a normal bolus is given for a meal high in protein and fat concentrations, circulating insulin levels rise rapidly and may peak before the carbohydrates are absorbed. This mismatch in insulin and blood glucose levels can result in postprandial hypoglycemia. Therefore, a dual wave bolus, as a combination of the normal and square wave bolus techniques, can be introduced. Using this technique, half of the insulin dose is given (over a short period of time) at the onset of the meal, and the remainder over a 2-4 h period. The profile of a dual wave bolus is modeled as a function of time, f(t), in Eq. (4) over a period of 3 h (Fig. 1(a)-(c)).

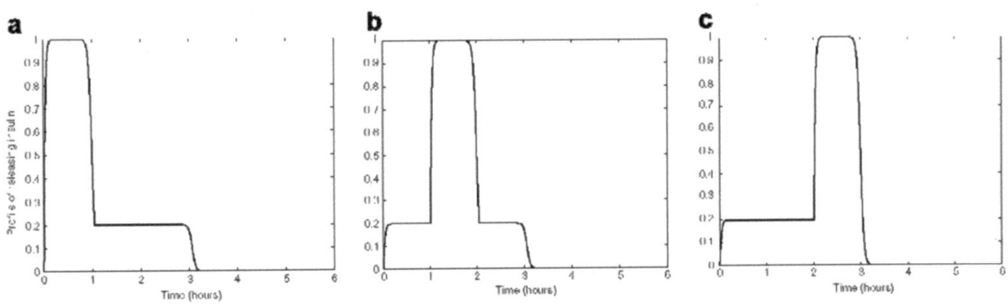

Fig. 1. Profile of insulin release by the pump *f*(*t*), for 3h: HLL release; (b)LHL release; (c) LLH release, where *H* stands for high amount release of insulin and *L* stands for its low amount per hour *f*(*t*) is normalized so that *H*=*L*

S No	Parameter	Description	Value	Unit
1	G_b	Base line value of glucose concentration in plasma	118	mg dl^{-1}
2	G_c	Glucose threshold concentration in plasma	100-107	mg dl^{-1}
3	I_b	Baseline value of insulin concentration in plasma	7	μU ml^{-1}
4	l_1	The insulin dependent rate of tissue glucose uptake	10	Min^{-1}
5	l_2	Scaling factor determining TDD of insulin	Variable	min^{-1} μU mg^{-1}
6	l_3	The rate of decay for insulin in plasma	0.264	min^{-1}
7	p_1	The rate of spontaneous decrease of glucose uptake	0.0107	min^{-1}
8	p_2	The rate of insulin - dependent increase in tissue glucose uptake due to insulin concentration excess over its baseline	0.007	min^{-2} μU ml^{-1}

Table 1. Description and values of the model parameters obtained from the published literature

This particular work is published in Applied Mathematics and computation, 2007, pages 1476 - 1483 and has been cited by Kato, R, Munkhjargal, M and Takahashi, D "An autonomous drug release system based on chemo- mechanical energy conversion "Organic Engine" for feedback control of blood glucose", Biosensors and Bioelecetronics in 2010 Vol 26(4), pages 1455 - 1459.

2.7 Future work

More advanced mathematical models can be formulated to explain the effects of obesity on diabetes, effects of exercise on management of type 2 diabetes. Parameters involving glucose sensors can be added to the insulin pump model for a better programmed insulin delivery by insulin pump.

3. References

[1] D. Araujo-Vilar, C.A. Rega-Liste, D.A. Garcia-Estevez, F. Sarmiento-Escalona, V. Mosquera-Tallon, J. Cabezas-Cerrato, Minimal model of glucose metabolism: modified equations and its application in the study of insulin sensitivity in obese subject, Diabetes Res. Clin. Pract. 39 (1998) 129–141.

[2] R.N. Bergman, L.S. Phillips, C. Cobelli, Physiologic evaluation of factors controlling glucose tolerance in man, J. Clin. Invest. 68 (1981) 1456–1467.

[3] B.W. Bode, R.D. Steed, P.C. Davidson, Reduction in severe hypoglycemia with long term continuous subcutaneous insulin infusion in type 1 diabetes, Diabetes Care 19 (1996) 324–327.

[4] A. Boutayeb, E.H. Twizell, K. Achouayb, A. Chetouani, A mathematical model for the burden of diabetes and its complications, BioMed. Eng. (2004), doi:10.1186/1475-925X-3-20, Online.

[5] A. De Gaetano, O. Arino, Mathematical modelling of the intravenous glucose tolerance test, J. Math. Biol. 40 (2000) 136–168.

[6] M. Derouich, A. Boutayeb, The effect of physical exercise on the dynamics of glucose and insulin, J. Biomech. 35 (2002) 911–917.

[7] Diabetes Control and Complications Trial Research Group, The effect of intensive treatment of diabetes on the development and progression of long-term complications in insulin-dependent diabetes mellitus, New. Engl. J. Med. 329 (1993) 977–985.

[8] T.M. Gross, D. Kayne, A. King, C. Rother, S. Juth, A bolus calculator is an effective means of controlling postprandial glycemia in patients on insulin pump therapy, Diabetes Technol. Ther. 5 (2003) 365–369.

[9] A.P. Harmel, R. Mathur, Davidson's Diabetes Mellitus: Diagnosis and Treatment, fifth ed., 2004.

[10] W.B. Saunders, A.E. Kitabchi, J.N. Fisher, G.A. Burghen, M.S. Gaylord, N.M. Blank, Evaluation of a portable insulin infusion pump for outpatient management of brittle diabetes, Diabetes Care 2 (1979) 421–424.

[11] R. Linkeschova, M. Raoul, U. Bott, M. Berger, M. Spraul, Less Severe hypoglycemia, better metabolic control and improved quality of life in type 1 diabetes mellitus with continuous subcutaneous insulin infusion (CSII) therapy; an observational study of 100 consecutive patients followed for a mean of 2 years, Diabetes Med. 19 (2002) 746–751.

[12] R.S. Parker, F.J. Doyle, N.A. Peppas, A model-based algorithm for blood glucose control in type I diabetic patients, IEEE Trans. BioMed. Eng. 46 (1999) 148–157.

[13] L. Perko, Differential Equations and Dynamical Systems, Springer-Verlag, New York, 1996.

[14] J.C. Pickup, M.C. White, H. Keen, J.A. Parsons, K.G. Alberti, Long-term continuous subcutaneous insulin infusion in diabetics at home, Lancet 2 (1979) 870–873.

[15] J. Pickup, H. Keen, Continuous subcutaneous insulin infusion at 25 years: evidence base for the expanding use of insulin pump therapy in type 1 diabetes, Diabetes Care 25 (2002) 593–598.

[16] G. Pillonetto, G. Sparacino, C. Cobelli, Numerical non-identifiability regions of the minimal model of glucose kinetics: superiority of Bayesian estimation, Math. Biosci. 184 (2003) 53–67.

[17] W. Regittnig, Z. Trajanoski, H.J. Leis, M. Ellmerer, A. Wutte, G. Sendlhofer, L. Schaupp, G.A. Brunner, P. Wach, T.R. Pieber, Plasma and interstitial glucose dynamics after intravenous glucose injection, Diabetes 48 (1999) 1070–1081.

[18] Report of the expert committee on the diagnosis and classification of diabetes mellitus, Diabetes Care 20 (1997) 1183–1197.

[19] The UK Prospective Diabetes Study (UKPDS) Group, Intensive blood glucose control with sulphonylureas or insulin compared withconventional treatment and risk of complications in patients with type 2 diabetes (UKPDS33), Lancet 352 (1998) 837–853.

[20] G. Toffolo, E. Breda, M.K. Cavaghan, D.A. Ehrmann, K.S. Polonsky, C. Cobelli, Quantitative indexes of b-cell function duringgraded up and down glucose infusion from C-peptide models, Am. J. Physiol. Endocrinol. Metab. 280 (2001) E2–E10.

[21] I.M. Tolic´, E. Mosekilde, J. Sturis, Modelling the insulin–glucose feedback system: the significance of pulsatile insulin secretion, J. Theor. Biol. 207 (2000) 361–375.

[22] J. Unger, A primary care approach to continuous subcutaneous insulin infusion, Clin. Diabetes 17 (1999) 113–127.

[23] Management of Type 2 Diabetes, N ENGL J MED 358;3, 2008.

[24] Himsworth/ H. 1. and 5er/ R. B./ Insulin sensiti<e and insulin insensiti<e types of diabetes mellitus/ Clinical Science/ 4 D1F3FH 11F.